Mosby's **Textbook for**
Nursing Assistants

Mosby's Textbook for Nursing Assistants

Sheila A. Sorrentino, *R.N., B.S.N., M.A., Ph.D.*

Director of Career Education and Training
Heartland Community College
Normal, Illinois

THIRD EDITION

with 650 illustrations

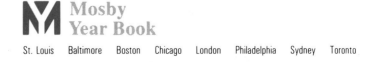

Mosby
Year Book

St. Louis   Baltimore   Boston   Chicago   London   Philadelphia   Sydney   Toronto

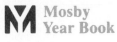
Mosby
Year Book
Dedicated to Publishing Excellence

Executive editor: Richard A. Weimer
Assistant editors: Rina Steinhauer, Mary Beth Ryan
Project manager: Patricia Tannian
Production editor: Ann E. Rogers
Book design: Susan Lane

Photography: Rick Brady
Third edition art: Jack Tandy
Cover illustration: © Thomas Moore

THIRD EDITION

Printed in the United States of America

Mosby–Year Book, Inc.
11830 Westline Industrial Drive
St. Louis, Missouri 63146

Library of Congress Cataloging in Publication Data

Sorrentino, Sheila A.
    Mosby's textbook for nursing assistants / Sheila A. Sorrentino. —
3rd ed.
        p.   cm.
    Includes index.
    ISBN 0-8016-4728-2
    1. Nurses' aides. 2. Care of the sick. I. Title. II. Title:
Textbook for nursing assistants.
    [DNLM: 1. Nurses' Aides. 2. Nursing Care. WY 193 S714m]
RT84.S67   1991
610.73—dc20
DNLM/DLC
for Library of Congress   91-22746
                                                              CIP

GW/CD/VH 10 9 8 7 6 5 4

To my nephew
Kyle Anthony
  Because Santa Claus made him so cute

Preface

The third edition of *Mosby's Textbook for Nursing Assistants*, a resource for nursing assistant education, incorporates the Omnibus Budget Reconciliation Act of 1987 (OBRA) guidelines for nursing assistant education. As with previous editions, this book focuses on safe and effective functioning when giving care and when working in health care settings. Emphasis continues to be placed on nursing assistant skills and functions and the psychosocial approach to care. Throughout the book, caring, understanding, respect for the individual, personal choice, and dignity of person are attitudes that are conveyed to the nursing assistant.

The textbook presents the accepted functions of nursing assistants, as well as those functions they may be asked to perform if given the necessary education, training, and supervision. Because facilities vary in their use of nursing assistants, the responsibilities and limitations of nursing assistants are emphasized throughout the text. Chapter 2 (The Nursing Assistant) specifically deals with the legal and ethical aspects of their role.

The textbook is intended for use in nursing assistant education programs conducted by community colleges, technical colleges, high schools, vocational-career centers, hospitals, long-term care facilities, home care agencies, and other agencies providing nursing assistant education. *Mosby's Textbook for Nursing Assistants* is organized to allow for variations in curriculum structure and program length. The order of presentation of chapters or chapter sections can be determined by the instructor. For example, an instructor may chose to begin a course with infection control, body mechanics, bedmaking, and giving a bed bath. The appropriate chapters and sections of this book can be assigned for reading in the above order without jeopardizing content or learning. Or an instructor may choose to present the measurement of vital signs early in the course.

Organization of the third edition is similar to previous editions in that basic nursing concepts and learning strategies were considered:

- Nursing assistants need to be aware of and understand their work environment and the individuals in that environment.

- An understanding of body structure and function and normal growth and development is helpful in developing desirable attitudes toward individuals and in performing psychomotor skills safely and competently.
- Learning proceeds from the simple to the complex. Those concepts and procedures integral to other activities and functions (safety, body mechanics, and medical asepsis) are presented early. Psychomotor skills that are easy to learn and basic to the role of nursing assistants are then presented; these include bedmaking, personal care, certain urinary and bowel elimination procedures, measuring intake and output, serving food trays, and feeding patients. More complex content is then presented. Measuring vital signs, the application of heat and cold, and care of surgical patients are more complex in regard to learning and safe practice—these may not be considered nursing assistant functions in all facilities.
- The book encompasses the life span with content and precautions regarding care of infants, children, and the elderly integrated throughout the textbook where appropriate.
- The basic needs described by Abraham Maslow are emphasized.
- The patient is presented as an individual with physical, psychological, social, and spiritual needs.
- The influence and importance of cultural heritage to activities of daily living and responses to illness are presented where appropriate.

Mosby's Textbook for Nursing Assistants is comprehensive and serves as a reference for nursing assistants as they expand their skills and knowledge. Chapters focusing on growth and development, safety, the patient having surgery, vision and hearing problems, rehabilitation, care of the elderly, common health problems, sexuality, the home health care assistant, and basic emergency care demonstrate the book's comprehensiveness. Two new chapters in the third edition enhance the book's comprehensiveness. One new chapter deals with Alzheimer's disease and other dementias, and the other new chapter focuses on the care of mothers and newborns.

Along with the two new chapters and the integration of OBRA standards throughout the text, other highlights of the third edition of *Mosby's Textbook for Nursing Assistants* include:

- A full-color format.
- Content relating to telephone answering skills.
- Improved readability. Constant attention was given to the reading level and vocabulary. Except for medical terms, which are defined throughout the text, the vocabulary is basic with common terms. The readability of the text has been improved without compromising professionalism, caring, and sensitivity.
- Chapter 9 (Preventing Infection) has been broadened to include gloving, gowning, wearing a mask, and the infection precaution standards outlined by the Centers for Disease Control. Information about universal precautions has been integrated throughout the text and the various procedures.
- AIDS, hepatitis, and other communicable diseases have been added to the Common Health Problems chapter.
- The Medical Terminology chapter has been moved to the end of the book for ease of reference.

The third edition of *Mosby's Textbook for Nursing Assistants* includes new and updated color illustrations and photographs, which are used throughout the book to enhance the student's understanding of the material presented. Other important features include learning objectives and key terms with definitions at the beginning of each chapter, as well as review questions and answers to evaluate learning at the end of each chapter.

As with the previous editions, there are many people who contributed in some way to the second edition of *Mosby's Textbook for Nursing Assistants*. Helen Chigaros, R.N., nursing assistant instructor at Kankakee Community College and her students merit special acknowledgment for their advice, suggestions, and support. Others deserving of my thanks and appreciation include:

Relda Kelly for writing the third edition of the workbook to accompany the textbook.

Stephanie Vaughn for developing the instructor reference materials.

Sally Flesch from Black Hawk College in Moline, Illinois for being a consultant, advisor, and friend.

Ann Rogers for her production efforts.

And Richard Weimer, executive editor at Mosby–Year Book, for his dedication to this book and for being my friend.

Sheila A. Sorrentino

Contents

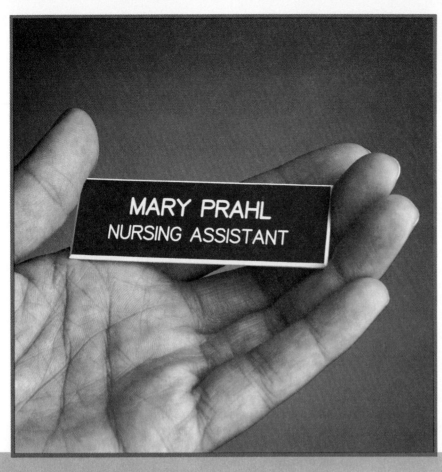

MARY PRAHL
NURSING ASSISTANT

Introduction to Health Care Facilities

1

OBJECTIVES

- Define the key terms listed in this chapter
- Describe the types, purposes, and organization of health care facilities
- Identify the members of the health team and nursing team
- Describe the nursing service department
- Know the differences between RNs, LPNs, and nursing assistants
- Explain how the nursing assistant is a member of the nursing team
- Describe six programs that pay for health care
- Explain how diagnostic related groups affect Medicare and Medicaid payments

acute illness A sudden illness from which the patient is expected to recover

chronic illness An illness, slow or gradual in onset, for which there is no known cure; the illness can be controlled, and complications can be prevented

functional nursing A method of organizing nursing care; nursing personnel are given specific tasks to do for all assigned patients

health team A variety of workers who work together to provide health care for patients

home health agency An agency that provides nursing care and assistance to patients in their homes

hospice A health care facility or program for persons dying of terminal illness

hospital A health care facility where ill and injured persons are given health care, including medical and nursing care

licensed practical nurse (LPN) An individual who has completed a 1-year nursing program and has passed the licensing examination for practical nurses

long-term care facility A health care facility in which individuals live and are given nursing care; nursing facility or nursing home

mental health hospital A hospital for persons who are mentally ill

nursing assistant An individual who gives simple, basic nursing care under the supervision of a registered nurse or an LPN; also called nurse's aide, nursing attendant, patient care assistant, health care assistant, and orderly

nursing facility A long-term care facility or nursing home

nursing team Individuals who provide nursing care—registered nurses, LPNs, and nursing assistants

orderly A male nursing assistant

primary nursing A method of organizing nursing care; a registered nurse is responsible for the total care of patients on a 24-hour basis

registered nurse (RN) An individual who has studied nursing for 2, 3, or 4 years and has passed a licensing examination

team nursing A method of organizing nursing care; an RN serves as a team leader; RNs, LPNs, and nursing assistants are assigned to care for certain patients

There are many different types of health care facilities for people with health problems. These include hospitals, long-term care facilities, mental health hospitals, community centers, home health agencies, and hospices. Others include physicians' offices, clinics, centers for the handicapped, and homes for the mentally retarded. There are also facilities for alcoholics, drug abusers, single mothers, and others needing health care.

This chapter deals with the basic purposes of health care facilities and with the types of facilities that commonly employ nursing assistants. The organization of health care facilities, the nursing team, and insurance programs are also included.

HEALTH CARE FACILITIES

Health care facilities serve the needs of individuals requiring health care. They offer many services ranging from the simple to the complex. Some offer a specific type of service. The many people working in these facilities each have special talents, knowledge, and skills. All work on behalf of the patient—the focus of care.

Purpose

Health care facilities have similar purposes and services. The *detection and treatment of disease* is the primary purpose of most facilities. Diagnostic testing, physical examinations, surgery, emergency care, and medications are some methods used to detect and treat disease. Nurses are involved in disease detection by observing signs and symptoms. They participate in disease treatment by giving nursing care and carrying out therapeutic measures ordered by the doctor. Because you will assist the nurse, you will also be involved in the observation and care of patients (Fig. 1-1).

The *promotion of health* includes both physical and mental health. Health is promoted by teaching and counseling people to stay healthy, change unhealthful habits, eat a proper diet, and get proper exercise. Individuals are also taught the signs and symptoms that warn of serious illness.

A great deal of research is taking place in the *prevention of disease*. Great advances have been made in preventing such diseases as polio, smallpox, and tuberculosis. Heart disease and cancer are among the leading causes of death today. Scientists are looking for the causes and cures of these diseases and for ways to prevent them. Nursing and other health care personnel play valuable roles in research and in the prevention of disease.

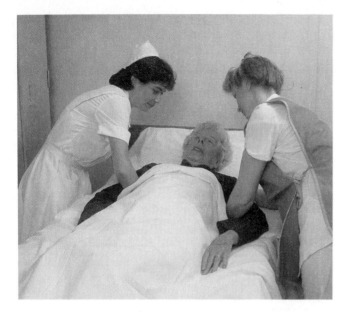

Fig. 1-1 A nursing assistant helping an RN give patient care.

Rehabilitation, sometimes called restorative care, helps individuals return to their highest possible level of physical and psychological functioning. In the past, rehabilitation primarily focused on people who were physically handicapped because of a birth injury, birth defect, or physical injury. Rehabilitation now recognizes that a person can have difficulty functioning psychologically, as well as physically, in everyday activities and at work. Rehabilitation helps individuals learn or relearn the skills needed to live, work, and enjoy life.

Rehabilitation begins when the patient is admitted to the health care facility. Many health care workers are involved in helping the person become as independent as possible. The person is taught and encouraged to function without help.

Many health care facilities provide educational experiences for students. The students may be studying to become nurses, doctors, x-ray and laboratory technicians, dieticians, or nursing assistants. These students are concerned with the same purposes the health care facilities are. They assist in disease detection and treatment, health promotion, disease prevention, and rehabilitation.

These purposes are all interrelated and are difficult to separate. One example is a patient who enters a hospital emergency room with severe chest pain and difficulty in breathing. An examination of the patient and laboratory test results lead the doctor to diagnose the patient as having had a heart attack. The patient is then admitted to the hospital for treatment. During the course of treatment, the patient is given health teaching and counseling about the causes of a heart attack and about health habits that need changing. The teaching and counseling are done to promote

health and to prevent another heart attack. The patient is probably afraid of dying and worried about being unable to lead an active life. A rehabilitation program is planned in which activity begins slowly; activity may progress to jogging or swimming. More teaching and counseling are provided about diet, medication, life-style, and activity. The patient and family are encouraged to talk about their fears and concerns and are given help in finding ways to cope. Thus a successful rehabilitation program helps promote the patient's health and may prevent another heart attack.

Types of Health Care Facilities

Nursing assistants work in many types of health care facilities. Some are employed in doctors' offices to perform basic functions and to help with clerical duties. Nursing assistants may work in private homes to care for homebound patients. Most nursing assistants are employed in the facilities discussed in the following sections.

Hospitals *Hospitals* vary in size from small community hospitals with 25 to 50 beds to large medical centers with more than 500 beds (Fig. 1-2). Most large hospitals are in major cities or are associated with colleges and universities. Hospital services are varied and extensive. Services include emergency care, surgery, x-ray procedures and treatments, laboratory testing, respiratory therapy, physical therapy, occupational therapy, and speech therapy.

People of all ages are hospitalized. They are hospitalized to have babies, for mental health problems, to have surgery, to heal broken bones, to diagnose and treat medical problems, or to die. The hospital stay may last days, weeks, or months depending on the patient's condition and illness.

Patients can have acute, terminal, or chronic illnesses. An *acute illness* is one that begins suddenly

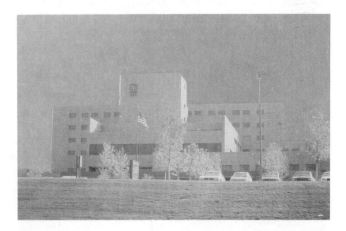

Fig. 1-2 Community hospital. (Courtesy of Mercy Hospital, Davenport, Iowa.)

and from which the patient is expected to recover. A *terminal illness* eventually results in death (see Chapter 30). A *chronic illness* begins slowly and has no cure. The illness can be controlled, and complications can be prevented with proper treatment.

Long-term care facilities *Long-term care facilities*, often called nursing homes, provide health care services to individuals who cannot care for themselves at home but who do not need hospital care. Medical, nursing, food, recreational, rehabilitative, and social services are provided.

Individuals in long-term care facilities are called residents, not patients, because the facility is either their temporary or permanent home. Most residents are elderly, with chronic disease, poor nutrition, or poor health. Long-term care facilities are designed to meet the special needs of the elderly (Fig. 1-3). Some residents may become well enough to return home; others require nursing care until death.

Long-term care facilities and the needs of residents are discussed in Chapter 7. Throughout this book, the term *nursing facility* will be used when referring to long-term care facilities.

Mental health hospitals *Mental health hospitals* specialize in the care of mentally ill individuals. These patients may have difficulty dealing with events in life. Some are dangerous to themselves or others because of the way they think and behave. Patients may be hospitalized for a short time or for life. The term "psychiatric hospital" was used in the past to refer to a mental health hospital.

Home health agencies *Home health agencies* care for patients in their homes. The agency may be part of a city or county public health department or may be sponsored by a hospital or private business. Services range from providing health teaching and supervision to a mother of a newborn, to providing bedside nursing care to a homebound patient. Home health care is an alternative to a nursing facility for some elderly

persons and for those who are dying. Besides nursing care, agencies may provide social activities, physical therapy, and food services. Home health care and the role of the nursing assistant are discussed in Chapter 31.

Hospices A *hospice* is a special program for those who are dying. The physical, emotional, social, and spiritual needs of the patient and family are provided for in a setting that allows a great deal of freedom. Children and pets usually can visit at any time, and the patient's family and friends can participate in giving care. A hospice may be a separate facility or part of a hospital; hospice care can also be provided in the patient's home.

HOW A HEALTH CARE FACILITY IS ORGANIZED

Health care facilities have a governing or controlling body called the board of trustees or board of directors. The board makes sure that the facility provides adequate and safe care at the lowest possible cost. The board makes policies for the facility and delegates the management of the facility to an administrator. The administrator reports directly to the board. A group of directors assists the administrator in operating and managing the facility.

The directors or department heads are responsible for specific areas. The director of business affairs may be responsible for the payroll department, patient billing, laundry and housekeeping, public relations, the admitting office, the personnel office, and the purchasing department. The medical director supervises the activities of the medical staff, which includes doctors and possibly residents and interns. A director of ancillary services may be responsible for the x-ray department, social services, the pharmacy, and spiritual care.

The director of nursing is responsible for the entire nursing staff and for the activities involved in providing safe nursing care to patients. The nursing service department is discussed later in this chapter. Figure 1-4 shows a typical organizational chart of a health care facility.

The Health Team

The *health team* involves a variety of workers whose skills and knowledge are directed to the total care of the patient. In the past, the health team was made up of the patient, doctor, and nurse. Today many workers provide services with the overall goal of providing quality patient care. Members of the health team work together to meet the patient's needs.

Because many health care workers are involved in the care of one patient, coordination of care is essential. The nursing staff is usually responsible for the coordination of care, with an RN in the key leadership

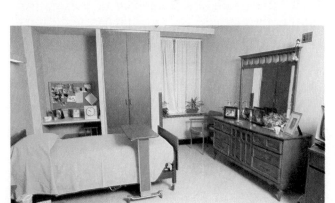

Fig. 1-3 Room of a modern long-term care facility.

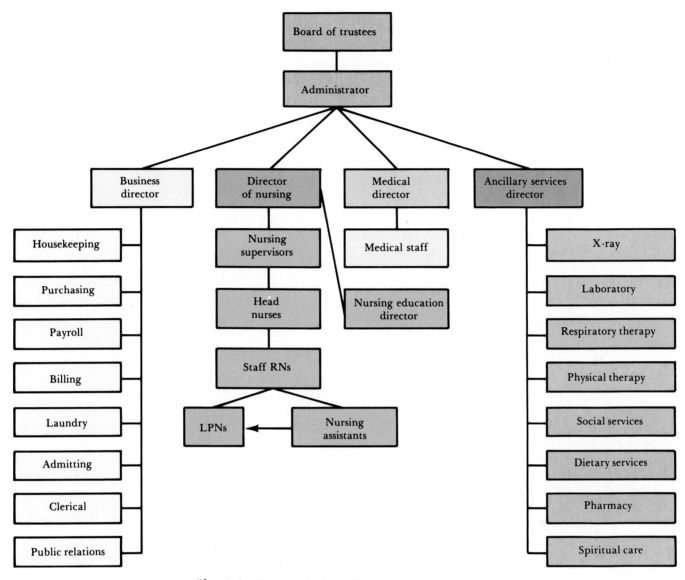

Fig. 1-4 The organizational chart of a health care facility.

position. Figure 1-5 shows the patient as the focus of all the health care workers.

Nursing Service

Nursing service is a major department in a health facility. The director of nursing is an RN, who may have a bachelor's or master's degree in nursing. Nursing supervisors assist the director in managing and carrying out the responsibilities of the nursing department. Nursing supervisors are also RNs and may have college degrees.

The nursing supervisors may be responsible for a particular shift or nursing area. The nursing areas may be surgical nursing units, medical nursing units, intensive care units, maternity departments, pediatric units, operating and recovery rooms, an emergency department, or a mental health nursing unit. Each area has a head nurse. Head nurses are responsible for all patient care and the actions of nursing personnel in their areas. Head nurses report to the nursing supervisors.

RNs are assigned to each nursing area. They provide nursing care and assign and supervise the work of LPNs and nursing assistants. The staff RN reports to the head nurse, and the LPN reports to the staff RN. The nursing assistant reports to the RN or LPN supervising his or her work.

A nursing education department is also part of nursing service. A director of nursing education reports to the director of nursing. The director of nursing education is an RN, who may have a bachelor's or master's degree in nursing. RNs may be hired as nursing education instructors. The instructors plan and present educational sessions to nursing personnel so that current and safe patient care can be provided.

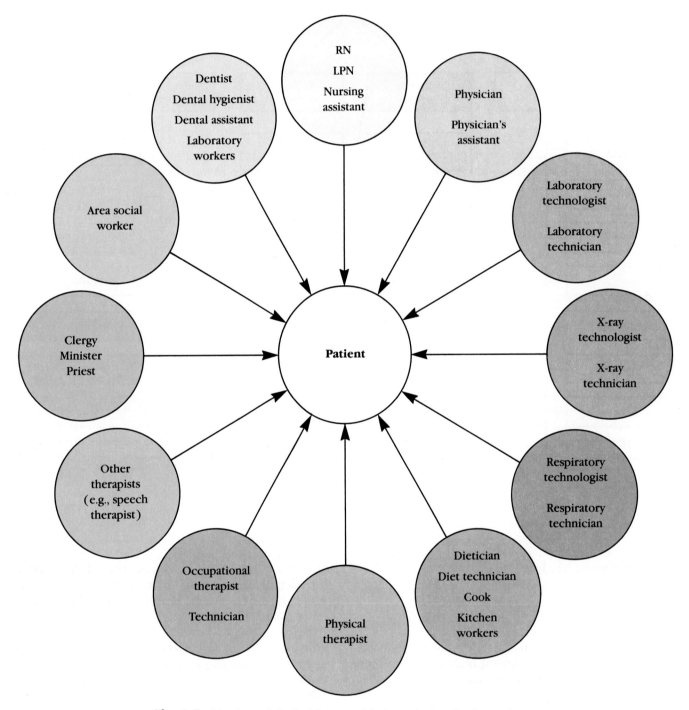

Fig. 1-5 Members of the health team with the patient as the focus of care.

Methods of Organizing Nursing Care

Nursing care has been organized in several ways for safe and effective care. The number of patients to be cared for, the available staff, and the cost are factors that influence how nursing care is organized. The three most common methods are presented.

Functional nursing involves assigning each member of the nursing team specific functions or tasks to do for all patients. One RN may give all medications. Another RN may change all dressings and give all treatments. LPNs may give all the baths, take all vital signs, and weigh all patients. Nursing assistants may be asked to make all beds, pass all drinking water, and feed patients who cannot feed themselves. Functional nursing is uncoordinated and fragmented. Disadvantages to the patient are many. They include interrupted rest, having to learn several names and titles of nursing personnel, waiting to have total care completed, and frequent interruptions.

Team nursing is a popular and efficient method. The team is led by an RN who determines the amount and kind of care required by each patient. The team leader assigns other RNs, LPNs, and nursing assistants to care for specific patients. Assignments are made according to the patients' needs and the capabilities of the team members. The team members report back to the team leader about any observations made and the patient care given.

Primary nursing is a popular method of organizing nursing care. It involves total and comprehensive patient care. The primary nurse is an RN who is responsible for the patient's care on a 24-hour basis. Other RNs and LPNs give care when the primary nurse is off duty. The RN assesses, plans, implements, and evaluates patient care. The RN gives bedside nursing care and teaches and counsels the patient and family. The RN also plans the patient's discharge. If necessary, home care or admission to a nursing facility is arranged. Patient satisfaction and quality of care are increased with this method. "My nurse" is a phrase often used by patients when primary nursing is used.

THE NURSING TEAM

The *nursing team* involves RNs, LPNs, and nursing assistants. Each has different roles and responsibilities as a result of the amount and kind of education received. All are concerned with the physical, social, emotional, and spiritual needs of patients.

Registered Nurses

A *registered nurse* studies for 2 years at a community college, 2 or 3 years in a hospital-based diploma program, or 4 years at a college or university. Nursing and the biological, social, and physical sciences are studied. On completing the program of study, the graduate takes a licensing examination offered by a state board of nursing. The licensing examination must be passed for the nurse to become *registered* and receive a license to practice. Registered nurses in the United States must be licensed by the state in which they practice.

RNs assess, plan, implement, and evaluate nursing care. The RN identifies the patient's nursing problems and develops a plan of care. The RN then carries out the plan of care and evaluates its effectiveness on the patient's condition. Patients are helped to become more independent and are taught ways to stay or become healthy. The patient and family are instructed by RNs at the bedside or in classrooms.

The doctor's orders are carried out by the RN. The RN may delegate the responsibility of carrying out the doctor's orders to an LPN or a nursing assistant. RNs are not allowed to diagnose diseases or illnesses or to prescribe treatments or medications.

RNs work as staff nurses, head nurses, supervisors, directors of nursing, and instructors. The opportunities available to an RN depend on the amount and type of education, professional abilities, and experience.

Licensed Practical Nurses

Licensed practical nurses complete 1 year of study in a hospital-based nursing program, community college, vocational school, or technical school. Some public high schools offer 2-year practical nursing programs. In the classroom and clinical settings, the study of nursing is emphasized. Students also study body structure and function, basic psychology, arithmetic, and communication skills. Graduates take a licensing examination for practical nursing. When the test is passed, the individual receives a license to practice and the title of *licensed practical nurse*. Like the RN, the practical nurse must have a license to practice nursing.

LPNs work under the supervision of RNs, licensed physicians, and licensed dentists. An LPN's responsibilities and functions are more limited than an RN's because the LPN has less education in the biological, physical, and social sciences. The LPN can function with little supervision when the patient's needs are simple and the patient's condition is stable. The LPN assists the RN in providing care when the patient is acutely ill and when complex procedures are required.

Nursing Assistants

Nursing assistants are employed in health facilities to assist nurses in providing patient care. Nurse's aide, nursing attendant, patient care assistant, and health care assistant are titles used to refer to the nursing assistant. A male nursing assistant may be called an *orderly*. Under the direct supervision of RNs and LPNs, nursing assistants give simple, basic nursing care. The nursing assistant as a member of the nursing team is discussed in greater detail in Chapter 2.

In 1987 the Congress of the United States passed the Omnibus Budget Reconciliation Act. The law is commonly called "OBRA." This federal law applies to all 50 states. The law requires training for nursing assistants (nurse aides) working in nursing facilities. It also requires "competency evaluation." This means that nursing assistants must prove that they have the knowledge and skills necessary to give safe care. Competency evaluation involves a written test and a skills test. Nursing assistant training and competency evaluation are discussed in greater detail in Chapter 2.

Some nursing assistant courses are conducted by community colleges, technical schools, and high school vocational programs. Others are offered by nursing education departments in health care facilities.

You may wish to continue your education to become an RN or LPN. Community colleges and 4-year colleges and universities in your area can help you select the best program to meet your needs, abilities, and financial situation.

PAYING FOR HEALTH CARE

Hospital care and long-term care are very costly and can financially ruin a patient and family. Even after the patient returns home, bills may continue for doctors' visits, medicines, medical supplies, and home care services.

Most people cannot afford large medical bills. Some avoid medical care because they cannot pay. Others make sure doctor bills are paid even if they must go without food or needed medicine. Worry, fear, and emotional upset are often experienced by those who face the problem of paying for health care. If the patient has insurance, part or all of the health care costs are usually covered.

Insurance Programs

Private and government insurance programs pay for part or all of a person's health care costs. The basic programs are described in general terms.

1. *Private insurance plans* are purchased by individuals and families. Depending on the plan, the insurance company pays for some or all health care costs.
2. *Group insurance plans* cover individuals belonging to a group. Often employers offer health insurance to employees under group coverage. The insurance premium may be paid by the employee, the employer, or the employee and

employer. Premiums are lower with group plans than with private insurance plans.
3. A *health maintenance organization* (HMO) provides health care services for a prepaid fee. The set fee is paid at intervals such as every month, every 3 months, or every year. For the fee, individuals receive all of the needed services offered by the organization. Some need only an annual physical examination, but others require hospitalization. Whatever services are used, the cost is covered by the prepaid fee. HMOs emphasize disease prevention and maintaining health. Keeping someone healthy costs far less than treating illness.
4. A *preferred provider organization* (PPO) is a group of doctors or a hospital that provides health care at reduced rates. Usually the arrangement is made between the PPO and a company. The company's employees are given reduced rates for the services used.
5. *Medicaid* is a health insurance program sponsored by the federal and state governments. The benefits, regulations, and eligibility requirements vary from state to state. People older than 65, the blind, the disabled, and low-income families are usually eligible. Medicaid usually pays for hospital services, doctor fees, x-ray and laboratory tests, home care, family planning, dental and eye care, immunization and well-child clinics, and rehabilitation. There is no insurance premium to pay.
6. *Medicare* is a health insurance plan administered by the Social Security Administration of the federal government. Benefits are available for persons age 65 and older. Younger people who are disabled may also be eligible. Monthly premiums are paid by those who are insured. Medicare has two parts. Part A pays for some hospital costs up to certain amounts during a specified time period (see the section on diagnostic related groups). Long-term care and home care are included if certain regulations are met. Part B pays for some medical expenses such as physicians' office visits, diagnostic tests, and treatments. If ordered by the doctor, such things as physical therapy and rental of hospital equipment for home care may be covered by Part B. The benefits and regulations surrounding Medicare are very complex and change often. Your local Social Security office can provide information and answer questions.

Diagnostic Related Groups

Diagnostic related groups (DRGs) were legislated by Congress in 1983 to reduce Medicare and Medicaid costs. Before DRGs, Medicare and Medicaid paid for a certain percentage of actual hospital costs. The amount was determined *after* the hospital stay. Under the DRG system, Medicare and Medicaid payments have been determined *before* the person is hospitalized.

A diagnostic related group consists of specific diagnoses. For a DRG, the government has determined the length of stay and the cost of treating illnesses in the specific category. The hospital is paid the predetermined amount for Medicare and Medicaid patients. If the costs for treating the patient are less than the DRG amount, the hospital keeps the extra money. If the costs are greater than the DRG amount, the hospital takes the loss.

DRGs have had a great effect on health care. Hospitals want to avoid financial loss from lengthy patient stays. Therefore patients are being discharged earlier

than in the past. These patients are often still quite ill. Additional care in nursing facilities or home care is often required.

SUMMARY

This chapter has introduced various types of health care facilities, their general purposes and organization, and the health care workers involved in patient care. Insurance programs that pay for health care were also presented.

Whatever the size of the facility, the focus of care is still the patient. All members of the health team work on behalf of the patient. You have an important place on the health team as RNs and LPNs supervise your work.

REVIEW QUESTIONS

Circle the best *answer.*

1 Helping an individual return to the best possible physical and psychological functioning is known as
   a Detection and treatment of disease
   b Promotion of health
   c Rehabilitation
   d Disease prevention

2 The governing body of a health care facility is called the
   a Director of nursing
   b Health team
   c Board of trustees
   d Nursing team

3 A health care facility for dying patients is called
   a A hospice
   b A long-term care facility
   c An extended care facility
   d A hospital

4 The nursing team includes all of the following *except*
   a Registered nurses
   b Physicians
   c Nursing assistants and orderlies
   d Licensed practical nurses

5 Which provides total and comprehensive nursing care?
   a Functional nursing
   b Primary nursing
   c Team nursing
   d Hospice care

6 These statements are about insurance programs. Which is *false?*
   a Preferred provider organizations (PPOs) provide health care at reduced rates
   b Health maintenance organizations (HMOs) provide health care for a prepaid fee

   c Medicare and Medicaid are government programs for anyone in need
   d Diagnostic related groups (DRGs) affect Medicare and Medicaid payments

Circle T *if the answer is true and* F *if the answer is false.*

T F **7** Rehabilitation begins when the person is ready to be discharged from the health care facility.

T F **8** The director of nursing is responsible for the entire nursing staff and the activities involved in providing safe nursing care.

T F **9** Nursing supervisors are RNs or LPNs.

T F **10** The nursing assistant is a member of both the health team and the nursing team.

T F **11** Primary nursing offers greater patient satisfaction and quality care than does team nursing.

T F **12** An LPN functions under the supervision of an RN, licensed physician, or licensed dentist.

T F **13** An RN can diagnose a patient's health problems and prescribe the appropriate treatment.

T F **14** A nursing assistant assists RNs and LPNs in providing nursing care to patients.

Answers

14 True	**7** False
13 False	**6** c
12 True	**5** b
11 True	**4** b
10 True	**3** a
9 False	**2** c
8 True	**1** c

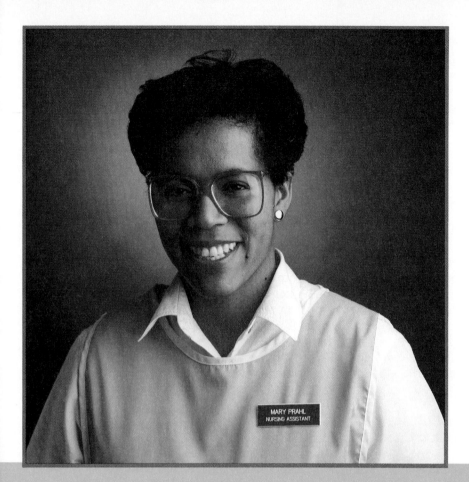

The Nursing Assistant

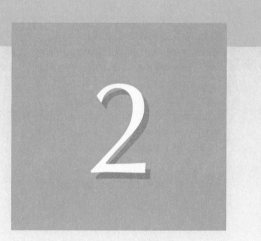

2

OBJECTIVES

- Describe your role as a nursing assistant, and list the functions you can and cannot perform
- Explain why a job description is important
- Describe the qualities and characteristics of a successful nursing assistant
- Identify good health and personal hygiene practices
- Describe how you should dress for work
- Describe nursing assistant training and competency evaluation programs as required by OBRA
- Identify the information contained in the nursing assistant registry and other OBRA requirements
- Describe the ethical behavior of a nursing assistant
- Explain how you can prevent negligent acts
- Give examples of false imprisonment, defamation, assault, and battery
- Describe how to protect the right to privacy
- Identify the role of the nursing assistant in relation to preparing and signing wills
- Describe how the nursing assistant can work well with others to plan and organize work

assault Intentionally attempting or threatening to touch a person's body without the person's consent

battery Unauthorized touching of a person's body without the person's consent

civil law Laws concerned with the relationships between people; private law

crime An act that is a violation of a criminal law

criminal law Laws concerned with offenses against the public and society in general; public law

defamation Injuring a person's name and reputation by making false statements to a third person

empathy The ability to see things from another person's point of view

ethics Knowledge of what is right and wrong conduct

false imprisonment Unlawful restraint or restriction of a person's movement

invasion of privacy A violation of a person's right not to have his or her name, photograph, or private affairs exposed or made public without giving consent

law A rule of conduct made by a government body

legal That which pertains to a law

libel Defamation through written statements

malpractice Negligence by a professional person

negligence An unintentional wrong in which a person fails to act in a reasonable and careful manner and causes harm to a person or to the person's property

slander Defamation through oral statements

tort A wrong committed against a person or the person's property

will A legal statement of how a person's property is to be distributed after the person's death

S tudying to become a nursing assistant is very interesting and exciting. You will learn about things you may have wondered about. How can a bed be made with a person in it? How can a person receive a complete bath in bed? What is heard through a stethoscope when a blood pressure is taken? How do body organs function, and how are they related to each other?

But first you need to understand the roles and responsibilities of nursing assistants. You may be told to do something that is not within the role of a nursing assistant. Therefore you need to know which functions you can and cannot perform. You must also know what is right and wrong behavior and what your legal limitations are in order to safely perform your job. Equally important is an understanding of the qualities and characteristics of a good nursing assistant and how to work effectively with others.

THE ROLES OF A NURSING ASSISTANT

You will perform simple and basic nursing functions under the supervision of a nurse. Your work will be supervised most of the time by RNs and occasionally by LPNs. To help nurses provide safe and effective care, you must understand that nursing is a scientific and personal service given to patients. You will be concerned mainly with assisting nurses in giving patient care. Often you will perform simple functions without a nurse physically present. At other times you will actually help a nurse give bedside nursing care. The following rules should help you understand your role.

1. You are an assistant to the nurse.
2. A nurse determines and supervises your work.
3. You do not decide what should or should not be done for a patient.
4. If you do not understand directions or instructions, you must ask the nurse for clarification before going to the patient.
5. Perform no function or task that you have not been prepared to do or that you do not feel comfortable performing without a nurse's supervision.

FUNCTIONS AND RESPONSIBILITIES

Nursing assistant functions and responsibilities vary among health facilities. *Responsibility* is the duty or obligation to perform some act or function, as well as being able to answer for one's actions. The procedures in this textbook have been performed by nursing assistants. Some are more advanced than others. You will find that the functions and responsibilities of nursing assistants are greater in nursing facilities than in hospitals. Usually, the more nurses in a facility, the simpler and more basic the tasks performed by nursing assistants.

Nursing assistants perform functions and procedures relating to personal hygiene, safety, nutrition, exercise, and elimination needs. Related functions include lifting and moving patients, observing patients, helping promote physical comfort, and collecting specimens (Fig. 2-1). You may also assist with the admission and discharge of patients, and measure temperatures, pulses, respirations, and blood pressures.

Your training may prepare you to perform certain procedures. However, your employer may not allow nursing assistants to perform some of those procedures. Other facilities may have nursing assistants perform procedures and tasks that you did not learn.

There are certain functions, procedures, and tasks that nursing assistants never perform. It is extremely important that you understand what you *cannot* do as a nursing assistant.

Never give medications. This includes medications given orally, rectally, by injection, or directly into the bloodstream through an intravenous line. There have been instances when a nurse has brought a medication to a patient's room while the patient was in the bathroom or busy with some activity. The nurse then instructed the nursing assistant to give the medication to the patient later. In this situation (and other similar situations) the nursing assistant should respectfully but firmly refuse to follow the nurse's direction. Otherwise the nursing assistant would be performing a function and responsibility that is beyond the scope of nursing assistants.

Never insert tubes or objects into body openings or remove them from the body. You must not insert tubes into the patient's bladder, esophagus, trachea, nose, ears, bloodstream, or body openings that have been surgically created. Exceptions to this rule are procedures in this textbook that you will study and practice with your instructor's supervision.

Never take oral or telephone orders from physicians. You might answer the telephone or be near a doctor who wants to give you an order. You should politely give your name and title, ask the doctor to wait, and promptly find a nurse to speak with the doctor.

Never perform procedures that require sterile technique. With sterile technique, all objects that will be in contact with the patient's body are free of all microorganisms. Sterile technique and procedures require skills, knowledge, and judgment beyond the training you will receive. You may assist the nurse during a sterile procedure. However, you will not perform the procedure yourself.

Never tell the patient or family the patient's diagnosis or medical or surgical treatment plans. The physician is responsible for informing the patient and family about the diagnosis and treatment. Nurses may fur-

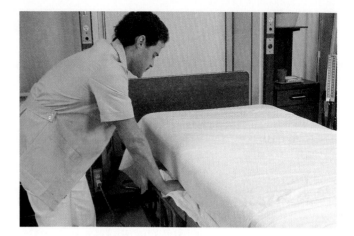

Fig. 2-1 A nursing assistant performing the simple nursing function of making a bed.

ther clarify what the doctor has told the patient and family.

Never diagnose or prescribe treatments or medications for patients. Only doctors can diagnose and prescribe.

Never supervise other nursing assistants. Nurses are responsible for supervising the work of nursing assistants. You will not be trained or paid to supervise the work of others. Supervising other nursing assistants can have serious legal consequences.

Never ignore an order or request to do something that you cannot do or that is beyond the scope of nursing assistants. Promptly explain to the nurse why you cannot carry out the order or request. The nurse will assume you are doing what you were told to do unless you explain otherwise. Patient care cannot be neglected.

Always request a written job description from an employer. The job description lists your responsibilities and the functions that you may be asked to perform. Before accepting a job you should inform your employer of any functions you do not know how to do. Also advise the employer of functions you are opposed to doing for moral or religious reasons. Have a clear understanding of what is expected of you before accepting a job. Do not accept a job that requires you to function beyond your educational limitations or perform acts that are against your moral or religious principles. A sample job description for nursing assistants follows.

No one can force you to perform a function, task, or procedure that is beyond the scope of a nursing assistant. Many times a nursing assistant's job will be threatened for refusal to follow the orders of a nurse. Often the nursing assistant will obey out of fear. That is why you must understand the roles and responsibilities of nursing assistants. You also need to know which functions you can safely perform, the things you should never do, and your job description. Understanding the ethical and legal aspects of your role as a nursing assistant is equally important.

JOB DESCRIPTION*

JOB TITLE: Nursing Assistant
DEPARTMENT: Nursing
JOB SUMMARY: The nursing assistant provides patient care under the direction of the charge nurse, and assists the nursing team in maintaining the nursing and patient units.
SUPERVISOR: Charge nurse
QUALIFICATIONS: 1 High school education preferred but must have at least a grade school education.
2 Documentation of a formal nursing assistant course, or orientation and passage of the competency evaluation.
3 Willingness to learn and work under close supervision.
4 Ability to work with others as a member of the health team.
5 Ability to communicate intelligently with the geriatric patient.
6 Genuine interest in patients and co-workers as demonstrated by timeliness and working when scheduled, including weekends and holidays.

Responsibilities

1 Patient care
   a Treats patients with respect at all times.
   b Provides personal care such as baths, showers, oral hygiene, skin care, hair care, fingernail and toenail care, monitoring fluid intake and output, and toileting care.
   c Assists the male patient to shave daily.
   d Assists in serving and feeding patients.
   e Passes fresh drinking water each shift.
   f Uses safety measures for patients and self when using body mechanics, side-rails, collapsible tubs, etc.
   g Assists with restorative nursing procedures: good body alignment, bed positioning, range-of-motion exercises, transferring patients with the use of a gait belt, etc.
   h Follows the bowel or bladder training program established for a patient.
   i Assists the patient to the bathroom as necessary.
   j Attends scheduled therapy sessions for better understanding of a patient's needs and progress.
   k Encourages and assists the patient to attend all therapies and programs ordered by the doctor (for example, physical therapy).

Continued.

QUALITIES AND CHARACTERISTICS

Caring about others is a common trait of members of the health team. Caring enough to want to make the life of a person happier, easier, or less painful is an essential characteristic of a nursing assistant. There are certain traits, attitudes, and manners that allow one to perform the job well. These are called "qualities and characteristics."

Along with caring, the following qualities and characteristics are necessary for you to function effectively (Fig. 2-2).
   1. *Dependability.* The patient and members of the nursing team rely on you to report to work when scheduled and to be on time. They also depend on you to perform duties and tasks as assigned and to keep obligations and promises.
   2. *Consideration.* You need to be considerate of the patient's physical and emotional feelings.

Patients must be treated gently and with kindness.
   3. *Cheerfulness.* You need to greet and converse with patients and others in a pleasant manner. You cannot be moody, bad tempered, sarcastic, or unhappy when caring for patients.
   4. *Empathy.* Empathy is the ability to see things from the patient's point of view—to put yourself in the patient's position. How would you feel if you had the patient's problem?
   5. *Trustworthiness.* Patients and co-workers have placed their confidence in you. They believe you will keep patient information confidential and not gossip about patients, co-workers, physicians, or members of the health team.
   6. *Respectfulness.* The patient has rights, values, beliefs, and feelings. Although these may dif-

JOB DESCRIPTION—cont'd

l   Assists the patient to follow through and practice activities or exercises learned in the therapy programs.

m Assists in mental rehabilitation programs, especially 24-Hour Reality Orientation.

n   Plans and organizes care so that patients can attend activities or therapies as scheduled.

o   Assists in transferring patients to activity programs.

p   Makes regular rounds to all patients and provides necessary care.

q   Answers call lights promptly and provides or obtains the necessary care.

r   Observes and reports unusual symptoms, changes, accidents, and injuries, to the charge nurse.

s   Uses and maintains assignment cards under the supervision of the charge nurse.

t   Participates in patient care conferences.

u   Reports to the charge nurse before going off duty.

v   Performs other duties as directed by the supervisor.

2 Departmental

a   Makes beds and cleans units on a daily basis as assigned by the charge nurse.

b   Cares for soiled and clean linen and patients' personal laundry according to procedure.

c   Follows established cleaning schedule for drawers, closets, clean and dirty utility rooms, and nurses' station.

d   Cleans and cares for equipment and utensils as assigned by the charge nurse.

3 Personal

a   Wears the official uniform.

b   Maintains good standards of cleanliness and grooming.

c   Completes the nursing assistant orientation program and successfully passes the examination.

d   Attends staff meetings and staff development programs as required.

e   Is able to interpret the "Resident's Rights" to the patient and family.

4 Physical demands

Must have good physical health and be willing and able to be on his or her feet and be active during the entire work shift.

I HAVE READ AND UNDERSTAND THE JOB DESCRIPTION AS STATED. THE JOB DESCRIPTION IS SATISFACTORY AS STATED. I AGREE TO ACCEPT THE POSITION OF NURSING ASSISTANT AS DESCRIBED.

Signature _____ Date _____

*Adapted from "Nursing Assistant Job Description." Courtesy Americana Health Care Center, Kankakee, Illinois.

fer from yours, you must not criticize or condemn the patient. The patient is treated with respect and dignity at all times. Also show respect for supervisors and co-workers.

7. *Courtesy*. You need to be polite and courteous to patients, families, visitors, and co-workers. People are addressed by title and name ("Mrs. Johnson" or "Dr. Wilson.") Other courteous acts include explaining to the patient what is going to be done before performing a procedure, saying "please" and "thank you," and not interrupting others unnecessarily.

8. *Conscientiousness*. You must be careful, alert, and exact in following orders and instructions. You must give thorough care with knowledge and skill, and give your best possible effort.

9. *Honesty*. You must be truthful, sincere, and

genuine, and show a true interest in the patient. The amount and kind of care given, your observations, and any errors are to be reported truthfully and accurately.

10. *Cooperation*. You must be willing to help and work with others. Cooperation is shown by getting along well with others and taking that "extra step" during busy and stressful times.

11. *Enthusiasm*. Enthusiasm is evident if you are eager, interested, and excited about your work. What you are doing is important. If you are enthusiastic, you will want to gain more self-confidence, skill, and knowledge.

12. *Self-awareness*. Being self-aware means that you know your own feelings, strengths, and weaknesses. You need to understand yourself before you can understand your patients.

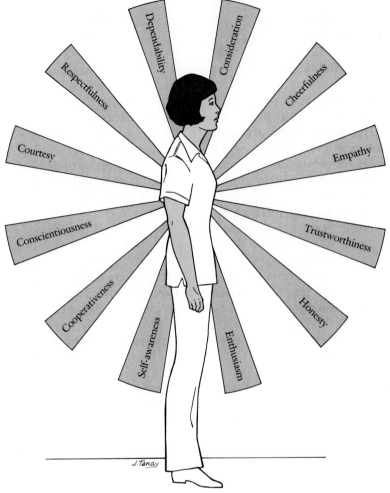

Fig. 2-2 The qualities and characteristics of a successful nursing assistant.

PERSONAL HEALTH, HYGIENE, AND APPEARANCE

The health team serves as an example to others. Patients, families, and visitors expect the health team to set a healthy example. A patient has reason to question a nurse or doctor who chain smokes, especially when the patient is told to stop smoking. As a member of the nursing team you also set an example for others. Your personal health, appearance, and hygiene deserve careful attention.

Your Health

Feeling and looking healthy are important to you as a person, to your patients, and to your employer. Patients and employers have placed their trust in you. They believe that you will provide conscientious and effective care. To fulfill this trust you must be physically and mentally healthy. Otherwise you cannot function at your best.

Diet Good nutrition involves eating a balanced diet from the four basic food groups. Dairy products, fish and meats, fruits and vegetables, and breads and cereals should be in your daily diet. Begin your day with a good breakfast. To maintain your weight, the number of calories taken in must balance your energy needs. To lose weight, caloric intake must be less than energy needs. Avoid excess sweets, salty foods, and crash diets.

Sleep and rest Adequate sleep and rest are needed to stay healthy and do your job well. Most people need 7 to 8 hours of sleep daily. However, the amount varies with each person. Fatigue, lack of energy, and irritability mean that you need more rest and sleep.

Body mechanics You will bend; carry heavy objects; and lift, move, and turn patients. These activities cause stress and strain on your body. You need to have good posture and learn to use your muscles effectively. Posture and body mechanics are discussed in Chapter 10.

Exercise Exercise is important for muscle tone, circulation, and weight control. There are also psychological benefits from exercise. Walking, running, swimming, and biking are excellent forms of exercise. You will feel better physically and more alert mentally when you exercise regularly. Do not begin a vigorous exercise program until you have consulted your physician.

Your eyes Consider for a moment what it would be like if you could not see. Loss of vision would require major changes in the way you live, work, and travel. Your eyes deserve special care and respect. Have your eyes examined and wear glasses or contact lenses as prescribed. Make sure you have enough light when reading or doing fine work.

Good vision is necessary in your work as a nursing assistant. Along with reading instructions, you will measure blood pressures and temperatures. These procedures involve fine measurements. Inaccurate readings can place your patient in danger.

Smoking Smoking has been linked to lung cancer, chronic lung diseases, and many heart and circulatory disorders. If you smoke, remember that cigarette smoke can be offensive to others. Smoke only in areas where smoking is allowed, and never smoke in or near a patient's room. Smoke odors stay on hands, clothing, and hair. Therefore handwashing and good personal hygiene are essential. Wash your hands immediately after smoking and before giving patient care.

Drugs Drug abuse is a major problem in society. People can become physically and psychologically dependent on drugs. Drugs affect thinking, feeling, behavior, and functioning. Accidents, suicides, divorce, crime, and other tragic and violent events have been linked to drug abuse. Individuals who are dependent on drugs may go to any length to obtain them.

Drugs that have an undesirable effect on your mind and body will lessen your ability to work effectively. Working under the influence of drugs places your patients in danger. You should take only drugs prescribed by a doctor and only in the manner prescribed.

Alcohol At first, alcohol may produce feelings of well-being and stimulation. However, alcohol is a drug that has a depressant effect on the brain. Thinking, balance, coordination, and mental alertness are affected. Some people are physically or psychologically dependent on alcohol. These individuals have alcoholism—an illness that can be treated and controlled with the individual's desire and cooperation.

Moderate alcohol use is socially accepted by many people and religious groups. However, because alcohol affects your mind and body, you must never report to work under the influence of alcohol or drink alcohol while on the job. The safety of your patients, co-workers, and yourself must be considered.

Hygiene You must pay careful attention to your personal cleanliness. Preventing offensive body and breath odors is important. You should bathe daily, use a deodorant or antiperspirant, brush your teeth after meals, and use a mouthwash regularly. Your hair should be clean and styled in an attractive and simple way. Fingernails should be clean, short, and neatly shaped.

Special hygiene measures are necessary during menstrual periods. Be sure to change tampons or sanitary napkins frequently, especially if flow is heavy. The genital area should be washed with soap and water at least twice a day. Handwashing is a necessary practice after going to the bathroom, changing tampons or napkins, and washing the genital area.

Foot care prevents odors and infection. Feet should be bathed daily and dried thoroughly between the toes. Cut toenails straight across after bathing or soaking them in water.

Appearance Good health and personal hygiene practices will help you look and feel well. The following practices and suggestions will help you to look neat, clean, and professional (Fig. 2-3).

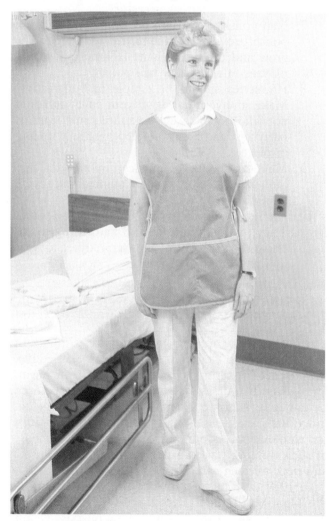

Fig. 2-3 A well-groomed nursing assistant. Note the hairstyle, length and fit of the uniform, and shoes.

1. Uniforms should fit well and be modest in length and style.
2. Make sure your uniforms are clean, pressed, and mended. Wear a clean uniform daily.
3. Underclothes should be clean, fit properly, and be changed every day. Because of perspiration, you may want to change underclothing more often during hot, humid weather and after vigorous exercise.
4. Jewelry should not be worn while on duty. Most facilities let employees wear wedding rings; engagement rings may be allowed. Large rings and bracelets can scratch patients. Necklaces, bracelets, and earrings can easily be pulled off by confused or combative patients, causing you physical injury.
5. Stockings and socks should be clean, well-fitting, and changed daily. Do not roll stockings down or wear round garters. These practices interfere with circulation in the legs.
6. Shoes should be comfortable, give needed support, and fit properly. Clean and polish shoes often to keep them white and neat. Wash laces and replace them as necessary.
7. Nail polish should not be worn. Chipped nail polish provides a place for microorganisms to grow and multiply. Some facilities allow employees to wear clear nail polish.
8. Hairstyles should be simple and attractive. Make sure your hair is off your collar and does not fall in your face. Use simple pins, combs, barrettes, and bands to keep long hair up and in place.
9. Makeup should be modest in amount and moderate in color. Avoid a painted and severe appearance.
10. Perfumes and colognes should not be worn. They may be offensive and nauseating to patients. Some facilities allow employees to wear lightly scented colognes.

NURSING ASSISTANT TRAINING AND COMPETENCY EVALUATION

The care given by nursing assistants is very important to the health and welfare of patients. Safe, effective, quality care is essential to protect patients from harm. Until recently, nursing assistant training was required by law only in some states. The laws required that individuals learn basic nursing knowledge and skills for employment as nursing assistants. The purpose of such training was to protect patients from unsafe and poor nursing care.

In 1987 the Congress of the United States passed the Omnibus Budget Reconciliation Act (OBRA). This law applies to all 50 states. One purpose of this law is to improve the quality of care given to residents of nursing facilities. The law requires education and competency evaluation for all nursing assistants employed in nursing facilities. The requirement is to ensure that nursing assistants have the necessary knowledge and skills to give safe care.

The Training Program

Now every state must have a nursing assistant training and competency evaluation program. The training program must be at least 75 hours of instruction. Sixteen of the hours must be supervised practical training. Such training occurs in a laboratory or clinical setting. The student actually performs nursing care and procedures on another individual. This practical training (also called a clinical practicum or clinical experience) is supervised by a nurse. Usually the nurse is the course instructor.

The training program includes the knowledge and skills needed by nursing assistants to perform their roles and responsibilities. Areas to be studied include communication, infection control, safety and emergency procedures, residents' rights, basic nursing skills, personal care skills, feeding techniques, and skin care. Students also learn how to transfer, position, turn, dress, and ambulate residents, and how to perform range-of-motion exercises. They also learn the signs and symptoms of common diseases and conditions and how to care for cognitively impaired residents (those who have problems with thinking and memory).

Competency Evaluation

The competency evaluation program includes a written test and a skills test. The *written* test involves multiple-choice questions. Each question has 4 possible answers. Only 1 answer is correct. The test is made up of about 75 questions. The *skills* evaluation involves the demonstration of nursing skills. You will have to perform certain skills learned in your training program.

Preparation for the competency evaluation began the first day of your training program. You will learn the basic nursing content areas and skills you need to know for giving safe, quality care. If you listen, pay attention, study hard, and practice safe and effective care, you should do well on both the written and skills tests.

The written and skills competency evaluations are taken after you complete your training program. Your instructor or supervisor can help you in determining where to take the tests and in completing the required application form. There is also a fee for the competency evaluation. This fee must be sent with your application. You will be notified about the location and time of the tests after your application has been processed.

The nursing assistant is given a registration number after successfully completing the competency evaluation. This number is given by the state in which the nursing assistant took the tests. If the first attempt was unsuccessful, the individual can retake the competency evaluation. OBRA requires that individuals be given three opportunities to successfully complete the evaluation.

Nursing Assistant Registry

OBRA requires each state to establish a nursing assistant registry. The registry is an official record or listing of persons who have successfully completed a nursing assistant training and competency evaluation program. The registry contains the following information about each nursing assistant.

1. Full name, including maiden name and any married names
2. Last known home address
3. Registration number and its expiration date
4. Date of birth
5. Last known employer, date hired, and date employment was terminated
6. Date the competency evaluation was passed
7. Information about findings of abuse, neglect, or dishonest use of property. Such information includes the nature of the offense and evidence supporting the finding. If a hearing was held, the date and its outcome are included. The individual has the right to include a statement disputing the finding. All of this information must remain in the registry for at least 5 years.

Registry information can be requested by any nursing facility or agency needing the information. The nursing assistant also receives a copy of all information relating to him or her in the registry. The copy is provided when first included in the registry and when information is changed or added. The nursing assistant can correct information if it is inaccurate.

Other OBRA Requirements

OBRA also requires retraining and a new competency evaluation program for nursing assistants who have not worked for 2 consecutive years (24 months). For example, imagine you completed a training and competency evaluation. After working as a nursing assistant, you quit your job. You were either not employed or you worked in some other field for 2 or more years. Then you decided to work as a nursing assistant again. According to OBRA, you would have to take another training and competency evaluation program. This is to ensure that you have current knowledge and skills to give safe care. It does not matter how long you worked as a nursing assistant. What matters is how long you did *not* work.

Regular in-service education and performance reviews are other OBRA requirements. Nursing facilities must regularly provide educational programs to nursing assistants. The work of each nursing assistant must also be regularly evaluated. These are ways to help ensure that nursing assistants have the knowledge and skills to give your patients safe, effective care.

ETHICAL AND LEGAL CONSIDERATIONS

As a nursing assistant, you will often be in situations in which you must decide what you should and should not do or what you can and cannot do. These questions may involve ethical considerations, or they may be of a legal nature. What would you do in the following situations?

1. A patient asks you to witness the signing of a will.
2. A nurse tells you to "tie down" Mr. Elliott because he keeps trying to get out of bed.
3. A friend's boss is one of your patients. The friend asks you to explain what is wrong with the patient.
4. A nurse has told you to give Mrs. Andrews an enema. Mrs. Andrews refuses to let you perform the procedure.
5. You are helping Sue Jones, RN, with a patient. She tells you to leave the door to the room open so that she can see when Dr. James arrives.

The following discussion will help you to decide what to do in these and other situations.

Ethics

Ethics is the discipline concerned with what is right and wrong conduct. It involves morals and making choices or judgments about what should or should not be done. An ethical person behaves and acts in the right way.

Each professional group has a code of ethics. The code consists of rules, or standards of conduct, that members of the group are to follow. The American Nurses' Association has a code of ethics for RNs, and the National Federation of Licensed Practical Nurses has code of ethics for LPNs. You should develop your own personal code of ethics. Consider the following rules of conduct for nursing assistants.

1. Respect each patient as an individual.
2. Perform no act that is not within the legal scope of the nursing assistant.
3. Perform no act for which you have not been adequately prepared.
4. Take no drug without the prescription and supervision of a physician.
5. Carry out the directions and instructions of the nurse to your best possible ability.
6. Be loyal to your employer and co-workers.
7. Act as a responsible citizen at all times.
8. Recognize the limits of your role and knowledge.
9. Keep patient information confidential.
10. Consider the patient's needs to be more important than your own.

Legal Considerations

Legal considerations relate to laws. A *law* is a rule of conduct made by a government body such as Congress or a state legislature. Laws protect the public welfare and are enforced by the government.

Criminal laws are concerned with offenses against the public and against society in general. A violation of a criminal law is called a *crime*. A person found guilty of a crime will be fined or sent to prison. Murder, robbery, rape, and kidnapping are examples of crimes.

Civil laws are concerned with the relationships between people. Examples of civil laws are those that pertain to contracts and nursing practice. An individual found guilty of breaking a civil law will usually have to pay a sum of money to the injured person.

Torts

Tort comes from a French word meaning *wrong*. Torts fall under the category of civil law. A tort is committed by an individual against another person or the person's property. Torts may be intentional or unintentional. The torts common to health care will be presented.

Negligence is an unintentional wrong. The negligent person fails to act in a reasonable and careful manner and thereby causes harm to the person or property of another. The person at fault failed to do what a reasonable and careful person would have done, or did what a reasonable and careful person would not have done. The negligent person may have to pay damages (that is, a sum of money) to the injured party.

Malpractice refers to negligence by professionals. A person is considered to be a professional because of training, education, and the type of service provided. Nurses, doctors, lawyers, and pharmacists are examples of professional people.

Some common examples of negligent acts committed by nursing assistants are:

1. The side rails are left down on the bed of a confused patient. The patient falls out of bed and breaks a hip.
2. A patient is burned because a nursing assistant applied a warm water bottle that was too hot.
3. A patient's dentures break after being dropped by the nursing assistant.
4. A patient complains to the nursing assistant of chest pain and difficulty breathing. The complaints are not reported to the nurse, and the patient dies of a heart attack.
5. A patient puts on the signal light, and the nursing assistant does not answer the light for several minutes. The patient goes into shock because of sudden, severe bleeding.

As a nursing assistant, you are legally responsible (*liable*) for your own actions. What you do or do not do can lead to a lawsuit if harm results to the person or property of another. At times a nurse may direct you to do something that is beyond the legal scope of your role or something for which you have not been prepared. Giving medications is an example. You may be told not to worry, that the nurse will take full responsibility if anything happens. The nurse will be held liable as your supervisor, but in no way are you relieved of personal liability. *You are responsible for your own actions.*

Although you function under the direction and supervision of a nurse, at times you have a right and a duty to refuse to follow the nurse's directions. You should refuse to follow the nurse's order if:

1. You are asked to do something that is beyond the legal scope of your role.
2. You have not been prepared to perform the function safely.
3. You know that the act or procedure may cause harm to the patient.
4. The nurse's directions or orders are unethical, illegal, or against the policies of the facility.
5. Directions are unclear or incomplete.

You can protect your patients and yourself from negligent acts by using common sense. Ask yourself whether what you are doing is safe for the patient.

Defamation is injuring the name and reputation of a person by making false statements to a third person. *Libel* is making false statements in writing or through drawings. *Slander* is making false statements orally. You can protect yourself from defamation by never making false statements about a patient, co-worker, or any other person. The following are some examples of defamation.

1. Implying or suggesting that an individual has a venereal disease
2. Stating that a patient is insane
3. Implying or suggesting that a person is corrupt or dishonest in dealing with others

Assault and battery are intentional torts. They may result in both civil and criminal charges. *Assault* is intentionally attempting or threatening to touch a person's body without the person's consent. The individual is placed in fear of bodily harm. Threatening to "tie down" or restrain an uncooperative patient is an example of assault.

Battery is the actual unauthorized touching of a person's body without the person's consent. Consent is the important factor in assault and battery. The patient must give consent for any procedure, treatment, or other act that involves touching the body. The patient has the right to withdraw consent at any time.

Consent is more than the patient's verbal okay or signature on a form. For the patient's consent to be valid, it must be *informed* consent. Informed consent recognizes a person's right to decide what will be done to his or her body and who will be allowed to touch his or her body. Consent is considered to be informed when the patient clearly understands the reason for a treatment, what will be done, how it will be done, who will do it, and the expected outcomes. The patient also must understand the treatment alternatives and the consequences of not having the treatment. The responsibility of informing the patient rests with the physician.

You can protect yourself from being accused of battery. Explain to the patient what is to be done and get a consent from the patient. The consent may be verbal; or it may be a gesture, such as a nod, turning over for a backrub, or holding out an arm so that the pulse can be taken.

False imprisonment is the unlawful restraint or restriction of a person's freedom of movement. Threat of restraint or actual physical restraint constitutes false imprisonment. This is an intentional tort.

The following are common examples of false imprisonment.
1. Preventing a person who wants to leave the health care facility from doing so
2. Using restraints on a patient unnecessarily

Invasion of privacy is another tort. Every person has the right not to have his or her name, photograph, or private affairs exposed or made public without having given consent. A violation of this right is an invasion of privacy. You must treat patients with respect and ensure their privacy. Only health workers involved in the patient's care should see, handle, or examine the patient's body. You can ensure the patient's right to privacy by exercising the following precautions.
1. Make sure the patient is covered when being moved in corridors.
2. Screen the patient as in Figure 2-4, or close the door when giving care. Also close drapes and window shades as appropriate.
3. Expose only the body part involved in a treatment or procedure.
4. Do not discuss the patient or the patient's treatment with anyone except the nurse supervising your work. "Shop talk" is a common cause of invasion of privacy.
5. Ask visitors to leave the room when care must be given. Only personnel involved in the person's care should be present when care is given.
6. Keep information contained in the individual's medical record confidential (see Chapter 3).
7. Do not open the person's mail. Individuals have the right to send and receive mail unopened.
8. Allow the individual to visit with others and to use the telephone in private.

Wills

A *will* is a legal statement of how an individual wishes to have property distributed after his or her death. There is no ethical or legal reason you cannot witness the signing of a will if asked to do so. You may also refuse to be a witness without fear of legal liability.

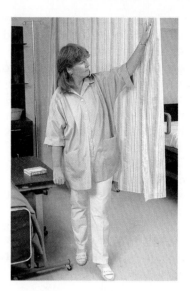

Fig. 2-4 A nursing assistant protecting the patient's privacy by pulling the curtain around the patient's bed.

A patient may ask you to help prepare a will. You must politely refuse such a request. Explain that you do not have the knowledge or legal ability to prepare a will. Ask a nurse to speak to the patient about contacting a lawyer.

Do not witness a patient's will if you have been named in the will. To do so would prevent you from receiving that which had been left to you. As a witness, you must be prepared to testify that the patient was of sound mind at the time the will was signed. Also be prepared to testify that the patient stated that the document being signed was the patient's last will. Be sure to tell your supervisor that you were a witness to a patient's will.

WORKING WITH OTHERS

You are a member of both the nursing and health teams. You will work closely with RNs, LPNs, and other nursing assistants. Your ability to work well with others will influence how well you function as a nursing assistant and the quality of care given to your patients. Besides the ethical and legal considerations just discussed, the following guidelines will help you to work well with others.
1. Understand the roles, functions, and responsibilities in your job description.
2. Develop the desired qualities and characteristics of a nursing assistant.
3. Report to work on time.
4. Call the facility if you cannot report to work. Call as soon as possible, and give the reason for your absence.
5. Practice good personal health and hygiene measures.
6. Take pride in your appearance and follow the dress code of the facility.
7. Act in an ethical and legal manner at all times.
8. Follow the directions and instructions of the

nurse who is supervising your work.
9. Question unclear instructions and things you do not understand.
10. Report patient complaints and your observations to the nurse promptly.
11. Help others willingly when asked.
12. Do not waste supplies and equipment.
13. Do not use the telephone, supplies, or equipment for your personal use.
14. Follow the rules and regulations of the facility in which you are employed.
15. Be accurate in measuring, reporting, and recording.
16. Tell the nurse when you are leaving and when you return to the nursing unit.
17. Do not discuss your personal problems with patients.

Planning and Organizing Your Work

Working well with others includes working in an organized and efficient way. You will be assigned to give nursing care to patients and to perform routine tasks on the nursing unit. Some assignments must be completed by a certain time. Other tasks or functions need to be done by the end of the shift. Planning and organizing your work to give safe, thorough care and to make good use of your time is important. The following guidelines will help you to plan and organize your work.

1. Discuss priorities with the RN or LPN when you receive your assignment.
2. Know the routine of your shift and nursing unit.
3. List care or procedures that must be performed on a schedule. Some patients need to be turned or offered the bedpan every 2 hours.
4. Estimate how much time is needed for each patient, procedure, and task.
5. Identify which tasks and procedures can be done while patients are eating, visiting, or involved in activities or therapies.
6. Plan care around meal times, visiting hours, and therapies. If employed in a nursing facility, you must also consider daily recreation and social activities.
7. Identify situations in which you will need help from a co-worker. Ask a co-worker to help you, and tell the person the approximate time when you will need help.
8. Schedule any equipment or rooms if necessary. Some facilities have only one shower or bathtub to a nursing unit. You will need to schedule the room for your patients' use.
9. Review the procedures to be performed and gather the necessary supplies beforehand.

SUMMARY

This chapter has presented many important considerations about your role as a nursing assistant. You have learned about what you can and cannot do both legally and ethically. The important qualities and characteristics of nursing assistants and their health, hygiene, and personal appearance have been presented. The nursing assistant training and competency evaluation program, registry, and other OBRA requirements were explained. Working well with others was also discussed.

What you do and how you do it will affect yourself, your patients, and your co-workers. All will be affected both personally and legally. You have an important role, and you are a special person for wanting to be a nursing assistant. Use common sense, and act in a reasonable and careful manner. Respect the rights of your patients, and enjoy your work!

REVIEW QUESTIONS

Circle T *if the answer is true and* F *if the answer is false.*

T F **1** You perform simple and complex procedures under the supervision of a nurse.

T F **2** You must perform all tasks and procedures as directed by the nurse.

T F **3** Nursing assistants make decisions about what should be done for patients.

T F **4** All health care facilities allow nursing assistants to perform the same procedures and tasks.

T F **5** You should have a written job description before employment.

T F **6** Nursing assistants never give medications unless directed to do so by an RN.

T F **7** Nursing assistants do not take verbal or telephone orders from physicians.

T F **8** The nursing assistant is responsible for informing the patient about the diagnosis and treatment decided on by the doctor.

T F **9** A nursing assistant shows empathy by feeling sorry for patients.

T F **10** You must show respect for the values, beliefs, and feelings of patients.

T F **11** The nursing assistant should take drugs only under the advice and supervision of a doctor.

T F **12** Alcohol must never be consumed while on duty.

T F **13** A nursing assistant's uncorrected eye problems can affect the patient's safety.

T F **14** Bathing should not be done during menstrual periods.

T F **15** Jewelry is part of your uniform.

T F **16** You can wear pastel nail polish while on duty.

T F **17** You must pass a training program and a competency evaluation program to be employed in a nursing facility.

T F **18** The nursing assistant registry is private and confidential.

T F **19** Competency evaluation involves a written test and a skills test.

T F **20** Only your name and address are included in the registry.

T F **21** Laws are ethical standards of what is right and wrong conduct.

T F **22** A person who breaks a law may be sent to prison or made to pay a sum of money.

T F **23** Negligence occurs when a patient is not reasonable about receiving treatment.

T F **24** Nursing assistants are always responsible for their own actions.

T F **25** Defamation is the unauthorized touching of another person.

T F **26** Assault is attempting or threatening to touch another person without that person's consent.

T F **27** False imprisonment is the illegal restraint of another person's movement.

T F **28** A patient has the right to have the information about treatment and care kept private and confidential.

T F **29** A nursing assistant cannot witness the signing of a will.

T F **30** Nursing assistants can use the telephone and supplies of a facility for personal use.

T F **31** If unable to report to work, you should call and give the employer the reason for your absence.

T F **32** An RN or LPN plans and organizes your work.

Answers

32 False	16 False
31 True	15 False
30 False	14 False
29 False	13 True
28 True	12 True
27 True	11 True
26 True	10 True
25 False	9 False
24 True	8 False
23 False	7 True
22 True	6 False
21 False	5 True
20 False	4 False
19 True	3 False
18 False	2 False
17 True	1 False

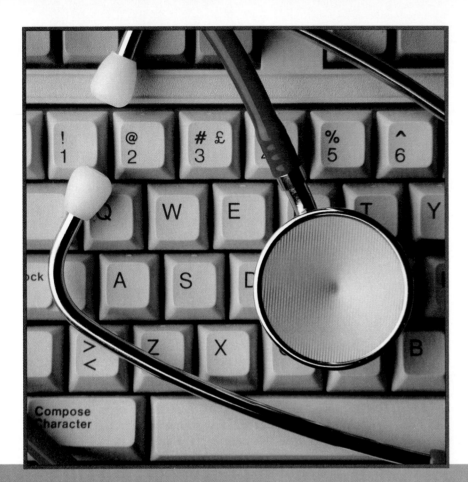

Communicating in the Health Care Facility

OBJECTIVES

- Define the key terms listed in this chapter
- Explain the purpose of communication among members of the health team
- Describe five rules for communicating effectively
- Explain the purpose, parts, and information found in the patient's record
- Describe the legal and ethical responsibilities of nursing assistants who have access to patient records
- Identify information that can be collected about a patient using sight, hearing, touch, and smell
- List the information that should always be included when reporting to the nurse
- Explain the differences between end-of-shift reports and patient care conferences
- List the 15 basic rules for recording
- Describe the purpose of the nursing care plan and the Kardex
- Explain how computers are used in health care
- Describe the rules for answering the telephone

chart Another term for the patient's record

communication The exchange of information; a message sent is received and interpreted by the intended person

Kardex A type of card file that summarizes information found in the patient's record; includes medications, treatments, diagnosis, routine care measures, and special equipment used by the patient

nursing care plan A written guide that gives direction about the nursing care a patient should receive

objective data Information that can be seen, heard, felt, or smelled by another person; signs

observation Using the senses of sight, hearing, touch, and smell to collect information about the patient

patient record A written account of the patient's illness and response to the treatment and care given by the health team; commonly called a chart

recording Writing or charting patient care and observations

reporting A verbal account of patient care and observations

signs Objective data

subjective data That which is reported by the patient and cannot be observed by using the senses; symptoms

symptoms Subjective data

Health team members must communicate with one another for coordinated and effective patient care. Information must be shared about what has been done and what needs to be done for the patient. Information about the patient's response to treatment must also be shared.

Consider this example of communication among the health team. The doctor orders an x-ray examination of Mrs. Bailey's stomach. Because the stomach must be empty to get a clear x-ray film, Mrs. Bailey cannot have breakfast until she returns from the radiology department. A nurse tells the dietary department not to send the patient's breakfast until notified. Mrs. Bailey goes for the x-ray examination and is brought back to her room. An x-ray technician tells the nurse that the patient may have breakfast. The nurse orders the meal, and a member of the dietary department brings the tray to the nursing unit. You are told that Mrs. Bailey's tray may be served, and you take it to her. When she has finished eating, you remove the tray and observe how much

she has eaten of each food on the tray. You report your observations to the nurse, who then records the information in Mrs. Bailey's record. Because health team members communicated with one another, Mrs. Bailey's care was coordinated and effective.

You will communicate with members of the health team. However, you will have more direct and frequent communication with the nursing team. You need to understand the basic elements and rules of communication. Then you can learn ways to communicate patient information to the health team.

COMMUNICATION

Communication is the exchange of information—a message sent is received and interpreted by the intended person. For communication to be effective, words must have the same meaning for both the sender and the receiver of the message. The words "small," "moderate," and "large" are often used in health care. Unfortunately, the words mean different things to different people. Is small the size of a dime or the size of a half dollar? In health care, differences in meaning can have serious consequences. Try to avoid words that have more than one meaning.

Using words familiar to people you communicate with is important. You will learn medical terminology as you study and gain experience as a nursing assistant. If a nurse or health team member uses an unfamiliar term, ask for an explanation. If you do not understand the message sent to you, communication will not have occurred. Likewise, remember not to use terms that are unfamiliar to your patients.

Try to be brief and concise when communicating. Do not add unrelated or nonessential information. You must stay on the subject, avoid wandering in thought, and not get wordy. Being brief and concise reduces the possibility of omitting important details.

Information should be presented in a logical and orderly manner. Organize your thoughts so that you can present them logically and in sequence. Think about what happened step by step, and present the information to the nurse in that way.

You need to present facts and be specific when giving information. The receiver should have a clear picture of what you are communicating. Asking for clarification or for more information should not be necessary. Telling the nurse that a patient's temperature is 100.2° F is more specific, factual, and descriptive than saying the "temperature is up."

THE PATIENT'S RECORD

The *patient's record* (chart) is a written account of the patient's illness and response to treatment and care.

The primary purpose of the patient's record is to provide a way for the health team to communicate information about the patient. The record is permanent and can be retrieved many years later if the patient's health history is needed. The record is a legal document. It can be used in court as evidence of the patient's problems, treatment, and care.

The record has many forms organized into sections for easy use. The record includes the patient's history, results of the physical examination, doctor's orders, and doctor's progress notes. Also included are the graphic sheet, x-ray examination reports, IV therapy record, respiratory therapy record, consultation reports, surgery and anesthesia reports, and admission sheet. Each page must be stamped with the patient's name, room number, and other identifying information. This helps prevent errors and improper placement of records.

Members of the health team record information on the forms for their department and service. The information is then available to other health team members who need to know what care has been provided and the patient's response (Fig. 3-1).

Health care facilities have policies about the contents of patient records and about who may have access to them. Policies may state how often health workers need to make a recording and who can record on the specific forms. There will also be policies about acceptable abbreviations, correcting errors, the color of ink to use, and how to sign entries. You need to know the policies of your facility as they relate to patient records.

Some facilities do not allow nursing assistants to write in patient records. Those facilities believe that recording patient information is a nurse's responsibility. Others rely on nursing assistants to record observations and care. General guidelines for recording are presented later in the chapter.

Usually all professional health workers involved in the patient's care have access to the patient's record. Those not directly involved usually cannot review the patient's record. Cooks, laundry and housekeeping personnel, and office clerks have no need to see patient records. Some facilities do not let nursing assistants read patient charts. In such instances the nurse shares necessary patient information with the nursing assistants.

If you have access to patient records, you have an ethical and legal responsibility to keep patient information confidential. Also remember that only members of the health team involved in the patient's care need to read the chart. Therefore, if you have a friend, relative, or acquaintance in the facility, and you are not involved in that patient's care, you have no right to review that person's chart. To review the chart would be an invasion of privacy.

Many facilities allow patients to see their records if they make such a request. You should know your employer's policy regarding patients seeing their charts. If a patient asks you for the chart, report the request to the nurse. The nurse will then be responsible for dealing with the patient's request.

The following parts of the patient's record relate to your work as a nursing assistant.

The Admission Sheet

The admission sheet is completed when the person is admitted to the health care facility. It contains identifying information about the patient—legal name, birth date, age, sex, current address, marital status, Social Security number, religion, occupation, employer, and insurance coverage. The patient's nearest relative and the name and number of the person to notify in an emergency are found on the admission sheet. Some facilities include the patient's diagnosis, date and time of admission, and the physician's name. An identification number, given to each patient admitted to the facility, is included on the admission sheet.

You might use the admission sheet to learn background information about a patient. You might also use it to fill out other forms that require some of the same information. If you use the admission sheet to fill out other forms, the patient does not have to answer the same question several times.

The Graphic Sheet

The graphic sheet is used to record patient measurements and observations that are made every shift or 4 to 5 times per day (Fig. 3-2). Information may include the patient's blood pressure, temperature, pulse, respirations, height and weight, and the time of the doctor's visit. Some graphic sheets have places to chart the patient's intake and output, appetite at each meal, routine care, and bowel movements.

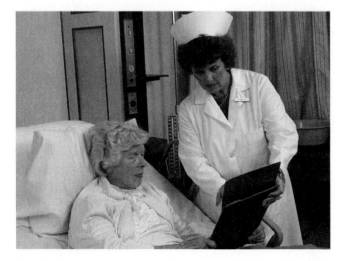

Fig. 3-1 A nurse reviewing a chart to learn more about the patient.

Date	8/21/84		8/22/84		8/23/84		8/24/84		8/25/84		8/26/84		8/27/84	
	HD	PO	HD	PO	HD	PO	HD	PO	HD	PO	HD	PO	HD	PO
	1		2		3		4		5		6		7	

Temperature	AM		PM		AM		PM		AM		PM		AM		PM		AM		PM		AM		PM		AM		PM		AM		PM	
Time	8	12	4	8	8	12	4	8	8	12	4	8	8	12	4	8	8	12	4	8	8	12	4	8	8	12	4	8

(Temperature graph: range 96° to 106°, plotted around 99°–100° early, dipping to ~98° on 8/22, peak ~100.5° on 8/25, declining to ~98° by 8/27.)

Pulse	84	86	88	86	84	80	82	86	86	84	88	84	80	78	78	82	88	96	86	84	80	82	78	74	76	78	76	74
Respirations	20	20	22	22	20	20	22	22	22	20	22	20	20	18	18	20	22	24	22	20	20	22	18	16	18	20	20	18
Blood pressure	128/74	130/80	126/80	126/72	118/70	116/74	118/76	120/80	124/80	128/80	130/84	120/80	116/70	116/74	126/80	120/82	114/70	110/68	120/82	124/80	116/72	120/84	124/80	118/76	110/70	120/74	120/76	114/72

Weight	130 lbs	129 lbs	129 lbs	129½ lbs	130 lbs	130 lbs	130 lbs

Intake	11-7	7-3	3-11	11-7	7-3	3-11	11-7	7-3	3-11	11-7	7-3	3-11	11-7	7-3	3-11	11-7	7-3	3-11	11-7	7-3	3-11
Oral	100	950	760	50	1200	900	200	1120	875												
IV & Subq.	—	—	—	—	—	—	—	—	—												
Other																					
TOTAL	100	950	760	50	1200	900	200	1120	875												
Output	650	710	250	500	830	625	700	850	480												
Urine																					
Emesis																					
TOTAL	650	710	250	500	830	625	700	850	480												
24 Hour intake	1810			2150			2195														
24 Hour output	1610			1755			2030														
Bowel movement	—	—	—	✓	—	—	✓	—	—	—	—	—	✓	—	—	✓	—	—	—	—	—
Doctor visited	—	9 A	—	—	920/A	—	—	10 A	—	—	1130/A	—	—	8 A	—	—	1020/A	—	—	12 N	—

Fig. 3-2 A sample graphic sheet.

Nurses' Notes

Nurses' notes are a written description of nursing care given, the patient's response to care, and signs and symptoms that the nurse observed about the patient's condition (Fig. 3-3). They are used to record information about special treatments and medications that were given. Patient teaching and counseling, procedures performed by the physician, and visits by health team members are also recorded in the nurses' notes.

If you have access to nurses' notes, you can use them to better understand the patient's care and response. Some facilities allow nursing assistants to chart in the nurses' notes.

Flow Sheets

A flow sheet is used to record measurements or observations made at frequent intervals. For example, a patient's blood pressure, pulse, and respirations may be taken every 15 minutes or more often. The graphic sheet does not have enough room for frequent measurements. A flow sheet designed for this purpose does. The intake and output record kept at the bedside is another type of flow sheet; it is discussed in Chapter 16.

Date	Time		Signature
8/23/84	3⁴⁰/PM	Pt. complained of incisional pain. Pointed to incision and described pain as "throbbing." Holding pillow over incisional area. Skin warm and dry with perspiration noted on forehead. No new drainage noted on dressing; dressing intact. ————	S. Smith, R.N.
8/23/84	3⁴⁵/PM	BP 138/88, P 90, R 22. Demerol 100 mg IM in RVG for incisional pain. Pt. positioned in left side-lying position. Back massage given. ————	S. Smith, R.N.
8/23/84	4⁰⁰/PM	BP 132/84, P 84, R 20. Pt. stated pain "going away." Appears more relaxed and resting with more comfort. ————	S. Smith, R.N.

Nurses' Notes

NAME:
SOCIAL SECURITY NUMBER:
IDENTIFICATION NUMBER:
ROOM AND BED NUMBER:
PHYSICIAN NAME:

Fig. 3-3 A sample of nurses' notes.

REPORTING AND RECORDING OBSERVATIONS

Reporting and recording are ways in which communication takes place among health team members. Both are accounts of what has been done for and observed about the patient. *Reporting* is the verbal account of patient care and observations. *Recording* or *charting* is the written account.

Observations

Observation is using the senses of sight, hearing, touch, and smell to collect information about the patient. When you look at a patient you will observe such things as the way the patient is lying, sitting, or walking. You will also observe if the patient's skin is flushed or pale, and if there are any reddened or swollen body areas. You will listen to the patient breathe, talk, and cough, and you will use a stethoscope to listen to the heartbeat. By touching the patient you can collect information about skin temperature and feel if the skin is moist or dry. You will also use the sense of touch to take the patient's pulse. The sense of smell is used to detect body, wound, and breath odors and unusual odors from urine and bowel movements.

Information observed about a patient is called objective data. *Objective data (signs)* are those things you can see, hear, feel, or smell. You can feel a pulse and you can see what a patient has vomited. However, you cannot feel or see the patient's pain or nausea. The things a patient tells you about that you cannot observe through your senses are *subjective data (symptoms)*.

There are many other things you will observe about your patients. More specific observations are discussed as they relate to the procedures and patient care presented throughout this book. The following box lists the basic observations you need to make and report to the nurse.

You should make notes of your observations. They will be valuable later when you report to the nurse.

BASIC OBSERVATIONS OF THE PATIENT

A Ability to respond
1 Is the patient easy or difficult to arouse?
2 Is the patient able to give his or her name, the time, and the location when asked?
3 Can the patient identify others accurately?
4 Can the patient answer questions correctly?
5 Can the patient speak clearly?
6 Are instructions followed appropriately?
7 Is the patient calm, restless, or excited?
8 Is the patient conversing, quiet, or talking a lot?

B Movement
1 Can the patient squeeze your fingers with each hand?
2 Can the patient move arms and legs?
3 Are the patient's movements shaky or jerky?

C Pain or discomfort
1 Where is the pain located? (Ask the patient to point to the pain.)
2 Does the pain go anywhere else?
3 What is the duration of the pain?
4 How does the patient describe the pain?
  a Sharp
  b Severe
  c Knifelike
  d Dull
  e Burning
  f Aching
  g Comes and goes
  h Depends on position
5 Has medication been given?
6 Did medication help relieve the pain? Is pain still present?
7 Is the patient able to sleep and rest?
8 What is the position of comfort?

D Skin
1 Is the skin pale or flushed?
2 Is the skin cool, warm, or hot?
3 Is the skin moist or dry?
4 What color are the lips and nails?
5 Are there any sores or reddened areas?

E Eyes, ears, nose, and mouth
1 Is there drainage from the eyes?
2 Are the eyelids closed?
3 Are the eyes reddened?
4 Does the patient complain of spots, flashes, or blurring?
5 Is the patient sensitive to bright lights?
6 Is there drainage from the ears?
7 Can the patient hear? Is repeating necessary? Are questions answered appropriately?
8 Is there drainage from the nose?
9 Can the patient breathe through the nose?
10 Is there breath odor?
11 Does the patient complain of a bad taste in the mouth?

F Respirations
1 Do both sides of the patient's chest rise and fall with respirations?
2 Is there noisy breathing?
3 Is there difficulty breathing?
4 What is the amount and color of sputum?
5 What is the frequency of the patient's cough? Is it dry or productive?

G Bowels and bladder
1 Is the abdomen firm or soft?
2 Does the patient complain of gas?
3 What is the amount, color, and consistency of bowel movements?
4 Does the patient have pain or difficulty urinating?
5 What is the amount of urine?
6 What is the frequency of urination?
7 What is the frequency of bowel movements?

H Appetite
1 Does the patient like the diet?
2 How much of the food on the tray is eaten?
3 What are the patient's food preferences?
4 How much liquid was taken?
5 What are the patient's liquid preferences?
6 How often does the patient drink liquids?
7 Is the patient experiencing nausea?
8 What is the amount and color of material vomited?
9 Does the patient have hiccups?
10 Is the patient belching?

I Activities of daily living
1 Can the patient perform personal care without help?
  a Bathing
  b Brushing teeth
  c Combing and brushing hair
  d Shaving
2 Does the patient use the toilet, commode, bedpan, or urinal?
3 Is the patient able to feed self?
4 Is the patient able to walk?
5 What amount and kind of assistance is needed?

If you carry a note pad and pen in your pocket, you can note your observations when they are made (Fig. 3-4).

Reporting

The nursing assistant reports about patient care and observations to the nurse. Reports must be prompt, thorough, and accurate. Always tell the nurse the patient's name, room and bed number, and the time your observations were made or the care was given. Report only those things that you observed or did yourself. Reports are given as often as the patient's condition requires or as often as requested by the nurse. Use your written notes to give a specific, concise, and descriptive report (Fig. 3-5).

The nurse gives a report at the end of the shift to nursing personnel of the oncoming shift (end-of-shift report). Information is shared about the care that has been given and the care that must be given to patients. Information about the patient's condition is also included. Some facilities require that all members of the nursing team hear the end-of-shift report as they come on duty. Others require that nursing assistants perform routine tasks while RNs and LPNs hear the report.

Recording

If allowed to record on the patient's chart, you have an even greater responsibility to communicate clearly and thoroughly. You should follow these basic rules when recording.

1. Always use ink.
2. Include the date and the time whenever a recording is made.
3. Make sure writing is legible and neat.
4. Use only the abbreviations approved by the facility in which you are employed (see Chapter 32).
5. Use correct spelling, grammar, and punctuation.
6. Never erase if you make an error. Cross out the incorrect part, write "error" over it, and rewrite the part.
7. Sign all entries with your name and title as required by facility policy (for example, Jane Bates, NA).
8. Do not skip lines. Draw a line through the blank space of a partially completed line to prevent others from recording in a space with your signature.
9. Make sure each form on which you are writing is stamped with the patient's name and other identifying information.
10. Record only what you have observed and done yourself.
11. Never chart a procedure or treatment until it has been completed.
12. Be accurate, concise, and factual. Do not record judgments or interpretations.
13. Record in a logical and sequential manner.
14. Be descriptive. Avoid terms that have more than one meaning.
15. Use the patient's exact words whenever possible. Use quotation marks to show that the statement is a direct quote.

NURSING CARE PLANS

The *nursing care plan* is a written guide that gives direction about the care a patient should receive. The plan consists of patient problems identified by the nurse and the actions nursing personnel will take to help the patient solve the problem. The nurse responsible for the patient's care develops the care plan. Some nurses welcome suggestions from nursing assistants when developing nursing care plans.

A care plan is developed for each patient. You can use the nursing care plan as a guide to the individualized care of a patient.

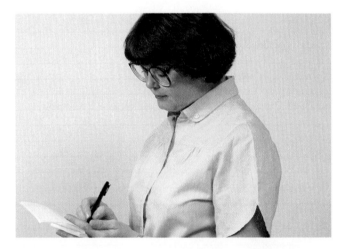

Fig. 3-4 A nursing assistant writing down observations.

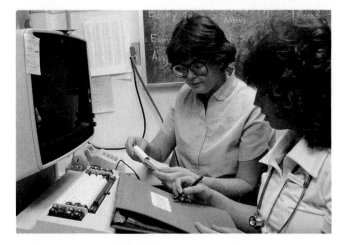

Fig. 3-5 A nursing assistant using notes when reporting.

Diet:

Activities:	Bath:	Travel:	Position:
___ Complete bed rest ___ Bed rest ___ Bathroom privileges ✓ Up ad lib	___ Bed bath ___ Partial ✓ Bathe self ___ Tub ___ Shower	___ Wheelchair ___ Stretcher ✓ Ambulatory ___ Walker ___ Cane ___ Crutches	

Side rails:	Oxygen:	Special equipment:
___ Constantly ___ Nights only ✓ Side rail release	___ Liters per minute ___ PRN ___ Constantly ___ Tent ___ Catheter ___ Mask ___ Cannula	

Prosthesis:	Special privileges:	
___ Dentures ✓ Eye glasses ___ Contact lenses ___ Hearing aid ___ Limb ___ Other	May shampoo hair as desired	Allergies: None known

Date	Medications	Date	Treatments
8/21	Tagamet 300 mg qid — 9-1-5-9 — po	8/21	Vital signs — qid
8/21	Mylanta 10 ml po 90 min pc + HS		Fluids
		8/21	Intake and output
		8/21	Hematest stools for occult blood
8/22	HS Med Dalmane 30 mg po		
PRN 8/22	Tylenol tabs 2 po q4h — headache		IVs
		8/21	D5W 1000 ml q8h

Room	Name	Age	Diagnosis	Doctor
333-1	Bailey, Laura	46	Duodenal ulcer	J. Wilson

Fig. 3-6 A sample Kardex.

Forms for nursing care plans vary in each facility. Often the care plan is included in the patient's record or in a Kardex.

THE KARDEX

The *Kardex* is a type of card file used in some health care facilities. For each patient there is a card that contains some of the information found in the patient's record. The Kardex is basically a summary of the current medications and treatments ordered by the doctor, the patient's current diagnosis, routine care measures, and special equipment needs. The Kardex is a quick, easy source of patient information (Fig. 3-6).

MEDICAL TERMINOLOGY AND ABBREVIATIONS

Medical terminology and abbreviations are commonly used when communicating in health care. The terms seem strange and confusing at first. They also seem difficult to learn and remember. You will learn medical words and abbreviations as you study to become a nursing assistant. Soon you will find yourself understanding and using them. You will continue to learn them as you work and gain experience.

Medical terms and abbreviations are presented throughout this book. Chapter 32 deals only with medical terminology and abbreviations. If a word or phrase is used that you do not understand, be sure to ask a nurse to explain its meaning. Otherwise, effective communication will not have occurred. You may also want to purchase a medical dictionary so that you can look up and learn new words.

COMPUTERS IN HEALTH CARE

As in other businesses and professions, the use of computers is a growing trend in health care. Information systems have been developed that collect, send, record, and store information. The information can be retrieved when needed. Patient records and care plans are on computer in many facilities. Instead of recording on the patient's chart, health team members enter information into the computer (Fig. 3-7). Using a computer is easier, faster, and more efficient than writing on the chart. Using the computer to record observations is also more accurate, legible, and reliable.

Departments such as x-ray, the laboratory, dietary, and pharmacy communicate with the nursing unit by computer. Instead of sending a typed report by messenger for the patient's record, the information is entered into the computer. The information can be accessed at the computer in the nurses' station. These systems provide communication links between the various departments. The systems have reduced the

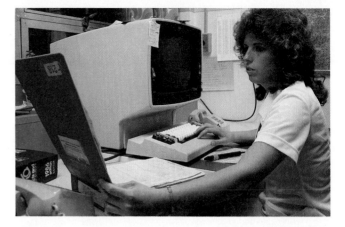

Fig. 3-7 A nurse entering information into a computer.

amount of clerical work and telephone calls between departments. Information is communicated with greater speed and accuracy.

Computers are also used to monitor certain measurements such as blood pressures, temperatures, heart rates, and heart function. The computer recognizes normal and abnormal measurements. When the abnormal is sensed, an alarm alerts the nursing staff. Monitoring by computer is accurate and increases early detection of life-threatening events.

Computers help save time. The quality and safety of patient care are increased. There are fewer things omitted from the patient's record and fewer errors made in recording. Records are more complete, and personnel are more efficient.

Because of the vast amount of information that can be stored and the easy access to the computer, the patient's right to privacy must be protected. Only certain individuals are allowed to use the computer. They have their individual codes to access the computer files. Nursing assistants are usually not allowed to use the computer. If you are allowed access, you must follow the ethical and legal considerations relating to privacy, confidentiality, and defamation (see Chapter 2).

Using a computer is easy and fun. If you have the opportunity to use the computer in your place of employment, take advantage of the opportunity. Eventually all health care facilities will have computerized information systems. Knowing how to use computers is an additional skill that makes you a good person to employ.

PATIENT CARE CONFERENCES

A patient care conference involves health team members sharing information and ideas about the patient's care (Fig. 3-8). The purpose is to develop or revise a patient's nursing care plan so that effective care can be provided. Nursing assistants are usually included in the conference and are encouraged to share suggestions and observations.

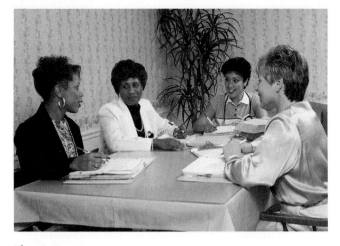

Fig. 3-8 Members of the health team having a patient care conference.

TELEPHONE COMMUNICATIONS

Clerical personnel are hired to answer telephones on nursing units and in facilities. However, other health team members may need to answer a ringing phone. Often it is necessary to answer the phone in a patient's room. Good telephone communication skills are essential. The caller cannot see you. But much information is given by your tone of voice, how clearly you speak, and your attitude. When answering the phone you must be as professional as you would be if you were speaking to the other person face-to-face.

Most facilities have policies about how telephones should be answered. You need to follow the policies where you work. The following guidelines can help you be professional and courteous when answering phones at work or at home.

1. Answer the call on the second ring if possible. This avoids excessive ringing of phones, which can disturb patients. It also tells the caller that personnel are efficient.
2. Do not answer the phone in a rushed or hasty manner. Take a deep breath before answering to avoid sounding breathless to the caller.
3. Give a courteous greeting, identify the area, and give your name. For example: "Good morning. Three center. Sandy Hill." Or: "Good afternoon. Mr. Weimer's room. Tara Willis speaking."
4. Have a pencil and paper ready when you answer the phone. This lets you take a message for other health workers or for the patient.
5. Write down the caller's name. This way, you will not have to ask the caller to repeat his or her name later during the call.

6. Get the correct spelling of the caller's name. This lets you address the caller correctly and give correct messages.
7. Collect the following information when taking a message: the caller's name, date and time of the call, telephone number, and the message.
8. Repeat the message and telephone number back to the caller. This helps you make sure you have the right information.
9. Ask the caller to "Please hold" if necessary. You may have to place a caller on hold if you are taking another call, if another line is ringing, or if you cannot complete the conversation. However, find out who is calling first, then ask if the caller can hold. You do not want to put a caller with an emergency on hold.
10. Do not lay the phone down or cover the receiver with your hand when you are not speaking to the caller. The caller may overhear confidential conversations.
11. Return to a caller on hold within 30 seconds. It is impolite to keep a caller on hold. Ask if the caller can wait longer or if the call can be returned.
12. Do not give confidential information to any caller. Remember that patient information is confidential. Refer such calls to a nurse.
13. Transfer the call if appropriate. Tell the caller that you are going to transfer the call. Give the name of the department if appropriate. Give the caller the phone number in case the call gets disconnected or the line is busy.
14. End the conversation politely. Thank the person for calling and say good-bye.
15. Give the message to the appropriate person.

SUMMARY

Communication among health team members is essential for effective and coordinated patient care. Verbal and written communication should be factual, concise, understandable, and presented in a logical order. Reports, the nursing care plan, the Kardex, patient records, and patient care conferences are ways in which health team members communicate with one another. Good telephone answering skills are also important when communicating in health care.

The traditional patient record presented in this chapter is being replaced in many facilities with computers. Regardless of the type of patient record used, remember that the patient's record is a legal document that contains highly personal and confidential information.

REVIEW QUESTIONS

Circle T *if the answer is true and* F *if the answer is false.*

T F **1** Health team members communicate to provide effective and coordinated patient care.

T F **2** The patient's chart is destroyed after the patient leaves the health care facility to protect the patient's right to privacy.

T F **3** The patient's chart cannot be used in a lawsuit because of the right to privacy.

T F **4** Nursing assistants generally have access to the charts of all patients in the facility.

T F **5** Information is collected about the patient by using sight, hearing, touch, and smell.

T F **6** Subjective data are signs observed by using the senses.

T F **7** The nursing care plan summarizes the medications and treatments ordered by the doctor.

T F **8** The end-of-shift report and the patient care conference have the same purpose.

T F **9** Patient care conferences are held to develop or revise the patient's nursing care plan.

Circle the best *answer.*

10 When communicating, you should do all of the following *except*
a Use terms that have more than one meaning
b Be brief and concise
c Present information logically and in sequence
d Give facts and be specific

11 These statements are about patient records. Which is *false?*
a The record is used to communicate information about the patient.
b The record is a written account of the patient's illness and response to treatment.
c The record is a written account of care given by the health team.
d Anyone working in the facility can read the patient's record.

12 A patient's blood pressure is measured 4 times a day. Where should the blood pressure be recorded?
a Admission sheet
b Graphic sheet
c Flow sheet
d Nurses' notes

13 Where does the nurse describe the nursing care given?
a Nursing care plan
b Nurses' notes
c Graphic sheet
d Kardex

14 When recording information you should do all of the following, *except*
a Use ink
b Include the date and time
c Erase if you make an error
d Sign all entries with your name and title

15 These statements are about recording. Which is *false?*
a Use the patient's exact words when possible.
b Record only what you have observed and done yourself.
c Do not skip lines.
d To save time, chart a procedure before it is completed.

16 The nursing care plan
a Is written by the physician
b Consists of actions nursing personnel should take to help a patient
c Is the same for all patients
d Is also called the Kardex

17 These statements are about computers in health care. Which is *false?*
a Computers are used to collect, send, record, and store information.
b The patient's privacy must be protected.
c Computers link one department to another.
d All employees can use the computer.

18 You answer the patient's phone. How should you answer?
a "Good morning. Mr. Klein's room."
b "Good morning. Third floor."
c "Hello."
d "Good morning. Mr. Klein's room. Betsy Simpson speaking."

Answers

18	d	9	True
17	d	8	False
16	b	7	False
15	d	6	False
14	c	5	True
13	b	4	False
12	b	3	False
11	d	2	False
10	a	1	True

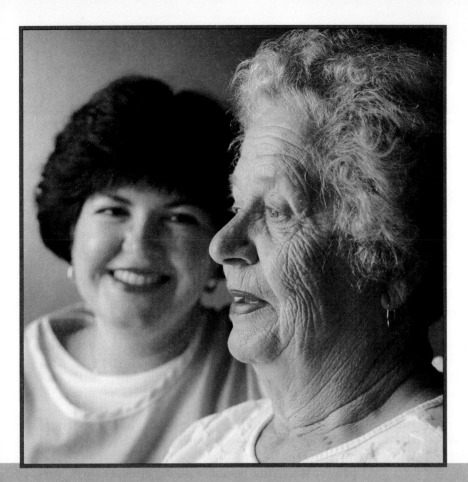

Understanding Your Patients

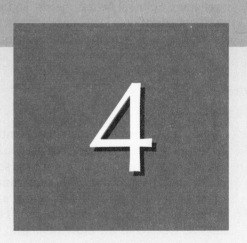

4

OBJECTIVES

- Define the key terms listed in this chapter
- Identify the parts that make up the whole person
- Describe the basic needs identified by Abraham Maslow
- Explain how culture and religion influence health and illness
- Identify the psychological and social effects of illness
- Describe individuals cared for in health care facilities
- Identify patient rights as outlined in the American Hospital Association's *A Bill of Rights*
- Identify the elements needed for effective communication
- Describe how nursing assistants use verbal and nonverbal communication
- Identify six communication barriers
- Explain why family and visitors are important to patients
- Identify the courtesies nursing assistants should give to patients and visitors

body language Facial expressions, gestures, posture, and body movements that send messages to others

culture The values, beliefs, habits, likes, dislikes, customs, and characteristics of a group that are passed from one generation to the next

esteem The worth, value, or opinion one has of a person

geriatrics The branch of medicine concerned with the problems and diseases of old age and the elderly

need That which is necessary or desirable for maintaining life and mental well-being

nonverbal communication Communication that does not involve words

obstetrics The branch of medicine concerned with the care of women during pregnancy, labor, and childbirth, and for the 6 to 8 weeks after birth

pediatrics The branch of medicine concerned with the growth, development, and care of children ranging in age from the newborn to the adolescent

psychiatry The branch of medicine concerned with the diagnosis and treatment of people with mental health problems

religion Spiritual beliefs, needs, and practices

self-actualization Experiencing one's potential

verbal communication Communication that uses the written or spoken word

The patient is the most important person in the health care facility. Age, religion, nationality, education, occupation, and life-style are some factors that make each patient a unique individual. The patient must be treated as a human being, as a person who is valuable, important, and special. The patient must also be treated as an individual who can think, act, and make decisions.

You will care for many patients. You must remember that each patient is a person. You need to understand the fears, needs, and rights of the patient. This chapter will help you understand and communicate with the patients you will serve, help, and care for.

THE PATIENT AS A PERSON

In the busy world of health care it is often easy to forget that the patient lying in the bed is a person who lives, works, loves, and has fun. Things are done to and for the patient. The patient is told what to eat and when to eat, sleep, bathe, have visitors, sit in a chair, walk, and use the bathroom. The fact that the

patient once tended to these activities without help is easily forgotten. No wonder patients often complain that doctors, nurses, nursing assistants, and other health workers treat them as things rather than as people.

Too often the patient is viewed and referred to as a physical disease or problem, such as "The appendectomy in 310" rather than "Sally Jones in 310." Most patients receive care for physical problems. However, to effectively care for patients, you must be aware of the whole person.

The whole person consists of physical, social, psychological, and spiritual parts. The parts are woven together and cannot be separated (Fig. 4-1). Each part relates to and depends on the others. As a social being, a person speaks and communicates with others. Physically, the brain, mouth, tongue, lips, and throat structures must function for speech. Communication is also highly psychological because it involves the thinking and reasoning abilities of the mind. To consider only the physical part is to ignore the patient's ability to think, make decisions, and interact with others. It also ignores the fact that the patient is a living person with experiences, joys, sorrows, and needs.

NEEDS

A *need* is that which is necessary or desirable for maintaining life and mental well-being. According to Abraham Maslow, a famous psychologist, certain ba-

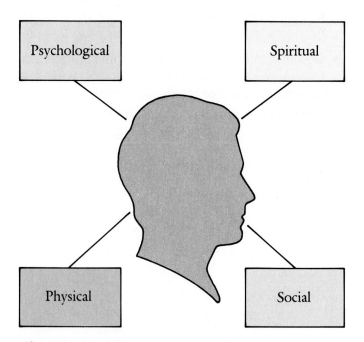

Fig. 4-1 A person is a physical, psychological, social, and spiritual being. The parts overlap and cannot be separated.

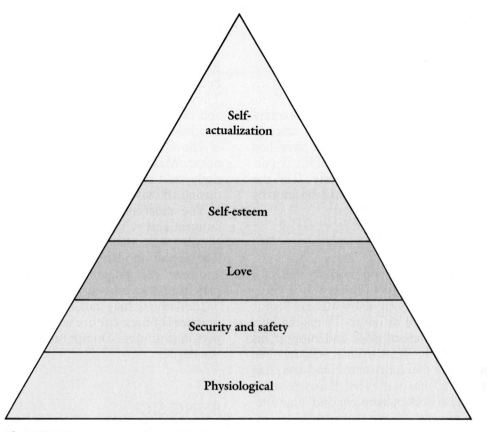

Fig. 4-2 Basic needs for life as described by Maslow. These needs, from the lowest to the highest level, are physiological needs, the need for safety and security, the need for love and belonging, the need for esteem, and the need for self-actualization.

sic needs must be met if a person is to survive and function. These needs are arranged in order of importance. The lower level needs must be met before the higher level needs. These basic needs, from the lowest level to the highest, are physiological or physical needs, the need for safety and security, the need for love and belonging, esteem needs, and the need for self-actualization (Fig. 4-2). People normally meet their own needs every day. When they are unable to meet their basic needs it is usually because of disease, illness, or injury. When ill, they usually seek help from doctors, nurses, and other health team members.

Physiological Needs

Human beings share certain physiological needs with other forms of life such as animals, fish, and plants. The physical needs required for life are oxygen, food, water, elimination, and rest. These needs are the most important for survival. They must be met before higher level needs.

An individual will die within minutes without oxygen. People can survive longer without food or water but will begin to feel weak and ill within a few hours. If the kidneys or intestines are not functioning nor-

mally, poisonous wastes build up in the bloodstream. If the problem is not corrected, the person will die. Without enough rest and sleep, an individual will become exhausted.

You will assist nurses to help patients meet their physical needs. You need to develop a true appreciation of these physical needs. Most people take them for granted until a problem develops. How do you feel when you have difficulty breathing or when you feel a choking sensation? How do you react when you are thirsty, hungry, or unable to get enough sleep?

The Need for Safety and Security

Safety and security needs relate to the need for shelter, clothing, and protection from harm or danger. Problems from inadequate shelter or clothing are often dealt with by health workers. Frostbite is common during the winter because of inadequate clothing and shelter.

Many people feel that certain medical and nursing procedures are harmful or dangerous. This is not surprising because many procedures involve frightening equipment, require entering the body, and cause pain or discomfort. Patients feel safer and more secure if they know why a procedure is to be done, how it will be performed, and the sensations they can expect to feel.

The Need for Love and Belonging

The need for love and belonging relates to love, closeness, affection, belonging, and meaningful relationships with others. There have been many cases in which patients have had slow recoveries or have died because of lack of love and belonging. This is particularly true of children and the elderly. The patient's need for love and belonging can be met by family, friends, and health workers.

The Need for Esteem

Esteem is the worth, value, or opinion one has of a person. Esteem needs relate to thinking well of yourself and of being thought well of by others. People often lack esteem when ill or injured. Imagine how a father feels when he cannot work and support his family because of an illness. A woman who has had a breast removed may feel unattractive and less than whole. A person who has had facial burns or a leg amputation may also feel incomplete and unattractive.

The Need for Self-Actualization

Self-actualization means experiencing one's potential. It involves learning, understanding, and creating to the limit of a person's capacity. This is the highest need. Rarely, if ever, is this need totally met. Most people constantly try to learn and understand more. The need for self-actualization can be postponed and life will continue.

CULTURE AND RELIGION

Culture is defined as the characteristics of a group of people—the values, beliefs, habits, likes, dislikes, and customs—that are passed from one generation to the next. The patient's culture influences health beliefs and practices. Culture also influences behavior during illness.

You will care for people from different cultural backgrounds. Besides caring for Americans of various nationalities, you may care for people from other cultures and countries. These people have family practices, food preferences, hygiene habits, and clothing styles that are different from your own. The person may also speak and understand a foreign language. Some cultural groups have beliefs about the causes and cures of illnesses. They may perform certain rituals aimed at ridding the body of disease.

Religion relates to spiritual beliefs, needs, and practices. Like culture, an individual's religion influences health and illness practices. Religions may have beliefs and practices relating to diet, healing, days of worship, birth, and death.

Most Americans are of the Jewish, Protestant, or Roman Catholic faiths. Many people find religion to be a source of comfort and strength during illness. They may wish to observe certain religious practices and may appreciate a visit from their spiritual leader or adviser. If a patient requests a visit from a member of the clergy, promptly report the request to the nurse. Make sure the patient's room is neat and orderly, and place a chair by the bed. Ensure privacy during the visit.

You must show respect and accept the patient's cultural and religious background. When you meet people from other cultures or religions, take advantage of the opportunity to learn about their beliefs and practices. This will help you to understand your patient and give better care.

Individuals may not follow all of the beliefs and practices of their culture or religion. Remember, each person is unique. Do not judge patients by your own standards.

BEING SICK

If people had a choice between staying healthy or becoming ill, surely health would be selected. Unfortunately, people do become ill and injured. Besides physical problems caused by illness, the sick person experiences some psychological and social effects.

The patient may be unable to perform normal activities such as working, going to school, preparing meals, doing house or yard work, and participating in sports or hobbies. Daily activities bring personal satisfaction, worth, and contact with others. Most people feel frustrated and angry when unable to perform them. These feelings may become even greater if others must perform routine functions for the patient.

Sick people have many fears and anxieties. There is fear of death, disability, chronic illness, and loss of function. Some can explain why they are afraid. Others keep their feelings to themselves because they fear being laughed at for being afraid. A patient with a broken leg may be afraid of having a limp or of not walking again. A patient having surgery might be afraid that cancer will be found. These fears and anxieties are normal and expected. You need to appreciate how patients are affected by illness. Thinking about how you would feel and react if you had the patient's illness and problems will help you to have empathy for the patient.

Sick people are generally expected to behave in a certain way. They are expected to see a doctor, stay in bed, and rely on others for care and comfort. These dependent behaviors are accepted so that the person can get well. When recovery is delayed or does not occur, the normal psychological and social effects of illness intensify.

PATIENTS YOU WILL CARE FOR

Patients are grouped in health facilities according to problems, needs, and age. Areas may be designated for children, patients with medical problems, those having surgery, and people with mental health problems. Nursing personnel in each area are familiar with the patients' problems. They have the knowledge and skill to give the best care possible. The areas also have equipment and supplies to meet the patients' needs.

Obstetrical Patients

Obstetrics is the branch of medicine concerned with the care of women during pregnancy, labor, and childbirth, and during the 6 to 8 weeks after birth. Obstetrical patients are seen usually in clinics or physicians' offices during pregnancy. When labor begins these women usually go to a hospital and are admitted to the obstetrical (maternity) department.

Pregnancy, labor, and childbirth are normal and natural events. The process is usually without problems or complications. However, complications can occur at any time from the beginning of pregnancy through the 6 to 8 weeks after childbirth.

Newborns

Newborns are generally cared for in the nursery next to the maternity department. Nursing personnel care for the newborns and take them to their mothers at feeding times. Most hospitals have "rooming-in" programs that allow the mother to care for the infant in the mother's room. Similar programs allow the mother to care for the baby during the day; at night the newborn is cared for in the nursery.

Pediatric Patients

Pediatrics is the branch of medicine concerned with the growth, development, and care of children ranging in age from the newborn to the adolescent. Pediatric patients may be healthy or sick. Children may be seen in clinics, doctors' offices, or at home. When hospitalized, children are admitted to a pediatric unit. The unit is specially designed and equipped to meet the needs of children and parents. The child's physical, safety, and emotional needs are major concerns of nursing personnel (Fig. 4-3).

Medical Patients

Medical patients are usually adults with illnesses, diseases, or injuries that do not require surgery. They

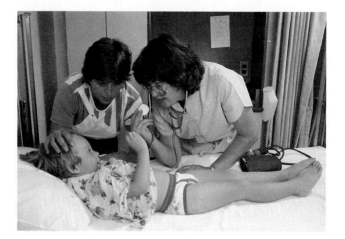

Fig. 4-3 The nursing assistant giving care to a sick child.

may have acute, chronic, or terminal illnesses. Examples are infections, strokes, or heart attacks. Various therapies, medications, and treatments help these patients meet their basic needs.

Surgical Patients

Surgical patients are those who are being prepared for or who have had surgery. Surgeries range from simple to very complex procedures. An appendectomy is a simple surgery. Open-heart and brain surgery are complex procedures.

The needs of preoperative patients usually involve physical preparation and teaching about what to expect in the postoperative period. Patients are also helped to deal with their fears and anxieties about the need for and the outcome of the operation. The needs of postoperative patients relate to relieving pain and discomfort, preventing complications, and adjusting to body changes caused by surgery. Chapter 23 deals with patients having surgery.

Psychiatric Patients

Psychiatry is the branch of medicine concerned with the diagnosis and treatment of people with mental health problems. These patients may be treated in physicians' offices, clinics, general hospitals, or psychiatric hospitals. Their problems vary from mild to severe mental and emotional disorders. Some function normally but need help making some decisions or coping with life stresses. Others are severely disturbed. They cannot perform simple functions such as eating, bathing, or dressing. Special precautions and treatments may be necessary if patients are dangerous to themselves or others.

Geriatric Patients

Geriatrics is the branch of medicine concerned with the problems and diseases of old age and the elderly.

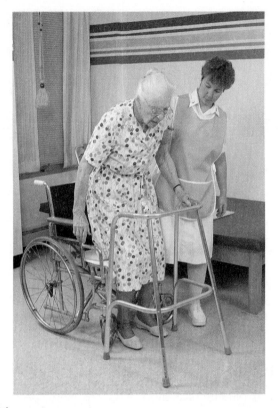

Fig. 4-4 This elderly person lives in a nursing facility.

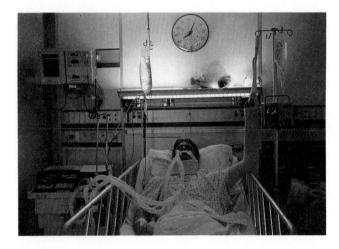

Fig. 4-5 A general view of the design and equipment in a coronary care unit.

Aging is a normal process, not an illness or disease. Many elderly people enjoy good health. Others suffer from acute or chronic illnesses or from degenerative diseases common in the elderly.

Some body changes normally occur because of the aging process. There are also social and psychological changes. The physical, psychological, and social changes of aging are presented in Chapter 7. Sometimes the changes are so severe that the person may have to reside in a nursing facility (Fig. 4-4).

Patients in Special Care Areas

Some patients have special problems, are seriously ill, or are in life-and-death situations. They need special care and equipment. Special care units are designed and equipped to treat and prevent life-threatening problems and complications. These special care areas include intensive care units, coronary care units (Fig. 4-5), surgical intensive care units, neonatal intensive care units, kidney dialysis units, burn units, and emergency rooms. The nurses in these areas have had special education and training. They are prepared to meet the patient's complex needs and to operate the sophisticated equipment.

PATIENT AND RESIDENT RIGHTS

In 1973 the American Hospital Association (AHA) issued *A Patient's Bill of Rights*. The idea of patient rights came about when people demanded more information about their health problems and treatment. They also demanded better care at lower costs and greater involvement in decisions about their care and treatment. Patients were not willing to be viewed as helpless and unknowing people who accepted the doctor's advice without question.

A Patient's Bill of Rights has an ethical and legal basis. The right to privacy and informed consent are involved. Although the relationship between the physician and the patient is emphasized, there are important messages for the health team. The basic points of *A Patient's Bill of Rights* are presented in Table 4-1.

The Omnibus Budget Reconciliation Act of 1987 (OBRA) outlines the rights of residents in nursing facilities. They are presented in Chapter 7.

COMMUNICATING WITH THE PATIENT

Several elements are necessary for effective communication between you and the patient. First, you must understand and respect your patient as a person. Second, the patient must be viewed as more than a disease or an illness; the patient is a physical, psychological, social, and spiritual human being. Third, you must appreciate the problems and frustrations the patient is experiencing as a result of being sick. Fourth, you need to recognize and respect the patient's rights. Finally, you must accept and respect the patient's religion and culture.

The rules for communication discussed in Chapter 3 apply when you are communicating with patients.

1. Use words that have the same meaning to both you and the patient.
2. Avoid using medical terminology and other words that are unfamiliar to the patient.
3. Communicate in a logical and orderly manner; do not allow your thoughts to wander.

TABLE 4-1   Patient Rights

Right	Explanation
Consideration and respect	To be treated as a person and be given kind and thoughtful care. Personal values, beliefs, cultural practices, and personality are considered when planning and providing care.
Information	To receive information from the doctor about the diagnosis, treatment, and prognosis in terms the patient can understand. Unfamiliar medical terminology is avoided. An interpreter is needed if the patient does not understand or speak English. The nearest relative or legal guardian is informed of the patient's diagnosis, treatment, and prognosis if it is considered unwise to tell the patient.
Informed consent	To receive information and explanations about any treatments or procedures. The doctor must provide information about treatment purpose, risks, alternatives, and probable length of incapacitation. The patient should be told the name of the person who will perform the treatment or procedure. (Informed consent is discussed in Chapter 2.)
Refusing treatment	To refuse treatment. The patient does not have to consent to each treatment or procedure recommended by the doctor. The doctor must inform the patient of the risks to life and health involved in refusing the treatment.
Privacy	To have the patient's body, record, care, and personal affairs kept private. The right to privacy is still protected after death. (The right to privacy is discussed in Chapter 2.)
Confidentiality	To expect that information will be shared with other health workers in a wise and careful manner. All health workers must recognize the confidential nature of patient information. (Some patients are very sensitive about their health problems and personal relationships.)
Hospital services	To expect that the hospital can provide needed services. After immediate needs are met, the patient may be transferred to another facility that is better equipped to handle the patient's problems and needs. The patient is to be informed of the reason for the transfer and of other alternatives.
Information on the hospital's relationship to educational and health care institutions	To be informed of any relationships with schools and other health care facilities. Patients have the right to know about these relationships and to know the names of students or other persons providing or involved in their care.
Information on research and human experimentation	To receive information and explanations about research for making an informed decision about participating. The patient's consent must be obtained before involvement in human experimentation or research. The patient may refuse to participate.
Continuing care	To be informed of the care needed after discharge. The patient must be given written information about the times and locations of appointments with doctors.
The patient's bill	To examine bills and receive an explanation of the items in the bill. This right exists even if the bill is to be paid by an insurance company or the government.
Hospital rules and regulations	To be informed of any rules and regulations applying to conduct as a patient. The patient and family may be given a pamphlet that explains the rules and regulations.

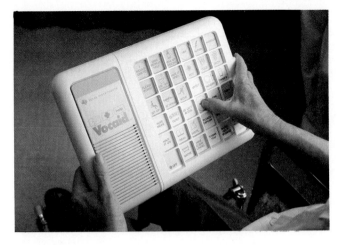

Fig. 4-6 A patient using an electronic talking aid.

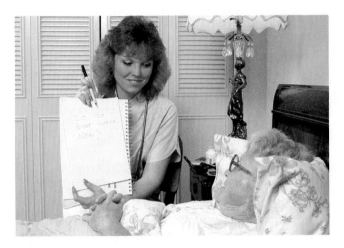

Fig. 4-7 The nursing assistant writing a note to a patient who has a hearing difficulty.

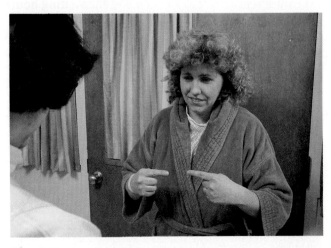

Fig. 4-8 A patient using sign language to communicate.

4. Be specific and factual when presenting information.

Verbal and nonverbal methods of communication are used when relating to patients. You need to understand how to use both methods for effective communication with your patients.

Verbal Communication

Words are used in *verbal communication*. The words may be spoken or written. Verbal communication is used to converse with patients, to find out how they are feeling physically and emotionally, and to share information with them.

Most verbal communication involves the spoken word. You need to control the loudness and tone of your voice, speak clearly and distinctly, and avoid using slang or vulgar words. Shouting, whispering, and mumbling cause ineffective communication.

The written word is used when patients cannot speak or hear. If a patient cannot speak, provide a way for the patient to send messages. A Magic slate, paper and pencil, or an electronic talking aid (Fig. 4-6) can be used. Write messages to communicate with deaf patients or those with severe hearing problems (Fig. 4-7). Deaf patients may use sign language to communicate (Fig. 4-8).

Communication between you and the patient should be kept on a professional level. You should not become personally involved or develop friendships with patients.

Nonverbal Communication

Nonverbal communication does not involve words. Gestures, facial expressions, posture, body movements, touch, and smell are examples of how messages can be sent and received without words. Nonverbal messages are considered to be a more accurate reflection of a person's feelings. They are usually involuntary and difficult to control. A patient may say one thing but act in a different way. Therefore you need to watch the patient's eyes, the way hands are held or moved, gestures, posture, and other actions.

Touch Touch is a very important form of nonverbal communication. Comfort, caring, love, affection, and reassurance can be conveyed by touch. Touch means different things to different people. The meaning depends on the person's age, culture, sex, and life experiences. Although some people do not like to be touched, do not be afraid to use touch to convey caring and warmth. Often it is comforting to patients to have their hands held.

Body Language Patients send messages to you through their *body language*. Posture, gestures, and body movements are involved in body language. A person with slumped posture is probably not feeling well or happy. A patient may deny having pain but may protect the affected body part by standing, lying, or sitting in a certain way.

You also send messages to the patient by the way you act and move. Your facial expressions, the way you stand or sit, how you walk, and how you look at the patient are some of the ways you communicate with the patient. Your body language should show interest and enthusiasm about your work and caring and respect for the patient. Be sure to control body language in relation to odors from excretions or the patient's body. Many odors are beyond the patient's control. The patient's embarrassment and humiliation will increase if you react to the odor.

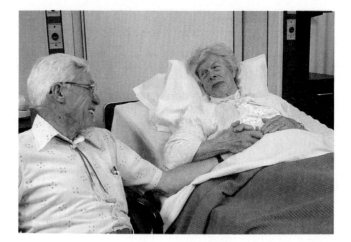

Fig. 4-9 A patient visiting with family.

Barriers to Effective Communication

Communication may fail to occur for many reasons. You and the patient must use and understand the same language. If you do not, messages will not be accurately interpreted.

Changing the subject is another barrier to communication. Either you or the patient may change the subject when the topic being discussed causes one or both to be uncomfortable. Avoid changing the subject whenever possible.

Giving your opinion usually tells the patient that you are judging the patient's values, behavior, or feelings. Let patients express their feelings and concerns without adding your opinion, making a judgment, or jumping to conclusions.

Some nursing assistants talk a lot when patients are silent or speak infrequently. The excessive talking is usually due to nervousness and being uncomfortable with silence. Silences have meaning. Acceptance, rejection, fear, or the need for quiet and time to think may be conveyed by silence.

Listening is very important for effective communication. Communication will be blocked if you fail to listen to your patients with interest and sincerity. Do not pretend to listen. This causes inappropriate responses to the patient and conveys a lack of interest and caring. You may also miss important complaints of pain, discomfort, or other abnormal sensations that must be reported to the nurse.

Pat answers such as "Don't worry," "Everything will be okay," and "Your doctor knows best" block communication. These make patients feel that their concerns, feelings, and fears are being ridiculed and are not important to you or the nursing team.

THE PATIENT'S FAMILY AND VISITORS

Family, relatives, and friends can help meet the patient's needs for safety and security, love and belonging, and esteem. They can offer support and comfort and can lessen feelings of loneliness. Some

also help with the patient's care. They may help with such things as meals, bathing, and brushing and combing hair. Often a patient's recovery is influenced by the presence or absence of significant family members or friends.

The patient should be allowed to visit with family and friends in private and without unnecessary interruptions (Fig. 4-9). Sometimes care must be given when visitors are present. You should politely ask them to leave the room and show them where they can wait comfortably. Do not expose the patient's body in front of visitors. Promptly notify the visitors when they may return to the room.

Family and visitors must be treated with courtesy and respect. They may be very concerned and frightened about the patient's condition. They also need the support and understanding of the nursing team. However, you should not discuss the patient's condition with them. Refer their questions to the nurse responsible for the patient's care.

Visitors often have questions about visiting rules. The number of visitors allowed and the visiting hours vary among facilities. Often they depend on the patient's age or condition. Parents of a hospitalized child are usually allowed to visit as often and as long as they desire. The family of a patient in a critical care unit may be restricted as to the time and length of visits. Dying patients are usually allowed to have family members present at the bedside constantly. You need to know the visiting policies of your facility and the special considerations allowed for individual patients. Visitors may also have questions about the location of the chapel, gift shop, business office, lounge, or cafeteria. You must know the location, special rules, and hours of these facilities.

Sometimes a family member or friend can have a negative effect on the patient. If the patient becomes upset or is becoming tired because of a visitor, report your observations to the nurse. The nurse can then speak with the visitor about the patient's needs.

SUMMARY

People are physical, psychological, spiritual, and social human beings. They have certain basic needs necessary for life: physiological needs, the need for safety and security, love and belonging, esteem, and self-actualization. When people cannot meet their own needs, they usually seek the services of a doctor or other health workers.

Culture and religion influence the lives of most people. Beliefs, values, habits, diet, and health and illness practices may relate to a person's culture or religion. Try to become aware of the beliefs and practices of the major cultural and religious groups in your community.

Being sick affects a person physically, psychologically, and socially. How a person handles illness is influenced by religion, culture, family, the patient's basic personality, the seriousness of the illness, and the speed of recovery. The patient may have many

fears and anxieties about illness, basic needs, and being able to function normally again. You need to have empathy for your patients if you are to provide effective care.

Patients are usually grouped in health care facilities according to problems, needs, and age. These patients may have different problems, but all have the same basic needs and the same rights. Verbal and nonverbal communication is used by patients and health workers. You need to be aware that the strongest and truest messages are usually sent nonverbally. Observe facial expressions, gestures, and body language for clues about the patient's feelings. Try to control your own nonverbal communication so that you do not send the patient negative messages. Use touch to communicate understanding, comfort, and caring to your patients. Avoid blocking communication by being aware of the common barriers to effective communication.

Finally, remember that family members and visitors are important to the patient. They can help meet the patient's basic needs and influence recovery. Treat them with respect and courtesy.

REVIEW QUESTIONS

Circle T *if the answer is true and* F *if the answer is false.*

T F **1** A person is a physical, psychological, social, and spiritual being.

T F **2** Physiological needs are the most essential for survival.

T F **3** Food, clothing, and shelter are physical needs.

T F **4** Love and belonging are not important to the sick person.

T F **5** Esteem means love, closeness, affection, and meaningful relationships with others.

T F **6** Self-actualization is the need to learn, create, and understand to the limit of a person's capacity.

T F **7** The patient's cultural background will probably influence health and illness practices.

T F **8** Dietary practices may be influenced by both culture and religion.

T F **9** A patient's religious and cultural practices are not allowed in the health care facility.

T F **10** Fears and anxieties about being sick are normal reactions.

T F **11** An obstetrical patient is one who is pregnant, in labor, giving birth, or who has given birth during the previous 6 to 8 weeks.

T F **12** Pediatrics is concerned only with sick children.

T F **13** The psychiatric patient has some type of mental health problem.

T F **14** Geriatric patients suffer from a disease commonly known as aging.

T F **15** The patient has the right to expect considerate and respectful care.

T F **16** Patients have the right to receive information about their diagnoses, treatment, and prognoses from their doctors.

T F **17** Patients cannot refuse treatment if the doctor believes it is necessary.

T F **18** The right to privacy is protected after death.

T F **19** The patient has the right to refuse to participate in research and human experimentation.

T F **20** Verbal communication involves the written or spoken word.

T F **21** Verbal communication is the truest reflection of a person's feelings.

T F **22** Messages can be sent by facial expressions, gestures, posture, body language, and touch.

T F **23** Touch means different things to different people.

T F **24** Verbal communication will not occur if the sender and the receiver use and understand different languages.

T F **25** Changing the subject promotes communication because more interests and concerns of the patient are discussed.

T F **26** You should offer an opinion when the patient is expressing fears and concerns.

T F **27** You should talk when the patient is silent.

T F **28** Listening is essential for effective communication.

T F **29** Pat answers, such as, "Don't worry," encourage the patient to express feelings and concerns.

T F **30** Family and friends can help the patient meet basic needs.

T F **31** Patients and visitors should be allowed privacy when visiting.

T F **32** Visitors should be politely asked to leave the room when care must be given.

Answers

1 True	**12** False	**23** True
2 True	**13** True	**24** True
3 True	**14** False	**25** False
4 False	**15** True	**26** False
5 False	**16** True	**27** False
6 True	**17** False	**28** True
7 True	**18** True	**29** False
8 True	**19** True	**30** True
9 False	**20** True	**31** True
10 True	**21** False	**32** True
11 True	**22** True	

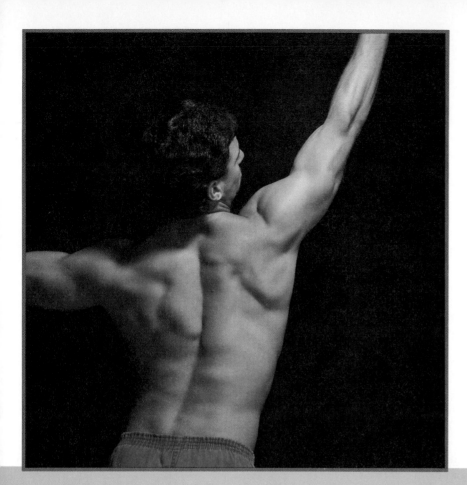

Body Structure and Function

5

OBJECTIVES

- Define the key terms listed in this chapter
- Identify the basic structures of the cell, and explain how cells divide
- Describe four types of tissue
- Identify the structures of each body system
- Describe the functions of each body system

artery A blood vessel that carries blood away from the heart

capillary A tiny blood vessel; food, oxygen, and other substances pass from the capillaries to the cells

cell The basic unit of body structure

digestion The process of physically and chemically breaking down food so that it can be absorbed for use by the cells

hemoglobin The substance in red blood cells that carries oxygen and gives blood its color

hormone A chemical substance secreted by the glands into the bloodstream

menstruation The process in which the lining of the uterus breaks up and is discharged from the body through the vagina

metabolism The burning of food for heat and energy by the cells

organ Groups of tissues with the same function

peristalsis Involuntary muscle contractions in the digestive system that move food through the alimentary canal

respiration The process of supplying the cells with oxygen and removing carbon dioxide from them

system Organs that work together to perform special functions

tissue Group of cells with the same function

vein A blood vessel that carries blood back to the heart

NOTE: Students are responsible for only those terms mentioned in the text. Additional terms used in labeling figures throughout this chapter are for illustrative purposes only.

You will care for people who need help meeting their basic needs. Their bodies cannot work at peak efficiency because of illness, disease, or injury. You will be directed to provide care and perform procedures to promote comfort, healing, and recovery. A basic knowledge of the body's normal structure and function will help you understand certain signs and symptoms, reasons for care, and purposes of procedures. This knowledge should result in safer and more efficient patient care.

CELLS, TISSUES, AND ORGANS

The basic unit of body structure is the *cell*. Each cell of the body has the same basic structure. However, the functions, size, and shape of cells may be different

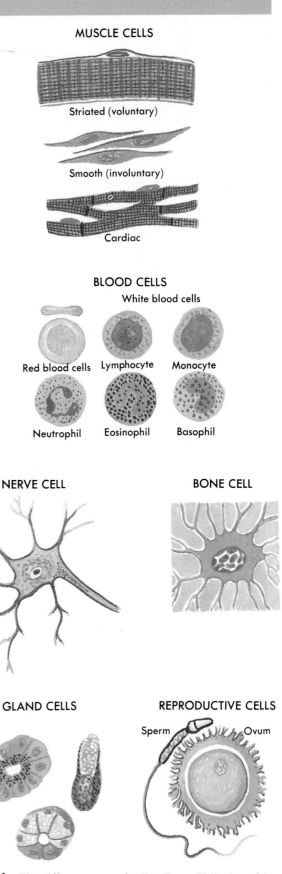

Fig. 5-1 The different types of cells. (From Thibodeau GA: *Anatomy and physiology*, St Louis, 1987, Mosby–Year Book.)

(Fig. 5-1). Cells are so small that a microscope is needed to see them. Cells need food, water, and oxygen to live and perform their functions.

The cell and its basic structures are shown in Figure 5-2. The *cell membrane* is the outer covering that encloses the cell and helps the cell hold its shape. The *nucleus* is the control center of the cell; it directs the cell's activities. The nucleus is in the center of the cell. The *cytoplasm* is the portion of the cell that surrounds the nucleus. Cytoplasm contains many smaller structures that perform cell functions. The *protoplasm,* which means "living substance," refers to all of the structures, substances, and water within the cell. Protoplasm is a semiliquid substance much like an egg white.

Chromosomes are threadlike structures within the nucleus. Each cell has 46 chromosomes. Chromo-

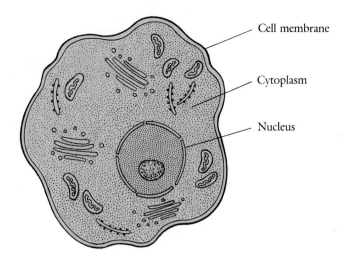

Cell membrane

Cytoplasm

Nucleus

Fig. 5-2 Parts of a cell.

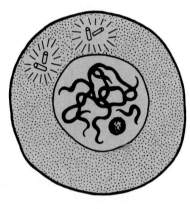

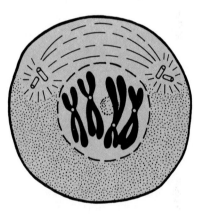

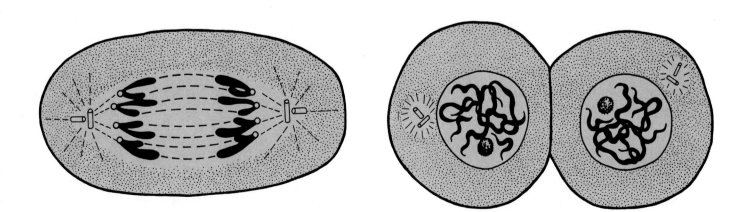

Fig. 5-3 Cell division.

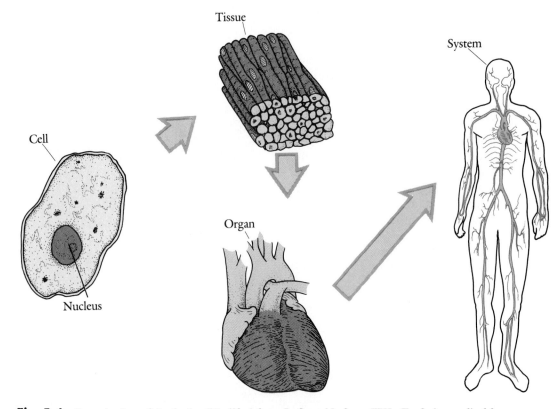

Fig. 5-4 Organization of the body. (Modified from Lafleur M, Starr WK: *Exploring medical language: a student-directed approach*, ed 2, St Louis, 1989, Mosby–Year Book.)

somes contain *genes*. Genes control the physical and chemical traits inherited by children from their parents. Inherited traits include height, sex, and the color of eyes and skin.

Besides controlling cell activities, the nucleus is responsible for cell reproduction. Cells reproduce by dividing in half. The process of cell division is called *mitosis*. Cell division is necessary for growth and repair of body tissues. During the process of mitosis, the 46 chromosomes arrange themselves in 23 pairs. As the cell divides, the 23 pairs of chromosomes are pulled in half. The two new cells are identical, and each contains 46 chromosomes (Fig. 5-3).

The cells are the building blocks of the body. Groups of cells with similar functions combine to form *tissues*. The body has four basic types of tissue:

1. *Epithelial tissue* covers the internal and external surfaces of the body. Tissue that lines the nose, mouth, respiratory tract, stomach, and intestines is epithelial tissue. Skin, hair, nails, and glands are included in this category.
2. *Connective tissue* anchors, connects, and supports other body tissues. Connective tissue is found in every part of the body. Bones, tendons, ligaments, and cartilage are connective tissue. Blood is a form of connective tissue.
3. *Muscle tissue* allows the body to move by stretching and contracting. There are three types of muscle tissue (see p. 55).

4. *Nerve tissue* receives and carries impulses to the brain and back to body parts.

Groups of tissues form *organs*. An organ performs one or more functions. Examples of organs include the heart, brain, liver, lungs, and kidneys. *Systems* are formed by organs that work together to perform special functions (Fig. 5-4).

THE INTEGUMENTARY SYSTEM

The *integumentary system*, or skin, is the largest system of the body. *Integument* means covering. The skin is the natural covering of the body. The skin is made up of epithelial, connective, and nerve tissue, as well as oil and sweat glands. There are two skin layers: the epidermis and the dermis (Fig. 5-5). The *epidermis* is the outer layer; it contains living and dead cells. The dead cells were once deeper in the epidermis and were pushed upward as other cells divided. The dead cells constantly flake off and are replaced by living cells. Living cells also eventually die and flake off. Living cells of the epidermis contain *pigment*. The pigment gives the skin its color. There are no blood vessels and few nerve endings in the epidermis. The *dermis* is the inner layer of the skin and is made up of connective tissue. Blood vessels, nerves, sweat and oil glands, and hair roots are found in the dermis.

Oil and *sweat glands, hair,* and *nails* are considered appendages of the skin. The entire body, except the

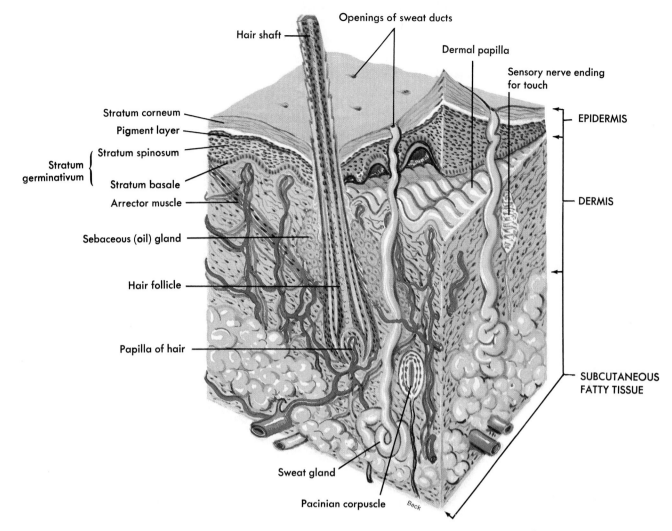

Hair shaft

Openings of sweat ducts

Dermal papilla

Sensory nerve ending for touch

Stratum corneum

Pigment layer

Stratum spinosum

Stratum germinativum {

Stratum basale

Arrector muscle

Sebaceous (oil) gland

Hair follicle

Papilla of hair

Sweat gland

Pacinian corpuscle

EPIDERMIS

DERMIS

SUBCUTANEOUS FATTY TISSUE

Beck

Fig. 5-5 Layers of the skin. (From Thibodeau GA: *Anatomy and physiology*, St Louis, 1987, Mosby–Year Book.)

palms of the hands and soles of the feet, is covered with hair. The hair of the nose, eyes, and ears protects these organs from dust, insects, and other foreign objects. Nails protect the tips of fingers and toes. Nails help fingers pick up and handle small objects. Sweat glands help the body regulate temperature. Sweat consists of water, salt, and a small amount of wastes. Sweat is secreted through pores in the skin. The body is cooled as sweat evaporates. Oil glands lie near the hair shafts. They secrete an oily substance into the space near the hair shaft. Oil travels to the skin surface, helping to keep the hair and skin soft and shiny.

The skin performs many important functions. It serves as a protective covering for the body. Bacteria and other substances are prevented from entering the body. The skin prevents excessive amounts of water from leaving the body and protects the organs from injury. Nerve endings in the skin sense both pleasant and unpleasant stimulation. There are nerve endings over the entire body. The body is protected because

cold, pain, touch, and pressure can be sensed. The skin helps regulate body temperature. Blood vessels dilate (widen) when temperature outside the body is high. More blood is brought to the body surface for cooling during evaporation. When blood vessels constrict (narrow), heat is retained by the body because less blood reaches the skin.

THE MUSCULOSKELETAL SYSTEM

The musculoskeletal system provides the framework for the body and allows the body to move. This system also protects and gives the body shape. Besides bones and muscles, the system includes ligaments, tendons, and cartilage.

Bones

The bony framework of the body consists of 206 bones (Fig. 5-6). There are four types of bones:

1. *Long bones* bear the weight of the body. The bones of the legs are long bones.

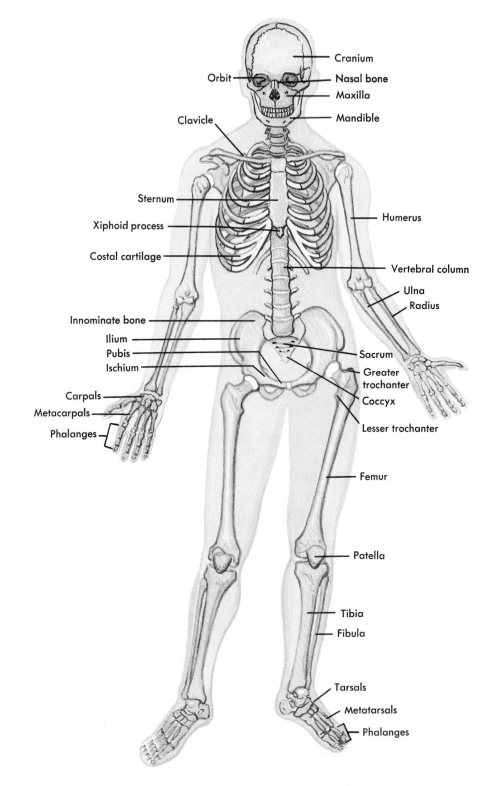

Fig. 5-6 Bones of the body. (From Glanze WD, Anderson KN, and Anderson LE: *Mosby's medical, nursing, and allied health dictionary*, ed 3, St Louis, 1990, Mosby–Year Book.)

2. *Short bones* allow skill and ease in movement. Bones in the wrists, fingers, ankles, and toes are short bones.
3. *Flat bones* protect the organs of the body. These bones include the ribs, skull, pelvic bones, and shoulder blades.
4. *Irregular bones* are the vertebrae in the spinal column. They allow various degrees of movement and flexibility.

Bones are hard, rigid structures that are made up of living cells. They are covered by a membrane called *periosteum*. Periosteum contains blood vessels that supply bone cells with oxygen and food. Inside the hollow centers of the bones is a substance called *bone marrow*. Blood cells are manufactured in the bone marrow.

Joints

The point at which two or more bones meet is called a *joint*. Joints allow movement. Connective tissue at the end of long bones is called *cartilage*. Cartilage cushions the joint so that the ends of the bones do not rub together. The *synovial membrane* lines the joints. The membrane secretes *synovial fluid*. Synovial fluid acts as a lubricant to allow the joint to move smoothly. Bones are held together at the joint by strong bands of connective tissue called *ligaments*.

There are three types of joints (Fig. 5-7). The *ball-and-socket* joint is made up of the rounded end of one bone and the hollow end of another bone. The rounded end of one fits into the hollow end of the other. Movement is possible in all directions. The joints of the hips and shoulders are ball-and-socket joints. The elbow is a *hinge joint;* movement is in one direction. The *pivot joint* allows turning from side to side. The skull is connected to the spine by a pivot joint. Joint movement is discussed further in Chapter 18.

Muscles

There are more than 500 muscles in the human body (Figs. 5-8 and 5-9). Some are voluntary, and others are involuntary. *Voluntary* muscles can be consciously controlled. Muscles that are attached to bones (*skeletal muscles*) are voluntary. Arm muscles do not work unless you move your arm; likewise for leg muscles. Skeletal muscles are *striated*, that is, the muscles appear striped or streaked. *Involuntary muscles* work automatically and cannot be consciously controlled. Involuntary muscles control the action of the stomach, intestines, blood vessels, and other body organs. Involuntary muscles are also called *smooth muscles*. They are smooth in appearance, not streaked or striped. *Cardiac muscle* is found in the heart. Although it is an involuntary muscle, it has the striated appearance of skeletal muscle.

Muscles perform three important body functions: the movement of body parts, the maintenance of posture, and the production of body heat. Strong, tough connective tissues called *tendons* connect muscles to bones. When muscles contract (shorten), tendons at each end of the muscle cause the bone to move. There are many tendons in the body; the Achilles tendon is shown in Figure 5-9. Some muscles are constantly contracted in order to maintain the body's posture. When muscles contract, they burn food for energy, resulting in the production of heat. The greater the muscular activity, the greater the amount of heat produced in the body. Shivering is a way in which the body produces heat when exposed to cold. The shivering sensation is the result of rapid, general muscle contractions.

THE NERVOUS SYSTEM

The nervous system controls, directs, and coordinates body functions. There are two main divisions of the nervous system: the *central nervous system* (CNS) and the *peripheral nervous system*. The central nervous system consists of the *brain* and *spinal cord* (Fig. 5-10). The peripheral nervous system involves the *nerves* throughout the body (Fig. 5-11). Nerves carry mes-

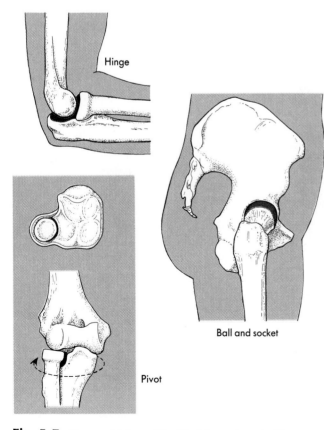

Hinge

Pivot

Ball and socket

Fig. 5-7 Types of joints. (Modified from Austrin M: *Young's learning medical terminology step by step*, ed 7, St Louis, 1991, Mosby–Year Book.)

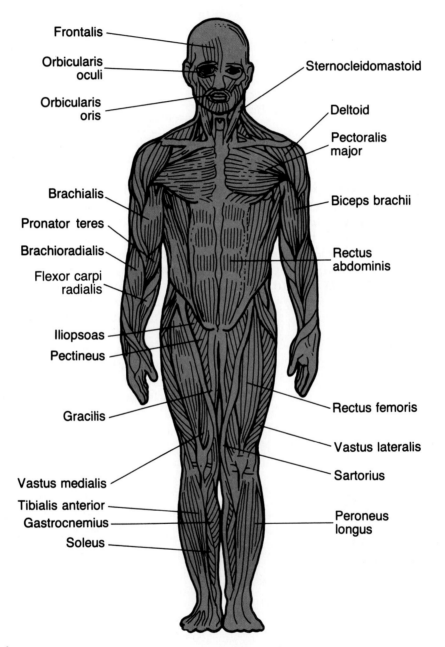

Fig. 5-8 Anterior view of the muscles of the body. (From Austrin M: *Young's learning medical terminology step by step*, ed 7, St Louis, 1991, Mosby–Year Book.)

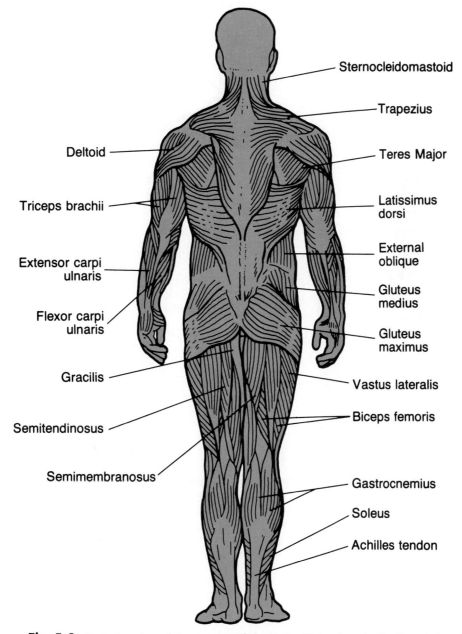

Fig. 5-9 Posterior view of the muscles of the body. (From Austrin M: *Young's learning medical terminology step by step*, ed 7, St Louis, 1991, Mosby–Year Book.)

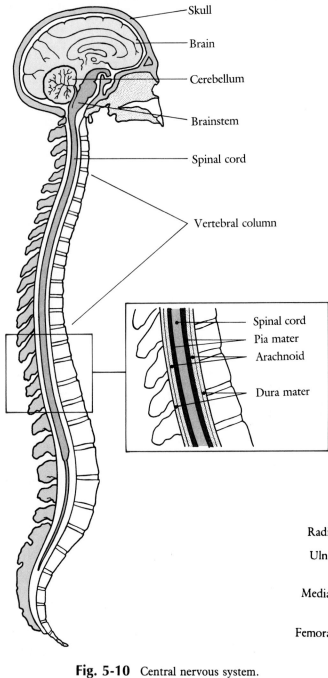

Fig. 5-10 Central nervous system.

Fig. 5-11 Peripheral nervous system. (From Austrin M: *Young's learning medical terminology step by step*, ed 7, St Louis, 1991, Mosby–Year Book.)

sages or impulses to and from the brain. The nerves are connected to the spinal cord. The nerve cell *(neuron)* is the basic unit of the nervous system (Fig. 5-12). Threadlike projections from the cytoplasm of the neuron are called *nerve fibers.* Nerve fibers that bring impulses to the cell are called *dendrites.* Fibers that carry impulses away from neurons are called *axons.* A neuron usually has only one axon. Dendrites may be short or as long as 3 feet.

Receptors or *end-organs* are inside and outside of the body. Each receptor is attached to a neuron by a dendrite. A stimulus is received by the receptor and travels to the brain. Such stimuli include heat, cold, touch, smell, hearing, vision, balance, hunger, and thirst. If the body or body part must respond to the stimulus, the brain sends an impulse through the neurons to the proper muscles and glands.

Nerves are easily damaged and take a long time to heal. Some nerve fibers have a protective covering called a *myelin sheath.* The myelin sheath also insulates the nerve fiber. Nerve fibers covered with my-

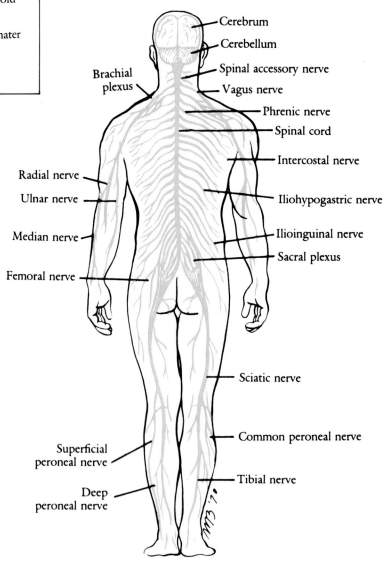

elin can conduct impulses faster than those fibers without the protective covering.

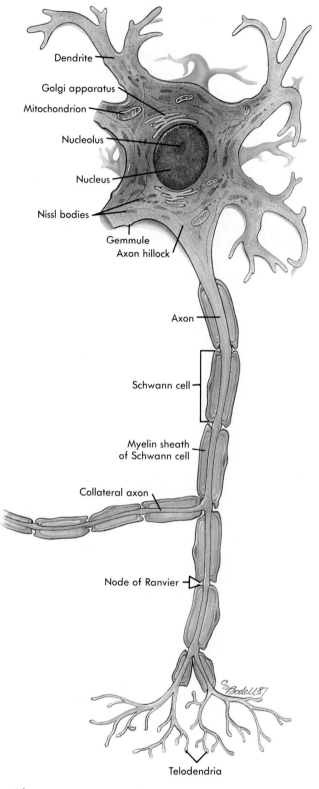

Dendrite

Golgi apparatus

Mitochondrion

Nucleolus

Nucleus

Nissl bodies

Gemmule
Axon hillock

Axon

Schwann cell

Myelin sheath
of Schwann cell

Collateral axon

Node of Ranvier

Telodendria

Fig. 5-12 A neuron. (From Seeley RR, Stephens TD, and Tate P: *Anatomy and physiology*, St Louis, 1989, Mosby–Year Book.)

The Central Nervous System

The central nervous system consists of the brain and spinal cord. The brain is covered by the skull. The three main parts of the brain are the *cerebrum*, the *cerebellum*, and the *brainstem* (Fig. 5-13).

The cerebrum is the largest part of the brain and is the center of thought and intelligence. The cerebrum is divided into two halves called the right and left *hemispheres*. The right hemisphere controls the movement and activities of the left side of the body. The left hemisphere controls the body's right side. The outside of the cerebrum is called the *cerebral cortex*. The cerebral cortex controls the highest functions of the brain. Reasoning, memory, the conscious, speech, voluntary muscle movement, vision, hearing, sensation, and other activities are controlled by the cerebral cortex.

The cerebellum regulates and coordinates body movements. The smooth movements of voluntary muscles and balance are made possible because of control by the cerebellum. Injury to the cerebellum results in jerky movements, loss of coordination, and muscle weakness.

The brainstem connects the cerebrum to the spinal cord. There are three important structures within the brainstem: the *midbrain, pons,* and *medulla.* The midbrain and pons relay messages between the medulla and the cerebrum. The medulla is located directly below the pons. Heart rate, breathing, the size of blood vessels, swallowing, coughing, and vomiting are some body functions controlled by the medulla. The brain is connected to the spinal cord at the lower end of the medulla.

The spinal cord lies within the spinal column. The cord is about 18 inches long. Pathways that conduct messages to and from the brain are contained within the cord.

The brain and spinal cord are covered and protected by three layers of connective tissue called *meninges.* The outer layer, which lies next to the skull, is a tough covering called the *dura mater.* The middle layer is called the *arachnoid,* and the inner layer is the *pia mater.* The space between the middle and inner layers is called the *arachnoid space.* The space is filled with fluid called *cerebrospinal fluid.* It circulates around the brain and spinal cord. Cerebrospinal fluid protects the central nervous system by cushioning shocks that could easily injure structures of the brain and spinal cord.

The Peripheral Nervous System

The peripheral nervous system involves twelve pairs of *cranial nerves* and 31 pairs of *spinal nerves.* Cranial

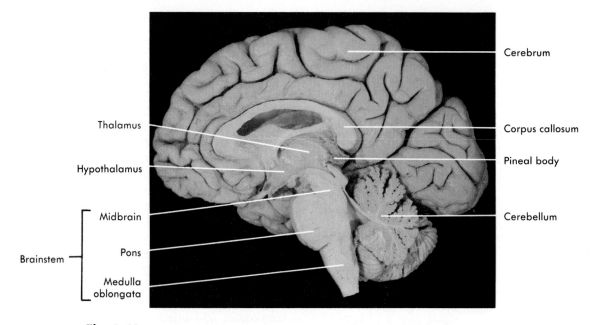

Fig. 5-13 The brain. (From Seeley RR, Stephens TD, and Tate P: *Anatomy and physiology*, St Louis, 1989, Mosby–Year Book.)

nerves conduct impulses between the brain and the head, neck, chest, and abdomen. They conduct impulses for smell, vision, hearing, pain, touch, temperature, pressure, voluntary muscle control, and involuntary muscle control. Spinal nerves carry impulses from the skin, extremities, and the internal body structures not supplied by cranial nerves.

Some peripheral nerves with special functions form the *autonomic nervous system*. This system controls involuntary muscles and certain body functions. The functions include the heartbeat, blood pressure, intestinal contractions, and glandular secretions. These functions occur automatically without conscious effort. The autonomic nervous system is divided into the *sympathetic nervous system* and the *parasympathetic nervous system*. These divisions balance one another. The sympathetic nervous system tends to speed up functions, whereas the parasympathetic nervous system slows them down. When you are angry, frightened, excited, or exercising, the sympathetic nervous system is stimulated. The parasympathetic system is activated when you relax or when the sympathetic system has been under stimulation for too long.

The Sense Organs

The five major senses are sight, hearing, taste, smell, and touch. Receptors for taste are in the tongue and are called *taste buds*. Receptors for smell are in the nose. Touch receptors are found in the dermis, especially in the toes and fingertips.

The eye Receptors for vision are located in the eyes. The eye is a delicate organ that can be easily injured. Bones of the skull, eyelids and eyelashes, and tears protect the eyes from injury. Eye structures are shown in Figure 5-14. The eye has three layers. The *sclera*, the white of the eye, is the outer layer. The sclera is made of tough connective tissue. The second layer is the *choroid*. Blood vessels, the *ciliary muscle*, and the *iris* make up the choroid. The iris gives the eye its color. The opening in the middle of the iris is the *pupil*. Pupil size varies with the amount of light entering the eye. The pupil constricts (narrows) in bright light and dilates (widens) in dim or dark places. The inner layer of the eye is called the *retina*. Receptors for vision and the nerve fibers of the optic nerve are contained in the retina.

Light enters the eye through the *cornea*. The cornea is the transparent part of the outer layer that lies over the eye. Light rays pass to the *lens*, which lies behind the pupil. The light is then reflected to the retina and carried to the brain by the optic nerve.

The *aqueous chamber* separates the cornea from the lens. The chamber is filled with a fluid called *aqueous humor*. The fluid helps the cornea keep its shape and position. The *vitreous body* is behind the lens. The vitreous body is a gelatin-like substance that supports the retina and maintains the shape of the eye.

The ear The ear is a sense organ that functions in hearing and balance. The ear is divided into the *external ear*, *middle ear*, and *inner ear*. Ear structures are shown in Figure 5-15.

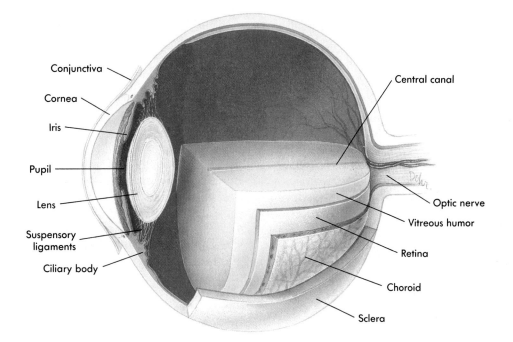

Fig. 5-14 The eye. (From Seeley RR, Stephens TD, and Tate P: *Anatomy and physiology,* St Louis, 1989, Mosby–Year Book.)

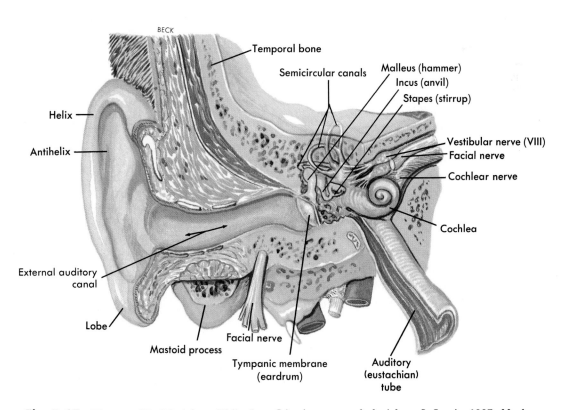

Fig. 5-15 The ear. (Modified from Thibodeau GA: *Anatomy and physiology,* St Louis, 1987, Mosby–Year Book.)

The external ear (outer part) is called the *pinna* or *auricle*. Sound waves are guided through the external ear into the *auditory canal*. Many glands in the auditory canal secrete a waxy substance called *cerumen*. The auditory canal extends about 1 inch to the *eardrum*. The eardrum *(tympanic membrane)* separates the external and middle ear.

The middle ear is a small space that contains the *eustachian tube* and three small bones called *ossicles*. The eustachian tube connects the middle ear and the throat. Air enters the eustachian tube so that there is equal pressure on both sides of the eardrum. The ossicles amplify sound received from the eardrum and transmit the sound to the inner ear. The three ossicles are called the *malleus*, which looks like a hammer; the *incus*, which resembles an anvil; and the *stapes*, which is shaped like a stirrup.

The inner ear consists of the *semicircular canals* and the *cochlea*. The cochlea, which looks like a snail shell, contains fluid. The fluid carries sound waves received from the middle ear to the *auditory nerve*. The auditory nerve then carries the message to the brain.

The three semicircular canals are involved with balance. They sense the head's position and changes in position, and send messages to the brain.

THE CIRCULATORY SYSTEM

The circulatory system is made up of the blood, heart, and blood vessels. The heart pumps blood through the blood vessels. The circulatory system performs many important functions. Blood carries food, oxygen, and other substances to the cells. Blood also removes waste products from cells. Regulation of body temperature is aided by the blood and blood vessels. Heat from muscle activity is carried by the blood to other body parts. Blood vessels in the skin dilate if the body needs to be cooled. They constrict if heat should be kept in the body. The circulatory system also produces and carries cells that defend the body from disease-causing germs.

The Blood

The blood consists of blood cells and of a liquid called *plasma*. Plasma, which is mostly water, carries blood cells to other body cells. Plasma also carries other substances needed by body cells for proper functioning. Food (proteins, fats, and carbohydrates), hormones (see the endocrine system, page 75), and chemicals are among the many substances carried in the plasma. Waste products are also carried in the plasma.

Red blood cells are called *erythrocytes*. They give the blood its red color because of a substance in the cell called *hemoglobin*. As red blood cells circulate through the lungs, hemoglobin picks up oxygen. The hemoglobin carries oxygen to the cells. When the blood appears bright red, hemoglobin in the red blood cells is saturated with oxygen. As blood circulates through the body, oxygen is given to the cells. The cells release carbon dioxide (a waste product), which is picked by the hemoglobin. Red blood cells saturated with carbon dioxide make the blood appear dark red.

There are about 25 trillion (25,000,000,000,000) red blood cells in the body. About 4½ to 5 million are in a cubic milliliter of blood (the size of a tiny drop). These cells live for 3 or 4 months. They are destroyed by the liver and spleen as they wear out. Bone marrow produces new red blood cells. About one million new red blood cells are produced every second.

White blood cells, called *leukocytes*, are colorless. They protect the body against infection. There are 5000 to 10,000 white blood cells in a cubic milliliter of blood. At the first sign of infection, white blood cells rush to the site of the infection and begin to multiply rapidly. The number of white blood cells increases when there is an infection in the body. White blood cells are also produced by the bone marrow. They live about 9 days.

Platelets (thrombocytes) are necessary for the clotting of blood. They are also produced by the bone marrow. There are about 200,000 to 400,000 platelets in a cubic milliliter of blood. A platelet survives for about 4 days.

The Heart

The heart is a muscle that pumps blood through the blood vessels to the tissues and cells. The heart lies in the middle to lower part of the chest cavity toward the left side (Fig. 5-16). The heart is hollow and has three layers (Fig. 5-17). The outer layer is the *pericardium;* it is a thin sac covering the heart. The *myocardium* is the second layer. This layer is the thick muscular portion of the heart. The *endocardium* is the inner layer. The endocardium is the membrane lining the inner surface of the heart.

The heart has four chambers (see Fig. 5-17). Upper chambers receive blood and are called the *atria*. The *right atrium* receives blood from body tissues. The *left atrium* receives blood from the lungs. Lower chambers are called ventricles. Ventricles pump blood. The *right ventricle* pumps blood to the lungs for oxygen. The *left ventricle* pumps blood to all parts of the body.

Valves are located between the atria and ventricles. The valves allow blood to flow in one direction. They prevent blood from flowing back into the atria from the ventricles. The *tricuspid valve* is between the right atrium and right ventricle. The *mitral valve (bicuspid valve)* is between the left atrium and left ventricle.

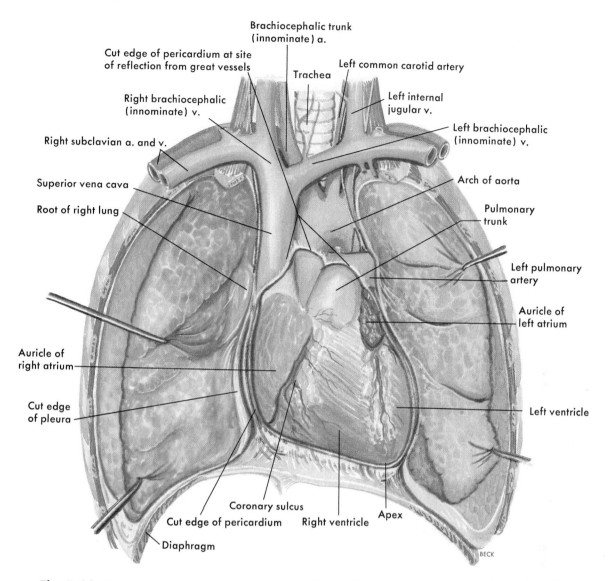

Brachiocephalic trunk
(innominate) a.

Cut edge of pericardium at site
of reflection from great vessels

Trachea

Left common carotid artery

Right brachiocephalic
(innominate) v.

Left internal
jugular v.

Right subclavian a. and v.

Left brachiocephalic
(innominate) v.

Superior vena cava

Arch of aorta

Root of right lung

Pulmonary
trunk

Left pulmonary
artery

Auricle of
left atrium

Auricle of
right atrium

Cut edge
of pleura

Left ventricle

Coronary sulcus

Cut edge of pericardium

Right ventricle

Apex

Diaphragm

BECK

Fig. 5-16 Location of the heart in the chest cavity. (From Thibodeau GA: *Anatomy and physiology*, St Louis, 1987, Mosby–Year Book.)

The are two phases of heart action: systole and diastole. During *diastole*, the resting phase, heart chambers fill with blood. During *systole*, the working phase, the heart contracts. Blood is pumped through the blood vessels when the heart contracts.

The Blood Vessels

Blood flows to body tissues and cells through the blood vessels. There are three groups of blood vessels: arteries, capillaries, and veins. *Arteries* carry blood away from the heart. Arterial blood is rich in oxygen. The *aorta* is the largest artery. The aorta receives blood directly from the left ventricle. The aorta branches off into other arteries that carry blood to all parts of the body (Fig. 5-18). These arteries branch

off into smaller parts within the tissues. The smallest branch of an artery is an *arteriole*. Arterioles connect with blood vessels called *capillaries*. Capillaries are very tiny vessels. Food, oxygen, and other substances pass from capillaries into the cells. Waste products, including carbon dioxide, are picked up from cells by the capillaries. Waste products are carried back to the heart by the veins.

Veins return blood to the heart. They are connected to the capillaries by *venules*. Venules are small veins. Venules begin branching together to form veins. The many branches of veins also branch together as they near the heart to form two main veins (Fig. 5-18). The two main veins are the *inferior vena cava* and the *superior vena cava*. Both empty into the right atrium. The inferior vena cava carries blood from the legs

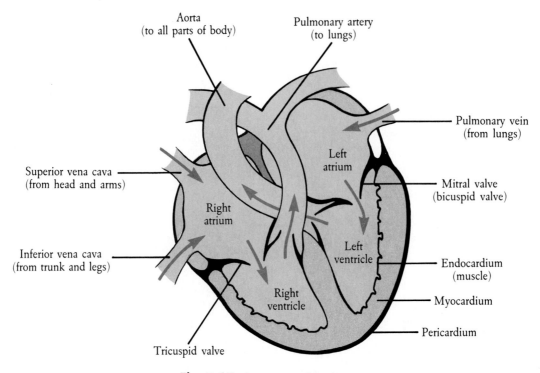

Fig. 5-17 Structures of the heart.

and trunk. The superior vena cava carries blood from the head and arms. Venous blood is dark red in color because it contains little oxygen and a great deal of carbon dioxide.

Blood flow through the circulatory system is diagrammed in Figure 5-17 and can be summarized as follows. Venous blood, poor in oxygen, empties into the right atrium. Blood flows through the tricuspid valve into the right ventricle. The right ventricle pumps blood into the lungs to pick up oxygen. Oxygen-rich blood from the lungs enters the left atrium. Blood from the left atrium passes through the mitral valve into the left ventricle. The left ventricle pumps the blood to the aorta, which branches off to form other arteries. The arterial blood is carried to the tissues by arterioles and to the cells by capillaries. The cells and capillaries exchange oxygen and nutrients for carbon dioxide and waste products. Capillaries connect with venules. Venules carry blood that contains carbon dioxide and waste products. The venules form veins. Veins return blood to the heart.

THE RESPIRATORY SYSTEM

Oxygen is necessary for survival. Every cell requires oxygen. Air contains about 20% oxygen, enough to meet the body's needs under normal conditions. The respiratory system brings oxygen into the lungs and eliminates carbon dioxide. The process of supplying the cells with oxygen and removing carbon dioxide from them is called *respiration*. Respiration involves *inhalation* (breathing in) and *exhalation* (breathing out). The terms *inspiration* (breathing in) and *expiration* (breathing out) are also used. The respiratory system is shown in Figure 5-19.

Air enters the body through the *nose*. The air then passes into the *pharynx* (throat), a tube-shaped passageway for both air and food. Air passes from the pharynx into the *larynx*. The larynx is commonly called the voice box. A piece of cartilage called the *epiglottis* acts like a lid over the larynx. The epiglottis prevents food from entering the airway during swallowing. During inhalation the epiglottis lifts up to let air pass over the larynx. Air passes from the larynx into the *trachea*, commonly called the windpipe. The trachea divides at its lower end into the *right bronchus* and *left bronchus*. Each bronchus enters a lung. On entering the lungs, the bronchi further divide several times into smaller branches called *bronchioles*. Eventually the bronchioles subdivide and end in tiny one-celled air sacs called *alveoli*. Alveoli look like small clusters of grapes. They are supplied by capillaries. Oxygen and carbon dioxide are exchanged between the alveoli and capillaries. Blood in the capillaries picks up oxygen from the alveoli. Then the blood is returned to the left side of the heart and pumped to the rest of the body. Alveoli pick up carbon dioxide from the capillaries for exhalation.

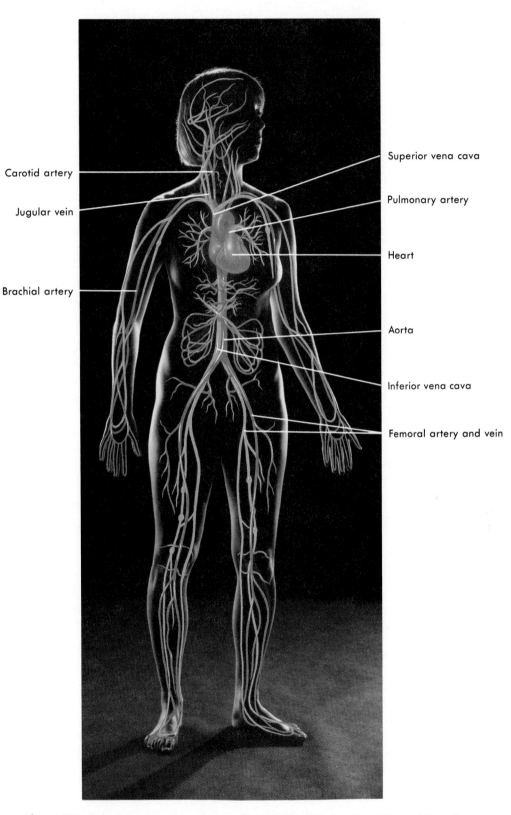

Carotid artery

Jugular vein

Brachial artery

Superior vena cava

Pulmonary artery

Heart

Aorta

Inferior vena cava

Femoral artery and vein

Fig. 5-18 Arterial and venous systems. (From Seeley RR, Stephens TD, and Tate P: *Anatomy and physiology*, St Louis, 1989, Mosby–Year Book.)

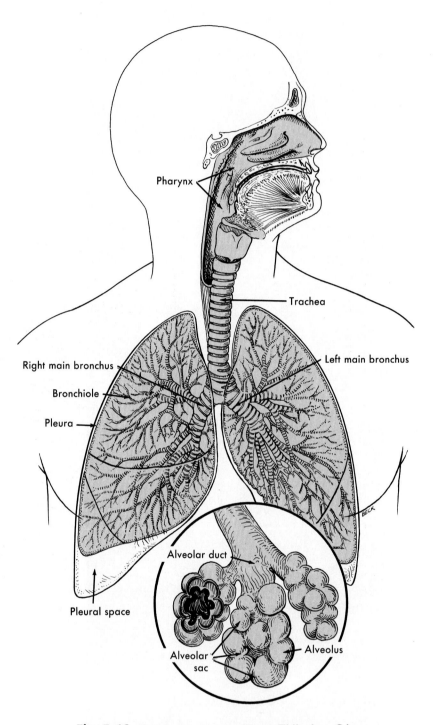

Fig. 5-19 Respiratory system. (From Thibodeau GA: *Anatomy and physiology*, St Louis, 1987, Mosby–Year Book.)

The lungs are spongy tissues filled with alveoli, blood vessels, and nerves. Each lung is divided into lobes. The right lung has three lobes, and the left lung has two. The lungs are separated from the abdominal cavity by a muscle called the *diaphragm*. Each lung is covered by a two-layered sac called the *pleura*. One layer is attached to the lung and the other to the chest wall. The pleura secretes a very thin fluid that fills the space between the layers. The fluid prevents the layers from rubbing together during inhalation and exhalation. A bony framework consisting of the ribs, sternum, and vertebrae protects the lungs.

THE DIGESTIVE SYSTEM

The digestive system breaks down food physically and chemically so that it can be absorbed for use by the cells. This process is called *digestion*. The digestive system is also called the *gastrointestinal system*. The system also eliminates solid wastes from the body. The digestive system consists of the *alimentary canal* (also called the *GI tract*) and the accessory organs of digestion (Fig. 5-20). The alimentary canal is a long tube extending from the mouth to the anus. The mouth, pharynx, esophagus, stomach, small intestine, and large intestine are the major parts of the alimentary canal. The accessory organs of digestion are the teeth, tongue, salivary glands, liver, gallbladder, and pancreas.

Digestion begins in the *mouth*. The mouth is also called the *oral cavity*. The oral cavity receives food and prepares it for digestion. Using chewing motions, the *teeth* cut, chop, and grind food into smaller particles for digestion and swallowing. The *tongue* aids in chewing and swallowing. *Taste buds* on the tongue's surface contain nerve endings. Taste buds allow sweet, sour, bitter, and salty tastes to be distinguished. *Salivary glands* in the oral cavity secrete *saliva*. Saliva moistens food particles for easier swallowing and begins the digestion of food. During swallowing, the tongue pushes food into the pharynx.

The *pharynx* is a muscular tube known as the throat. The act of swallowing is continued as the pharynx contracts. Contraction of the pharynx pushes food into the *esophagus*. The esophagus is a musuclar tube about 10 inches long. It extends from the pharynx to the stomach. Involuntary muscle contractions called *peristalsis* move food down the esophagus into the stomach.

The *stomach* is a muscular, pouchlike sac located in the upper left portion of the abdominal cavity. Strong stomach muscles stir and churn food to break it up into even smaller particles. The stomach is lined with a mucous membrane containing glands that secrete *gastric juices*. Food is mixed and churned with the gastric juices to form a semiliquid substance called

chyme. Through peristalsis, the chyme is pushed from the stomach into the small intestine.

The *small intestine* is about 20 feet long and is divided into three parts. The first part is called the *duodenum*. In the duodenum, more digestive juices are added to the chyme. One of the juices is called *bile*. Bile is a greenish liquid produced by the *liver* and stored in the *gallbladder*. Juices from the *pancreas* and small intestine are also added to the chyme. The digestive juices chemically break down food so that it can be absorbed.

Peristalsis moves the chyme through the two remaining portions of the small intestine: the *jejunum* and the *ileum*. Tiny projections called *villi* line the small intestine. The villi absorb the digested food into the capillaries. Most of the absorption of food takes place in the jejunum and ileum.

Some chyme remains undigested. The undigested chyme passes from the small intestine into the *large intestine*. The large intestine is also called the *large bowel* or *colon*. The colon absorbs most of the water from the chyme. The remaining semisolid material is called *feces*. Feces consist of a small amount of water and solid wastes, and some mucus and germs. These are the waste products of digestion. Feces pass through the colon into the *rectum* by peristalsis. Feces pass out of the body through the *anus*.

THE URINARY SYSTEM

Wastes are removed from the body through the respiratory system, the digestive system, and the skin. The digestive system rids the body of solid wastes. The lungs rid the body of carbon dioxide. Water and other substances are contained in sweat. There are other waste products in the blood as a result of body cells burning food for energy. The functions of the urinary system are to remove waste products from the blood and to maintain water balance within the body. The structures of the urinary system are shown in Figure 5-21.

The *kidneys* are two bean-shaped organs located in the upper abdomen. They lie against the muscles of the back on each side of the spine. They are protected by the lower edge of the rib cage.

Each kidney consists of over a million tiny *nephrons* (Fig. 5-22). The nephron is the basic working unit of the kidney. Each nephron contains a *convoluted tubule*, which is a tiny coiled tubule. Each convoluted tubule has a *Bowman's capsule* at one end. The capsule partially surrounds a cluster of capillaries called a *glomerulus*. Blood passes through the glomerulus and is filtered by the capillaries. The fluid portion of the blood is squeezed into the Bowman's capsule. The fluid then passes into the tubule. Most of the water and other necessary substances are reabsorbed by the

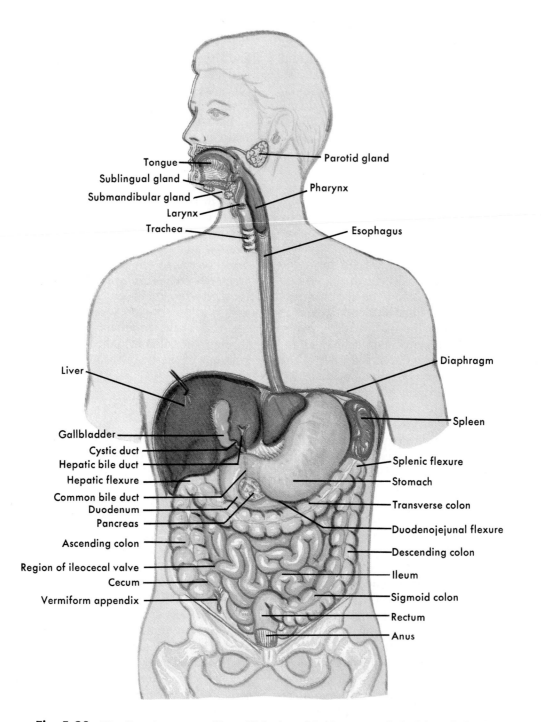

Fig. 5-20 The digestive system. (From Thibodeau GA: *Anatomy and physiology*, St Louis, 1987, Mosby–Year Book.)

blood and recirculated in the body. The rest of the fluid and the waste products form *urine* in the tubule. Urine flows through the tubule to a *collecting tubule*. All of the collecting tubules within the millions of nephrons drain into the *renal pelvis* within the kidney.

A tube, called the *ureter*, is attached to the renal pelvis of the kidney. Each ureter is about 10 to 12 inches long. The ureters carry urine from the kidneys to the *bladder*. The bladder is a hollow muscular sac situated toward the front in the lower part of the abdominal cavity. Urine is stored in the bladder until the desire to urinate is felt. The need to urinate usually occurs when there is about half a pint (250 ml)

of urine in the bladder. Urine passes from the bladder through the *urethra*. The opening at the end of the urethra is the *meatus*. Urine passes from the body through the meatus. Urine is a clear yellowish fluid.

THE REPRODUCTIVE SYSTEM

Human reproduction is the result of the union of a sex cell from the female and a sex cell from the male. The structures of the male and female reproductive systems are different. The differences allow for the process of reproduction.

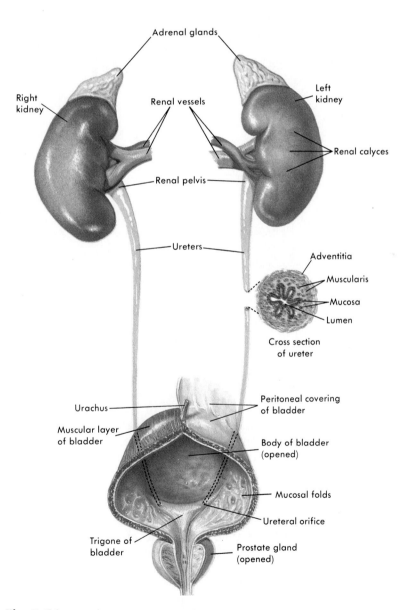

Fig. 5-21 Urinary system. (From Glanze WD, Anderson KN, and Anderson LE: *Mosby's medical, nursing, and allied health dictionary*, ed 3, St Louis, 1990, Mosby–Year Book.)

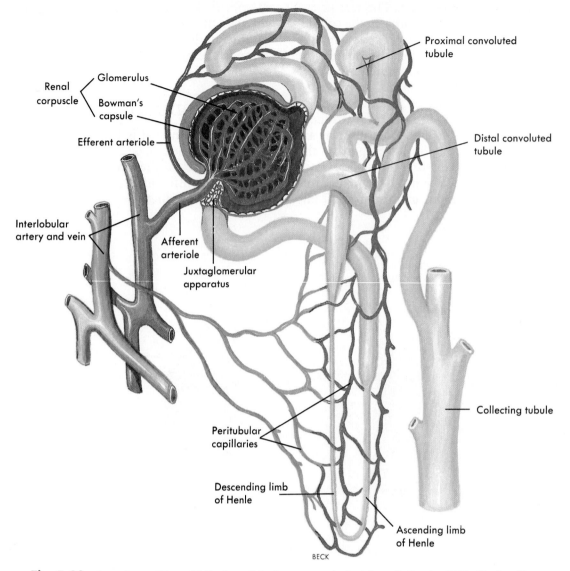

Fig. 5-22 A nephron. (From Thibodeau GA: *Anatomy and physiology*, St Louis, 1987, Mosby–Year Book.)

The Male Reproductive System

The structures of the male reproductive system are shown in Figure 5-23. The *testes (testicles)* are the sex glands of the male. Sex glands are also called *gonads*. The two testes are oval or almond-shaped glands. Male sex cells are produced in the testes. Male sex cells are called *sperm* cells. *Testosterone*, the male hormone, is also produced in the testes. This hormone is necessary for the functioning of the reproductive organs and for the development of the male's secondary sex characteristics (see Chapter 6). The testes are suspended between the thighs in a sac called the *scrotum*. The scrotum is made of skin and muscle.

Sperm travel from the testis to the *epididymis*. The epididymis is a coiled tube located on top and to the side of the testis. From the epididymis, sperm travel through a tube called the *vas deferens*. Eventually each vas deferens joins a *seminal vesicle*. The two seminal vesicles store sperm and produce *semen*. Semen is a fluid that carries sperm from the male reproductive tract. The ducts of the seminal vesicles unite to form the *ejaculatory duct*. The ejaculatory duct passes through the prostate gland.

The *prostate gland*, shaped like a doughnut, lies just below the bladder. The gland secretes fluid into the semen. As the ejaculatory ducts leave the prostate they join the *urethra*, which also runs through the prostate. The urethra is the outlet for both urine and semen; the urethra is contained within the penis.

The *penis* is located outside of the body and is composed of *erectile* tissue. When the man becomes

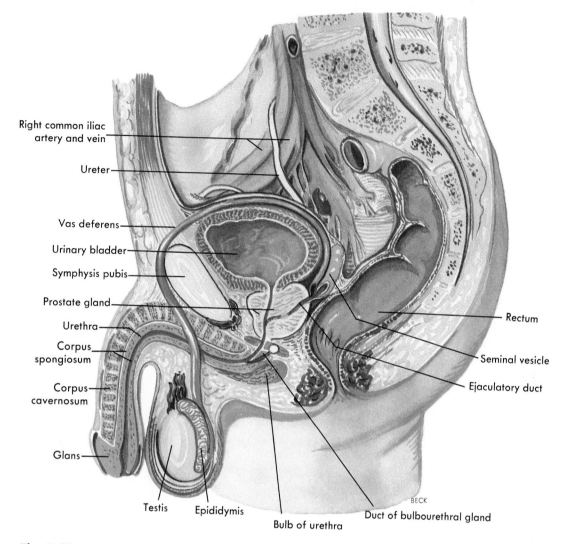

Right common iliac
artery and vein

Ureter

Vas deferens

Urinary bladder

Symphysis pubis

Prostate gland

Urethra

Corpus
spongiosum

Corpus
cavernosum

Glans

Testis   Epididymis

Bulb of urethra

Rectum

Seminal vesicle

Ejaculatory duct

Duct of bulbourethral gland

BECK

Fig. 5-23 Male reproductive system. (From Thibodeau GA: *Anatomy and physiology*, St Louis, 1987, Mosby–Year Book.)

sexually excited, blood fills the erectile tissue, causing the penis to become enlarged, hard, and erect. The erect penis can enter the vagina of the female reproductive tract. The semen, which contains sperm, is then released into the female vagina.

The Female Reproductive System

The structures of the female reproductive system are shown in Figure 5-24. The female gonads are two almond-shaped glands called *ovaries*. Each ovary is located on either side of the uterus in the abdominal cavity. The ovaries contain the *ova* or eggs. Ova are the female sex cells. One ovum (egg) is released monthly during the woman's reproductive years. The release of an ovum from an ovary is called *ovulation*. The ovaries also secrete the female hormones *estrogen* and *progesterone*. These hormones are responsible for

the functioning of the reproductive system and the development of secondary sex characteristics in the female (see Chapter 6).

When an ovum is released from an ovary, it travels through a *fallopian tube*. There are two fallopian tubes, one on each side. The tubes are attached at one end to the uterus. The ovum travels through the fallopian tube to the *uterus*. The uterus is a hollow muscular organ shaped like a pear. The uterus is in the center of the pelvic cavity behind the bladder and in front of the rectum. The main part of the uterus is the *fundus*. The neck or narrow section of the uterus is the *cervix*. Tissue lining the uterus is called the *endometrium*. Many blood vessels are contained in the endometrium. If sex cells from the male and female unite into one cell, that cell implants into the endometrium, where it grows into a baby. The uterus

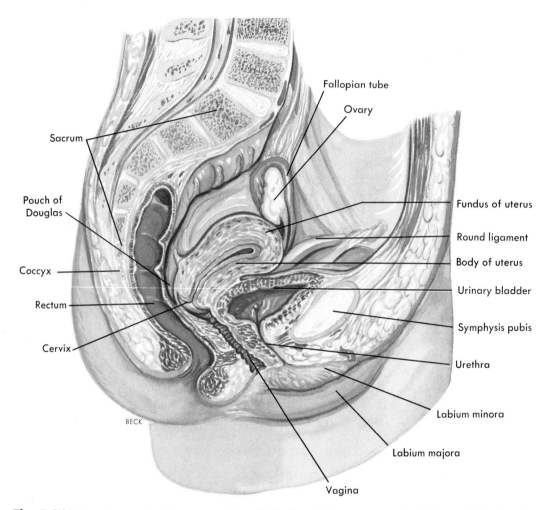

Fig. 5-24 Female reproductive system. (From Thibodeau GA: *Anatomy and physiology*, St Louis, 1987, Mosby–Year Book.)

serves as a place for the unborn baby to grow and receive nourishment.

The cervix of the uterus projects into a muscular canal called the *vagina*. The vagina opens to the outside of the body and is located just behind the urethra. The vagina receives the penis during sexual intercourse and serves as part of the birth canal. Glands in the vaginal wall keep it moistened with secretions. The external vaginal opening is partially closed by a membrane called the *hymen*.

The external genitalia of the female are referred to as the *vulva* (Fig. 5-25). The *mons pubis* is a rounded fatty pad over a bone called the *symphysis pubis*. The mons pubis is covered with hair in the adult female. The *labia majora* and *labia minora* are two folds of tissue on each side of the vaginal opening. The *clitoris* is a small organ composed of erectile tissue. The clitoris becomes hard when sexually stimulated.

The *mammary glands* (*breasts*) are considered organs of reproduction because they secrete milk after childbirth. The glands are located on the outside of

the chest. They are made up of glandular tissue and fat (Fig. 5-26). The milk drains into ducts that open onto the nipple.

Menstruation The endometrium is rich in blood to nourish the cell that grows into an unborn baby (*fetus*). If pregnancy does not occur, the endometrium breaks up and is discharged through the vagina to the outside of the body. This process is called *menstruation*. Menstruation occurs about every 28 days. Therefore, it is also called the *menstrual cycle*.

The first day of the cycle begins with menstruation. Blood flows from the uterus through the vaginal opening. Menstrual flow usually lasts 3 to 7 days. Ovulation occurs during the next phase of the cycle. An ovum matures in an ovary and is released. Ovulation usually occurs on or about the fourteenth day of the cycle. Meanwhile, estrogen and progesterone (the female hormones) are secreted by the ovaries. These hormones cause the endometrium to thicken for possible pregnancy. If pregnancy does not occur, the

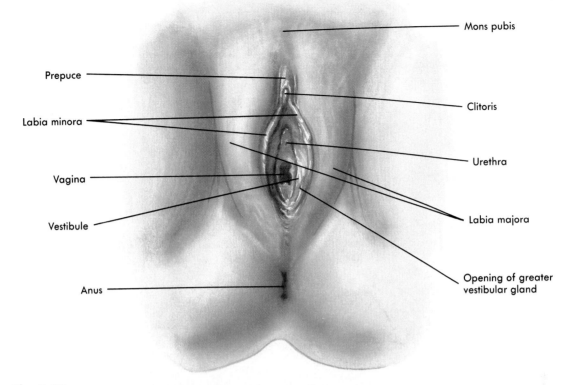

Fig. 5-25 External female genitalia. (From Seeley RR, Stephens TD, Tate P: *Anatomy and physiology*, St Louis, 1989, Mosby–Year Book.)

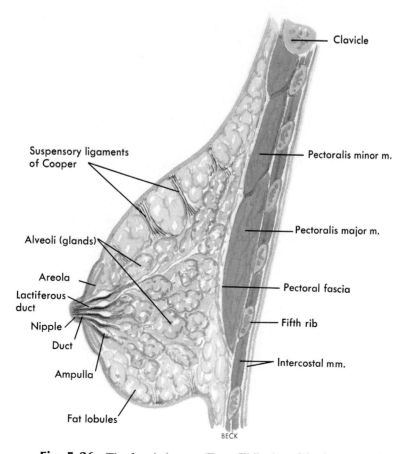

Fig. 5-26 The female breast. (From Thibodeau GA: *Anatomy and physiology*, St Louis, 1987, Mosby–Year Book.)

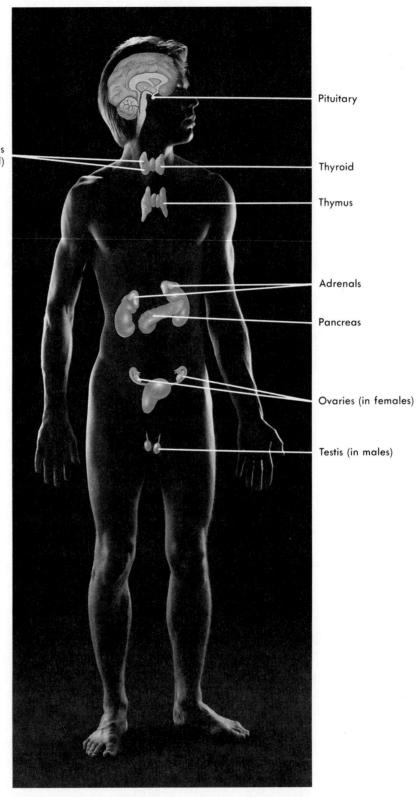

Fig. 5-27 Endocrine system. (From Seeley RR, Stephens TD, and Tate P: *Anatomy and physiology*, St Louis, 1989, Mosby–Year Book.)

hormones decrease in amount. Blood supply to the endometrium decreases because of the decrease in hormones. The endometrium breaks up and is discharged through the vagina. Another menstrual cycle begins.

Fertilization

For reproduction to occur, a male sex cell (sperm) must unite with a female sex cell (ovum). The uniting of the sperm and ovum into one cell is called *fertilization*. A sperm contains 23 chromosomes, and an ovum contains 23 chromosomes. When the two cells unite, the fertilized cell contains 46 chromosomes.

During intercourse, millions of sperm are deposited in the vagina. Sperm travel up the cervix, through the uterus, and into the fallopian tubes. If a sperm and an ovum unite in a fallopian tube, fertilization occurs and results in pregnancy. The fertilized cell travels down the fallopian tube to the uterus. After a short time, the fertilized cell implants in the thick endometrium and grows during pregnancy.

THE ENDOCRINE SYSTEM

The endocrine system is made up of glands called the *endocrine glands* (Fig. 5-27). The endocrine glands secrete chemical substances called *hormones* into the bloodstream. Hormones regulate the activities of other organs and glands in the body.

The *pituitary gland* is called the *master gland*. About the size of a cherry, it is located at the base of the brain behind the eyes. The pituitary gland is divided into the anterior pituitary lobe and the posterior pituitary lobe. The *anterior pituitary lobe* secretes important hormones. *Growth hormone* is needed for the growth of muscles, bones, and other organs. Adequate amounts of growth hormone are needed throughout life to maintain normal sized bones and muscles. Growth will be stunted if a baby is born with deficient amounts of the growth hormone. Too much of the hormone causes excessive growth.

Thyroid stimulating hormone (TSH) is also secreted by the anterior pituitary lobe. The thyroid gland requires thyroid stimulating hormone for proper functioning. *Adrenocorticotropic hormone* (ACTH) is another hormone secreted by the anterior lobe. This hormone stimulates the adrenal gland. The anterior lobe also secretes hormones that regulate the growth, development, and function of the male and female reproductive systems.

The *posterior pituitary lobe* secretes *antidiuretic hormone* (ADH) and *oxytocin*. Antidiuretic hormone prevents the kidneys from excreting excessive amounts of water. Oxytocin causes the uterine muscles to contract during childbirth.

The *thyroid gland*, shaped like a butterfly, is located in the neck in front of the larynx. *Thyroid hormone*

(TH) is secreted by the thyroid gland. Thyroxine is another term for thyroid hormone. Thyroid hormone regulates *metabolism*. Metabolism is the burning of food for heat and energy by the cells. Too little thyroid hormone results in slowed body processes, slowed movements, and weight gain. Too much of the hormone causes increased metabolism, excess energy, and weight loss. If a baby is born with deficient amounts of thyroid hormone, physical and mental growth will be stunted.

The *parathyroid glands* secrete *parathormone*. There are four parathyroid glands. Two are located on each side of the thyroid gland. Parathormone regulates the body's use of calcium. Calcium is needed for the proper functioning of nerves and muscles. Insufficient amounts of calcium cause *tetany*. Tetany is a state of severe muscle contraction and spasm. If untreated, tetany can cause death.

There are two *adrenal glands*. An adrenal gland is located on the top of each kidney. The adrenal gland has two parts: the *adrenal medulla* and the *adrenal cortex*. The adrenal medulla secretes *epinephrine* and *norepinephrine*. These hormones stimulate the body to quickly produce energy during emergencies. Heart rate, blood pressure, muscle power, and energy all increase. The adrenal cortex secretes three groups of hormones that are essential for life. The *glucocorticoids* regulate metabolism of carbohydrates. They also control the body's response to stress and inflammation. The *mineralcorticoids* regulate the amount of salt and water that is absorbed and lost by the kidneys. The adrenal cortex also secretes small amounts of male and female sex hormones.

The *pancreas* secretes *insulin*. Insulin regulates the amount of sugar in the blood available for use by the cells. Insulin is needed for sugar to enter the cells. If there is too little insulin, sugar cannot enter the cells. If sugar cannot enter the cells, excess amounts of sugar build up in the blood. This condition is called *diabetes mellitus*.

The *gonads* are the glands of human reproduction. Male sex glands (testes) secrete *testosterone*. Female sex glands (ovaries) secrete *estrogen* and *progesterone*.

SUMMARY

The human body is made up of several systems. Each system has its own structures and functions. The body systems are related to and dependent on each other for proper functioning and survival. Injury to or disease of one part of the system affects the entire system and the whole body. You may need to refer to this chapter as you study other chapters in this book and as you learn basic nursing procedures. Each procedure involves the patient's body and your body. You need to have a basic understanding of the body's structure and function to give safe and effective care.

REVIEW QUESTIONS

Circle the best *answer.*

1   The basic unit of body structure is the
    a   Cell
    b   Neuron
    c   Nephron
    d   Ovum
2   Organs are formed by groups of
    a   Cells
    b   Tissues
    c   Systems
    d   Chromosomes
3   The outer layer of the skin is called the
    a   Dermis
    b   Epidermis
    c   Integument
    d   Myelin
4   Which is *not* a function of the skin?
    a   Providing the protective covering for the body
    b   Regulating body temperature
    c   Sensing cold, pain, touch, and pressure
    d   Providing the shape and framework for the body
5   Which part allows movement?
    a   Bone marrow and periosteum
    b   Synovial membrane
    c   Joints
    d   Ligaments
6   Skeletal muscles
    a   Are under involuntary control
    b   Appear smooth
    c   Are under voluntary control
    d   Appear striped and smooth
7   Muscles are connected to bones by
    a   Cartilage
    b   Ligaments
    c   Nerve fibers
    d   Tendons
8   The basic unit of the nervous system is the
    a   Brain
    b   Spinal cord
    c   Neuron
    d   Nephron
9   Which is *not* a main part of the brain?
    a   Cerebrum
    b   Pons
    c   Brainstem
    d   Cerebellum
10 The highest functions of the brain take place in the
    a   Cerebral cortex
    b   Medulla
    c   Brainstem
    d   Spinal nerves

11 Besides hearing, the ear is involved with
    a   Regulating body movements
    b   Balance
    c   Smoothness of body movements
    d   Controlling involuntary muscles
12 The liquid part of the blood is the
    a   Hemoglobin
    b   Red blood cell
    c   Plasma
    d   Alveolus
13 Which part of the heart pumps blood to the body?
    a   Right atrium
    b   Right ventricle
    c   Left atrium
    d   Left ventricle
14 Which carry blood away from the heart?
    a   Capillaries
    b   Veins
    c   Venules
    d   Arteries
15 Oxygen and carbon dioxide are exchanged
    a   In the bronchi
    b   Between the alveoli and capillaries
    c   Between the lungs and the pleura
    d   In the trachea
16 The process of digestion begins in the
    a   Mouth
    b   Stomach
    c   Small intestine
    d   Colon
17 Food is made easier to swallow by
    a   Bile
    b   Gastric juices
    c   Chyme
    d   Saliva
18 Most food absorption takes place in the
    a   Stomach
    b   Small intestine
    c   Colon
    d   Large intestine
19 Urine is formed by the
    a   Jejunum
    b   Kidneys
    c   Bladder
    d   Liver
20 Urine passes from the body through
    a   The ureters
    b   The urethra
    c   The anus
    d   Nephrons
21 The male sex gland is called the
    a   Penis

b Semen
c Testis
d Scrotum
22 The male sex cell is the
a Semen
b Ovum
c Gonad
d Sperm
23 The female sex gland is the
a Ovary
b Fallopian tube
c Uterus
d Vagina
24 The discharge of the lining of the uterus is called
a The endometrium
b Ovulation
c Fertilization
d Menstruation
25 The endocrine glands secrete substances called
a Hormones
b Mucus
c Semen
d Insulin
26 The "master gland" of the body is the
a Endocrine gland
b Pituitary gland
c Thyroid gland
d Adrenal gland

Answers

26 b	18 b	9 b
25 a	17 d	8 c
24 d	16 a	7 d
23 a	15 b	6 c
22 d	14 d	5 c
21 c	13 d	4 d
20 b	12 c	3 b
19 b	11 b	2 b
	10 a	1 a

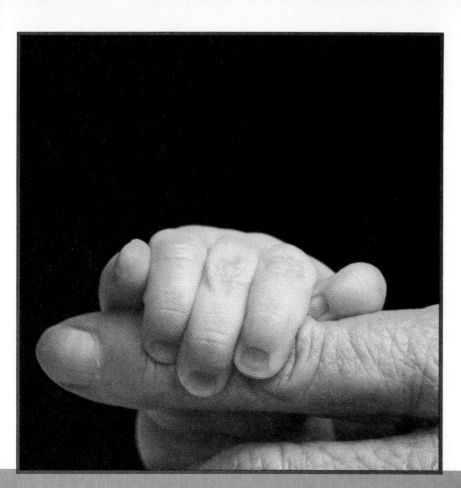

Growth and Development

6

OBJECTIVES

- Define the key terms listed in this chapter
- Understand six principles of growth and development
- Identify the stages of growth and development
- Identify the normal age ranges for each stage of growth and development
- Identify the developmental tasks of the infant, toddler, and preschooler
- Describe the normal growth and development of the infant, toddler, and preschooler
- Identify the developmental tasks of middle childhood, late childhood, and adolescence
- Describe the normal growth and development of middle childhood, late childhood, and adolescence
- Identify the developmental tasks of young, middle, and late adulthood
- Describe the normal growth and development of young and middle adulthood

development Changes in a person's psychological and social functioning

developmental task That which the individual must accomplish during a stage of development

growth The physical changes that can be measured and that occur in a steady, orderly manner

menarche The time when menstruation first begins

menopause The time when menstruation stops

primary caregiver The individual in the child's environment who is mainly responsible for providing or assisting with the child's basic needs

puberty The period during which the reproductive organs begin to function and secondary sex characteristics appear

reflex An involuntary movement

You will care for people in different stages of development. A basic understanding of growth and development will help you give better care. You will also have a better understanding of the needs of patients. This chapter presents the basic changes that occur in normal, healthy individuals from birth through old age.

Human growth and development is presented in eight stages. Approximate age ranges and normal characteristics are given for each stage. Only basic descriptions are given. Because the stages overlap, it is difficult to see clear-cut endings and beginnings of the stages. You need to be aware that there are variations in the rate of growth and development among individuals.

Growth and development theories have generally involved the traditional two-parent family. In our changing society, many households have only one parent. Single-parenthood is common today because of the high divorce rate and because many unmarried mothers keep their babies. Though single mothers keep their babies, often the children are raised by a relative while the mother works or attends school. Also, many divorced fathers gain custody of their children. Because of these changes, the term "primary caregiver" is used in this chapter where "mother" or "father" would have been used. The *primary caregiver* is that individual in the child's environment who is mainly responsible for providing or assisting with the child's basic needs. The primary caregiver may be a mother, father, grandparent, aunt, uncle, or court-appointed guardian. The words "parent" and "parents" are used in this chapter. However, another primary caregiver may be in the parent role.

PRINCIPLES

Growth is the physical changes that can be measured and that occur in a steady and orderly manner. Growth can be measured in height and weight. Growth can also be measured in the changes in physical appearance and body functions that occur as a person grows older.

Development relates to changes in psychological and social functioning. A person behaves and thinks in certain ways in different stages of development. A 2-year-old thinks in simple terms and needs a primary caregiver to meet many basic needs. A 40-year-old thinks in complex ways and can meet most basic needs without the help of others.

Growth and development affect the entire person. Although separately defined, growth and development overlap, are dependent on each other, and occur at the same time. For example, an infant cannot say simple syllables (development) until the physical structures involved in speech are strong enough (growth). The basic principles of growth and development are:

1. Growth and development occur from the moment of fertilization until death.
2. The process proceeds from the simple to the complex. A baby learns to sit before standing, to stand before walking, and to walk before running.
3. Growth and development occur in specific directions. The first direction is from the head to the foot. Babies learn to hold up their heads before they learn to sit and then to stand. The second direction is from the center of the body outward. Babies control shoulder movements before they control hand movements.
4. There is a sequence, order, and pattern to growth and development. Certain *developmental tasks* must be accomplished during each stage. A stage cannot be skipped. Each stage lays the foundation for the next stage.
5. The rate of growth and development is uneven rather than occurring at a set pace. Children have growth spurts. Some children develop rapidly, and others develop slowly.
6. Each stage of growth and development has its own characteristics and developmental tasks.

INFANCY (BIRTH TO 1 YEAR)

Infancy is the first year of life. This period is characterized by rapid physical, psychological, and social growth and development. The developmental tasks of infancy have been identified as:

1. Learning to walk
2. Learning to eat solid foods
3. Beginning to talk and communicate with others
4. Beginning to have emotional relationships with primary caregivers, brothers, and sisters
5. Developing stable sleep and feeding patterns

The *neonatal period* of infancy is the first 4 weeks after birth. A baby may be called a *neonate* or a *newborn* during this time.

The average newborn is 19 to 21 inches long and weighs 7 to 8 pounds at birth. Boys are usually longer and weigh more than girls. The birth weight usually doubles by the age of 5 to 6 months and triples by the first birthday. Babies are usually 20 to 30 inches long at the end of the first year.

The newborn's head is large in proportion to the rest of the body. The skin is wrinkled, and the baby is red in appearance. The extremities seem short compared with the trunk, and the abdomen is large and round. Eyes are a deep blue. The newborn has fat, pudgy cheeks, a flat nose, and a receding chin (Fig. 6-1).

The newborn's central nervous system is not well developed. Movements are uncoordinated and generally without purpose. Babies can see at birth, although vision is not clear. Infants seem attracted to bright objects, especially red ones. Babies hear well. They are startled by loud noises and soothed by soft sounds. Babies respond better to female voices than to male voices. Infants react to touch, and the senses of smell and taste are developed.

Certain *reflexes*, involuntary movements, are normally present in the newborn. These reflexes eventually disappear as the central nervous system develops. The *Moro reflex (startle reflex)* occurs when an infant is frightened by a loud noise or sudden movement. The arms are thrown apart, the legs extend, and the head is thrown back. The *rooting reflex* is stimulated by touching the infant's cheek at or near the mouth. The baby's head turns in the direction of the touch. The rooting reflex is necessary for feeding; it helps guide the baby's mouth to the nipple. The *sucking reflex* is produced by touching the cheeks or side of the lips.

The *grasping reflex* occurs when the palm of an infant's hand is stimulated, causing the fingers to close around the object (Fig. 6-2). This reflex begins to subside around the second month and disappears by the third month.

Infants sleep most of the time during the first few weeks of life. They awaken when hungry and fall asleep right after eating. The time between feedings becomes longer as infants grow and develop. Infants also stay awake more and sleep less as growth and development occur.

Body movements of newborns are uncoordinated and purposeless. They are generally involuntary. As the central nervous system and muscular system de-

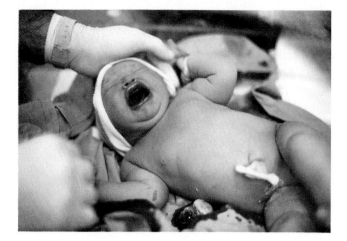

Fig. 6-1 A newborn.

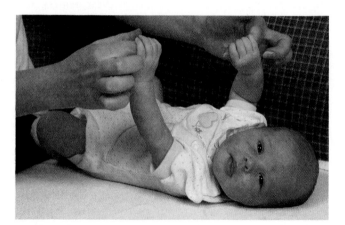

Fig. 6-2 The grasping reflex.

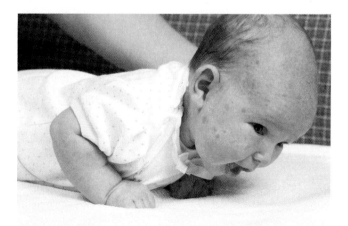

Fig. 6-3 The 1-month-old can lift the head when lying on the stomach.

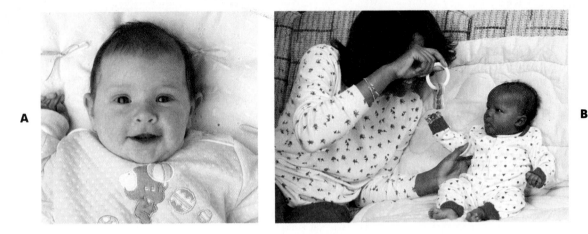

Fig. 6-4   A 2-month-old child. **A,** Child smiles. **B,** Child follows objects with the eyes.

velop, infants develop specific, voluntary, and coordinated movements. Newborns cannot hold their heads up. At 1 month, infants can hold their heads up when held and can lift and turn their heads when lying on their stomachs (Fig. 6-3). Two-month-old infants can smile and follow objects with their eyes (Fig. 6-4). The grasping reflex is diminishing in the 2-month-old infant.

Three-month-old infants can raise their heads and shoulders when lying on their stomachs (Fig. 6-5). They can sit for a short while when supported and can hold a rattle. The grasping reflex has disappeared. Infants 4 months of age should be able to roll over. They can sit up if supported and may sleep all night. The Moro and rooting reflexes have disappeared, and tears are shed when crying. A rattle can be held with both hands, objects are put in the mouth, and the infant babbles when spoken to. At 5 months, infants can grasp objects and play with their toes. Teeth begin to come through (Fig. 6-6).

Six-month-old infants usually have two lower front teeth and begin to chew and bite finger foods. They

can hold a bottle for feeding and can sit alone for a short time (Fig. 6-7). At 7 months the upper teeth begin to erupt. Babies respond to their names, can say "dada," and show a fear of strangers. At age 8 months, infants may be able to stand when holding onto something. They react to the word "no." Infants at this age do not like to be dressed or have diapers changed. Nine-month-old infants crawl and right- or left-handedness becomes evident (Fig. 6-8). More upper teeth appear.

At 10 months, infants can walk around while holding on to furniture (Fig. 6-9). They understand the words "bye-bye," "mama," and "dada." They smile when they look into a mirror. Infants at 11 months of age may begin to take steps and can hold a crayon. At 1 year of age infants should begin to walk. They can hold a cup for drinking. One-year-olds know more words, can say "no," and shake their heads for "no."

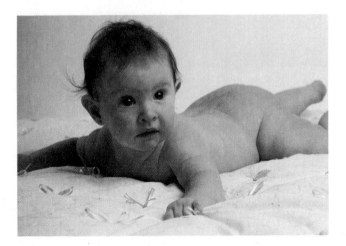

Fig. 6-5   The 3-month-old child can raise the head and shoulders.

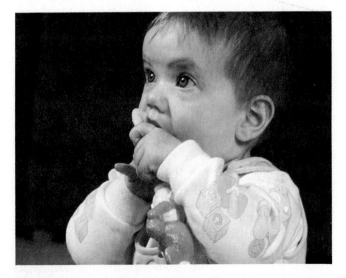

Fig. 6-6   The 5-month-old child puts objects into the mouth as teeth begin to erupt.

During the first 6 months, the infant's diet is mainly breast milk or formula. Solid foods are usually added during the fifth or sixth month. These solid foods are usually strained fruits and vegetables. Junior foods are added during the eighth and ninth months. A 1-year-old can eat table foods.

THE TODDLER (1 TO 3 YEARS)

Physical growth during the second year of life is not as rapid as during infancy. The developmental tasks during this period have been identified as:

1. Tolerating separation from the primary caregiver
2. Gaining control of bowel and bladder function
3. Using words to communicate with others
4. Becoming less dependent on the primary caregiver

The toddler years have been described as the "terrible two's." The ability to move about and walk increases, as does the child's curiosity. Toddlers get into anything and everything. Whatever can be reached is touched, smelled, and tasted. As toddlers become more coordinated, they develop the ability to climb. They soon learn that things look different and can be seen better from above than from below. The toddler's new and increasing skills allow exploration of the environment. The child ventures farther away from the primary caregiver. The toddler also discovers that some things can be done without the primary caregiver's help. By the age of 3 years the toddler can run, jump, climb, ride a tricycle, and walk up and down stairs.

Hand coordination also increases, giving toddlers new skills. The need to feel, smell, and taste things is reflected in their increasing ability to feed themselves. They progress from eating with their fingers to using a spoon (Fig. 6-10). Toddlers can drink from cups. Hand coordination also allows toddlers to scribble, build towers with blocks, string beads, and turn pages in books.

Toilet training is a major developmental task for toddlers. Bowel and bladder control is related to development of the central nervous system. Children must be psychologically and physically ready for toilet training. Toddlers are usually ready around 18 to 20 months. The process begins with bowel control. Bowel control is easier because the number of bowel movements per day is fewer than the number of times children urinate. By the age of 2, toddlers are usually capable of bladder control during the day. By 3 years of age, toddlers achieve bladder control during the night.

Speech and language skills increase. Speech becomes clearer, and vocabulary increases. Words are learned by imitating others. Toddlers understand more words than they use. They are capable of 2- or

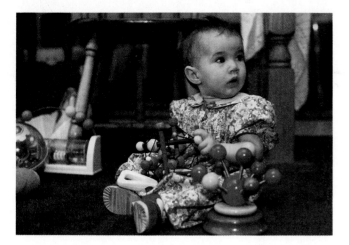

Fig. 6-7 A six-month-old child can sit alone for a short time.

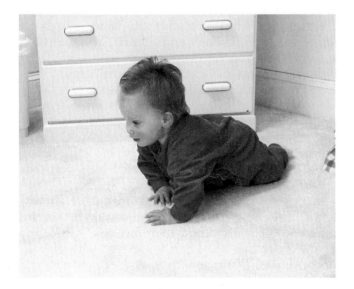

Fig. 6-8 A nine-month-old child is able to crawl.

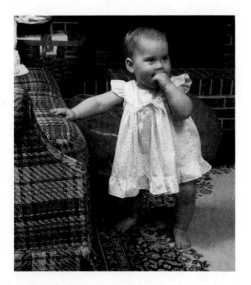

Fig. 6-9 A ten-month-old child can walk while holding onto furniture.

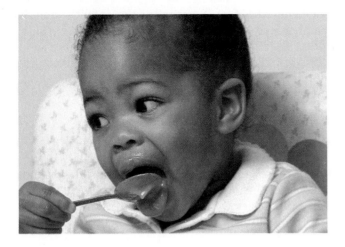

Fig. 6-10 A toddler is able to use a spoon.

3-word sentences. By 3 years of age, children can speak in short sentences.

The toddler's ability to play increases. The child plays alongside other children but does not play with them. There is no sharing of toys with others because the toddler is very possessive. The word "mine" is used frequently.

This stage of development may also be characterized by temper tantrums and use of the word "no." When disciplined the toddler often kicks and screams. The temper tantrum is the child's way of objecting to discipline. The use of the word "no" can be very frustrating to primary caregivers. Almost every request may be answered "no," even if the toddler is complying with the request.

Another developmental task is tolerating separation from the primary caregiver. As toddlers begin to explore their environments, they tend to venture away from their primary caregivers. However, when discomfort, frustration, or injury occur, they quickly return to primary caregivers or cry for their attention. If the primary caregiver is consistently present whenever needed, a child learns that the primary caregiver will be there and feels secure. Thus toddlers learn to tolerate brief periods of separation.

THE PRESCHOOLER (3 TO 6 YEARS)

The preschool years, also called early childhood, are from the ages of 3 to 6. Children grow taller but gain little weight during this stage. Preschoolers are thinner, more coordinated, and more graceful than toddlers. The developmental tasks of the preschool years include:

1. Increasing the ability to communicate and understand others
2. Performing self-care activities
3. Learning the differences between the sexes and developing sexual modesty

4. Learning right from wrong and good from bad
5. Learning to play with others
6. Developing family relationships

The 3-Year-Old

Three-year-olds become more coordinated. They can walk on tiptoe and balance on one foot for a few seconds. They can run, jump, and climb with ease and can draw circles and crosses. They can put on shoes, dress themselves, and manage buttons. Children this age can wash their hands and brush their teeth (Fig. 6-11). They can feed themselves, pour from a bottle, and help set the table without breaking dishes.

Most three-year-olds have vocabularies of about 1000 words, imitate new words, and ask questions constantly. They also talk constantly, even if no one is paying attention. Sentences are brief, usually only 3 or 4 words. Three-year-olds can name body parts, family members, friends, and animals. They like talking dolls and musical toys.

Play is important. They play in small groups with 2 or 3 other children and are able to share toys. They can play simple games and learn to follow simple rules. Three-year-olds may have imaginary playmates and may begin to imitate adults during play. Coloring books and crayons, scissors and paper, and playing "house" and "dress-up" are enjoyed by 3-year-olds (Fig. 6-12).

At 3 years old, children know that there are two sexes. They know that male and female bodies are different. They also know their own sex. Little girls may wonder how the penis works and why they do not have one. Little boys may wonder how girls can urinate without a penis.

Children 3 years of age begin to understand time. They may speak of the past, present, and future. "Yesterday" and "tomorrow" are still somewhat confusing. Children may be afraid of the dark and need a night-light in the bedroom.

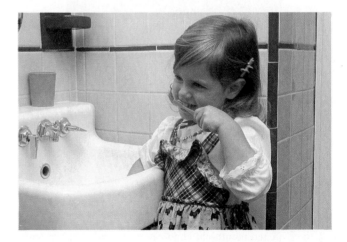

Fig. 6-11 A three-year-old has increased coordination.

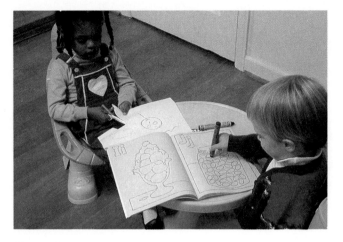

Fig. 6-12 Three-year-olds enjoy cutting paper and using coloring books and crayons.

Three-year-olds are less fearful of strangers. They can tolerate separation from primary caregivers for short periods. They are less jealous than toddlers are of a new baby. Things are done to please primary caregivers at this age.

The 4-Year-Old

Four-year-olds can hop, skip, and throw and catch a ball. Hand coordination also increases. They can lace shoes, draw faces, copy a square, and they try to print letters. They can bathe with some help and can usually tend to toileting needs with assistance.

Vocabulary increases to about 1500 words. The child continues to ask many questions and tends to exaggerate when telling stories. The 4-year-old can sing simple songs, repeat four numbers, count to three, and name a few colors.

Children 4 years of age may tend to physically attack others. They also tease, tattle, tell fibs, and may call other children names. They are more impatient and may blame an imaginary playmate when in trouble. Bragging, telling tales about family members, and showing off are seen in 4-year-olds. They can run simple errands and can play cooperatively with other children. Four-year-olds are proud of their accomplishments but have mood swings.

Children in this age-group enjoy playing "dress-up," wearing costumes, and telling and hearing stories. They like to draw and make things. Imagination, drama, and imitation of adults are seen in their play activities (Fig. 6-13). They play in groups of two or three and tend to be bossy. Children this age often play "doctor and nurse" as their curiosity about the opposite sex continues.

Four-year-olds have a strong preference for the primary caregiver of the opposite sex. Rivalries with brothers and sisters are seen, especially when younger children take the 4-year-old's possessions. Rivalries also occur when older children have more and different privileges. Family members are often the focus of the child's frustrations and aggressive behavior. Some 4-year-olds try to run away from home.

The 5-Year-Old

Coordination continues to develop. Five-year-olds can jump rope, skate, tie shoelaces, dress, and bathe. They can use a pencil well and copy diamond and triangle shapes. They can print a few letters and numbers and their first names. Drawings of people include the body, head, arms, legs, and feet.

The ability to communicate also increases. Vocabularly consists of about 2100 words. Sentences are 6 to 8 words. They ask fewer questions than before. However, questions are more meaningful. They may request definitions for unfamiliar terms and take part in conversations. Four or more colors, coins, days of the week, and months can be named. They specify what they draw and give detailed descriptions of their drawings.

Five-year-olds are more responsible and truthful, and they quarrel less than before. There is greater awareness of rules and an eagerness to do things the right way. They have manners, are independent, and can be trusted within limits. Five-year-olds have fewer fears but may have nightmares and dreams. They are also proud of their accomplishments.

Simple number and word games are enjoyable for 5-year-olds. Although they may cheat to win, they appreciate rules and try to follow them. They imitate adults during play and have a greater interest in watching television. They also enjoy activities with

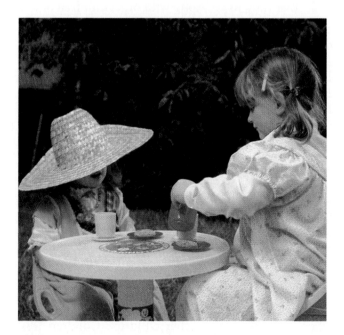

Fig. 6-13 Four-year-olds play "dress-up" and imitate adults.

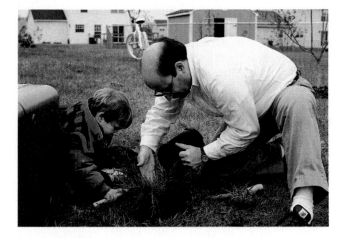

Fig. 6-14 Five-year-olds enjoy doing things with the parent of the same sex.

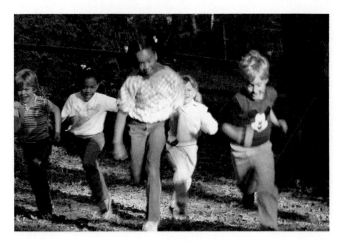

Fig. 6-15 Six-year-olds play with both sexes. They begin to prefer playing with children of the same sex.

the primary caregiver of the same sex (Fig. 6-14). Such activities include cooking, housecleaning, shopping, yard work, and sports.

The child of 5 years tolerates brothers and sisters well. Although younger children may be considered a nuisance, 5-year-olds are usually protective of them.

MIDDLE CHILDHOOD (6 TO 8 YEARS)

Preschoolers may have been to nursery school and kindergarten. However, middle childhood is the time for entering school. Children enter the world of peer groups, games, and learning. The developmental tasks of middle childhood are:

1. Developing the social and physical skills needed for playing games
2. Learning to get along with other children of the same age and background (peers)
3. Learning behaviors and attitudes appropriate to one's own sex
4. Learning basic reading, writing, and arithmetic skills
5. Developing a conscience and morals
6. Developing a good feeling and attitude about oneself

The 6-Year-Old

The 6-year-old grows about 2 inches in height and gains about 3 to 6 pounds. Baby teeth are lost, and replacement with permanent teeth begins. Children this age are very active and are skilled at running, jumping, skipping, hopping, and riding a bicycle. They seem to have a need to be constantly on the go. Sitting is tolerated for only a short time.

Six-year-olds enter the first grade and the world of school, activities, and other children. Children this age are often described as bossy, opinionated, charm-ing, argumentative, and as "know-it-alls." They have set ways of doing things and like to have their own way. They may have temper tantrums. Six-year-olds play well with children of both sexes. However, they begin to prefer playing with children of the same sex (Fig. 6-15). There is more sharing with others, and the child may have a "best friend." A child may cheat to win or may leave a game before it is over to avoid losing. Tattling is common.

Six-year-olds have a vocabulary of about 2500 words. They know the letters of the alphabet and begin to read and spell. They can communicate thoughts and feelings better than before.

Play interests range from rough play to quiet activities such as playing with cards, paints, clay, and checkers. Collections are started that consist of an assortment of odds and ends rather than specific things like stamps, rocks, or butterflies. More active play includes tag, hide-and-seek, playing with balls, skating, and playing in mud or sand.

The 7-Year-Old

Seven-year-olds grow about 2 inches in height. The average 7-year-old weighs about 49 to 56 pounds and is between 47 and 49 inches tall. Hand coordination increases. Children learn to write rather than print. They are quieter than 6-year-olds and spend much time alone. They are more serious, less stubborn, and more concerned about being well-liked. Seven-year-olds are more aware of themselves, their bodies, and the reactions of others. They do not like to be teased or criticized and are sensitive about how others treat them. They take pleasure in going to school, learning, and reading. They worry about the second grade being too hard. There are concerns about grades and what the teacher thinks about them. Reading skills increase, and the child can tell time.

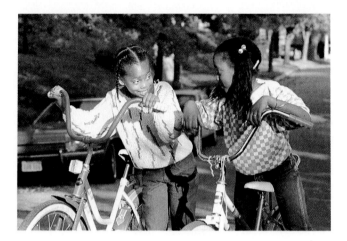

Fig. 6-16 Seven-year-olds enjoy biking.

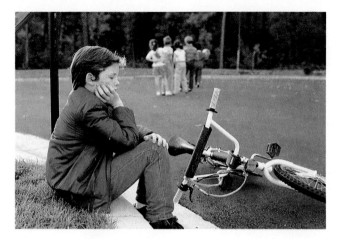

Fig. 6-17 Belonging to a peer group is important to the eight-year-old.

Play activities include swimming, biking, collecting and trading objects, playing ball, and working puzzles and magic tricks (Fig. 6-16). Children this age play in groups. However, boys prefer to play with boys and girls prefer to play with girls. They may join scouting groups, such as the "Cub Scouts" or "Brownies."

The 8-Year-Old

The 8-year-old enters the third grade. Growth in height and weight continues, and more permanent teeth appear. The child continues to be physically active. Movements are faster and more graceful.

Peer group activities and opinions are important to the 8-year-old. Being accepted and included in peer groups are important for the needs of love and belonging and esteem (Fig. 6-17). Children this age get along with adults. However, they prefer the fads, opinions, and activities of peer groups. Boys and girls continue to play separately. Their interests relate to group games, collections, television, and movies. An 8-year-old may belong to a "secret" club.

Eight-year-olds have been described as defensive, opinionated, practical, and outgoing. Advice is freely given to others. However, they do not accept criticism well. They often do household tasks such as vacuuming, cooking, and yard work, but they expect to be paid. They expect more privileges than younger brothers and sisters have.

The process of learning continues. They are curious about science, history, and other places and countries. They enjoy school, especially because it provides social opportunities with peers. Eight-year-olds become daring in the classroom. They may pass notes and throw spitballs or paper airplanes when they think the teacher is not looking. Despite these acts of mischief, they are mannerly, relate well to adults, and can participate in adult conversations. They are also friendly and affectionate.

LATE CHILDHOOD (9 TO 12 YEARS)

Late childhood is also called preadolescence. The person is between leaving childhood and dependency on others and entering adolescence. The developmental tasks of late childhood are similar to those of middle childhood. However, a preadolescent is expected to show more refinement and maturity in achieving the following tasks.

1. Becoming independent of adults and learning to depend on oneself
2. Developing and keeping friendships with peers
3. Understanding the physical, psychological, and social roles of one's sex
4. Developing moral and ethical behavior
5. Developing greater muscular strength, coordination, and balance
6. Learning how to study

Boys grow about 1 inch per year during this stage. Girls grow about 2 inches per year. Boys gain about 3½ to 4 pounds each year. Girls gain between 4 and 5 pounds each year. Girls are usually taller than boys during late preadolescence. Many permanent teeth erupt.

Body movements are more graceful and coordinated (Fig. 6-18). There is greater muscular strength and increased physical skill. Skill in team sports is very important to boys in late childhood.

Body changes occur as the onset of puberty approaches. In girls the pelvis becomes broader, fat appears on the hips and chest, and the budding of breasts occurs. Boys show fewer signs of maturing sexually during this time. Genital organs begin to grow in size. However, secondary sex characteristics, such as deepening of the voice or growth of facial hair, are not seen until about 13 or 14 years of age.

These children must receive factual sex education if it has not already been provided. Information about sex is shared among friends, although the information

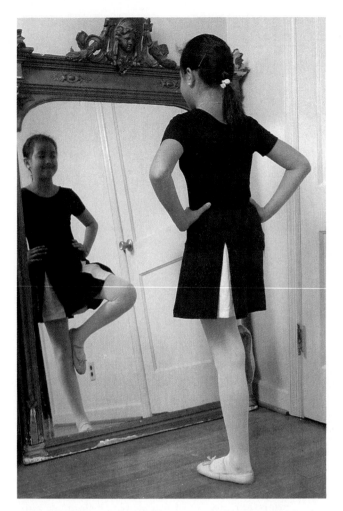

Fig. 6-18 Movements are smooth and graceful in late childhood.

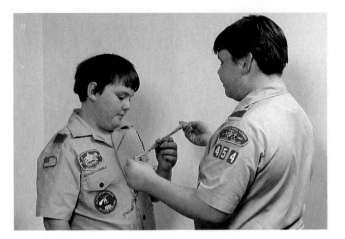

Fig. 6-19 Organized activities are important in late childhood.

and weaknesses of adults. They do not accept the standards and rules of adults without question. Rebellion against adults is common. Disagreements between parents and children increase, although the parents continue to be important for the child's development.

By the age of 12 the child uses about 7000 words in conversation and understands about 50,000 words in reading. Use of the dictionary, encyclopedia, and other reference books increases. Girls are generally better than boys are in the use of words, writing, and memorizing. Boys are often better in arithmetic. Interest in science, history, and geography continues in both sexes. Girls often enjoy reading romantic books and stories. Boys usually prefer science fiction, mysteries, and adventure stories.

is often incomplete and inaccurate. Parents and children may be uncomfortable discussing sex with each other and may avoid the subject. When children do ask questions, honest and complete answers should be given in terms the children can understand.

The peer group is the center of the preadolescent's activities. The group begins to affect the child's attitudes and behavior. Preference for companions of the same sex continues. Boys need to show their strength and toughness and may give each other nicknames. Membership in "secret" clubs continues to be important. Boys join organized team sports, scouting groups, and the YMCA (Fig. 6-19). Arguments between boys and girls are common, and boys often tease girls.

Associations between girls are stronger than those seen among boys. Writing and passing notes in class and talking on the telephone for long periods are frequent activities among girls.

Preadolescents become more aware of the mistakes

ADOLESCENCE (12 to 18 YEARS)

Adolescence is a time of rapid growth and psychological and social maturity. The stage begins with puberty. *Puberty* is the period during which the reproductive organs begin to function and the secondary sex characteristics appear. The age at the onset of puberty and the beginning of adolescence varies. Some girls may experience puberty as early as the age of 10. Others are 15 to 16 years old before the onset of puberty. Most girls reach puberty between the ages of 12 and 13. Most boys reach puberty around the age of 14.

Because the age of puberty varies, adolescence ranges from the ages of 12 to 18 years. The developmental tasks of adolescence include:

1. Accepting the changes in the body and appearance
2. Developing appropriate relationships with males and females of the same age

3. Accepting the male or female role appropriate for one's age
4. Becoming independent from parents and adults
5. Developing morals, attitudes, and values needed for functioning in society

The onset of puberty in girls is marked by *menarche*, the beginning of menstruation. Secondary sex characteristics appear. These include increase in breast size, the appearance of pubic and axillary (underarm) hair, slight deepening of the voice, and widening and rounding of the hips.

During late childhood, male sex organs begin to increase in size. This growth continues during adolescence. Puberty in boys is signaled by nocturnal emissions, commonly called "wet dreams." During sleep (nocturnal) the penis becomes erect and semen is released (emission). Other secondary sex characteristics appear. These include the appearance of facial hair and growth of a beard, pubic, and axillary hair; hair on the arms, chest, and legs; deepening of the voice; and increases in neck and shoulder size.

Adolescence is also marked by a growth spurt. Boys grow an average of 4 to 12 inches and gain 15 to 60 pounds. They usually stop growing between the ages of 18 and 21, although some continue to grow until about age 25. Girls grow an average of 2 to 8 inches and gain between 15 and 50 pounds. They usually stop growing between the ages of 17 and 18; some continue to grow until about age 21.

Adolescence is often described as the awkward stage. Awkwardness and clumsiness are due to the uneven growth of muscles and bones. The adolescent develops coordination and graceful body movements as the growth of muscles and bones evens out.

Teenagers often have difficulty accepting the changes in their appearance. Some girls are embarrassed about breast development, especially if breast size is very large or small. Some are embarrassed about wearing a brassiere. Others wear tight sweaters so that the breasts are more noticeable. Genital size may be a concern of boys. Height is also a problem to many teenagers. Boys do not like being short because it limits their participation in sports such as basketball and football. They do not like being significantly shorter than their peers. Tall girls may feel embarrassed about being different and taller than other girls and boys.

The emotional reactions of adolescents vary from high to low. Adolescents can be happy one moment and sad the next. Predicting their reaction to a particular comment or event is difficult. Teenagers can control their emotions better during the latter part of adolescence. Although older adolescents (15- to 18-year-olds) can still feel sad and become depressed, they can better control the time and place of their emotional reactions.

Adolescents need to become independent of adults, especially their parents. They must learn to function, make decisions, and act in a responsible manner without adult supervision. Many teenagers work toward this independence by having part-time jobs, babysitting, going to dances and parties, and dating. Joining school clubs and organizations, shopping without an adult, and staying home alone are other ways to work toward independence. However, the judgment and reasoning of teenagers is not always sound. They still need guidance, discipline, and emotional and financial support from parents. Arguments and disagreements with parents are common during this age, especially when restrictions and limitations are set on behavior and activities. Teenagers would rather be with their peers than do things with parents and other family members. Adolescents tend to confide in and seek advice from adults other than their parents.

The interests and activities of teenagers reflect their need to become independent, to develop relationships with the opposite sex, and to act like males or females. Both sexes have an increased interest in parties, dances, and other social activities. Clothing, makeup, and hairstyles become increasingly important. A teenager may babysit or get a part-time job to have extra money for clothes, makeup, and hair- and skin-care products. Parents and teenagers rarely agree about clothing styles. Teenagers may spend a lot of time experimenting with makeup and hairstyles. They may also spend a lot of time talking to friends on the phone, listening to music, and reading teen magazines (Fig. 6-20).

Dating begins during adolescence. Although the age when dating begins varies, there is usually a pattern of dating activities. "Crowd" dates are common in the seventh and eighth grades. They are usually related to school activities, such as a dance or basketball game. The same group of girls just happens to be with the same group of boys during these social

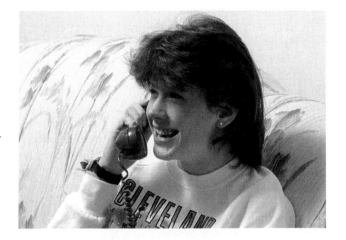

Fig. 6-20 Adolescents enjoy talking on the phone.

events. In the ninth grade, pairing off is common during crowd dating. The tenth grade is usually when boy-girl couples go to social events together and then join the crowd of other couples. The dating pattern progresses to double dating in the eleventh grade. Dates involve one couple during the twelfth grade, although there is some double dating.

Many difficult decisions and conflicts result as the adolescent matures physically, psychologically, and emotionally. Parents and teenagers often disagree about dating. Parents worry that dating will lead to sexual activities and pregnancy. Teenagers usually do not understand or appreciate their parents' concern. "Going steady" helps meet the teenager's need for security, love and belonging, and esteem. Teenagers sometimes have difficulty controlling their sexual urges and considering the consequences of being sexually active.

Adolescents begin to think about careers and what to do after high school graduation. Interests, skills, and talents are some factors that influence the choice of pursuing further education and getting a job. Adolescents also need to develop morals, values, and attitudes for living in society. They need to develop a sense about what is good and bad, right and wrong, and important and unimportant. Parents, peers, culture, religion, television, school and movies are among the many factors influencing teenagers. Drug abuse, unwanted pregnancy, alcoholism, and criminal acts are common problems of troubled adolescents.

YOUNG ADULTHOOD (18 TO 40 YEARS)

Psychological and social development continue during young adulthood. There is little physical growth. Adult height has been reached, and body systems are fully developed. Developmental tasks of young adulthood include:
1. Choosing education and an occupation
2. Selecting a marriage partner
3. Learning to live with the husband or wife
4. Becoming a parent and raising children
5. Developing a satisfactory sex life

Education and occupation are so closely related that they can rarely be separated. A young adult may choose to be a teacher, nurse, doctor, lawyer, computer programmer, nursing assistant, truck driver, mechanic, or one of many other occupations. Most jobs require specific knowledge and skills. The amount and kind of education needed depends on the career choice. Most adults find that employment opportunities are greater with adequate educational preparation. Employment is necessary for economic independence and for supporting a family.

Although some adults remain single, most marry at least once. The many reasons people get married

include love, emotional security, wanting a family, sex, wanting to leave an unhappy home life, social status, companionship, and money. Some marry to feel wanted, needed, and desirable. Many factors also influence the selection of a marriage partner. These factors include age, religion, interests, education, race, personality, and of course, love. Some marriages are happy and successful while others are not. There are no guarantees that a marriage will work. Therefore the two people will have to work together to build a marriage based on trust, respect, caring, and friendship.

The married couple must learn to live together. Habits, routines, meal preparation, and pastimes may need to be changed or adjusted to "fit" the other person's needs. The individuals must learn how to solve problems and make decisions together. They need to work toward the same goals. Open and honest communication helps create a successful marriage (Fig. 6-21).

Couples also need to develop a satisfactory sex life. There are variations to the frequency of sex, sexual desires, practices, and preferences. Understanding and accepting the other person's needs are necessary for a satisfying and intimate relationship.

Most couples decide to have children. With modern birth control methods, the number of children and when to have them can be planned. However,

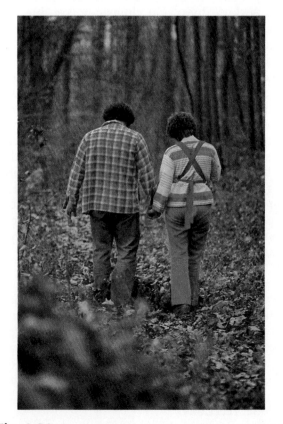

Fig. 6-21 Communication is necessary for a successful marriage and a satisfactory sex life.

many pregnancies are unplanned. Most couples have a child during the first few years of marriage; some wait several years before starting a family. Other couples decide not to have children. Some have difficulty or cannot have children because of physical problems in the husband or wife. Couples deciding to have children need to agree on child rearing practices and discipline methods. They will need to adjust to the child. They will also need to adjust to the child's need for time, energy, and parental attention.

MIDDLE ADULTHOOD (40 TO 65 YEARS)

This stage of development is more stable and comfortable. Children are usually grown and have moved away. Husbands and wives now have time to spend alone together. There are fewer worries about children and money. The developmental tasks of middle adulthood relate to the following:

1. Adjusting to physical changes
2. Having grown children
3. Developing leisure-time activities
4. Relating to aging parents

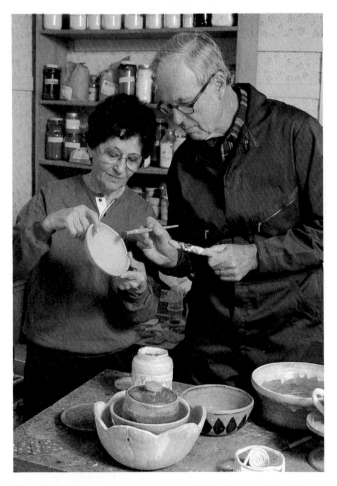

Fig. 6-22 Middle-age adults usually have more time for hobbies.

Several physical changes occur during middle adulthood. The changes may occur very gradually and go unnoticed, or they may be seen early. People in their early forties may feel energetic and able to function as they did in their twenties. However, energy and endurance begin to slow down. Weight control becomes a problem as metabolism and physical activities slow down. Facial wrinkles and grey hair appear. The need for eyeglasses is common. Hearing loss may begin. Menstruation stops between the ages of 42 and 55; this is called *menopause*. The ovaries stop secreting hormones, and the woman is no longer capable of having children. Many diseases and illnesses can develop. The disorders can become chronic or life threatening.

Children leave home for college, marry, move into homes of their own, and begin their own families. Adults in this stage have to cope with letting children go, being in-laws, and becoming grandparents. Parents must let children lead their own lives. However, they need to be available for emotional support in times of need.

Middle-aged adults often discover spare time when the demands of parenthood decrease. Hobbies and pastimes such as gardening, fishing, painting, golfing, volunteer work, and membership in clubs and organizations can be sources of pleasure (Fig. 6-22). Hobbies and pastimes become even more important after retirement and during later adulthood.

Middle-aged adults may have parents who are aging and developing poor health. Responsibility for aging parents may begin during this stage. Middle-aged adults often have to deal with the death of parents.

LATE ADULTHOOD (65 YEARS AND OLDER)

Many physical, psychological, and social changes occur during later adulthood. People in this stage of development are often referred to as the elderly.

Chapter 7 describes the changes that occur in the elderly, as well as the care they may require. The developmental tasks of the elderly are:

1. Adjusting to decreased physical strength and loss of health
2. Adjusting to retirement and reduced income
3. Coping with the death of a husband or wife
4. Developing new friends and relationships
5. Preparing for one's own death

SUMMARY

Growth and development continue throughout life and affect the whole person. There are eight stages, each with its own age range, characteristics, and developmental tasks. The developmental tasks of one stage must be accomplished before the next stage is entered. Although there is an orderly pattern to the process, the rate of growth and development varies among individuals.

The knowledge and understanding gained from this chapter can be applied in work and personal situations. Everyday life puts you in contact with people of different ages and levels of development.

A basic understanding of growth and development will help you better understand individuals. A 2-year-old's temper tantrum can be dealt with better. The changes of puberty and an adolescent's unpredictable behavior are more understandable. Perhaps you can be more sensitive to the worries, concerns, and needs of adults of different ages.

REVIEW QUESTIONS

Circle the best *answer.*

1 Changes in psychological and social functioning are called
   a Growth
   b Development
   c A reflex
   d A stage
2 Which is *false?*
   a Growth and development occur from the simple to the complex.
   b Growth and development occur in an orderly pattern.
   c Growth and development occur at specific rates.
   d Each stage has its own characteristics.
3 The stage of infancy is the first
   a 4 weeks of life
   b 3 months of life
   c 6 months of life
   d Year of life
4 Which reflexes are needed for feeding in the infant?
   a The Moro and startle reflexes
   b The rooting and sucking reflexes
   c The grasping and Moro reflexes
   d The rooting and grasping reflexes
5 Crawling begins at about
   a 5 months
   b 6 months
   c 7 months
   d 8 months
6 Solid foods are usually given to a baby during the
   a Fifth or sixth month
   b Seventh or eighth month
   c Nine or tenth month
   d Eleventh or twelfth month
7 Toilet training begins
   a During infancy
   b During the toddler years
   c When the primary caregiver is ready
   d At the age of 3

8 The toddler can
   a Use a spoon and cup
   b Ride a bike
   c Help set the table
   d Name parts of the body
9 Playing with other children begins during
   a Infancy
   b The toddler years
   c The preschool years
   d Middle childhood
10 Tattling, fibbing, and teasing are commonly seen at age
   a 3
   b 4
   c 5
   d 6
11 Loss of baby teeth usually begins at the age of
   a 4
   b 5
   c 6
   d 7
12 Which is *not true* of the 7-year-old?
   a The child learns to write.
   b The child spends a lot of time alone.
   c The child does not like school.
   d The child is able to tell time.
13 Peer group activities become more important at the age of
   a 6
   b 7
   c 8
   d 9
14 Most information about sex is exchanged between
   a Children and teacher
   b Teacher and parents
   c Parents and children
   d Members of a peer group
15 Reproductive organs begin to function and secondary sex characteristics appear during
   a Late childhood

b Preadolescence
c Puberty
d Early adulthood

16 Which is *false*?
  a Boys reach puberty earlier than girls.
  b Most girls reach puberty between the ages of 12 and 13.
  c Menarche marks the onset of puberty in girls.
  d A growth spurt occurs during adolescence.

17 Dating usually begins
  a During late childhood
  b With "crowd" dating
  c With "pairing off"
  d During late adolescence

18 Adolescence is a time when parents and children
  a Talk openly about sex
  b Express love and affection
  c Disagree
  d Do things as a family

19 Which is *not* a developmental task of young adulthood?
  a Adjusting to changes in the body and in physical appearance
  b Selecting a marriage partner
  c Choosing an occupation
  d Becoming a parent

20 Middle adulthood is from about
  a 25 to 35 years
  b 30 to 40 years
  c 40 to 50 years
  d 40 to 65 years

21 Middle adulthood is a time when
  a Families are started
  b Physical energy and free time are gained
  c Children are grown and leave home
  d People need to prepare for death

Answers

1 b	8 a	15 c
2 c	9 c	16 a
3 d	10 b	17 b
4 b	11 c	18 c
5 d	12 c	19 a
6 a	13 c	20 d
7 b	14 d	21 c

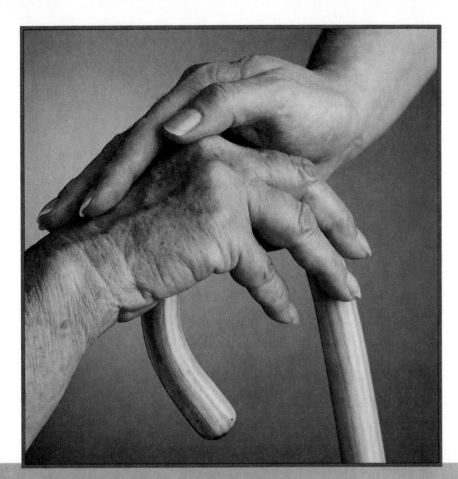

Care of the Elderly

7

dysphagia Difficulty (dys) in swallowing (phagia)
geriatrics The care of aging people
gerontology The study of the aging process
reality orientation A form of rehabilitation aimed at promoting or maintaining awareness of person, time, and place

The number of people older than 65 years of age is increasing every day. Individuals are living longer and are healthier than ever before. Today most people can expect to live into their 70s. In the 1900s most people died in their 50s. Many individuals in their 70s and 80s continue to live healthy and happy lives in their own homes.

Gerontology is the study of the aging process. *Geriatrics* is the care of the aged. Aging, or growing old, is a normal process. Normal changes occur in body structure and function. Because of these changes, the elderly have special needs. They are also at greater risk for illness, chronic diseases, and injuries.

PSYCHOLOGICAL AND SOCIAL EFFECTS OF AGING

Physical, psychological, and social changes occur as a person grows older. Graying hair, wrinkles, and slow movements are physical reminders of growing old. Retirement and the death of a spouse, relatives, and friends are social reminders. Society values youth and beauty. This emphasis can make growing old a painful process socially, psychologically, and physically.

Retirement

People traditionally retire at the age of 65. Some retire earlier. Others continue to work until the age of 70. Retirement is viewed as a reward for a lifetime of hard work. The individual has earned the right not to work and can now relax and enjoy life (Fig. 7-1). Travel, leisure, and doing whatever one wants are the "benefits" of retirement (Fig. 7-2). Many people enjoy retirement. Others are not so fortunate. Some must retire because of chronic disease or disability. Poor health and medical expenses can make enjoying retirement very difficult.

Working has social and psychological effects. Work helps meet the basic needs of love, belonging, and self-esteem. Personal satisfaction and usefulness result from working. There is the feeling of pride in a day's work or a job well done. Friendships develop, and day-to-day events are shared with co-workers.

Leisure activities, recreation, and companionship often involve co-workers. Some individuals rely on work for psychological and social fulfillment. Retirement can be difficult for them. Some retired people have part-time jobs or do volunteer work. Such activities promote usefulness and well-being.

Retirement usually means reduced financial income. The monthly social security check may be the only source of income. However, retirement and aging do not mean fewer expenses. There may still be rent or mortgage payments. Food, clothing, gas and electricity, water bills, and taxes are other expenses. Car expenses, home repairs, medicine, and health care are additional costs. So are entertainment and gifts for children and grandchildren. For many people, retirement causes severe financial problems. Some people plan for retirement through savings, investments, retirement plans, and insurance.

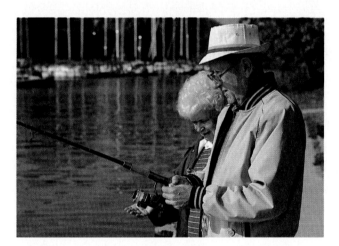

Fig. 7-1 A retired couple enjoying fishing together.

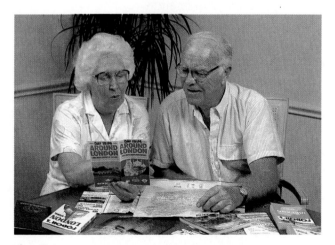

Fig. 7-2 An elderly couple planning a vacation.

Social Relationships

Social relationships change throughout life. Children have grown and left home and may have families of their own. Many live far away from their elderly parents. Elderly friends and relatives may have moved away, died, or are disabled. Many elderly people experience loneliness. Separation from children and the lack of companionship with people their own age are common causes of loneliness in the elderly (Fig. 7-3).

Many elderly people are able to adjust to these changes. Hobbies, church and community activities, and new friends help prevent loneliness. Being a grandparent can be a source of great love and enjoyment (Fig. 7-4). Being included in family activities helps prevent loneliness. It also allows the elderly person to feel useful and wanted (Fig. 7-5).

Some elderly individuals speak and understand a foreign language. They will have other social problems. Communication occurs with family and friends who speak the same language. These relatives and friends may move away or die. Greater loneliness and isolation for the foreign language speaking individual may result. The person may not have anyone to talk to and may not be understood by others. In addition, the person's cultural values and practices may not be understood or recognized.

Another social change experienced by some elderly people is being cared for by their children. Parents and children change roles. Instead of the parent caring for the child, the child cares for the parent. This role change and dependency on a child can make the elderly person feel more secure. However, others feel unwanted, in the way, and useless. Some feel a loss of dignity and self-respect. Tensions may develop between the child, parent, and other family members in the household. Tension can be caused by the lack of privacy and disagreements. Criticisms about housekeeping, childrearing, cooking, and friends are other common causes of tension.

Death of a Spouse

As a husband and wife grow older, the chances increase that one of them will die. Women live longer than men. Therefore becoming a widow will be a reality for many women.

A person may try to psychologically prepare for the death of a marriage partner. When death does occur, the loss of a spouse is devastating. No amount of preparation is ever enough for the emptiness and changes that result. The individual loses more than a husband or wife. A friend, lover, companion, and confidant are also lost. The grief felt by the surviving spouse may be very great. Serious physical and mental health problems can result. The surviving spouse may lose the will to live or attempt suicide.

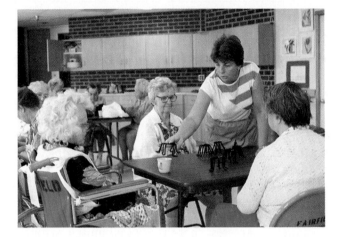
Fig. 7-3 Elderly people enjoying companionship with people their own age.

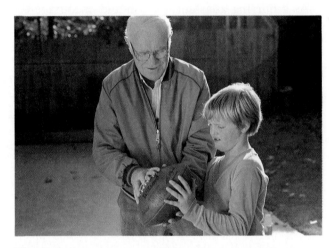
Fig. 7-4 An elderly man playing with a grandchild.

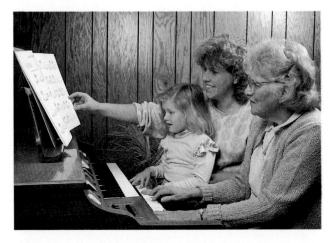
Fig. 7-5 An elderly woman is included in family activities.

PHYSICAL EFFECTS OF AGING

Certain physical changes are a normal part of the aging process and occur in all individuals (Table 7-1). The rate and degree of change vary with each person. Many changes are gradual and may go unnoticed for a long time. The physical changes of aging result in a slowing down of body processes. The energy level and the efficiency of the body decline. The normal changes of aging may be accompanied by changes caused by disease, illness, or injury.

The Musculoskeletal System

As aging progresses, there is gradual muscle atrophy (shrinking) and decreasing strength. Bones become brittle and can break easily. Joints become stiff and painful. These changes result in a gradual loss of height, loss of strength, and decrease in mobility. There is the possibility of developing a fracture (broken bone) from simply turning in bed.

As a nursing assistant, you should encourage the elderly person to be as active as possible. Range-of-motion exercises and diet can help slow down the rate of these changes. The diet should be high in protein, calcium, and vitamins. Because bones can break easily, the individual must be protected from injury. Measures to prevent falls must be practiced. The individual is turned and moved gently and carefully. A person may need support and assistance when getting out of bed and when ambulating.

The Cardiovascular System

The heart muscle becomes less efficient. Blood is pumped through the body with less force. These changes may not cause problems when the individual is resting. Activity, exercise, excitement, and illness increase the body's need for oxygen and nutrients. The heart may be unable to meet these needs.

Arteries lose their elasticity and become narrow. Less blood flows through them, causing poor circulation in many parts of the body. As a result, a weakened heart has to work harder to pump blood through the narrowed vessels.

The elderly person needs periods of rest during

TABLE 7-1 **Physical Changes During the Aging Process**

System	Changes	System	Changes
Musculoskeletal	Muscle atrophy Decreasing strength Bones become brittle and can break easily Joints become stiff and painful Gradual loss of height Decreased mobility		Fried and fatty foods are difficult to digest Loss of teeth Decreased peristalsis causing flatulence and constipation
Cardiovascular	Heart pumps with less force Arteries narrow and are less elastic Less blood flows through narrowed arteries	Integumentary	Skin becomes less elastic Fatty tissue layer of the skin is lost Folds, lines, and wrinkles appear Dry skin develops Increased sensitivity to cold Nails become thick and tough Whitening or graying hair Loss or thinning of hair
Respiratory	Respiratory muscles weaken Lung tissue becomes less elastic		
Urinary	Kidney function decreases Poisonous substances can build up in the blood Urine becomes concentrated Urinary incontinence may occur	Nervous	Vision and hearing decrease Decreased senses of taste and smell Reduced sense of touch and sensitivity to pain Reduced blood flow to the brain Progressive loss of brain cells Shorter memory Forgetfulness Slowed ability to respond Confusion Dizziness
Gastrointestinal	Decreased saliva production Difficulty in swallowing Decreased appetite Decreased secretion of digestive juices		

the day. Daily activities should be planned to avoid overexertion. The person should not walk long distances, climb many stairs, or carry heavy objects. Personal care items, the television, telephone, and other frequently used items should be in convenient locations. A moderate amount of daily exercise helps to stimulate circulation. Exercise also helps to prevent the formation of thrombi (blood clots) in the leg veins. Active or passive range-of-motion exercises are necessary if the individual is confined to bed. Some individuals have more severe cardiovascular changes. Doctors may order certain exercises and activity limitations.

The Respiratory System

Respiratory muscles weaken, and lung tissue becomes less elastic. Lung changes are not usually obvious at rest. However, difficulty in breathing (dyspnea) may occur with activity. The individual may not have enough strength to cough and clear the upper airway of secretions. Respiratory infections and diseases may develop. These can seriously threaten the elderly person's life.

Measures are necessary to promote normal breathing. Heavy bed linens should not cover the chest. They can prevent normal chest expansion. Turning, repositioning, and deep breathing help prevent respiratory complications that may result from bed rest. Breathing is usually easier in semi-Fowler's position (see Chapter 11). The individual should be as active as possible.

The Urinary System

During aging, kidney function decreases. A reduced blood supply causes the kidneys to atrophy (shrink). Poisonous substances can build up in the blood and cause serious health problems. Urine becomes more concentrated because the elderly usually do not drink enough fluids. Urinary incontinence may occur. Many elderly people have to go to the bathroom several times during the night.

The doctor may order increased fluid intake to promote kidney function. Intake should include water, fruit juices, and milk. Other beverages preferred by the individual should be provided. Most of the fluids should be ingested before 5:00 PM. This reduces the need to urinate during the night. Bladder training programs may be necessary for those with urinary incontinence. Indwelling catheters are sometimes needed.

The Gastrointestinal System

Many changes affect the gastrointestinal system in the elderly. Difficulty swallowing (*dysphagia*) often occurs because of decreases in the amount of saliva.

Taste and smell become dulled, causing a decrease in appetite. Secretion of digestive juices decreases. As a result, fried and fatty foods are difficult to digest and may cause indigestion. Loss of teeth and ill-fitting dentures make chewing difficult. This results in digestion problems. Certain foods are avoided because they are difficult to chew. Usually high-protein foods such as meat are avoided. Decreased peristalsis results in slower emptying of the stomach and colon. Flatulence and constipation are common because of decreased peristalsis (see Chapter 15).

Dry, fried, and fatty foods should be avoided. This helps the problems of difficulty in swallowing and indigestion. Good oral hygiene and denture care improve the ability to taste. People may not have natural teeth or dentures. Their food has to be pureed or ground. Avoiding high-fiber foods may be necessary even though they help prevent constipation. Foods high in fiber are difficult to chew and can irritate the intestines. High-fiber foods include apricots, celery, and fruits and vegetables with skins and seeds. Foods that provide soft bulk are often ordered for those with chewing difficulties or constipation. These foods include whole-grain cereals and cooked fruits and vegetables.

Aging requires certain dietary changes. Elderly people need fewer calories than younger people do. Energy levels and daily activity levels are lower. Additional fluids are needed to promote kidney function. Foods that prevent constipation and musculoskeletal changes need to be included in the diet. The diet should also include enough protein for tissue growth and repair. However, protein may be lacking in the diets of the elderly. Foods that are high in protein are generally the most expensive.

The Integumentary System

The skin loses its elasticity and fatty tissue layer. As a result, the skin sags. Folds, lines, and wrinkles appear. Dry skin develops because of decreases in oil and sweat glands. Skin breakdown and decubiti are dangers (see Chapter 13).

Loss of fatty tissues beneath the skin increases sensitivity to cold. Sweaters, lap blankets, socks, and extra blankets are often needed for warmth. Elderly people need to be protected from drafts and extreme cold. Thermostat settings may need to be higher than normal. Dry skin is easily damaged and causes itching. Daily showers or tub baths should be avoided. Usually a complete bath is taken twice a week. Partial baths are taken on the other days. This bathing schedule is sufficient to maintain hygiene. Only mild soaps are used. Often soap is not used on the arms, legs, back, chest, and abdomen. A lanolin-based lotion or a bath oil can be used to prevent drying and itching.

The nails become thick and tough. Feet usually have poor circulation. A nick or cut can lead to a serious infection. Amputation of a part of the foot or leg may be necessary to fight the infection. Nail and foot care are described in Chapter 13.

An elderly person may complain of cold feet. Socks should be put on. Hot water bottles and heating pads are not used because the risk of burns is great. Fragile skin, poor circulation, and decreased sensitivity to heat and cold increase the risk of burns.

White or gray hair is a common sign of aging. Men lose a lot of hair. Hair thins on both men and women. Thinning occurs on the head, in the pubic area, and under the arms. Hair tends to be more dry because of the decreased production of scalp oils. Brushing helps stimulate circulation and oil production. The frequency of shampooing depends on personal preference. Usually shampooing is less frequent than when younger. Shampooing should be done as often as necessary to maintain cleanliness and comfort.

The Nervous System

The loss of vision and hearing were discussed in Chapter 25. Loss of taste and smell are mentioned earlier in this chapter. Often the sense of touch and sensitivity to pain are also reduced in the elderly. Injuries and diseases that normally cause considerable pain may go unnoticed. They may cause only minor discomforts. Heat, cold, and pressure on bony areas may not be felt. Therefore the elderly must be protected from injury. Safety measures need to be practiced when applying heat or cold. The skin must be carefully inspected for signs of breakdown. Good skin care and the measures to prevent decubiti must be practiced.

Blood flow to the brain is reduced. There is also a progressive loss of brain cells. These changes affect personality and mental function. Memory is often shorter, and forgetfulness increases. The ability to respond is slowed. Confusion, dizziness, and fatigue may also occur. Elderly people often remember events in the distant past better than those in the recent past. Many elderly people keep mentally active and involved in current events. They show fewer personality and mental changes. Care of the confused person is described in the next section.

Less sleep is needed. Loss of energy and decreased blood flow cause fatigue. Usually the elderly rest or nap during the day. They usually go to bed early and get up early.

CONFUSION IN THE ELDERLY PERSON

Confusion in the elderly person can result from many causes. Diseases, infections, losses of hearing and sight, and reactions to medications are some major causes. Another is the physical changes that occur with aging. There is a reduced blood supply to the brain and the progressive loss of brain cells. These changes can result in personality and mental changes. The individual generally loses memory and the ability to make judgments. The person may not know people, the time, or the place. There may also be a gradual loss in the ability to perform activities of daily living. Changes in behavior are common. Anger, restlessness, depression, and irritability may occur.

Confusion is frightening and frustrating for the elderly person and the family. The problem may be temporary if caused by illness or medications. However, confusion caused by the physical changes of aging cannot be cured. There are measures to help improve the person's ability to function. *Reality orientation (RO)* promotes or maintains awareness of person, time, and place. Nursing care plans often include reality orientation for the elderly. Reality orientation can be used in the home, hospital, or nursing facility.

A reality orientation program generally consists of the following measures and activities.

1. Face the person and speak clearly and slowly.
2. Call the individual by name every time you are in contact with him or her. Know how the person prefers to be addressed (Mr., Mrs., Miss, Ms., first name, or a nickname).
3. State your name and show your name tag.
4. Tell the person the date and time each morning. Repeat the information as often as necessary during the day and evening.
5. Explain what you are going to do and why.
6. Give clear and simple answers to questions.
7. Ask clear and simple questions. Allow enough time for a response.
8. Give short, simple instructions.
9. Keep calendars and clocks with large numbers in the person's room (Fig. 7-6).
10. Encourage the individual to wear glasses and a hearing aid if needed.
11. Use touch to communicate (see Chapter 14).

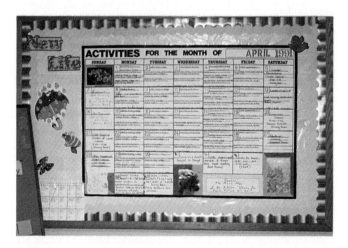

Fig. 7-6 A "reality board" is used as a part of reality orientation.

12. Allow the person to place familiar objects and pictures within view.
13. Provide newspapers and magazines. Read to the individual if appropriate.
14. Discuss current events with the person.
15. Allow the use of television and radio.
16. Maintain the day-night cycle. Open curtains, shades, and drapes during the day and close them at night. Use a night-light at night. Encourage the person to wear regular clothes during the day rather than gowns or pajamas.
17. Maintain a calm, relaxed, and peaceful atmosphere. Prevent loud noises, rushing, and congested hallways and dining rooms.
18. Maintain the routine set for the individual. Meals, bathing, exercise, television programs, and other activities are on a schedule. This promotes a sense of order and anticipation of what to expect.
19. Do not rearrange furniture or the person's belongings.
20. Encourage the person to participate in self-care activities.
21. Be consistent. The health team needs to follow the program developed for the individual.
22. Remind the person of holidays, birthdays, and other special events.

The confused person must be protected from injury. Dangerous situations may not be recognized. This is especially true if hearing and vision losses are present (see Chapter 25). Nutritional needs also require attention. The person may forget to eat regularly and to drink enough fluid. Chapter 16 describes how to assist in meeting food and fluid needs.

HOUSING ALTERNATIVES

Most elderly people live in their own homes. Some choose, or are forced, to give up their homes. Reduced income, taxes, home repairs, and the inability to do yard work are influencing factors. Some elderly people retire to warmer climates. Others find they no longer need the space of a large home when children are gone. One housing alternative is to live with children or other family members. There are several housing alternatives available to the elderly.

Apartments

Apartments have some advantages for the elderly. Maintenance, yard work, snow removal, and repair of major appliances are the landlord's responsibility. The elderly can still be independent. Personal belongings can be kept. However, rent payments can be costly. Utility bills are another expense. Many elderly individuals enjoy gardening and yard work (Fig. 7-7). Apartment living usually does not provide those opportunities.

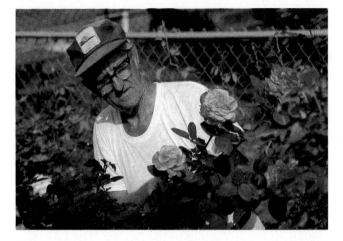

Fig. 7-7 This man is enjoying gardening. Apartment living usually does not provide opportunities for gardening or other yard work.

Residential Hotels

Some cities have residential hotels. Individuals can rent private rooms or efficiency apartments. Food services may include a dining room, cafeteria, or room service. Recreational activities and emergency medical services may be provided. Most hotels are close to shopping areas, churches, and other civic services. Residential hotels and apartments have similar disadvantages.

Senior Citizen Housing

State and federal funds have helped to build housing for senior citizens. An elderly person or couple can live independently in an apartment near people of the same age. The buildings have wheelchair access, handrails, elevators, and other safety measures. Apartments may be furnished. Appliances are arranged to meet the special needs of the elderly. Many services may be available. There is usually a dining room and a nurse or doctor on call. A daily telephone call is made to check on each tenant. Transportation is usually available to church, the doctor, or shopping areas. The elderly pay monthly rent. However, the rent is usually less than that for a regular apartment if government funds are involved.

Nursing Facilities

Nursing facilities are housing alternatives for the elderly who can no longer care for themselves. These are commonly called nursing homes. Nursing facilities offer different levels of care. Some merely provide room, food, and laundry services. Others provide nursing, rehabilitation, dietary, recreational, social, and religious services.

Nursing facilities may be privately owned or operated by the government. In either case, state and federal agencies monitor the care given. State and federal standards required by law must be followed. Periodic inspections may be expected or unannounced.

Some individuals remain in nursing facilities for the rest of their lives. Others stay until they are able to return to their own homes. The nursing facility is the person's temporary or permanent home. The surroundings are as home-like as possible (Fig. 7-8). The individual is referred to as a resident, not a patient.

Nursing facilities are designed to meet the special needs of the elderly. Physical changes of aging and the safety needs of the elderly are considered in the design and construction of the facility. The following features should be looked for in a nursing facility.

1. Elevators or a one-level building
2. Spacious and uncluttered areas
3. Handrails along hallways
4. Adequate lighting without shadows or glares
5. Floors that are carpeted or not heavily waxed
6. Pleasant landscaping
7. Variations in the use of colors
8. Acoustics for noise control
9. Ventilation for control of odors
10. Smoke detectors and a sprinkling system
11. Emergency exits
12. Windows with a pleasant view of the outdoors

Independent living units are a new trend. A wing of the facility has small apartments. Elderly people or couples live in the units. They perform self-care activities and take their own medications. Food services are available, and help is nearby if needed. However, each person takes care of himself or herself. Little supervision or assistance is needed.

Many hospitals now have long-term care units. These units are for individuals who still need skilled care but not to the extent required previously. At one time these patients were transferred to nursing facilities. Now they can receive skilled care on the long-term care unit. Some eventually go home. Others may go to nursing facilities.

Most nursing facilities receive Medicare or Medicaid funds. Such facilities must meet the requirements of the Omnibus Budget Reconciliation Act of 1987 (OBRA). Funding will not occur if the requirements are not met. Unannounced surveys are conducted to determine if nursing facilities are meeting OBRA requirements.

OBRA REQUIREMENTS

The Omnibus Budget Reconciliation Act of 1987 is concerned with the quality of life, health, and safety of residents. Nursing facilities must provide care in a manner and in an environment that maintains or improves each resident's quality of life, health, and safety. Nursing assistant training and competency evaluation are OBRA requirements (see Chapter 2). Many other requirements must be met as well.

Resident Rights

Residents of nursing facilities have certain rights under federal and state laws. Residents have rights as citizens of the United States. They also have rights relating to their everyday lives and care in a nursing facility. Nursing facilities must protect and promote resident rights. Residents must be able to exercise their rights without facility interference. Some residents are incompetent (not able) and cannot exercise their rights. Legal guardians exercise rights for them.

Nursing facilities must inform residents of their rights. They must be informed orally and in writing. Such information is given before or during admission to the facility. It must be given in the language used and understood by the resident.

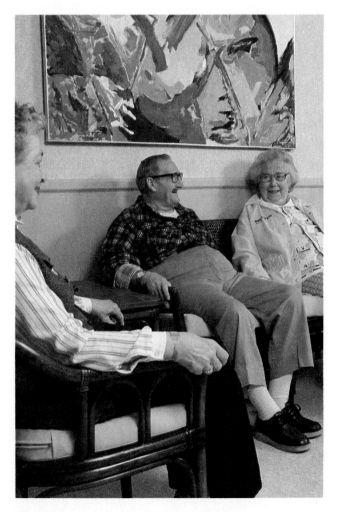

Fig. 7-8 The atmosphere of a nursing facility is similar to that of a home.

Privacy and confidentiality The rights to privacy and confidentiality were discussed in Chapter 2. They were also presented under the Patient's Bill of Rights in Chapter 4. OBRA also provides for privacy and confidentiality.

Residents have the right to personal privacy. The resident's body must not be exposed unnecessarily. Only those workers directly involved in care, treatments, or examinations should be present. The resident must give consent for others to be present. For example, a student may want to observe a procedure or treatment. The resident's consent is necessary for the student to be an observer. A resident also has the right to use the bathroom in private. Privacy should be maintained for personal care activities as well.

Residents also have the right to visit with others in privacy. They have the right to visit in an area where they cannot be seen or heard by others. The facility must try to provide private space when it is requested. Offices, chapels, dining rooms, meeting rooms, and conference rooms can be used if available.

The right to visit in privacy also involves telephone conversations (Fig. 7-9). Residents also have the right to send and receive mail without interference by others. Letters sent and received by the resident must not be opened by others without the resident's permission.

Information about the resident's care, treatment, and condition must be kept confidential. Medical and financial records are also confidential. The resident must give consent for them to be released to other facilities or individuals. However, consent is not needed for the release of medical records when the resident is being transferred to another facility. Records can also be released without the resident's consent when they are required by law or for insurance purposes.

Throughout this textbook you will be reminded to provide privacy. You will also be reminded to keep information about the person confidential. Providing for privacy and keeping medical and personal information confidential show respect for the individual. They also protect the person's dignity.

Personal choice OBRA requires that residents be free to choose their own physicians. They also have the right to participate in planning their own care and treatment. This means that residents have the right to choose activities, schedules, and care based on their personal preferences. For example, residents have the right to choose when to get up and go to bed, what to wear, how to spend their time, and what to eat (Fig. 7-10). They are also free to choose companions and visitors inside and outside of the nursing facility.

Personal choice is important for quality of life, dignity, and self-respect. The individual's personal preference is emphasized throughout this book. You will be reminded to allow the person's preferences whenever it is safely possible.

Disputes and grievances Residents have the right to voice concerns, questions, and complaints about treatment or care. The dispute or grievance may involve another resident. It may be about treatment or care that was not given. The facility must promptly try to correct the situation. The resident must not be punished in any way for voicing the dispute or grievance.

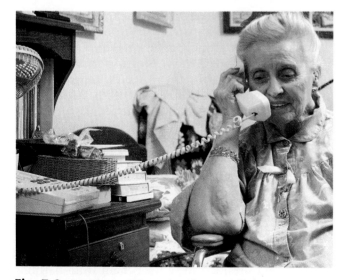

Fig. 7-9 Resident talking privately on a telephone.

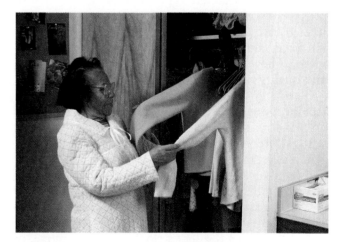

Fig. 7-10 Resident choosing what clothing to wear.

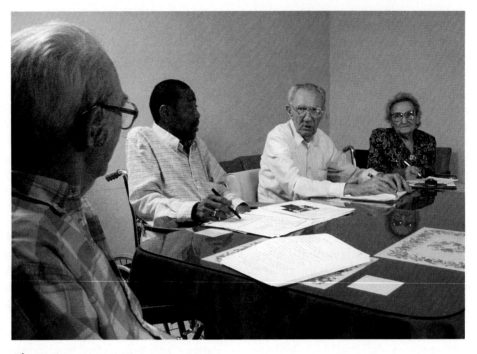

Fig. 7-11 Residents at a group meeting.

Participation in resident and family groups Residents have the right to participate in resident and family groups. This means that residents have the right to form groups (Fig. 7-11). And a resident's family has the right to meet with the families of other residents. These groups can discuss concerns and offer suggestions to improve the quality of life in the facility. They can also plan activities for residents and families. Or the groups can serve to provide support and reassurrance for group members. Residents also have the right to participate in social, religious, and community activities. They have the right to assistance in getting to and from activities of their choice.

Care and security of personal possessions Residents have the right to keep and use personal possessions. Available space and the health and safety of other residents can affect the type and amount of personal possessions allowed. A person's property must be treated with care and respect. Though the items may not have value to you, they are important to the resident. They also relate to personal choice, dignity, and quality of life.

The facility must take reasonable measures to protect the individual's property. Items should be labeled with the resident's name. And the facility must investigate reports of lost, stolen, or damaged items. Police assistance is sometimes necessary. The resident and family will probably be advised not to keep jewelry and other expensive items in the facility.

You must protect yourself and the facility from being accused of stealing a resident's property. Do not go through a resident's closet, drawers, purse, or other space without the person's knowledge and con-

sent. Have another worker with you and the resident or legal guardian present if it is necessary to inspect closets and drawers. The worker serves as a witness to your activities.

Freedom from abuse, mistreatment, and neglect OBRA states that residents have the right to be free from verbal, sexual, physical, or mental abuse. Elderly abuse is discussed later in this chapter.

Residents also have the right to be free from involuntary seclusion. Involuntary seclusion is separating the resident from others against his or her will. It can also mean keeping the person confined to a certain area or away from his or her room without consent. If the person is incompetent, involuntary seclusion occurs against the legal guardian's consent.

No one can abuse, neglect, or mistreat the resident. This includes facility staff, volunteers, staff from other agencies or groups, other residents, family, visitors, and legal guardians. Nursing facilities must have policies and procedures for investigating suspected or reported cases of resident abuse. Also, nursing facilities cannot employ individuals who have been convicted of abusing, neglecting, or mistreating other individuals.

Freedom from restraints Residents have the right not to have body movements restricted. Body movements can be restricted by the application of restraints or the administration of certain drugs. Some drugs can restrain the person because they affect mood, behavior, and mental function. Sometimes residents need to be restrained to protect them from harming themselves or others. A physician's order is necessary for restraints to be used. Restraints cannot be used for the convenience of the staff. Restraints are discussed in Chapter 8.

Quality of Life

OBRA requires that nursing facilities care for residents in a manner that promotes dignity, self-esteem, and physical, psychological, and emotional well-being. Protecting resident rights is one way to promote quality of life. Personal choice, privacy, participation in group activities, having personal property, and freedom from restraint show respect for the person.

The resident should also be spoken to in a polite and courteous manner (see Chapter 4). Giving good, honest, and thoughtful care will enhance the resident's quality of life.

Activities Activities are also important for a resident's quality of life. OBRA requires that nursing facilities provide activity programs that meet the interests and physical, mental, and psychosocial needs of each resident. Such activities must allow personal choice and promote physical, intellectual, social, and emotional well-being. Many facilities also provide religious services for spiritual health. You will be responsible for assisting residents to and from activity programs. You may also be assigned to help residents with activities.

Environment The environment of the facility must also promote quality of life. The environment must be clean and safe and be as home-like as possible. Allowing the resident to have personal possessions enhances quality of life by allowing personal choice and promoting a home-like environment. The safe environment is discussed in Chapter 8. The furniture and equipment in a resident's room are discussed in Chapter 11. Information relating to temperature and sound levels is also discussed.

ABUSE OF THE ELDERLY

Elderly abuse has become more evident in today's society. The abuser is usually a family member or a person caring for the elderly individual. There are different forms of abuse. The person may be intentionally harmed.

1. *Physical abuse* involves hitting, slapping, kicking, pinching, and beating. Physical injury and pain may result. The person may be deprived of needed medical services or treatment.
2. *Verbal abuse* can be described as the use of oral or written words or statements that speak badly of, sneer at, criticize, or condemn the resident. OBRA guidelines also include unkind gestures under verbal abuse.

3. *Involuntary seclusion* is confining the person to a specific area. Elderly people have been locked in closets, basements, attics, and other spaces.
4. *Financial abuse* is when the elderly person's money is used by another person.
5. *Mental abuse* relates to humiliation and threats of being punished or deprived of such things as food, clothing, care, a home, or a place to sleep.
6. *Sexual abuse* is when the person is harassed about sex or is attacked sexually. The person may be forced to perform sexual acts out of fear of punishment or physical harm.

Abused elderly people may be seen in their homes, hospitals, or nursing facilities. Often the abuse is unrecognized. There are many signs of elderly abuse. The abused person may show only some of the signs.

1. Living conditions are unsafe, unclean, or inadequate.
2. Personal hygiene is lacking. The individual is unclean, and clothes are dirty.
3. Weight loss has occurred. There are signs of poor nutrition and inadequate fluid intake.
4. There are frequent injuries. The circumstances behind the injuries are strange or seem impossible.
5. Old and new bruises are seen.
6. The person seems very quiet or withdrawn.
7. The person seems fearful, anxious, or agitated.
8. The individual does not seem to want to talk or answer questions.
9. The person is restrained or locked in a certain area for long periods of time. Toilet facilities, food and water, and other necessary items cannot be reached.
10. Private conversations are not allowed. The caregiver is present during all conversations.
11. The person seems anxious to please the caregiver.
12. Medications are not taken properly. Medications are not purchased, or too much or too little medication is taken.
13. Visits to the emergency room may be frequent.
14. The person may go from one doctor to another. Some people do not have a doctor.

OBRA and state laws require the reporting of elderly abuse. If abuse is suspected, it must be reported. Where and how to report suspected abuse varies in each state. If you do need to report suspected abuse, you must give as much information as possible. The reporting agency will take action based on the information given. They act immediately if there is a life-threatening situation. Sometimes the help of police or the courts is necessary.

Helping the abused elderly is not always easy or possible. The abuse may never be reported or recognized, or the investigating agency may be unable to gain access to the person. Sometimes the elderly are abused by their children. A victim may want to protect the child. Some victims are embarrassed or believe that the abuse is deserved. A victim may be afraid of what will happen. He or she may think that the present situation is better than no care at all. Some people fear they will not be believed if they report the abuse themselves.

Elderly abuse is an unfortunate situation. You may suspect that a person is being abused. If so, discuss the situation and your observations with your supervisor. Give the nurse as much information as possible. The nurse will then contact the appropriate members of the health team. The agency that investigates elderly abuse in your community will also be contacted.

SUMMARY

Aging is a normal process. Body functions slow down and become less efficient. Many individuals function independently. They enjoy life with a loving spouse, family, and friends. For others aging can be difficult, painful, and lonely. Loved ones may have died or moved away. The physical changes of aging, disease, and illness make even the most simple, everyday tasks difficult or impossible. Income may not cover monthly living expenses. There may be little or no money for medical bills and medicines. Leaving a life-long home for a nursing home is often the only alternative.

Many people dread having to live in a nursing home. However, OBRA serves to protect individuals who need to be in nursing facilities. Some of the many OBRA requirements relate to resident rights and the quality of life.

Some elderly are abused. Their needs and problems present additional concerns. You must be alert to the possibility that a person is being abused. You can help the victim by discussing the situation with a nurse as soon as possible.

You need to understand the physical, psychological, and social changes that accompany aging. Imagine yourself being old. Put yourself in the place of the elderly individual. The aged person depends on you for assistance in meeting basic needs. You can more effectively meet these needs if you can appreciate the person's situation. Patience, tolerance, and kindness are needed when working with the elderly. Their behaviors, habits, and body changes may seem unusual. However, they still need love and the companionship of others. You can help bring happiness and cheer to the elderly.

REVIEW QUESTIONS

Circle the best answer.

1 Retirement usually results in
  a Lowered income
  b Physical changes from aging
  c Companionship and usefulness
  d Financial security

2 Elderly people may experience loneliness because
  a Children may have moved away
  b Friends and relatives may have died or moved
  c Of difficulties in communicating with others
  d All of the above

3 When elderly people live with their children they often feel
  a Independent
  b Wanted and a part of things
  c Useless
  d Dignified

4 Death of a spouse results in the loss of a
  a Friend
  b Lover
  c Companion
  d All of the above

5 Changes occur in the musculoskeletal system during the aging process. Which is *false?*

  a Bones become brittle and can break easily.
  b Bed rest is needed because of loss of strength.
  c Joints become stiff and painful.
  d Range-of-motion exercises help to slow down the rate of the musculoskeletal changes.

6 Arteries lose their elasticity and become narrow. These changes result in
  a A slower heart rate
  b Lower blood pressure
  c Poor circulation to many parts of the body
  d A decrease in the amount of blood in the body

7 An elderly person has cardiovascular changes. Care should include all of the following *except*
  a Placing personal items in a convenient location
  b A moderate amount of daily exercise
  c Planning activities to avoid exertion
  d Walking long distances

8 Respiratory changes occur with aging. Which is *false?*
  a Heavy bed linens prevent normal chest expansion.
  b The individual should be turned and repositioned frequently if on bed rest.

c The side-lying position is best for breathing when there are respiratory changes.

d The person should be as active as possible.

9 The doctor has ordered an increased fluid intake for an elderly individual. You should

a Give most of the fluid before 5:00 PM

b Provide mostly water

c Start a bladder training program

d Insert an indwelling urinary catheter

10 The elderly should avoid dry foods because of

a Decreases in saliva

b Loss of teeth or ill-fitting dentures

c Decreased amounts of digestive juices

d Decreased peristalsis

11 Changes occur in the gastrointestinal system. The elderly individual should avoid

a Cooked fruits and vegetables

b Foods high in protein

c Apricots and celery

d All of the above

12 Changes occur in the skin. Care should include all of the following *except*

a Providing extra blankets for warmth

b Applying lotion

c Using soap daily

d Providing good skin care

13 An elderly person has cold feet. You should

a Provide socks

b Apply a hot water bottle

c Soak the feet in hot water

d Apply a heating pad

14 Reduced blood supply to the brain can result in

a Confusion

b Dizziness

c Fatigue

d All of the above

15 Changes occur in the nervous system. Which is *true?*

a More sleep is needed than when younger.

b Recent events are remembered better than past events.

c Sensitivity to pain is reduced.

d Confusion occurs in every elderly person.

16 The confused individual

a Loses the ability to make judgments

b Loses the ability to perform self-care

c May be angry, restless, or irritable

d All of the above

17 Reality orientation is needed. You should

a Call the individual by name

b Use touch

c Tell the person the date and time each morning

d All of the above

18 Which does *not* maintain the day-night cycle?

a Wearing regular clothes during the day

b Opening curtains and shades during the day

c Keeping bright lights on all the time

d Providing a clock and calendar

19 Which housing alternative does *not* allow the elderly to live independently?

a Apartments

b Residential hotels

c Senior citizen housing

d A nursing facility

20 You are working in a nursing facility. You must

a Open a resident's mail

b Choose what the resident will wear

c Provide for the resident's privacy

d Search the resident's closet and drawers

21 Who decides how a resident's hair should be styled?

a The resident

b The nurse

c The nursing assistant

d The family

22 Which statement is *false?*

a Residents can offer suggestions to improve the facility.

b Residents can be restrained to prevent them from leaving the facility.

c Residents must be free from abuse, neglect, and mistreatment.

d Allowing personal choice is important for the resident's quality of life.

23 Which is *not* a sign of elderly abuse?

a Stiff joints and joint pain

b Old and new bruises

c Poor personal hygiene

d Frequent injuries

24 You suspect a patient has been abused. What should you do?

a Tell the family.

b Call a state agency.

c Tell a nurse of your suspicion.

d Ask the patient if he or she has been abused.

Answers

24	c	16	d	8	c
23	a	15	c	7	d
22	b	14	d	6	c
21	a	13	a	5	b
20	c	12	c	4	d
19	d	11	c	3	c
18	c	10	a	2	d
17	d	9	a	1	a

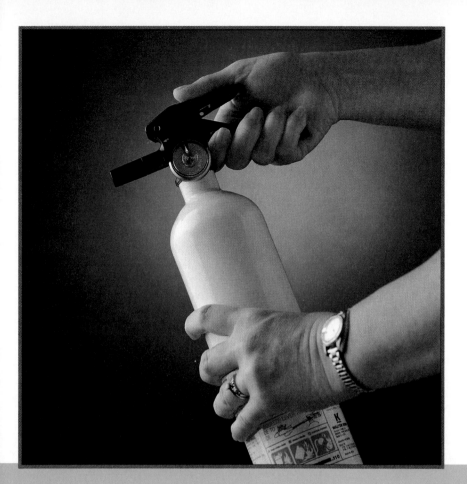

Safety in the Home and Health Care Facility

8

OBJECTIVES

- Define the key terms listed in this chapter
- Explain seven reasons why people may be unable to protect themselves
- Identify safety precautions when caring for infants and children
- Identify safety measures that prevent accidents in the home
- Identify common safety hazards in health care facilities
- Explain why a patient should be identified before receiving care and how to accurately identify a patient
- Describe the safety measures that prevent falls
- Explain the purpose of restraints and the safety rules for use
- Identify the information to report to the nurse when restraints are used
- Apply wrist and ankle, mitt, jacket, safety belt, and elbow restraints
- Describe common equipment-related accidents and how they can be prevented
- Identify the accidents and errors that need to be reported
- Describe the safety measures related to fire prevention and the use of oxygen
- Know what to do if there is a fire and how to use a fire extinguisher
- Give examples of natural and man-made disasters

coma A state of being completely unaware of one's surroundings and unable to react or respond to people, places, or things

disaster A sudden catastrophic event in which many people are injured and killed, and property is destroyed

ground That which carries leaking electricity to the earth and away from the electrical appliance

hemiplegia Paralysis on one side of the body

paraplegia Paralysis from the waist down

quadriplegia Paralysis from the neck down

suffocation Termination of breathing that results from lack of oxygen

Safety is a basic need. This need is present whether a person is driving a car, taking a walk, or being cared for at home or in a health care facility. People need to be safe from accidents and dangers. Homes and health care facilities are thought to be free of dangers and hazards. This is not true. Many accidental injuries occur in the home. Some cause death. Accidents also occur in health care facilities.

You are responsible for safe practices at home and in everyday activities. When caring for patients, you need to practice ordinary safety precautions and the other safety measures presented in this chapter.

THE SAFE ENVIRONMENT

A safe environment is one in which a person has a very low risk of becoming ill or injured. The person feels safe and secure both physically and psychologically. There is little risk of developing an infection, falling, being burned or poisoned, or suffering other injuries. The person is comfortable in relation to temperature, noise, and smells. There is enough lighting and room to move about safely. The person is not afraid and has few worries and concerns.

REASONS SOME PEOPLE CANNOT PROTECT THEMSELVES

There are many reasons why some people cannot protect themselves. Age, poor vision, and loss of hearing are some factors described in this section. You need to be aware of any factors that increase a patient's risk of an accident so that you can provide for the patient's safety.

Age

Children and the elderly need to be protected from injury. Infants are helpless and depend on others for protection. Young children have not learned what is safe and what is dangerous. They have the need to explore their surroundings, to put objects into their mouths, and to touch and feel new things. As a result they are in danger of falling, drinking poisonous fluids, choking, being burned, and having other accidents. These safety precautions must be practiced when caring for infants and children:

1. Do not leave infants or young children unattended. Children should not be left unattended in strollers, walkers, high chairs, infant seats, bathtubs, or wading pools. Children in cribs should be checked often.
2. Make sure crib side rails are up and locked in place.
3. Place safety plugs in electrical outlets (Fig. 8-1). The plugs prevent children from sticking their fingers or small objects into the openings.
4. Keep cords and electrical equipment out of the reach of children.
5. Keep one hand on a child lying in a crib, on a scale, or on a table if you need to look away for a moment (Fig. 8-2).
6. Childproof caps should be on medicine containers and household cleaners.
7. Do not let children play with toys that have loose parts, buttons, and sharp edges. The child can choke on or be cut by such toys.
8. Store household cleaners and medicines in locked storage areas that are beyond the reach of children (Fig. 8-3).
9. A child in a high chair should have the safety strap fastened to prevent falls.
10. Do not prop baby bottles on a rolled towel or blanket. Hold the baby and bottle during feedings.

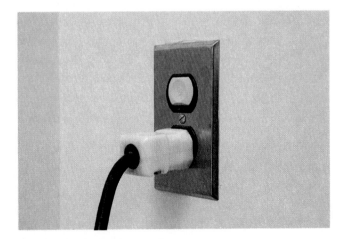

Fig. 8-1 Safety plug in an electrical outlet.

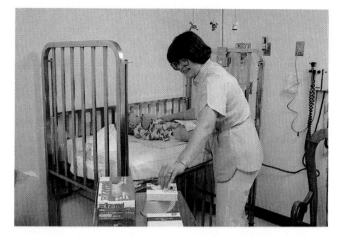

Fig. 8-2 One hand is kept on the child while the nursing assistant momentarily looks away.

11. Keep plastic bags and wraps away from children because of the danger of suffocation.
12. Use guardrails at the top and bottom of stairs to prevent small children from climbing up and down stairs.

Many elderly people are in danger of having accidents because of the changes in their bodies from aging. Movements are slower and less steady. Balance may be affected, causing the person to fall easily. The person may be unable to move quickly and suddenly to avoid dangerous situations. Other factors make the elderly prone to accidents and injuries. These include decreased sensitivity to heat and cold, poor vision, hearing difficulties, and a decreased sense of smell.

Awareness of Surroundings

People need to be aware of their surroundings to protect themselves from injury. Some patients are completely unaware of their surroundings. These patients are unconscious or in a *coma*. A person in a coma is unable to react or respond to people, places, or things. The patient must rely on others for protection.

Confusion and disorientation occur in some elderly people and in patients with certain diseases and injuries. These people have a reduced awareness of their surroundings. They may have difficulty understanding what is happening to and around them. Confused and disoriented people can be dangerous to themselves and others.

Vision

People with poor vision have difficulty seeing objects. They are often in danger of falling or tripping because of toys, furniture, or electrical cords in their paths. They may also have problems reading labels on medicine and other containers. Taking the wrong medicine, the wrong dose, or poisoning could result from the inability to read labels.

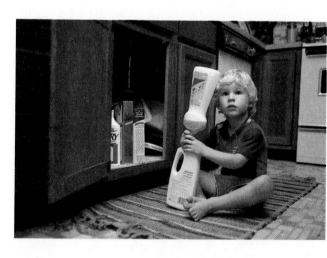

A

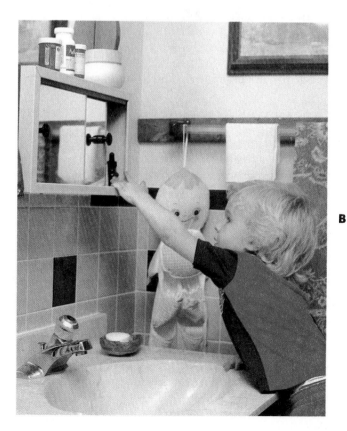

B

Fig. 8-3 **A,** Household cleaners are within a child's reach when placed in cabinets under the sink. They should be kept in high, locked cabinets that are not used to store food. **B,** The bathroom medicine chest holds many medicine containers. Like household products, they should be in high, locked places out of the reach of children.

Hearing

People with impaired hearing have problems hearing warning signals. Fire alarms, emergency vehicle sirens, and tornado sirens may not be heard. These people may not know that they should move to a safe place or out of the way of an emergency vehicle. They may have difficulty hearing oncoming cars and car horns.

Smell and Touch

Smell and touch can be affected by age and illness. If the sense of smell is reduced, there may be difficulty smelling smoke or gas. Individuals with a reduced sense of touch are easily burned. They have difficulty distinguishing between heat and cold.

Paralysis

Paraplegic patients are paralyzed from the waist down. *Quadriplegic* patients are paralyzed from the neck down. Patients with *hemiplegia* are paralyzed on one side of the body. These people may be unable to sense pain, heat, or cold. They may be aware of their surroundings and danger, but may be unable to move away from the danger.

Medications

Medications can have a variety of side effects on different people. Loss of balance, reduced awareness, confusion, disorientation, drowsiness, and loss of coordination are just some of the effects medications can have on people. These sensations may be new and frightening to the patient, causing the person to be fearful, uncooperative, and to act in unusual ways.

SAFETY IN THE HOME

Most accidents in the home can be prevented. Common sense and simple safety measures help eliminate some causes of accidental injuries. Nursing assistants employed by home health care agencies should check to see that measures have been taken to prevent accidents in the home. The nurse should be consulted if safety hazards are present.

Falls

Falls are the most common home accidents, especially among the elderly. Most falls occur in bedrooms and bathrooms. They are usually due to slippery floors, throw rugs, poor lighting, cluttered floors, furniture that is out of place, and slippery bathtubs and showers. The following measures can help prevent falls in the home.

1. Good lighting in rooms and hallways
2. Hand rails on both sides of stairs and in bathrooms
3. Wall-to-wall carpeting or carpeting that is tacked down. Avoid "throw rugs."
4. Nonskid shoes and slippers
5. Nonskid wax on hardwood, tiled, or linoleum floors
6. Floors kept uncluttered and free of toys and other objects that can cause tripping
7. Electric and extension cords kept out of the way
8. Rearranging furniture is avoided
9. Telephone and lamp at the bedside
10. Nonskid bathmats in tubs and showers

Burns

Burns are a leading cause of death in the United States, especially among children and the elderly. Common causes of home fires are smoking in bed, spilling hot liquids, children playing with matches, charcoal grills, fireplaces, and stoves (Fig. 8-4).

Safety measures to prevent burns in the home include:

1. Keeping matches out of the reach of children
2. Supervising the play of children and never leaving them at home alone
3. Teaching children fire prevention measures and the dangers of fire
4. Turning the handles of pots on stoves so that they do not point outward where people stand and walk (see Fig. 8-4)
5. Supervising the smoking of adults who are unable to protect themselves
6. Prohibiting smoking in bed
7. Keeping space heaters and materials that can catch on fire away from children

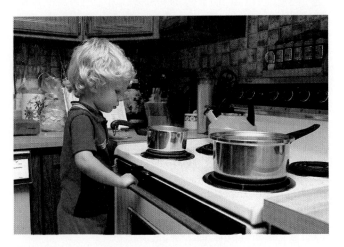

Fig. 8-4 This child is in danger of being burned from hot water. Other burns could result if the stove is hot. Pot handles should be turned inward.

Poisoning

Accidental poisoning is another major cause of death. Children are the most frequent victims. Aspirin and household products are the most common poisons. Poisoning in adults may be accidental from carelessness or poor vision when reading labels. Sometimes poisoning is a suicide attempt. Poisoning can be prevented by:

1. Having childproof caps on all medicine containers and household products
2. Labeling all medicine containers and household products clearly
3. Storing poisonous materials in a place that is high, locked, and out of the reach of children
4. Storing poisonous materials in their original containers and not in food containers
5. Keeping medicines out of purses where children may find them
6. Making sure there is adequate lighting so that labels can be read accurately

Suffocation

Suffocation is the termination of breathing that results from lack of oxygen. Death occurs if the person does not start breathing. Common causes of suffocation include choking on an object, drowning, inhaling gas or smoke, strangulation, and electrical shock. Safety measures to help prevent suffocation are:

1. Taking small bites of food and chewing food slowly and thoroughly
2. Having exhaust systems on cars checked regularly
3. Having gas odors promptly investigated by competent repairmen
4. Opening doors and windows if gas odors are noticed
5. Resting for at least 1 hour after eating and before strenuous activity or swimming
6. Making sure all electrical cords and appliances are in good repair

SAFETY IN THE HEALTH CARE FACILITY

Safety hazards also exist in health care facilities. The measures that promote safety in the home also apply in health care facilities. Additional safety measures are needed in the health care facility because similar and different kinds of dangers are present.

Identifying Your Patient

You will care for several different patients while on duty. Each has different treatments, therapies, and activity limitations. Patients must be protected from infections, falls, and accidents from equipment. Safety also involves giving care to the right patient.

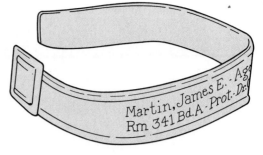

Fig. 8-5 Patient identification bracelet.

A patient's life and health can be threatened if the wrong care is given.

Hospitalized patients and residents of some nursing facilities receive identification (ID) bracelets when admitted to the facility. The person's name, room and bed number, age, religion, physician, the facility name, and other identifying information are on the bracelet (Fig. 8-5).

The ID bracelet is used to identify the patient before giving care. Some facilities have treatment cards for each treatment or therapy ordered by the doctor. To identify the patient, the identifying information on the treatment card is compared with that on the ID bracelet (Fig. 8-6). Comparing the treatment card and the ID bracelet helps ensure that care is given to the right patient. Assignment sheets can be used for the same purpose if treatment cards are not used.

You should also call the person by name while checking the ID bracelet. Calling the patient by name is a courtesy that should be given as the person is being touched and before care is given. However, calling the patient by name is not a reliable way to identify the patient. Confused, disoriented, drowsy, or hearing-impaired patients may answer to any name.

Residents of nursing facilities may not wear ID bracelets. The nursing facility is the resident's home. People do not wear ID bracelets in their homes. Therefore people living in nursing facilities do not need to wear ID bracelets. Some nursing facilities use an identification system that involves photographs. The resident's photograph is taken at the time of admission and placed in the individual's medical record for identification purposes. If you work in a facility that uses photographs for identification, you need to learn how to use the system safely.

Preventing the Spread of Microorganisms

The spread of infection is a major hazard in health care facilities. Infections are caused by microorganisms that are easily spread from one person to another. Illness increases a person's risk of developing

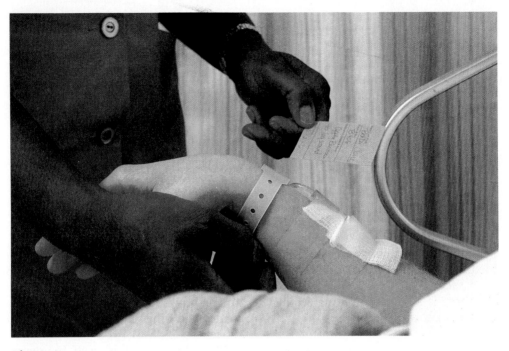

Fig. 8-6 The nursing assistant comparing the patient's ID bracelet with a treatment card to accurately identify the patient.

an infection. The infection adds to that individual's health problems. Chapter 9 describes how to prevent infection.

Preventing Falls

Falls are common safety problems in health care facilities. Besides those factors that affect the ability of patients to protect themselves, patients in health care facilities have other problems that can cause falls. Weakness from illness, a strange environment, new medications, and sleeping in a strange bed and room can increase the risk of falling.

The safety measures to prevent falls in the home apply to health care facilities. Additional safety measures may be needed for hospitalized patients, residents of nursing facilities, or persons receiving home care. Side rails, hand rails, and restraints are some safety devices used to prevent falls.

Side rails   Side rails are on the sides of hospital beds. They can be raised or lowered and are locked in place by levers, latches, or buttons. They protect the patient from falling out of bed. Patients can use side rails to move and turn in bed. Side rails can be half the length or the full length of the bed (Fig. 8-7). If the half length is used (see Fig. 12-17), there are usually two rails on each side. One is for the upper part of the bed and the other is for the lower part.

Side rails are necessary for patients who are unconscious, sedated with medication, confused, or dis-oriented. Side rails should be kept up at all times for these patients, except when giving bedside nursing care.

Many patients find the use of side rails embarrassing. They feel that they are being treated like children. Nurses are usually allowed to decide if side rails are needed for adults who are physically and mentally stable. Some facilities do not require side rails if the patient signs a statement releasing the facility from responsibility for falls. If a patient objects to the side rails, report the concern to the nurse. Patients must be protected physically, but their psychological need for esteem must also be protected.

Hand rails   Hand rails are in hallways (Fig. 8-8) and bathrooms in nursing facilities and hospitals. They provide support for patients who are weak or unsteady when walking. They also provide support for sitting down on or getting up from a toilet. Hand rails may be found along bathtubs for use in getting in and out of the tub. Hand rails are always found in stairways.

Other safety measures   You need to practice other safety measures to prevent patients from falling.
1. Keep the patient's bed in the lowest horizontal position, except when giving bedside nursing care. This way the distance from the bed to the floor is reduced if the patient falls or gets out of bed.
2. Have a night light on in the patient's room. The

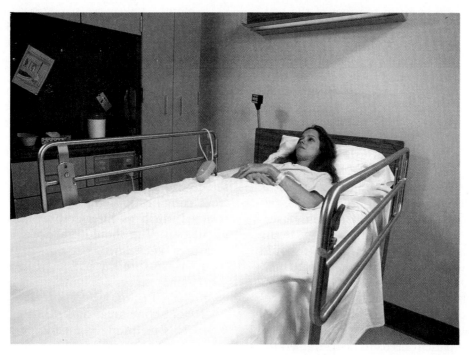

Fig. 8-7 Hospital bed with full-length side rails locked in the raised position.

patient can see on awakening and if it is necessary to get up during the night. Nursing personnel can see in the patient's room at night.

3. Keep floors free of spills and excess furniture.
4. Have patients wear nonskid shoes or slippers rather than soft bedroom slippers.
5. Make sure that crutches, canes, and walkers have nonskid tips, which prevent slipping or skidding on floors.
6. Keep the patient's signal light within reach at all times. The patient should be taught how to use the light and should be encouraged to call for help whenever help is needed. The signal light is described in Chapter 11.
7. Lock the wheels of beds, wheelchairs, and stretchers when transferring patients to or from them.
8. Use caution when turning corners, entering corridor intersections, and going through doors. You could bump into and injure a person coming from the opposite direction.

Restraints (Protective Devices)

Restraints, also called protective or safety devices, are used to protect patients from harming themselves or others. The patient may be confined to a bed or chair or may be prevented from moving a body part. Restraints are applied to the chest, waist, elbows, wrists, or ankles. They are made of either linen or leather. Restraints are used to prevent patients from:

1. Falling out of bed or from a chair, wheelchair, or stretcher

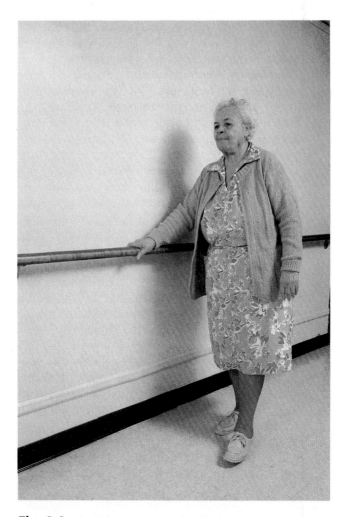

Fig. 8-8 An elderly woman using the hand rails for support when walking.

2. Crawling over side rails or the foot of the bed
3. Interfering with therapies. Restraints can prevent patients from pulling out tubes, removing dressings, or disconnecting equipment
4. Harming themselves or others. Some patients are confused or disoriented and do not know what they are doing. Others have violent behavior and can be dangerous to themselves and others

Remember the following about using restraints.

1. *Restraints are used to protect patients, not for the convenience of the staff.* Restraining a patient is often easier for the staff than providing the patient with the necessary supervision and observation. A restraint is used only when it is the best safety precaution for the patient. It should not be used to punish uncooperative patients.
2. *Restraints require a doctor's order.* OBRA and state laws protect individuals from being restrained unnecessarily. Health care facilities also have policies and procedures about using restraints. If a patient needs to be restrained for medical purposes, there must be a written doctor's order. The doctor is usually required by law to give the reason for the restraint. The order and its reason will be on the patient's Kardex. You need to know the laws and policies about using restraints where you work.
3. *Unnecessary restraint of a patient constitutes false imprisonment (see Chapter 2).* If you are told to apply a restraint, the need for it should be clearly evident and understood. If it is not, politely request an explanation. Nursing assistants who apply restraints unnecessarily may be charged with false imprisonment.
4. *The restrained patient's basic needs must be met by the nursing team.* The restraint should be snug and firm, but not tight. A tight restraint may interfere with circulation and breathing. The patient should be comfortable. Movement of the restrained part should be possible to a limited and safe extent. The patient and family should be given an explanation by the nurse about the need for and purpose of the restraint. The patient must be checked frequently.
5. *Restraints may have to be applied rapidly.* They must be applied with enough assistance to protect the patient and staff from injury. Patients who are in immediate danger of harming themselves or others need to be restrained quickly. Combative and agitated patients can injure themselves and the staff when the restraints are being applied. Enough staff members are needed to complete the task safely and efficiently.
6. *A patient may become more confused or agitated after being restrained.* Whether confused or alert, patients are aware of restricted body movements. The patient may try to get out of the restraint or may struggle or pull at the restraint. These behaviors are often misinterpreted as confusion. Confused patients may become more confused because they do not understand what is happening to them. The patient needs repeated explanations and reassurance. Spending time with the patient often has a calming effect.

Safety rules Though used to protect the patient, restraints can be dangerous. The patient must be observed frequently. The individual must be protected from complications that may result from being restrained, such as interferences with breathing and circulation. You should practice the following safety measures when caring for a restrained patient.

1. Make sure the patient is in good body alignment before applying the restraint (see Chapter 10).
2. Pad bony areas and skin that may be injured by a restraint. The padding protects the body parts from pressure and injury.
3. Apply the restraint securely enough to protect the patient but allow enough slack so that some movement of the restrained part is possible.
4. Make sure that the patient can breathe easily if a restraint has been applied to the chest.
5. Check the patient's circulation every 15 minutes if wrist or ankle restraints have been applied. You should feel a pulse at a pulse site below the restraint. Fingers or toes should be warm and pink.
6. Notify the nurse immediately if you cannot feel a pulse; if fingers or toes are cold, pale, or blue in color; or if the patient complains of pain, numbness, or tingling in the restrained part.
7. Tie restraints with a square knot (Fig. 8-9) or follow facility policy. A square knot is secure but easily released in an emergency.
8. Secure the restraint to the bed frame, not to the side rail (Fig. 8-10). Make sure the patient cannot reach the knot. Restraints are not secured to side rails because patients can reach them to release knots or buckles. Also, patients can be injured when side rails are raised and lowered.
9. Keep a pair of scissors handy for the staff but out of the patient's reach. In an emergency, cutting the tie is faster than untying the knot.
10. Remove the restraint and reposition the patient every 2 hours. Skin care is given and the restrained part is exercised at this time.
11. Make sure the patient receives food and fluids while restrained. Be sure to offer the bedpan and urinal at regular intervals.
12. Make sure the signal light is within the patient's reach at all times.

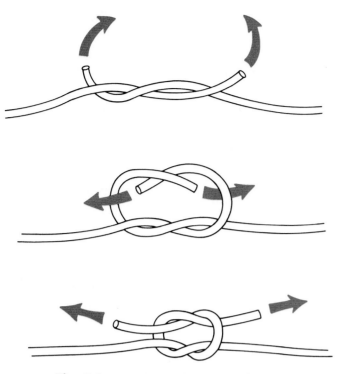

Fig. 8-9 Steps for making a square knot.

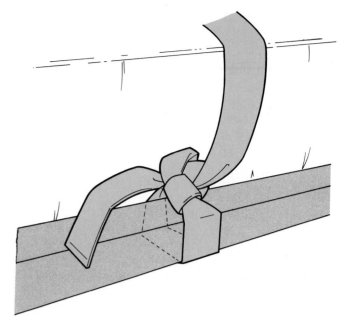

Fig. 8-10 The strap of a restraint is tied to the bed frame with a square knot or according to facility policy.

Reporting and recording Certain information about restraints must be included in the patient's record. You may be instructed to apply restraints or be assigned to care for a restrained patient. The following must be reported to the nurse:
1. The type of restraint applied
2. The time of application
3. The time of removal
4. The type of care given when the restraint was removed
5. The color and condition of the patient's skin
6. Whether or not a pulse is felt in the restrained extremity
7. Patient complaints of pain, numbness, or tingling in the restrained part

Wrist and ankle restraints Wrist and ankle restraints are also called hand and foot restraints. They are used to limit the movement of an arm or leg. Wrist and ankle restraints can be purchased or made as described in the box on p. 118.

Mitt restraints A patient's hands are placed in mitt restraints. They prevent use of the fingers but do not prevent hand or wrist movements. The arms can also be immobilized by securing the straps to the bed frame. Mitt restraints are thumbless and prevent the patient from scratching, pulling out tubes, or removing dressings. The patient may be given a hand

roll to grasp so that the fingers are kept in a normal position. (See the box on p. 119.)

Jacket restraints Jacket restraints are applied to the chest to protect the patient from falling out of bed or out of a chair. The patient's arms are put through the sleeves so that the vest crosses in front (Fig. 8-14). The vest should *never* cross in the back. The restraint is always applied over a gown, pajamas, or clothes.

The jacket restraint may have straps that lock in place. The lock is positioned so that it is face up and visible. This allows the lock to be seen and unlocked quickly in an emergency. The key to unlock the restraint should be visible in the patient's room. Patients who are restrained in chairs or wheelchairs may be in a dining room or lounge area. A key should be clearly visible in these areas or each member of the nursing team should carry one. (See the box on p. 120.)

Safety belt The safety belt (Fig. 8-15) is used for the same reasons as the jacket restraint. The belt is applied around the waist and secured to the bed or chair. The belt is applied over clothes, a gown, or pajamas. (See the box on p. 121.)

Elbow restraints Elbow restraints prevent infants and small children from bending their elbows. They prevent children from scratching and touching their

Text continued on p. 123.

APPLYING WRIST AND ANKLE RESTRAINTS

1 Collect the following equipment:
   a Thick gauze dressings
   b Roller bandage
   c Tape
2 Wash your hands.
3 Identify the patient. Check the ID bracelet and call the patient by name.
4 Explain the procedure to the patient.
5 Provide for privacy.
6 Make sure the patient is comfortable and in good body alignment (see Chapter 10).
7 Pad the wrist or ankle with the gauze dressing. Tape the dressing to secure it in place. Make sure it is not too tight.
8 Tie the roller bandage to the wrist or ankle using a clove hitch (Fig. 8-11).

9 Tie the ends to the bed frame under the mattress using a square knot or half bow (Posey) tie.
10 Check the pulse, color, and temperature of the restrained wrist or ankle every 15 minutes. Report your observations to the nurse.
11 Place the signal light within the patient's reach.
12 Unscreen the patient.
13 Wash your hands.
14 Remove the restraint every 2 hours and reposition the patient. Give skin care, perform range-of-motion exercises, and reapply the restraint.
15 Report your observations to the nurse.

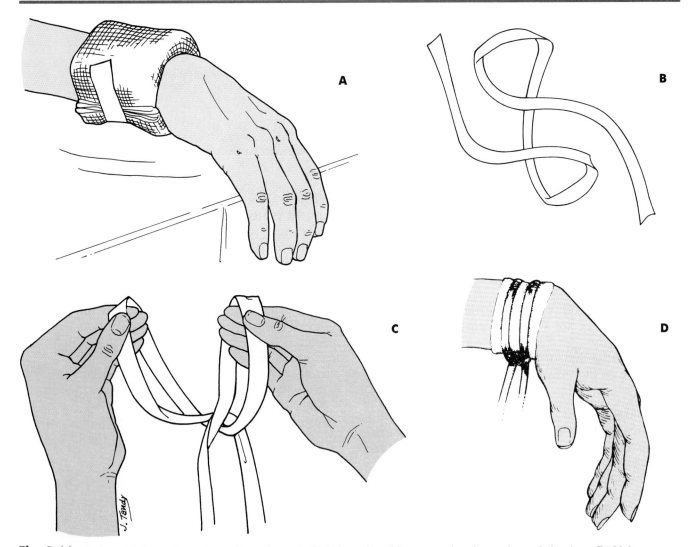

Fig. 8-11 A clove hitch can be made as shown here. **A,** Pad the wrist with a gauze dressing and tape it in place. **B,** Make a double loop. **C,** Pick up the loops. **D,** Slip the wrist through the two loops. (**D** is from Dison N: *Clinical nursing techniques,* ed 4, St Louis, 1979, Mosby–Year Book.)

APPLYING MITT RESTRAINTS

1 Collect the following equipment:
   a Two mitt restraints
   b Two washcloths
   c Tape
2 Make a hand roll as in Figure 8-12.
3 Wash your hands.
4 Identify the patient. Check the ID bracelet and call the patient by name.
5 Explain the procedure to the patient.
6 Provide for privacy.
7 Make sure the patient's hands are clean and dry.
8 Give the patient a hand roll to grasp so that the hand is in a natural position.
9 Apply the mitt restraint (Fig. 8-13).

10 Tie the straps to the bed frame under the mattress if the arm is to be immobilized.
11 Repeat steps 8, 9, and 10 for the other hand.
12 Place the signal light within the patient's reach.
13 Unscreen the patient.
14 Wash your hands.
15 Remove the restraint every 2 hours and reposition the patient. Give skin care, perform range-of-motion exercises, and reapply the restraint.
16 Report your observations to the nurse.

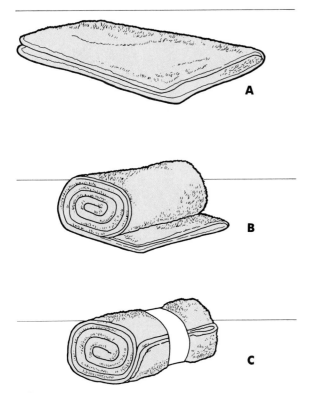

Fig. 8-12 Make a hand roll from a washcloth. **A,** Fold the washcloth in half. **B,** Roll up the washcloth. **C,** Tape the rolled washcloth.

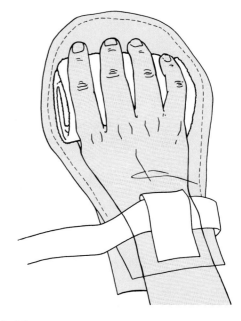

Fig. 8-13 Mitt restraint. Patient is holding a hand roll.

APPLYING A JACKET RESTRAINT

1 Get a jacket restraint in a size appropriate for the patient.
2 Get assistance if needed.
3 Wash your hands.
4 Identify the patient. Check the ID bracelet and call the patient by name.
5 Explain the procedure to the patient.
6 Provide for privacy.
7 Assist the patient to a sitting position (see page 148, *Raising a Patient's Head and Shoulders by Locking Arms With the Patient*).
8 Slip the patient's arms through the arm holes of the restraint with your free hand. The vest should cross in front.
9 Make sure there are no wrinkles in the front or back of the restraint.
10 Help the patient lie down.
11 Bring the ties through the slots.
12 Make sure the patient is comfortable and in good body alignment (see Chapter 10).
13 Tie the straps to the bed frame under the mattress or to the chair or wheelchair, or lock the straps in place.
14 Place the signal light within the patient's reach.
15 Unscreen the patient.
16 Wash your hands.
17 Remove the restraint every 2 hours and reposition the patient. Give skin care, perform range-of-motion exercises, and reapply the restraint.
18 Report your observations to the nurse.

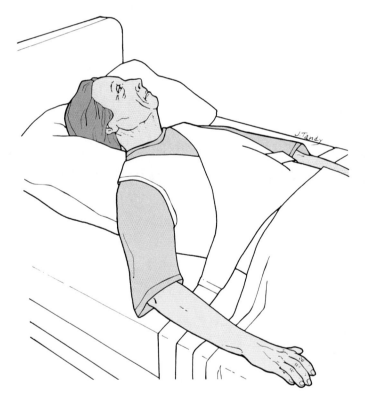

Fig. 8-14 Jacket restraint with the ties at the front.

APPLYING A SAFETY BELT

1 Obtain a safety restraint in a size appropriate for the patient.
2 Get assistance if needed.
3 Wash your hands.
4 Identify the patient. Check the ID bracelet and call the patient by name.
5 Explain the procedure to the patient.
6 Provide for privacy.
7 Assist the patient to a sitting position (see page 148, *Raising a Patient's Head and Shoulders by Locking Arms With the Patient*).
8 Place the belt around the front of the waist. Bring the ties to the back with your free hand.
9 Make sure there are no wrinkles in the front or back of the restraint.
10 Bring the ties through the slots.
11 Help the patient lie down.
12 Make sure the patient is comfortable and in good body alignment (see Chapter 10).
13 Tie the straps to the bed frame under the mattress or to the chair or wheelchair using a square knot, or according to facility policy.
14 Place the signal light within the patient's reach.
15 Unscreen the patient.
16 Wash your hands.
17 Remove the restraint every 2 hours and reposition the patient. Give skin care, perform range-of-motion exercises, and reapply the restraint.
18 Report your observations to the nurse.

A
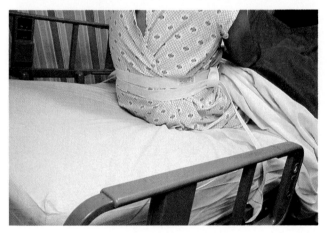

B
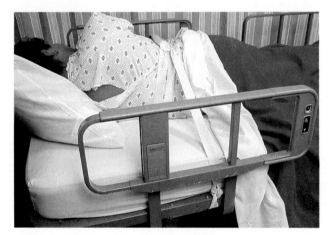

How to Use the Posey Quick-Release Tie

C
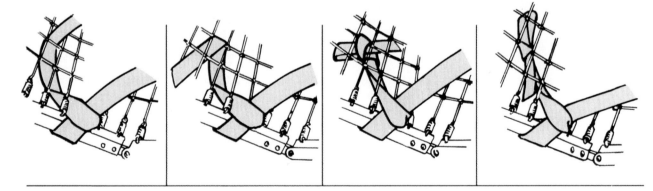

Fig. 8-15 A, B, Safety belt. **C,** The Posey quick-release tie.
(Courtesy of Posey, Arcadia, CA.)

APPLYING ELBOW RESTRAINTS

1 Collect the following equipment:
   a Two elbow restraints
   b Tongue depressors
   c Safety pins
2 Insert the tongue depressors into the slots (Fig. 8-16).
3 Wash your hands.
4 Identify the child. Check the ID bracelet and call the child by name.
5 Explain the procedure to the child and parents.
6 Provide for privacy.
7 Wrap the restraint around the child's elbow.
8 Tie the strings around the arm.
9 Pin the restraint to the child's shirt to prevent the restraint from sliding down the arm. The pins should point down and away from the child as in Figure 8-17.
10 Repeat steps 7, 8, and 9 to apply the other restraint.
11 Place the signal light within the child's or parents' reach.
12 Unscreen the child.
13 Wash your hands.
14 Remove the restraints every 2 hours. Give skin care, perform range-of-motion exercises, and reapply the restraints.
15 Report your observations to the nurse.

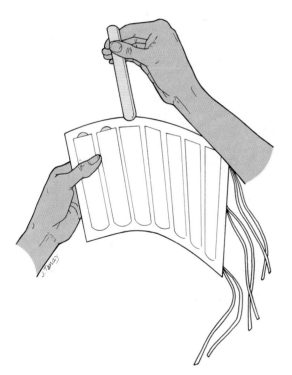

Fig. 8-16 Tongue depressors keep the elbow restraint rigid.

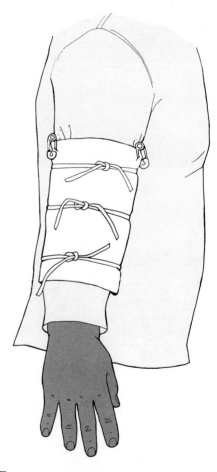

Fig. 8-17 An elbow restraint is secured to the shirt with safety pins. The pins should point down and away from the child.

incisions. A long-sleeved shirt is worn so that the restraint can be secured in place with safety pins. Both arms need to be restrained to achieve the desired effect. (See the box on p. 122.)

Accidents Due to Equipment

Glass and plastic equipment must be inspected before use. The equipment is checked for cracks, chips, and sharp or rough edges, which can easily cut, stab, or scratch patients. Damaged equipment should not be used or given to patients. Instead, take the item to the nurse, point out the defect, and discard the item as instructed.

Electrical equipment must function properly and be in good repair. Frayed cords (Fig. 8-18) and overloaded electrical outlets (Fig. 8-19) can cause electrical shocks that may result in death. Fires may also result. Frayed cords and equipment that does not function properly must be repaired by a trained individual.

Three-pronged plugs (Fig. 8-20) should be used on all equipment. Two prongs carry electrical current and the third prong is the ground. A *ground* carries leaking electricity to the earth and away from the piece of equipment. Leaking electricity can be conducted to a person, causing electrical shocks and possible death. Be sure to report if you receive a shock while using a piece of equipment. The item should be sent for repair.

Reporting Accidents and Errors

Accidents and errors must be reported immediately to your supervisor. This includes accidents involving patients, visitors, or staff. You must report errors in patient care. Such errors include giving a patient a wrong treatment, giving a treatment to the wrong patient, or forgetting to give a treatment. Breakage of items owned by the patient, such as dentures or eye glasses, must be reported. Loss of a patient's money or clothing must also be reported.

When reporting accidents or errors, you need to give the names of those involved and the date, time, and location of the accident or error. You also need to provide a complete description of what happened, including names of witnesses and any other requested information. Most facilities require written reports about the accident or error. These are called "incident reports."

FIRE SAFETY

Faulty electrical equipment and wiring, overloaded electrical circuits, and smoking are major causes of fire. Fire is a constant danger in homes and health care facilities. The entire health team is responsible

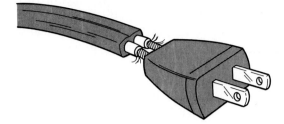

Fig. 8-18 A frayed electric wire.

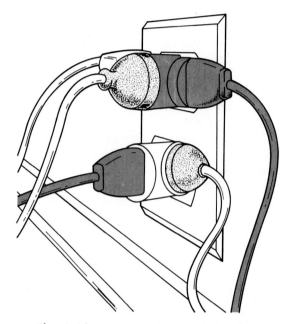

Fig. 8-19 An overloaded electrical outlet.

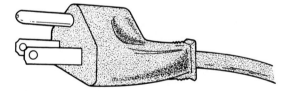

Fig. 8-20 A three-pronged plug.

for preventing fires and for acting quickly and responsibly in the event of a fire.

Fire and the Use of Oxygen

Three things are needed to start and maintain a fire: a spark or flame, a material that will burn, and oxygen. There is a certain amount of oxygen found in the air. However, some patients need more oxygen than is available in the air. Doctors order supplemental oxygen for these patients. Supplemental oxygen is supplied in portable oxygen tanks or through wall outlets (oxygen therapy is discussed in Chapter 22). Because oxygen is needed for fires, special safety precautions are practiced where oxygen is being given and stored.

1. "No Smoking" signs are placed on the patient's door and near the bed.
2. Patients and visitors are politely reminded not to smoke in the patient's room.
3. Smoking materials, (cigarettes, cigars, and pipes) matches, and lighters belonging to the patient are removed from the room.
4. Electrical equipment is turned off before being unplugged. Sparks occur when electrical appliances are unplugged while turned on.
5. Wool blankets and synthetic fabrics that cause static electricity are removed from the patient's room. The patient should wear a cotton gown or pajamas. Health care workers should wear cotton uniforms.
6. Electrical equipment is removed from the patient's room. This includes electric razors, heating pads, and radios.
7. Materials that ignite easily are removed from the patient's room. These include oil, grease, alcohol, and nail polish remover.

Fire Prevention

Fire prevention measures have been described in relation to children, burns in the home, equipment-related accidents, and the use of oxygen. These and other fire safety measures are summarized as follows:

1. Follow the fire safety precautions involved in the use of oxygen.
2. Smoke only in areas where smoking is allowed.
3. Be sure all ashes, cigars, and cigarettes are extinguished before emptying ashtrays.
4. Provide ashtrays to patients who are allowed to smoke.
5. Empty ashtrays into a metal container partially filled with sand or water. Do not empty ashtrays into plastic containers or wastebaskets lined with paper or plastic bags.
6. Supervise the smoking of patients who are unable to protect themselves. This includes confused, disoriented, and sedated patients.
7. Follow safety practices when using electrical equipment.
8. Supervise the play of children, and keep matches out of their reach.

What To Do if a Fire Occurs

Each health care facility has policies and procedures explaining what to do if there is a fire. You must know the policies and procedures for your facility.

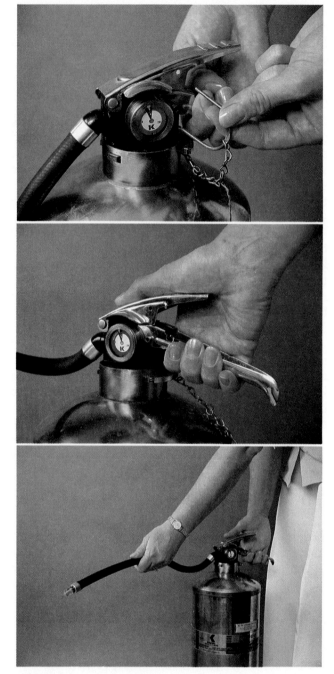

Fig. 8-21 **A,** The safety pin of the fire extinguisher is removed. **B,** The top handle is pushed down. **C,** The hose is directed at the base of the fire.

Also know the location of the fire alarms, fire extinguishers, and emergency exists. Fire drills are held periodically in all facilities so that the procedures can be practiced.

The following practices are usually carried out by the health team when there is a fire.

1. Sound the nearest fire alarm.

USING A FIRE EXTINGUISHER

1 Pull the fire alarm.
2 Get the nearest fire extinguisher.
3 Carry the extinguisher so that it is upright.
4 Take the extinguisher to the fire.

5 Remove the safety pin (Fig. 8-21, *A*).
6 Push the top handle down (Fig. 8-21, *B*).
7 Direct the hose at the base of the fire (Fig. 8-21, *C*).

2. Notify the switchboard operator of the exact location of the fire.
3. Move patients who are in the immediate area of the fire to a safe place.
4. Use a fire extinguisher on a small fire that has not spread to a larger area.
5. Turn off any oxygen or electrical equipment being used in the general area of the fire.
6. Close all doors and windows.
7. Clear equipment from all regular and emergency exits.
8. Do not use elevators if there is a fire.

You should be able to use a fire extinguisher. Fire departments often give demonstrations on how to use fire extinguishers to employees of health care facilities. These demonstrations are given once or twice a year. Some facilities require all employees to demonstrate use of a fire extinguisher.

There are different extinguishers for different kinds of fires: oil and grease fires; electrical fires; and paper and wood fires. A general procedure for using a fire extinguisher is presented in the box.

DISASTERS

A *disaster* is a sudden catastrophic event. Many people are injured and killed, and property is destroyed. Disasters may be natural, such as tornadoes, hurricanes, blizzards, earthquakes, volcanic eruptions, and floods. Man-made disasters include automobile, bus, train, and airplane accidents; fires; nuclear power plant accidents; riots; explosions; and wars.

Local communities and health care facilities have disaster plans. You should be familiar with the disaster plan where you work and the disaster plan of the community where you live and work.

Hospital disaster plans include policies and procedures to deal with great numbers of people who will be brought to the hospital for treatment. The plan generally provides for the discharge of patients who can go home. Certain personnel are assigned to the emergency department. Others are assigned to take extra equipment to the emergency area and to transport patients from the initial treatment area. Off-duty personnel may be called in to work.

SUMMARY

Most accidents can be prevented. Knowing the common safety hazards and accidents, knowing who needs protection, and using common sense are all necessary to promote safety. Remember that infants, young children, and the elderly are more likely to have accidents than are healthy people in other age-groups.

Similar accidents happen in homes and health care facilities. However, even older children, teenagers, and young and middle-aged adults have a greater risk of accidents when in health care facilities. Illness, medications, strange surroundings, and special equipment increase the risk of accidental injury. As a nursing assistant, you need to practice safety precautions, use side rails, and encourage patients to use hand rails.

The importance of identifying patients before giving care must be emphasized. The patient's life and health can be seriously threatened if the wrong care is given or if care is omitted. Use the ID bracelet to accurately identify the patient. Having two patients on the same nursing unit with the same last name is not uncommon. Some patients may even have the same first and last names.

If restraints are ordered, they must be used to protect the patient or to prevent the patient from harming others. The patient must be checked often to make sure that breathing and circulation are normal. Remember that the restrained patient depends on others for meeting basic needs. Also remember that you can be charged with false imprisonment if a patient is restrained unnecessarily.

Fire is a safety hazard. Safety precautions in relation to smoking and electrical equipment help prevent fires. Extra precautions are needed when oxygen is being used. Patients who smoke present additional fire safety concerns. Be sure you know where fire alarms, fire extinguishers, and emergency exits are located, as well as what to do if there is a fire. The safety precautions and measures that need to be taken for fires in the health care facility also apply to fire safety in the home.

REVIEW QUESTIONS

Circle T *if the answer is true and* F *if the answer is false.*

T F **1** A safe environment is one in which a person has a very small risk of becoming ill or injured.

T F **2** Young children are in danger of accidents because they have not learned what is safe and what is dangerous.

T F **3** Childproof caps are needed only on medicine containers.

T F **4** Household cleaners should be kept in locked storage areas out of the reach of children.

T F **5** Safety plugs in electrical outlets protect children from electrical shocks.

T F **6** Aging causes changes in the body that make an elderly person more likely to have accidents.

T F **7** A patient in a coma is safe from accidents.

T F **8** Smell, touch, sight, and hearing can be used to prevent accidents.

T F **9** A paraplegic is paralyzed on one side.

T F **10** Medications cause some accidents.

T F **11** Falls can be prevented by making sure there is adequate lighting.

T F **12** Patients should wear bedroom slippers to prevent skidding and slipping on floors.

T F **13** Supervising the play of children can prevent burns.

T F **14** People should not smoke in bed.

T F **15** Poisonous products should be clearly labeled and stored in their original containers.

T F **16** Poisonings occur in adults because of inadequate light when reading labels.

T F **17** Suffocation can be prevented by keeping electrical cords and appliances in good repair.

T F **18** The spread of infection is not a health hazard in health care facilities.

T F **19** Side rails are kept up at all times, even when giving care.

T F **20** Hand rails provide support when walking.

T F **21** The patient's ID bracelet is used to accurately identify the patient before giving care.

T F **22** Restraints are used only to prevent patients from harming themselves.

T F **23** Restraint of a patient unnecessarily is false imprisonment.

T F **24** Restraints should be applied so that they are tight.

T F **25** You should be able to feel a pulse in the wrist if the arm and hand are restrained.

T F **26** Square knots are used to secure the straps of a restraint to the side rails.

T F **27** Restraints are removed every 2 hours to reposition the patient and give skin care.

T F **28** Elbow restraints prevent children from scratching and touching incisions.

T F **29** Jacket restraints cross in front.

T F **30** The bed is kept in the lowest horizontal position except when giving bedside care.

T F **31** You should check glass and plastic equipment for damage.

T F **32** Two-pronged plugs are used to properly ground electrical equipment.

T F **33** Accidents or errors in giving care are reported to the nurse at the end of the shift.

T F **34** A spark or flame, a material that will burn, and oxygen are needed to start and maintain a fire.

T F **35** Smoking is not allowed where oxygen is being used.

T F **36** Wool blankets are used if a patient is receiving oxygen.

T F **37** You should supervise the smoking of a patient who is confused or sedated.

T F **38** Oxygen is turned off if it is being used in the area of a fire.

T F **39** You should close doors and windows when a fire alarm sounds.

T F **40** Many people are injured and killed and property is destroyed in a disaster.

Answers

		28 True		14 True	
		27 True		13 True	
40 True		26 False		12 False	
39 True		25 True		11 True	
38 True		24 False		10 True	
37 True		23 True		9 False	
36 False		22 False		8 True	
35 True		21 True		7 False	
34 True		20 True		6 True	
33 False		19 False		5 True	
32 False		18 False		4 True	
31 True		17 True		3 False	
30 True		16 True		2 True	
29 True		15 True		1 True	

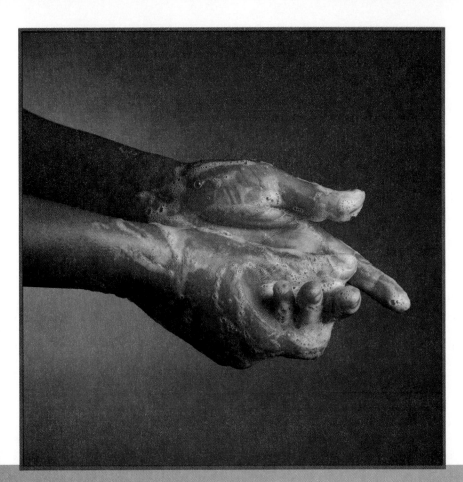

Preventing Infection

OBJECTIVES

- Define the key terms listed in this chapter
- Explain the difference between nonpathogens and pathogens
- Identify six requirements needed by microorganisms to live and grow
- Identify the signs and symptoms of an infection
- Describe six factors necessary for an infection to develop
- Explain the differences between medical asepsis, disinfection, and sterilization
- Describe practices of medical asepsis, two methods of sterilization, and how to care for equipment and supplies
- Explain the purpose of infection precautions and their effects on the patient
- Describe the types of infection precautions and the general rules for maintaining them
- Carry out infection precautions
- Perform the procedures in this chapter including gloving and bagging articles

asepsis   The absence of pathogens

autoclave   A pressurized steam sterilizer

carrier   A human being or animal that is a reservoir for microorganisms but that does not have the signs and symptoms of an infection

clean technique   Medical asepsis

communicable disease   A disease caused by pathogens that are easily spread; a contagious disease

contagious disease   Communicable disease

contamination   The process by which an object or area becomes unclean

disinfection   The process by which pathogens are destroyed

host   The environment in which microorganisms live and grow; reservoir

infection   A disease state that results from the invasion and growth of microorganisms in the body

infection precautions   Practices that limit the spread of pathogens; barriers are set up that prevent the escape of the pathogen

medical asepsis   The techniques and practices used to prevent the spread of pathogens from one person or place to another person or place; clean technique

microbe   A microorganism

microorganism   A small (micro) living plant or animal (organism) that cannot be seen without the aid of a microscope; a microbe

nonpathogen   A microorganism that does not usually cause an infection

normal flora   Microorganisms that usually live and grow in a certain location

pathogen   A microorganism that is harmful and capable of causing an infection

reservoir   The environment in which microorganisms live and grow; the host

sterile   The absence of all microorganisms

sterilization   The process by which all microorganisms are destroyed

Infection is a major safety and health hazard. Some infections are minor and cause short illnesses. Others are very serious and can cause death, particularly in infants and the elderly. The health team must protect patients and themselves from infection by preventing the spread of the cause of the infection.

MICROORGANISMS

A *microorganism* is a small (micro) living plant or animal (organism) that cannot be seen without a microscope. Microorganisms *(microbes)* are everywhere in the environment. They are in the air, food, mouth, nose, respiratory tract, stomach, intestines, and on the skin. They are in the soil and water and on animals, clothing, and furniture. Some microbes cause infections and are considered harmful. They are called *pathogens*. *Nonpathogens* are microorganisms that do not usually cause an infection.

Types of Microorganisms

There are five general types of microorganisms.
1. *Bacteria* are microscopic plant life that multiply rapidly. They consist of a single cell and are often called *germs*.
2. *Fungi* are plants that live on other plants or animals. Mushrooms, yeasts, and molds are common fungi.
3. *Protozoa* are microscopic one-celled animals.
4. *Rickettsiae* are microscopic forms of life found in the tissues of fleas, lice, ticks, and other insects. They are transmitted to humans by insect bites.
5. *Viruses* are extremely small microscopic organisms that grow in living cells.

Requirements of Microorganisms

Microorganisms need a reservoir to live and grow. The *reservoir* or *host* is the environment in which the microorganism lives and grows. The reservoir can be a human, a plant, an animal, the soil, food, water, or other material. The microorganism must receive *water* and *nourishment* from the reservoir. Most microbes need *oxygen* to live. Others cannot live in the presence of oxygen. A *warm* and *dark* environment is needed. Most microorganisms grow best at body temperature and are destroyed by heat and light.

Normal Flora

Normal flora refers to microorganisms that usually live and grow in a certain location. Certain microbes are found in the respiratory tract, in the intestines, on the skin, and in other sites outside the body. They are nonpathogenic when in or on a natural reservoir. If a nonpathogen is transmitted from its natural location to another site or host, it becomes a pathogen. *Escherichia coli* is a microorganism normally found in the large intestine. If the *E. coli* enters the urinary system, it can cause an infection.

INFECTION

An *infection* is a disease state resulting from the invasion and growth of microorganisms in the body. It may be localized in a specific body part or involve the whole body. The person with an infection has certain signs and symptoms. Some or all of the following may be present: fever, pain or tenderness, fatigue, loss of appetite, nausea, vomiting, diarrhea, rash, sores on mucous membranes, redness and swelling of a body part, and discharge or drainage from the infected area. Pathogenic microorganisms can be present without causing an infection. The development of an infection depends on several factors.

The Process of Infection

For an infection to develop, there must be a *source*. The source is a pathogen capable of causing disease. The pathogen must have a *reservoir* where it can grow and multiply. Humans and animals are reservoirs for microbes. If they do not have signs and symptoms of infection, they are *carriers*. Carriers can pass the

pathogen on to others. The pathogen must be able to leave the reservoir. In other words, it must have an *exit*. Exits in the human body are the respiratory, gastrointestinal, urinary, and reproductive tracts, breaks in the skin, and in the blood.

A pathogen that has left the reservoir must be *transmitted* to another host. Methods of transmission include direct contact, air, food, water, animals, and insects. Microbes can also be transmitted by eating and drinking utensils, dressings, and equipment for personal care and hygiene (Fig. 9-1). The pathogen must then enter the body through a *portal of entry*. Portals of entry are the same as the exits. Whether or not the pathogen grows and multiplies depends on the *susceptibility of the host*. The human body has the natural ability to protect itself from infection. A person's ability to resist infection is related to age, sex, nutritional status, fatigue, general health, medications, and the presence or absence of other illnesses.

MEDICAL ASEPSIS

Asepsis is the absence of all disease-producing microorganisms or the absence of pathogens. Because microbes are everywhere, there must be practices to achieve asepsis. These practices are known as *medical asepsis* or *clean technique*. Therefore medical asepsis is the techniques and practices used to prevent the spread of pathogenic microorganisms from one person or place to another person or place. Medical asepsis is different from disinfection and sterilization. *Disinfection* is the process by which pathogenic microorganisms are destroyed. *Sterilization* is the process in which *all* microorganisms are destroyed. *Sterile* means the absence of *all* microorganisms, both pathogenic and nonpathogenic.

Contamination is the process by which an object or area becomes unclean. In medical asepsis, an object or area is considered clean when it is free of pathogens. Therefore the object or area is contaminated if pathogens are present. Likewise, a sterile object or area is contaminated when pathogens or nonpathogens are present.

Common Aseptic Practices

Aseptic practices are followed in the home and the community. Some common ways to prevent the spread of microorganisms are:
1. Washing hands after urinating or having a bowel movement
2. Washing hands before handling or preparing food
3. Washing fruits and raw vegetables before eating or serving them
4. Providing individual toothbrushes, drinking glasses, towels, washcloths, and other personal care items for each family member

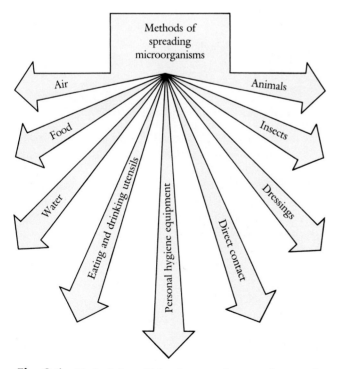

Fig. 9-1 Methods by which microorganisms can be spread.

5. Covering the nose and mouth when coughing, sneezing, or blowing the nose
6. Bathing, washing hair, and brushing teeth regularly
7. Washing cooking and eating utensils with soap and water after they have been used
8. Observing sanitation practices such as the disposal of garbage and the treatment of sewage

Handwashing

Handwashing with soap and water is the easiest and a most important way to prevent the spread of infection. The hands are used in almost every patient care activity. They are easily contaminated and can spread microorganisms if the worker does not practice handwashing before and after giving patient care. To properly wash your hands, you need to follow these rules:

1. Wash your hands under warm running water.
2. Hand-operated faucets are considered contaminated. Use a paper towel to turn water off at the end of the handwashing procedure (Fig. 9-2). The paper towel prevents the clean hand from becoming contaminated again. Some facilities consider hand controls to be clean. If hand controls are considered "clean," use a paper towel when turning the faucet on and off.
3. Bar soap is held during the entire procedure. When the procedure is completed, the soap is rinsed under running water. Then soap is dropped into the soap dish. Do not touch the soap dish during or after the handwashing procedure. Health care facilities usually have soap dispensers. Bar soap is used in home care.
4. Your hands and forearms are held lower than your elbows throughout the procedure. If your hands and forearms are held up, dirty water can run from the hands to the elbows, contaminating those areas.
5. Attention is given to those areas frequently missed during handwashing: the thumbs, knuckles, sides of the hands, little fingers, and underneath the nails. A nail file or orange stick is used to clean under the fingernails (Fig. 9-3).
6. A lotion should be used after handwashing to prevent chapping and drying of the skin.

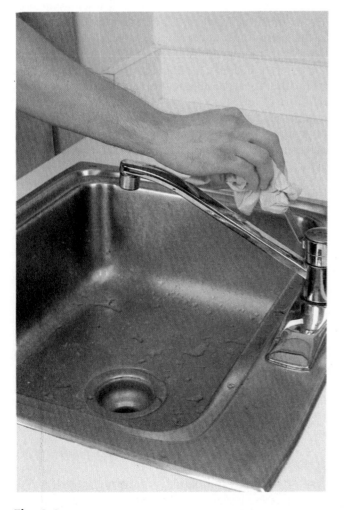

Fig. 9-2 A paper towel is used to turn the faucet off.

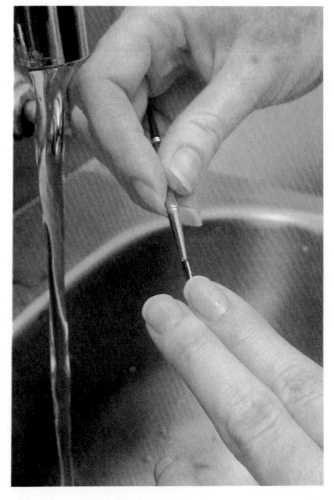

Fig. 9-3 An orange stick is used to clean under the fingernails.

HANDWASHING

1 Make sure that soap or detergent, paper towels, orange stick or nail file, and a wastebasket are available. Collect missing items.
2 Push your watch up 4 to 5 inches.
3 Stand away from the sink so that your clothes do not touch the sink. The soap and faucet must be within easy reach (Fig. 9-4).
4 Turn the faucet on, using a paper towel if this is a facility policy.
5 Adjust the water so that it feels warm and comfortable.
6 Toss the used paper towel into the wastebasket.
7 Wet your wrists and hands thoroughly under running water. Keep your hands lower than your elbows during the procedure (see Fig. 9-4).
8 Apply soap or detergent to your hands; rinse bar soap before it is used.
9 Rub your palms together to work up a good lather (Fig. 9-5).
10 Wash each hand and wrist thoroughly, and clean well between the fingers. Clean well under the fingernails by rubbing the tips of your fingers against your palms (Fig. 9-6).
11 Continue washing for 1 to 2 minutes, using friction and rotating motions.
12 Use a nail file or orange stick to clean under the fingernails (see Fig. 9-3).
13 Rinse your wrists and hands well. Water should flow from the arms to the hands.
14 Repeat steps 8 through 13.
15 Return soap to the soap dish (if bar soap is used).
16 Dry your wrists and hands with paper towels. Pat dry.
17 Turn off the faucet with the paper towels to avoid contaminating your hand.
18 Toss paper towels into the wastebasket.

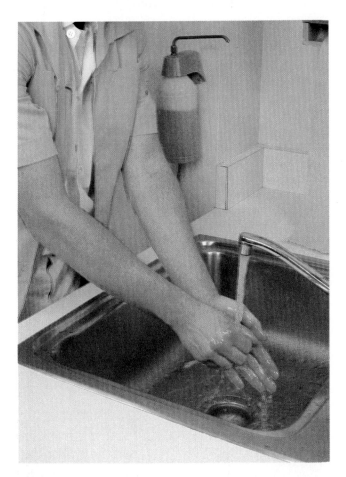

Fig. 9-4 The nursing assistant stands so that his uniform does not touch the sink. He can reach the soap and water. Hands are lower than the elbows.

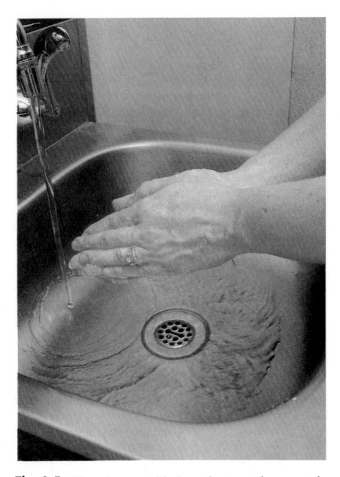

Fig. 9-5 The palms are rubbed together to work up a good lather.

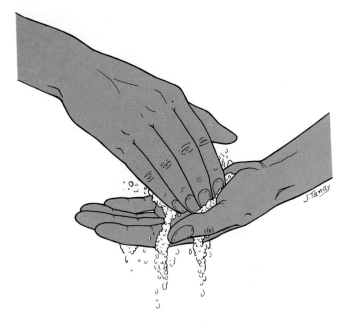

Fig. 9-6 The tips of the fingers are rubbed against the palms to clean underneath the fingernails.

Care of Supplies and Equipment

Most facilities have a central supply department that buys, disinfects, sterilizes, and distributes equipment. Much of the equipment is disposable. Disposable equipment is used once for an individual patient and then discarded. However, some disposable equipment can be used several times by a patient. Examples include disposable bedpans, urinals, wash basins, thermometers, water pitchers, and drinking cups. Disposable equipment helps reduce the spread of infection.

Larger and more expensive equipment is usually not disposable. It must be disinfected or sterilized before being used again by any patient. Before disinfection or sterilization, equipment is cleaned. Cleaning reduces the number of microbes to be destroyed and removes organic material. Organic material includes blood, pus, drainage from wounds, and body secretions or excretions. You should follow the general guidelines listed below when cleaning equipment.

1. Rinse the item in cold water first to remove organic material. Heat causes organic material to become thick, sticky, and hard to remove.
2. Use soap and hot water to wash the item.
3. Use a brush if necessary.
4. Rinse and dry the item.
5. Disinfect or sterilize the item.
6. Disinfect equipment used in the cleaning procedure.

Disinfection Disinfection is the process in which pathogenic microorganisms are destroyed. However, disinfection does not destroy spores. *Spores* are bacteria protected by a hard shell that forms around the microorganism. Spores are killed by extremely high temperatures. Disinfection methods usually do not destroy all spores.

Boiling water is a simple, inexpensive method. It can be done in the home. Small items can be disinfected by placing them in boiling water for at least 15 minutes.

Chemical disinfectants are usually used for cleaning instruments and equipment and for housekeeping. They are used to clean commodes, wheelchairs, stretchers, and furniture in the patient unit after a patient has been discharged. There are many types of chemical disinfectants. You should wear waterproof gloves when using a disinfectant to prevent skin irritation. Specific chemical disinfectants may have special precautions when being used or stored. Ask the nurse about procedures for a specific disinfectant.

Sterilization Sterilization procedures destroy all nonpathogens, pathogens, and spores. Extremely high temperatures are used. As stated earlier, microbes grow best at body temperature and are destroyed by heat.

You may learn to sterilize equipment when *steam under pressure* is the method used. An *autoclave* (Fig. 9-7) is a pressurized steam sterilizer used to sterilize metal objects such as surgical instruments, basins, bedpans, and urinals. Glass and surgical linens are also sterilized in autoclaves. Plastic and rubber items are not placed in autoclaves because they are destroyed by high temperatures. Pressure cookers used to prepare food can sterilize objects in the home. Steam under pressure usually sterilizes objects in 30 to 45 minutes.

Radiation, liquid chemicals, and a chemical gas may be used for sterilizing. Nursing assistants are generally not responsible for using these methods.

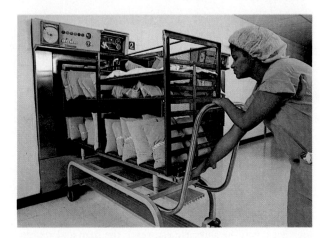

Fig. 9-7 An autoclave.

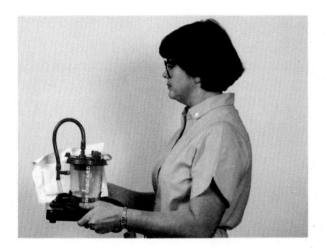

Fig. 9-8 Equipment is held away from the uniform.

Other Aseptic Measures

You should practice additional aseptic measures to prevent the spread of infection and microorganisms. These measures are essential in the health care facility to protect patients, visitors, and health workers. The measures can also be used in the home and in everyday activities.

1. Hold equipment and linens away from your uniform (Fig. 9-8).
2. Avoid shaking linens and other equipment, and use a damp cloth to dust furniture. These actions help prevent the movement of dust.
3. Clean from the cleanest area to the dirtiest. This prevents soiling a clean area.
4. Clean away from your body and uniform. If you dust, brush, or wipe toward yourself, microorganisms will be transmitted to your skin, hair, and uniform.
5. Pour contaminated liquids directly into sinks or toilets. Avoid splashing onto other areas.
6. Avoid sitting on a patient's bed. You will pick up microorganisms and transfer them to the next surface that you sit on.
7. Do not take equipment from one patient's room to use for another patient. Even if the item has not been used, do not take it from one room to another.

INFECTION PRECAUTIONS

Sometimes other measures are needed to prevent the spread of microorganisms. *Infection precautions* prevent the spread of pathogens from one area to another. Barriers are set up that prevent the escape of pathogens. The pathogens are kept within a specific area, usually the patient's room. The Centers for Disease Control (CDC) in Atlanta, Georgia have developed guidelines for infection precautions. Those guidelines are included in this section.

Instead of "infection precautions," you may hear the phrase "isolation techniques." The word "isolation" implies separating the patient from others. The pathogen, not the patient, is undesirable. Therefore CDC guidelines now use the phrase "infection precautions." However, "isolation" and "isolation techniques" are still used when describing infection precautions.

Purpose

Infection precautions prevent the spread of a *communicable* or *contagious disease*. Communicable diseases are caused by pathogens that are spread easily. Common communicable diseases are measles, mumps, chicken pox, syphilis, gonorrhea, and acquired immunodeficiency syndrome (AIDS) (see Chapter 25). Patients may have respiratory, wound, skin, gastrointestinal, or blood infections that are highly contagious. Infection precautions are indicated for these patients. Pathogens causing these infections are kept in a specific area.

Infection precautions are sometimes used to protect a patient. Age, weakness, illness, and certain medications make some patients very susceptible to infection. Their ability to fight an infection is reduced. If an infection develops, the consequences can be quite severe.

Clean Versus Dirty

Infection precautions are based on an understanding of "clean" and "dirty." "Clean" refers to those areas or objects that are uncontaminated. Uncontaminated areas are free of pathogens. Areas or objects considered "dirty" are those that are contaminated. If a "clean" area or object comes in contact with something "dirty," the object or area that was clean is now considered dirty. "Clean" and "dirty" also depend on the way in which the pathogen is spread.

The Patient's Room

When infection precautions are ordered, the patient is separated from others. The patient may be transferred to a private room. If necessary, a semiprivate room may be used. The room must have a sink with running water. The unit includes equipment and supplies for meeting basic needs (Fig. 9-9).

A cabinet, bedside stand, or cart is placed outside of the room. This is used to store the supplies needed for infection precautions. Needed supplies include gowns, gloves, masks, and plastic bags. Usually a sign is placed outside the room or on the door. It indicates the precautions being practiced.

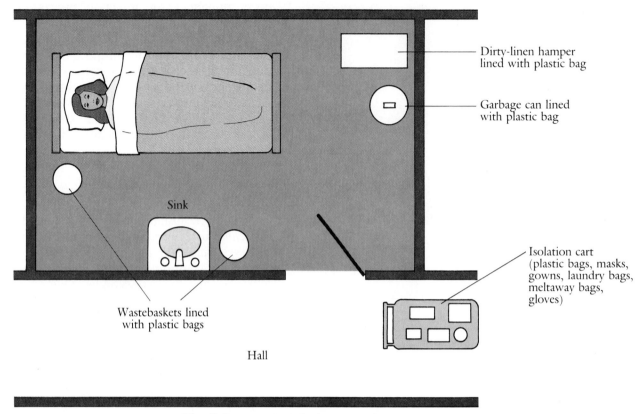

Fig. 9-9 Setup for infection precautions.

Types of Infection Precautions

The CDC has described seven categories of infection precautions (Table 9-1). Each category depends on how the pathogen is spread. Special procedures may be required. Gloves, masks, and gowns may be worn. Linens and equipment are bagged before leaving the patient's room. The special procedures are described later in this chapter.

You must understand how certain infections are spread (see Fig. 9-1). That will help you understand the different types of infection precautions. For example, enteric precautions prevent the spread of pathogens through fecal material. To spread the infection, the pathogen must be ingested orally. Oral ingestion usually occurs from contaminated hands. Hands are contaminated if they are not washed after touching fecal material. Hands are also contaminated if they touch bedpans or toilets contaminated with feces. Food, eating utensils, and drinking utensils can be contaminated by the hands. The pathogens are then ingested orally by eating and drinking. Pathogens may be spread by direct contact with a wound. They can also be spread by objects in contact with wound drainage. Dressings, linen, and the patient's clothing may be in contact with wound drainage.

Universal precautions Universal precautions were issued by the CDC in 1987. They were developed to prevent the spread of AIDS. The AIDS virus is spread through contact with the patient's blood. AIDS, hepatitis B, and other blood infections may be undiagnosed. Universal precautions prevent the spread of AIDS and other infections. Therefore universal precautions are used for *all* patients and residents of nursing facilities.

As a nursing assistant you will not insert needles into the patient's body or obtain blood for laboratory study. However, you may care for patients who have bleeding wounds. Their linens, gowns, pajamas, or clothing could become soiled with blood. Contact with blood may occur when giving oral hygiene to someone with bleeding gums. A patient can be nicked when being shaved. There may be blood or pathogens in urine, feces, vomitus, or respiratory or vaginal secretions. There are many other situations in which you could have contact with a patient's blood or body fluids.

Universal precautions involve setting up barriers to prevent contact with the patient's blood, body fluids, or body substances. These precautions are presented in the following box. *Remember; the Centers for Disease Control recommend the use of universal precautions for all patients and residents.* Your facility will have policies regarding universal precautions.

TABLE 9-1 **Infection Precautions**

Precaution	Indications	Practices
Strict	Communicable diseases spread by direct contact or through the air—smallpox, diphtheria, chicken pox, and infections caused by Staphylococcus and Strepto-coccus	Hands are washed on entering and leaving the room Gowns are worn by everyone entering the room Masks are worn by everyone entering the room Gloves are worn by everyone entering the room Linens, garbage, equipment, and other contaminated items are bagged and labeled
Contact	Prevents the spread of infection by close or direct contact—severe respiratory infections in infants and young children	Hands are washed on entering and leaving the room Masks are worn by everyone having direct contact with the patient Gowns are worn if soiling or patient contact is likely Gloves are worn if infected material will be touched Linens, garbage, equipment, and other contaminated items are bagged and labeled
Respiratory	Prevents the spread of pathogens through the air—measles, whooping cough (pertussis), and pneumonia caused by *Staphylococcus aureus*	Hands are washed on entering and leaving the room Gowns are not necessary Masks are worn for close contact Gloves are not worn Linens, garbage, equipment, and other contaminated items are bagged and labeled
AFB	Prevents the spread of acid-fast bacilli that cause tuberculosis	Hands are washed on entering and leaving the room Gowns are worn for direct patient contact Mask is worn if patient coughs and does not cover mouth Gloves are not worn Linens, garbage, equipment, and other contaminated items are bagged and labeled
Enteric	Prevents the spread of pathogens through feces—hepatitis, diarrhea	Hands are washed on entering and leaving the room Gowns are worn for direct patient contact Masks are not worn Gloves are worn by everyone having contact with the patient or the patient's urine, feces, bedpan, toilet, urinal, and linens Linens, garbage, equipment, and other contaminated items are bagged and labeled

Continued.

TABLE 9-1 **Infection Precautions—cont'd**

Precaution	Indications	Practices
Drainage/secretion	Prevents the spread of pathogens in wounds or wound drainage—staphylococcal and streptococcal infections, draining wounds	Hands are washed on entering and leaving the room Gowns are worn for direct contact with the wound or drainage Masks are not worn Gloves are worn for direct contact with the wound or drainage Linens, garbage, contaminated items, equipment used in dressing changes or in contact with the wound or drainage is bagged and labeled
Blood/body fluid	Prevents the spread of infection by direct or indirect contact with blood or body fluids—AIDS, hepatitis B, and syphilis	Hands are washed on entering and leaving the room Hands are washed immediately if contaminated with blood or body fluids Masks are not worn Gowns are worn if soiling with blood or body fluids is likely Gloves are worn when touching blood or body fluids Blood spills are promptly cleaned with a solution of 5.25% sodium hypochlorite diluted 1:10 with water Linens, garbage, equipment, and other contaminated items are bagged and labeled

NOTE: Blood/body fluid precautions require special handling of needles. However, nursing assistants do not use needles in patient care. Therefore needle handling is not included.

General Rules

Maintaining infection precautions can be difficult. Many different techniques may be ordered. Facility policies may be different from those in this text. The following rules are a guide for giving safe care to the patients requiring infection precautions.

1. Floors are contaminated. Any object that is on the floor or that falls to the floor is contaminated.
2. Floor dust is contaminated. Mops wetted with a disinfectant solution are used for cleaning. A wet mop keeps dust down.
3. Drafts should be prevented. Pathogens are carried in the air by drafts.
4. Paper towels are used to handle contaminated equipment and objects. This keeps the hands or gloves clean.
5. Items removed from the room are bagged.
6. Do not touch your hair, nose, mouth, eyes, or other body parts when caring for a patient in isolation.
7. If your hands become contaminated, they must not touch any clean area or object.
8. Wash your hands if they become contaminated.
9. Place clean items or objects on paper towels.
10. Do not shake linen.
11. Use paper towels to turn faucets on and off.
12. Tell the nurse if you have any cuts, open skin areas, a sore throat, vomiting, or diarrhea.

Special Procedures

Infection precautions require special procedures. Gloving, gowning, wearing a mask, and bagging articles removed from the area may be required. Special considerations are required for taking vital signs and collecting specimens.

Gloving Disposable gloves act as a barrier between the patient and the worker. They protect the worker from pathogens in the patient's blood, body fluids, and body substances. Patients are also protected from

UNIVERSAL PRECAUTIONS

Gloves are worn when touching blood, body fluids, body substances, and mucous membranes.

Gloves are worn when there are cuts, breaks, or openings in the skin.

Gloves are worn when there is possible contact with urine, feces, vomitus, dressings, wound drainage, soiled linen, or soiled clothing.

Masks, goggles, or face shields are worn when splattering or splashing of blood or body fluids is possible (Fig. 9-10). (This protects your eyes and the mucous membranes of your mouth.)

Gowns or aprons are worn when splashing, splattering, smearing, or soiling from blood or body fluids is possible.

Hands and other body parts must be washed immediately if contaminated with blood or body fluids.

Hands are washed immediately after removing gloves.

Hands are washed after contact with the patient.

Avoid nicks or cuts when shaving patients.

Handle razor blades and other sharp objects carefully to avoid injuring the patient or yourself.

Use resuscitation devices when mouth-to-mouth resuscitation is indicated (see Chapter 29).

Avoid patient contact when you have open skin wounds or lesions. Discuss the situation with your supervisor.

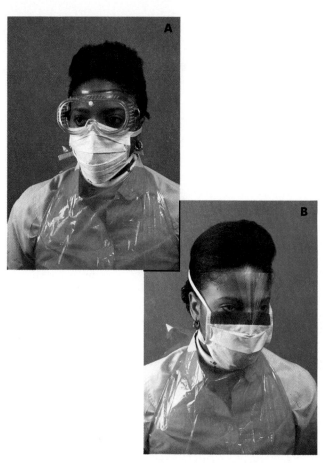

Fig. 9-10 A, Mask and goggles protect the eyes from splashing body fluids. **B,** A face shield protects the eyes and mucous membranes of the mouth. Note that a plastic apron is worn to protect the uniform from soiling.

microorganisms that may be on the worker's hands.

Disposable gloves are easy to put on. No special technique is required. However, you must be careful not to tear the gloves when putting them on. Carelessness, long fingernails, and rings can tear the gloves. Torn gloves must be discarded. Blood, fluids, and other substances can enter the glove through the tear. This contaminates the hand.

The following steps are important when removing gloves. When the gloves are removed, the inside part will be on the outside. The inside of the gloves is considered "clean."

1. When both hands are still gloved, be sure that only glove touches glove. The gloves should not touch skin on the wrists or arms.
2. Remove one glove by grasping it just below the cuff (Fig. 9-11, *A*).
3. Pull the glove down over your hand so that it is inside out (Fig. 9-11, *B*).
4. Hold the removed glove with your other gloved hand.
5. Reach inside the other glove with the first two fingers of your ungloved hand (Fig. 9-11, *C*).
6. Pull the glove down (inside out) over your hand and the other glove (Fig. 9-11, *D*).
7. Discard the gloves in the appropriate container.
8. Wash your hands.

Gowning Gowns keep clothing free from the patient's pathogenic microorganisms. Gowns also protect the patient from microorganisms that may be on the clothing of those entering the room. They also prevent soiling of clothing when giving care. Gowns are made of paper. They must be long enough and large enough to completely cover clothing. The sleeves are long with tight cuffs. The gown opens at the back, where it is tied at the neck and waist. The inside and the neck of the gown are considered "clean." The outside and waist strings are considered contaminated.

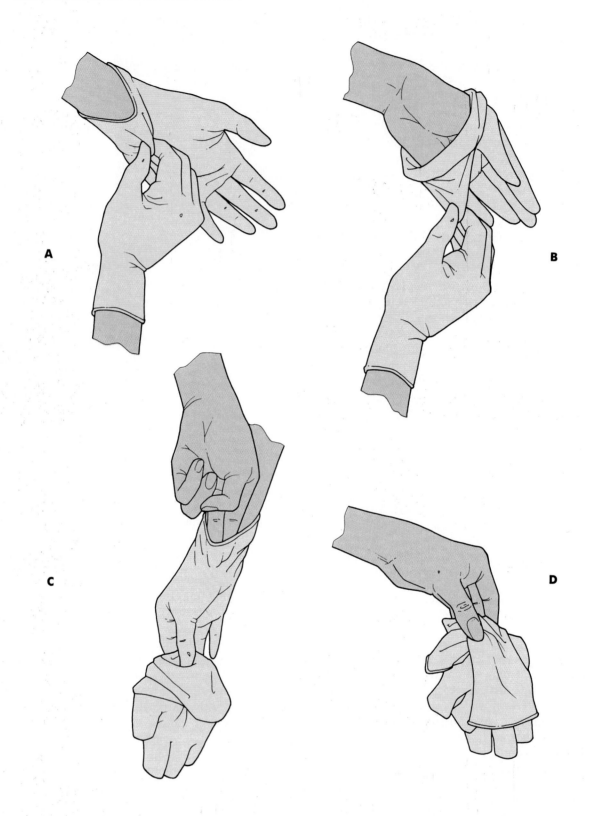

Fig. 9-11 Removing gloves. **A,** The glove is grasped below the cuff. **B,** The glove is pulled down over the hand. The glove is inside out. **C,** The fingers of the ungloved hand are inserted inside the glove. **D,** The glove is pulled down and over the hand and glove. The glove is inside out.

GOWNING TECHNIQUE

1 Remove your watch and all jewelry.
2 Roll up long sleeves of your uniform.
3 Wash your hands.
4 Pick up a clean gown. Hold it out in front of you so that it can unfold. Do not shake the gown.
5 Put your hands and arms through the sleeves of the gown as in Figure 9-12, *A*.
6 Make sure the gown completely covers the front of your uniform. The gown should be snug at the neck.
7 Tie the strings at the back of the neck (Fig. 9-12, *B*).
8 Overlap the back of the gown. Your uniform must be completely covered. The gown should be snug (Fig. 9-12, *C*) and should not hang loosely.
9 Tie the waist strings at the back.

10 Provide necessary patient care.
11 Remove the gown as follows:
    a Untie the waist strings.
    b Wash your hands.
    c Untie the neck strings. Do not touch the outside of the gown.
    d Pull the gown down from the shoulder.
    e Turn the gown inside out as it is removed. Hold the gown at the inside shoulder seams and bring your hands together (Fig. 9-12, *D*).
12 Roll up the gown away from you, keeping it inside out.
13 Discard the gown in the wastebasket.
14 Wash your hands.
15 Remove the face mask and discard it.
16 Wash your hands.
17 Open the door using a paper towel. Discard it in the wastebasket inside the room as you leave.

A
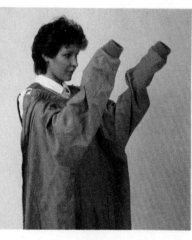

B
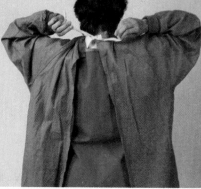

C
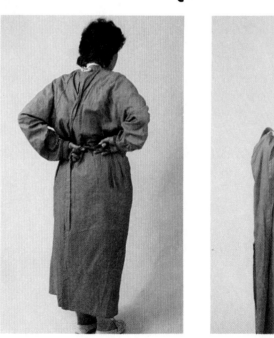

D
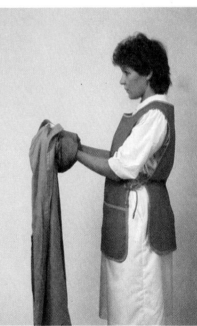

Fig. 9-12 Gowning technique. **A,** The arms and hands are put through the sleeves. **B,** The strings are tied at the back of the neck. **C,** The gown is overlapped in the back so that the entire uniform is covered. **D,** The gown is turned inside out as it is removed.

WEARING A FACE MASK

1 Wash your hands.
2 Pick up the mask by its upper ties. Do not touch the part that will cover your face.
3 Position the mask over your nose. Your nose and mouth must be covered (Fig. 9-13, *A*).
4 Place the upper strings over your ears. Tie the strings in the back toward the top of your head (Fig. 9-13, *B*).
5 Tie the lower strings at the back of your neck (Fig. 9-13, *C*). Make sure the lower part of the mask is under your chin. If you wear glasses, the mask should fit snugly over your nose and under the bottom edge of the glasses.
6 Mold the metal strip over the bridge of your nose.

7 Wash your hands.
8 Provide necessary care. Avoid coughing, sneezing, and unnecessary talking while wearing the mask.
9 Change the mask if it becomes moist or contaminated.
10 Remove the mask as follows:
   a Wash your hands.
   b Untie the lower strings.
   c Untie the top strings.
   d Hold the top strings and remove the mask.
   e Bring the strings together. The inside of the mask will fold together (Fig. 9-13, *D*). Avoid touching the inside of the mask.
11 Discard the mask in the wastebasket.
12 Wash your hands.

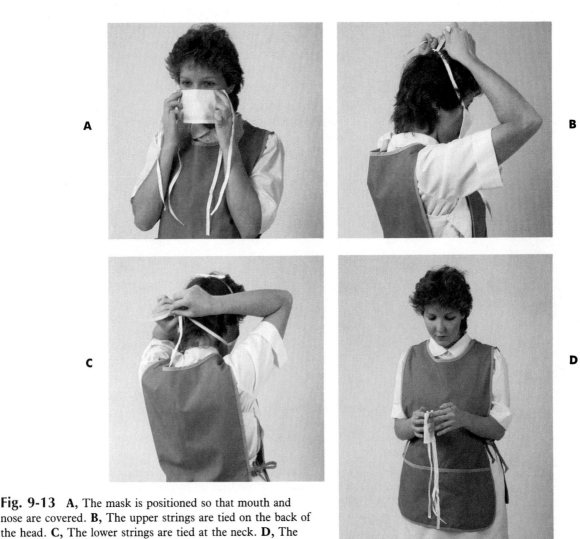

Fig. 9-13 **A,** The mask is positioned so that mouth and nose are covered. **B,** The upper strings are tied on the back of the head. **C,** The lower strings are tied at the neck. **D,** The strings of the face mask are brought together so that the inside of the mask will be folded together after being removed.

Some facilities use plastic aprons (see Fig. 9-10). Gowns are indicated when the arms and wrists must be protected from soiling or contact with blood or body fluids. Possible splashing or splattering indicate the need for gowns. Gowns and aprons are used once and then discarded. A wet gown is considered contaminated. If a gown becomes wet, it is removed and a dry one is put on.

Wearing a face mask Face masks prevent the spread of microorganisms from the respiratory tract. Masks may be worn by patients, visitors, or health care workers. Disposable masks are used. If a mask becomes wet or moist from breathing, it is considered contaminated. A new mask is applied when contamination occurs.

The mask should fit snugly over the nose and mouth. Hands are washed before putting on a mask and before undoing the ties. Only the ties are touched during removal. The front of the mask is considered contaminated.

Bagging articles Contaminated items are bagged before being removed from the patient's room. Plastic bags are used because they prevent leakage and microorganisms cannot go through them.

A single bag is usually adequate. Double bagging involves placing contaminated items in two bags. However, the CDC no longer recommends double bagging unless the outside of the bag is soiled. Two workers are needed for double bagging. One worker is inside the room and the other is at the doorway outside the room. The worker in the room places contaminated items into a bag. The bag is then sealed securely. The worker outside the room holds open another bag that is considered clean. A wide cuff is made on the clean bag to protect the hands from contamination (Fig. 9-14). The worker inside the room stands at the doorway and places the contaminated bag into the clean bag (Fig. 9-15).

The following guidelines apply to bagging articles:
1. Separate bags are used for linens, glass, dry garbage, wet garbage, and equipment being returned to the central supply department.
2. The contents of the bag (linens, dry garbage, wet garbage) are marked on the bag. Dry garbage consists of paper and disposable items. Dressings and leftover food are examples of wet garbage.
3. Flush leftover food (except bones) down the toilet, or put it in the wet garbage.
4. Seal each bag with string or tape.
5. Label the bag if required by facility policy.

Psychological Impact of Infection Precautions

The patient has needs for love, belonging, and self-esteem. Too often these needs go unmet when infection precautions are necessary. Visitors and health team members may need to put on a gown, mask, or gloves. The extra effort required before entering the

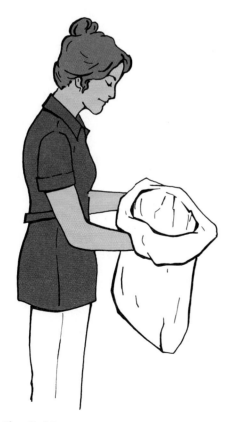

Fig. 9-14 A cuff is made on the clean bag.

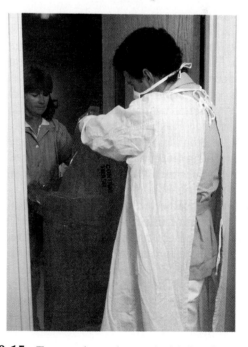

Fig. 9-15 Two nursing assistants double-bagging equipment. One nursing assistant is in the room inside the doorway. The other is outside the room. The "dirty" bag is placed inside the "clean" bag.

room, being unsure of what can and cannot be touched, and the fear of getting the disease often cause people to avoid the patient. Loneliness, feeling unloved and unwanted, and rejection can occur.

The patient's self-esteem can easily suffer. Besides being faced with illness, the individual knows that the disease is contagious and can be spread to others. The patient may feel dirty, unclean, and undesirable. Unfortunately, visitors and health care workers may unknowingly make the patient feel ashamed and guilty for having a contagious disease.

The nurse can help the patient, visitors, and the health team understand the need for infection precautions and their psychological effects on the patient. You can help meet the patient's need for love, belonging, and self-esteem. The following actions will be helpful.

1. Remember that it is the pathogen that is undesirable, not the patient.
2. Treat the patient with respect, kindness, and dignity.
3. Provide newspapers, magazines, and other reading materials.
4. Encourage the patient to telephone family and friends.
5. Provide a current television guide.
6. Organize your work so that you can stay in the room to visit with the patient.
7. Say hello from the doorway periodically.

SUMMARY

Preventing the spread of infection is the responsibility of every health worker. You must be conscientious about your work. Your employer and your patients assume that you will practice medical asepsis to prevent the spread of microorganisms and infection. One act of carelessness can spread microorganisms and endanger patient safety. The reverse is also true. You can develop the same infection as the patient if you do not practice medical asepsis or required infection precautions. The simple procedure of handwashing before and after patient contact significantly reduces the spread of microorganisms.

REVIEW QUESTIONS

Circle T *if the answer is true and* F *if the answer is false.*

T F **1** A pathogen can cause an infection.
T F **2** Microorganisms are not pathogenic in their natural environments.
T F **3** An infection results from the invasion and growth of microorganisms in the body.
T F **4** The source of an infection is a pathogen.
T F **5** A microorganism must enter the body of a susceptible host for an infection to develop.
T F **6** Sterilization is the same as clean technique.
T F **7** An item is sterile if nonpathogens are present.
T F **8** The hands and forearms should be held up during the handwashing procedure.
T F **9** You should clean under the fingernails when washing your hands.
T F **10** Disposable equipment helps reduce the spread of infection.
T F **11** Unused equipment in a patient's room can be used for another patient.

Circle the best *answer.*

12 A pathogen needs the following to grow *except*
a Water
b Nourishment
c Oxygen
d Light

13 Microorganisms grow best in an environment that is

a Warm and dark
b Warm and light
c Cool and dark
d Cool and light

14 The patient with an infection may have
a Fever, nausea, vomiting, rash, and/or sores
b Pain or tenderness, redness, and/or swelling
c Fatigue, loss of appetite, and/or a discharge
d All of the above

15 Microbes enter and leave the body through the
a Respiratory tract and/or breaks in the skin
b Gastrointestinal system and/or the blood
c Reproductive system and/or urinary system
d All of the above

16 The process of sterilization
a Destroys spores
b Is used to clean furniture
c Can be used for plastic and rubber items
d All of the above

17 You should do all of the following *except*
a Use a damp cloth to dust furniture
b Sit on the patient's bed
c Clean away from the body or uniform
d Clean from the cleanest area to the dirtiest

18 When cleaning equipment, you should
a Rinse the item in cold water before cleaning
b Wash the item with soap and hot water
c Use a brush if necessary
d All of the above

19 Which is used to sterilize equipment?
   a Handwashing
   b Boiling water
   c An autoclave
   d Chemical disinfectants
20 Infection precautions
   a Prevent infection
   b Destroy pathogens
   c Keep pathogens within a specific area
   d Destroy pathogens and nonpathogens
21 A "clean" area
   a Has been rinsed with water
   b Is contaminated with pathogens
   c Is free of pathogens
   d Has no obvious dirt
22 Universal precautions
   a Are used for all patients and residents
   b Prevent the spread of pathogens through the air
   c Require gowns, masks, and gloves
   d All of the above
23 Gloves are worn when in contact with the patient's
   a Blood
   b Body fluids
   c Body substances
   d All of the above
24 "Enteric precautions" prevent the
   a Patient from coming in contact with pathogens
   b Spread of pathogens found in wounds
   c Spread of pathogens through fecal material
   d Spread of pathogens through the air
25 Which statement about infection precautions is *false?*
   a Floors are contaminated.
   b Paper towels are used to handle contaminated objects.
   c Linens must be double bagged.
   d Hands are washed on entering and leaving the room.

26 Which part of the gown is "clean"?
   a The neck strings
   b The waist strings
   c The sleeves
   d The back
27 The face mask
   a Can be reused
   b Is considered clean on the inside
   c Is contaminated when it becomes moist
   d Should fit loosely over the nose and mouth so the person can breathe
28 Which does not reduce the psychological effects of infection precautions?
   a Treating the patient with respect, kindness, and dignity
   b Providing reading materials
   c Encouraging the patient to telephone family and friends
   d Finishing your work in the room quickly

Answers

1	True	15	d
2	True	16	a
3	True	17	b
4	True	18	d
5	True	19	c
6	False	20	c
7	False	21	c
8	False	22	a
9	True	23	d
10	True	24	c
11	False	25	c
12	d	26	a
13	a	27	c
14	d	28	d

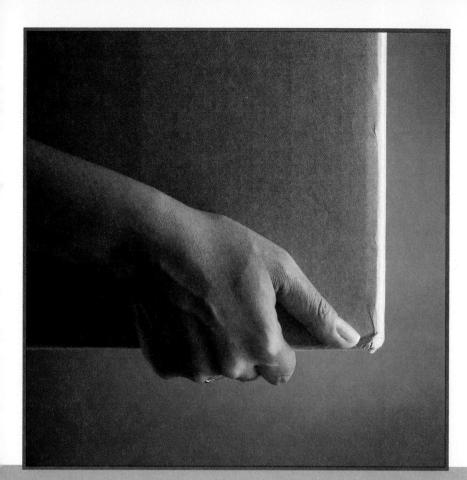

Body Mechanics

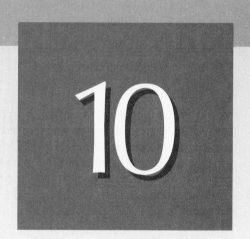

OBJECTIVES

- Define the key terms in this chapter
- Explain the purpose and rules of using good body mechanics
- Identify comfort and safety measures for lifting, turning, and moving patients in bed
- Explain the purpose of a transfer belt
- Identify the comfort and safety measures for using a stretcher to transport a patient
- Explain why good body alignment and position changes are important
- Identify the comfort and safety measures for positioning patients in bed
- Position patients in the five basic bed positions and in a chair
- Perform the procedures described in this chapter

base of support The area on which an object rests

body alignment The way in which body parts are aligned with one another; posture

body mechanics Using the body in an efficient and careful way

dorsal recumbent position The back-lying or supine position

Fowler's position A semi-sitting position; the head of the bed is elevated 45 to 60 degrees

friction The rubbing of one surface against another

gait belt A transfer belt

lateral position The side-lying position

logrolling Turning the patient as a unit in alignment with one motion

posture The way in which body parts are aligned with one another; body alignment

side-lying position The lateral position

Sims' position A side-lying position in which the upper leg is sharply flexed so that it is not on the lower leg and the lower arm is behind the patient

supine position The back-lying or dorsal recumbent position

transfer belt A belt used to hold onto a patient during a transfer or when walking with the patient; a gait belt

Y̲ou will move patients often. A patient may be moved or turned in bed or transferred from the bed to a chair, wheelchair, or stretcher. During these and other activities, you must use your body correctly to protect yourself from injury and to protect patients from the dangers of not being held or supported properly.

BODY MECHANICS

Body mechanics is using the body in an efficient and careful way. It involves using good posture, balance, and the strongest and largest muscles to perform work. Fatigue, muscle strain, and injury can result from improper use and positioning of the body during activity or rest. You must be concerned with the patient's and your own body mechanics.

The major movable body parts are the head, trunk, arms, and legs. *Posture*, or *body alignment*, is the way in which body parts are aligned with one another. Good body alignment (posture) allows the body to move and function with strength and efficiency. Good alignment is necessary when standing, sitting, or lying down.

The *base of support* is the area on which an object rests. The feet provide the base of support for humans. A good base of support is needed for balance. Balancing on one foot for a long time is difficult. You will have a wider base of support if you stand with your feet apart. The wider base of support makes you feel more balanced and stable. Therefore a wide base of support gives more balance and stability (Fig. 10-1).

The strongest and largest muscles are in the shoulders, upper arms, hips, and thighs. These muscles are used to lift and move heavy objects. If smaller and weaker muscles are used, strain and exertion is placed on them, causing fatigue and injury (Fig. 10-2, *A*). Use the strong thigh and hip muscles by bending your knees or squatting to lift a heavy object (Fig. 10-2, *B*). Avoid bending over from the waist when lifting. Bending from the waist involves the small back muscles. Holding items close to the body and base of support involves upper arm and shoulder muscles (Fig. 10-3). If the object is held away from the body, strain is placed on smaller muscles in the lower arms.

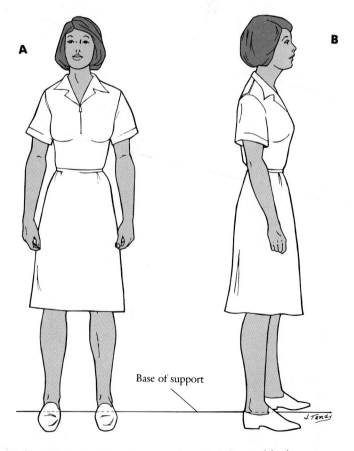

Fig. 10-1 **A,** Anterior view of an adult in good body alignment with feet apart for a wide base of support. **B,** Lateral view of an adult with good posture and alignment.

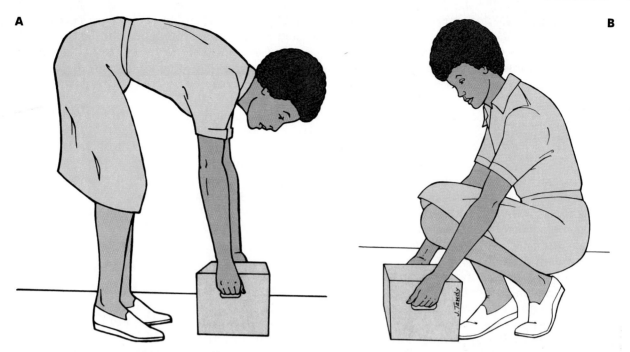

Fig. 10-2 **A,** Picking up a box using poor body mechanics. **B,** Picking up a box using good body mechanics.

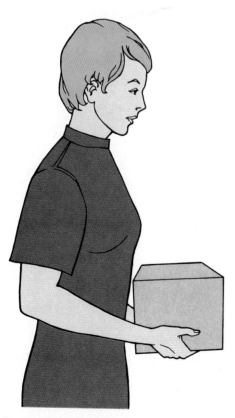

Fig. 10-3 The box is carried close to the body and base of support.

General Rules

You should use good body mechanics in your every-day activities. Cleaning, doing laundry, getting in and out of a car, picking up a baby, mowing the yard, and shoveling snow are some activities that require good body mechanics. The following rules will help you use good body mechanics for safe and efficient functioning when lifting and moving patients and heavy objects.

1. Make sure your body is in good alignment and that you have a wide base of support.
2. Use the stronger and larger muscles of your body. They are in the shoulders, upper arms, thighs, and hips.
3. Keep objects close to your body when lifting, moving, or carrying them.
4. Avoid unnecessary bending and reaching. If possible, have the height of the bed and overbed table level with your waist when giving care. Adjust the bed and table to the proper height (see Chapter 11).
5. Face the area in which you are working to prevent unnecessary twisting.
6. Push, slide, or pull heavy objects whenever possible rather than lifting them.
7. Use both of your hands and arms when lifting, moving, or carrying heavy objects.
8. Turn your whole body when you change the direction of your movement.
9. Work with smooth and even movements. Avoid sudden or jerky motions.

10. Get help from a co-worker to move heavy objects or patients whenever necessary.
11. Squat to lift heavy objects from the floor (see Fig. 10-2, *B*). Push against the strong hip and thigh muscles to raise yourself to a standing position.

LIFTING AND MOVING PATIENTS IN BED

Some patients can move and turn in bed by themselves. Others need help from at least one person for position changes. Patients who are unconscious, paralyzed, on complete bed rest, in a cast, or weak from surgery or disease need assistance. Sometimes 2 or 3 people are needed.

You must follow the rules of body mechanics when moving and lifting patients in bed. The patient must be protected from injury by being kept in good body alignment. The patient is positioned in good body alignment after being moved. Proper positioning is described on pages 167-169.

Friction must be reduced to protect the patient's skin. *Friction* is the rubbing of one surface against another. When moved in bed, the patient's skin rubs against the sheet. This can scratch and injure the skin. The patient is then at risk of an infection or decubitus ulcers (see Chapter 13). Reduce friction when moving patients in bed by rolling or lifting instead of sliding them. A cotton drawsheet (see Chapter 12) can be used as a *turning sheet* (lift or pull sheet) to move the patient in bed and reduce friction. A nurse may suggest sprinkling the patient's skin or sheets with talcum powder or cornstarch to help reduce friction.

Other comfort and safety measures need to be considered before moving patients in bed.
1. Consult the nurse for any limitations or restrictions in positioning or moving the patient. These may be ordered by the doctor or may be part of the care plan.
2. Decide how the patient will be moved and how many helpers you need.
3. Get enough co-workers to help you *before* beginning the procedure.
4. Keep the patient covered and screened to protect the right to privacy.
5. Protect any tubes or drainage containers connected to the patient.

Raising the Patient's Head and Shoulders

You may have to raise your patient's head and shoulders to tie the back of a gown, to turn or remove a pillow, or to give care. The head and shoulders can be easily and safely raised by locking arms with the patient. Help may be needed if a patient is heavy or difficult to move.

Moving the Patient Up in Bed

Many patients can have the head of their bed raised. However, that often causes them to slide down toward the middle and foot of the bed. They need to be moved up in bed to maintain good body alignment and comfort (Fig. 10-8). You can usually move children and light-weight adults up in bed without help. Some patients can assist with the procedure.

RAISING THE PATIENT'S HEAD AND SHOULDERS BY LOCKING ARMS WITH THE PATIENT

1 Wash your hands.
2 Identify the patient. Check the ID bracelet and call the patient by name.
3 Explain the procedure to the patient.
4 Provide for privacy.
5 Make sure the bed wheels are locked.
6 Raise the bed to its highest level or to where you can use good body mechanics.
7 Make sure the far side rail is raised. Lower the one near you.
8 Ask the patient to put the near arm under your near arm and behind your shoulder. His or her hand should rest on your shoulder. If you are standing on the right side, the patient's right hand will rest on your right shoulder (Fig. 10-4).
9 Put your arm near the patient under his or her arm near you. Your hand should be on the patient's shoulder.

10 Put your free arm under the patient's neck and shoulders (Fig. 10-5).
11 Help the patient pull up to a sitting or semi-sitting position on the count of "3" (Fig. 10-6).
12 Use the arm and hand that supported the neck and shoulders to straighten or remove the pillow, tie the gown, etc. (Fig. 10-7).
13 Help the patient lie down. Provide support with your locked arm. Support his or her neck and shoulders with your other arm.
14 Make sure the patient is comfortable and in good body alignment.
15 Place the signal light within reach.
16 Raise the side rail near you.
17 Lower the bed to its lowest position.
18 Unscreen the patient.
19 Wash your hands.

Moving the Patient up in Bed With Assistance

Assistance is needed when a patient cannot help with being moved up in bed. At least two people are needed to move heavy patients and those weak from surgery or disease. Be sure to ask for help before starting the procedure. Remember to cooperate if a co-worker asks you to help with care. See the box on p. 151.

Moving the Patient Up in Bed Using a Turning Sheet

With the help of a co-worker, you can easily and safely move a patient up in bed using a turning sheet. Friction is reduced, and the patient is lifted more evenly. A flat sheet folded in half or a drawsheet can be used for the turning sheet. The turning sheet is placed under the patient. It extends from the shoulders to above the knees. Certain patients should be moved up in bed with a turning sheet. They include those who are unconscious, paralyzed, recovering from spinal surgery, or who have spinal cord injuries.

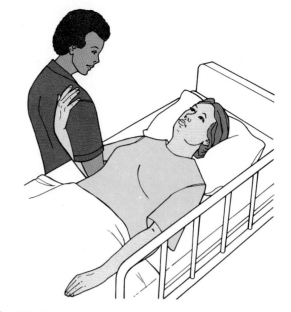

Fig. 10-4 Raise the patient's head and shoulders by locking arms with the patient. The patient's near arm is under the nursing assistant's near arm and behind the shoulder.

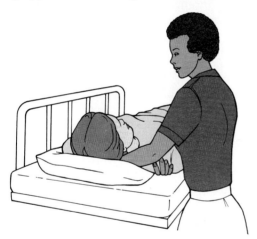

Fig. 10-5 The far arm of the nursing assistant is under the patient's neck and shoulders. The near arm is under the patient's near arm.

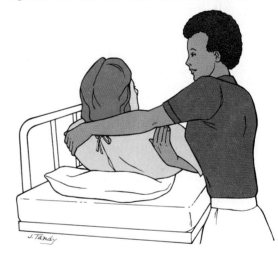

Fig. 10-6 The patient is raised to a semi-sitting position by locking arms.

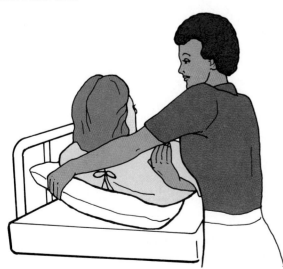

Fig. 10-7 The nursing assistant lifts the pillow while the patient is raised in a semi-sitting position.

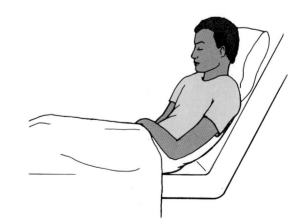

Fig. 10-8 A patient in poor body alignment after sliding down in bed.

Moving the Patient Up in Bed

1 Wash your hands.
2 Identify the patient. Check the ID bracelet and call the patient by name.
3 Explain the procedure to the patient.
4 Provide for privacy.
5 Make sure the bed wheels are locked.
6 Raise the bed to its highest level or to where you can use good body mechanics.
7 Lower the head of the bed to a level appropriate for the patient. The bed should be as flat as possible.
8 Place the pillow against the headboard if the patient can be without it. This prevents his or her head from hitting the headboard when being moved up.
9 Make sure the far side rail is raised. Lower the one near you.
10 Stand with your feet about 12 inches apart. Point the foot closest to the head of the bed toward the head of the bed. Face the head of the bed.
11 Bend your hips and knees and keep your back straight.
12 Place one arm under the shoulders and the other under the patient's thighs.
13 Ask the patient to grasp the head of the bed and to flex both knees as in Figure 10-9.
14 Explain that you will both move on the count of "3." Ask the patient to pull up with the hands and push against the bed with the feet. Explain what you will be doing.
15 Move the patient to the head of the bed on the count of "3." Shift your weight from your rear leg to your front leg (Fig. 10-10).
16 Put the pillow under the patient's head and shoulders. Lock arms with him or her to complete this step.
17 Straighten linens. Make sure the patient is comfortable and in good body alignment.
18 Place the signal light within reach.
19 Raise the side rail near you.
20 Raise the head of the bed to a level appropriate for the patient.
21 Lower the bed to its lowest position.
22 Unscreen the patient.
23 Wash your hands.

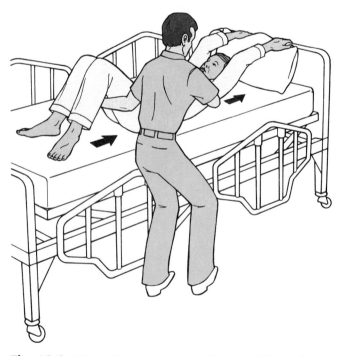

Fig. 10-9 The patient grasps the headboard and flexes the knees to assist in being moved up. The nursing assistant has one arm under the patient's shoulder and the other under the thighs.

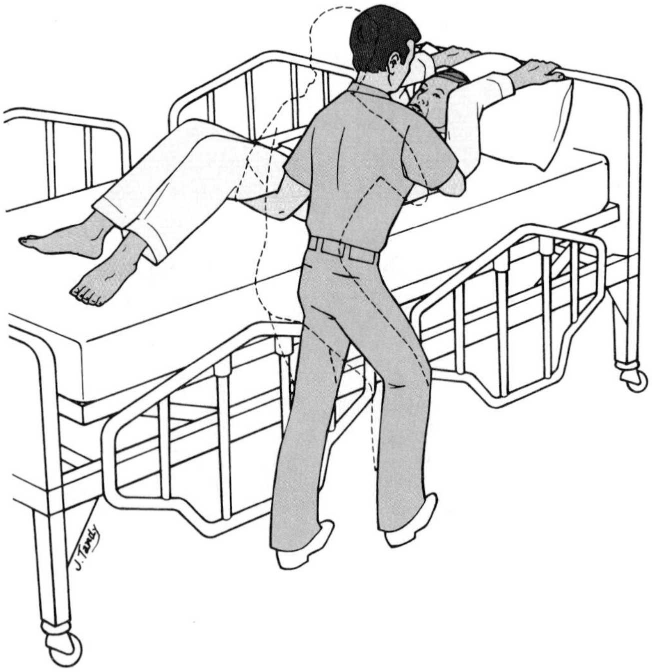

Fig. 10-10 The patient is moved up in bed as the nursing assistant's body weight is shifted from the rear leg to the front leg.

MOVING THE PATIENT UP IN BED WITH ASSISTANCE

1 Ask a co-worker to help you.
2 Wash your hands.
3 Identify the patient. Check the ID bracelet and call the patient by name.
4 Explain the procedure to the patient.
5 Provide for privacy.
6 Make sure the bed wheels are locked.
7 Raise the bed to its highest level or to where you can use good body mechanics.
8 Lower the head of the bed to a level appropriate for the patient. The bed should be as flat as possible.
9 Place the pillow against the headboard if the patient can be without it. This prevents his or her head from hitting the headboard when being moved up.
10 Stand on one side of the bed. Have your helper stand on the other.
11 Lower the side rails.
12 Stand with your feet about 12 inches apart. Point the foot nearest the head of the bed toward the head of the bed and face that direction.
13 Bend your hips and knees and keep your back straight.

14 Place one arm under the patient's shoulder and one arm under the buttocks. Your helper should do the same. Grasp each other's forearms.
15 Have the patient flex both knees (Fig. 10-11).
16 Explain that you and your helper will move on the count of "3." The patient should push against the bed with the feet if able.
17 Move the patient to the head of the bed on the count of "3." Shift your weight from your rear leg to your front leg (Fig. 10-12).
18 Repeat steps 12 through 17 if necessary.
19 Put the pillow under the patient's head and shoulders. Straighten linens. Make sure the patient is comfortable and in good body alignment.
20 Place the signal light within reach.
21 Raise the side rails.
22 Raise the head of the bed to a level appropriate for the patient.
23 Lower the bed to its lowest position.
24 Unscreen the patient.
25 Wash your hands.

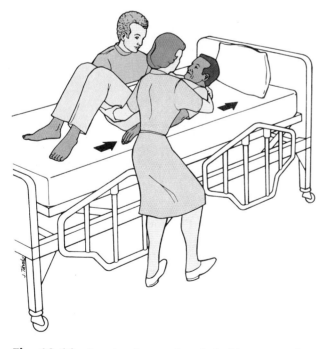

Fig. 10-11 A patient is moved up in bed by two nursing assistants. Each has one arm under the patient's shoulder and the other under the buttocks. They have locked arms under the patient. The patient's knees are flexed.

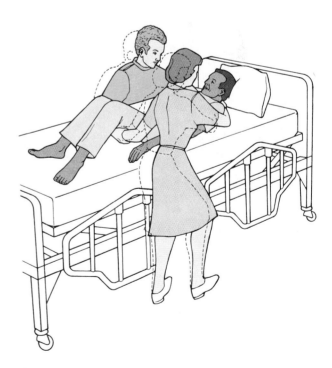

Fig. 10-12 A patient is moved up in bed as nursing assistants shift their weight from the rear leg to the front leg.

1 Ask a co-worker to help you.
2 Wash your hands.
3 Identify the patient. Check the ID bracelet and call the patient by name.
4 Explain the procedure to the patient.
5 Provide for privacy.
6 Make sure the bed wheels are locked.
7 Raise the bed to its highest level or to where you can use good body mechanics.
8 Lower the head of the bed to a level appropriate for the patient. It should be as flat as possible.
9 Place the pillow against the headboard if the patient can be without it. This prevents his or her head from hitting the headboard when being moved up.
10 Stand on one side of the bed and have your helper stand on the other side.
11 Lower the side rails.
12 Stand with your feet about 12 inches apart. Point the foot closest to the head of the bed toward the head of the bed and face that direction.
13 Roll the sides of the turning sheet up close to the patient (Fig. 10-13).
14 Grasp the rolled up turning sheet firmly near the patient's shoulders and buttocks.
15 Bend your hips and knees and keep your back straight.
16 Slide the patient up in bed on the count of "3" (Fig. 10-14). Shift your weight from your rear leg to your front leg.
17 Unroll the turning sheet.
18 Put the pillow under the patient's head and shoulders. Straighten linens. Make sure he or she is comfortable and in good body alignment.
19 Place the signal light within reach.
20 Raise the side rails.
21 Raise the head of the bed to a level appropriate for the patient.
22 Lower the bed to its lowest position.
23 Unscreen the patient.
24 Wash your hands.

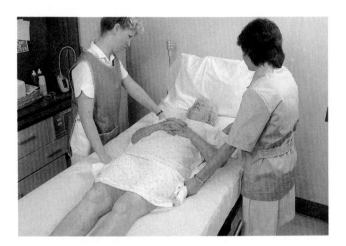

Fig. 10-13 The turning sheet is rolled up close to the patient.

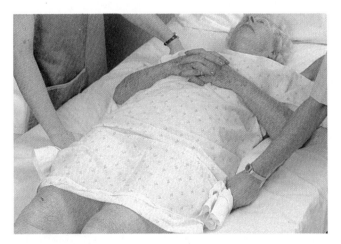

Fig. 10-14 Two nursing assistants move a patient up in bed with a turning sheet. The turning sheet is rolled close to the patient and held near the shoulders and buttocks.

Moving a Patient to the Side of the Bed

Patients are moved to the side of the bed for repositioning and for certain procedures such as a bed bath. A patient in the middle of the bed is moved to the side of the bed before being turned. Otherwise, after turning, the patient will be lying on the side of the bed rather than in the middle. A patient should lie in the middle of the bed to allow for good body alignment.

Sometimes you have to reach over the patient to give care. Good body mechanics can be used if reaching is minimized and if the patient is close to you.

The patient should be in the back-lying position when being moved to the side of the bed. The patient is moved in segments. This can be done by one person. Do not use this procedure for patients with spinal cord injuries or those recovering from spinal surgery. See the box on page 153.

Turning Patients

Patients are turned onto their sides to prevent the complications from bed rest and to receive care. Certain medical and nursing procedures require the side-lying position. Patients are turned toward or away from you. The direction depends on the patient's condition and the situation.

MOVING THE PATIENT TO THE SIDE OF THE BED

1 Wash your hands.
2 Identify the patient. Check the ID bracelet and call the patient by name.
3 Explain the procedure to the patient.
4 Provide for privacy.
5 Make sure the bed wheels are locked.
6 Raise the bed to its highest level or to where you can use good body mechanics.
7 Lower the head of the bed to a level appropriate for the patient. The bed should be as flat as possible.
8 Stand on the side of the bed to which you will move the patient.
9 Make sure the far side rail is raised. Lower the one near you.
10 Stand with your feet about 12 inches apart and with one foot in front of the other. Flex your knees.
11 Cross the patient's arms over the patient's chest.
12 Place your arm under the patient's neck and shoulders and grasp the far shoulder.

13 Place your other arm under the midback.
14 Move the upper part of the patient's body toward you. Rock backward and shift your weight to your rear leg (Fig. 10-15, A).
15 Place one arm under the patient's waist and one under the thighs.
16 Move the lower part of the patient's body toward you by rocking backward (Fig. 10-15, B).
17 Repeat the procedure for the legs and feet as in Figure 10-15, C. Your arms should be under his or her thighs and calves.
18 Make sure the patient is comfortable, in good body alignment, and positioned as directed by the nurse. Reposition the pillow under his or her head and shoulders.
19 Place the signal light within the patient's reach.
20 Raise the side rail near you.
21 Lower the bed to its lowest position.
22 Unscreen the patient.
23 Wash your hands.

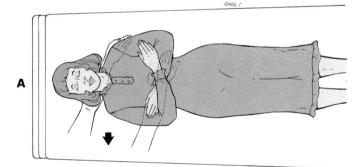

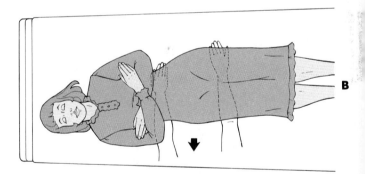

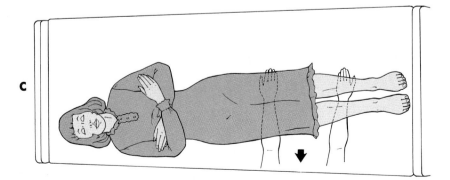

Fig. 10-15 **A,** The patient is moved to the side of the bed in segments. The upper part is moved first as the nursing assistant has one arm under the patient's neck and shoulders and the other under the middle of the back. **B,** The nursing assistant has one arm under the waist and the other under the thighs to move the patient's lower body to the side of the bed. **C,** The patient's legs and feet are moved to the side of the bed. The nursing assistant has one arm under the patient's thighs and the other under the calves.

TURNING THE PATIENT TOWARD YOU

1   Wash your hands.
2   Identify the patient. Check the ID bracelet and call the patient by name.
3   Explain the procedure to the patient.
4   Provide for privacy.
5   Make sure the bed wheels are locked.
6   Raise the bed to its highest level or to where you can use good body mechanics.
7   Lower the head of the bed to a level appropriate for the patient. The bed should be as flat as possible.
8   Stand on the side of the bed opposite to where you will turn the patient. Make sure the far side rail is up.
9   Lower the side rail near you.
10 Move the patient to the side near you.
11 Cross the patient's arms over the patient's chest. Cross the leg near you over the far leg.
12 Raise the side rail.
13 Go to the other side. Lower the side rail.
14 Stand with your feet 12 inches apart. Flex your knees and keep your back straight.
15 Place one hand on the far shoulder and the other on the far hip.
16 Roll the patient toward you gently (Fig. 10-16).
17 Make sure the patient is comfortable and in good body alignment (Fig. 10-17):
    a   Position a pillow against his or her back for support.
    b   Put a pillow under the head and shoulder.
    c   Place a pillow in front of the bottom leg. Place the top leg on top of the pillow in a flexed position.
    d   Support the arm and hand with a small pillow.
18 Place the signal light within reach.
19 Raise the side rail.
20 Lower the bed to its lowest position.
21 Unscreen the patient.
22 Wash your hands.

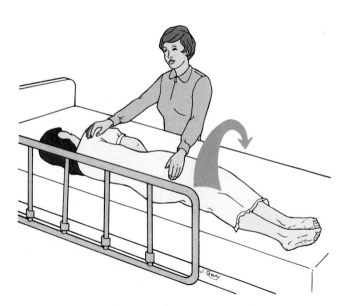

Fig. 10-16   The patient is turned toward the nursing assistant. The patient's arms and legs are crossed, and the nursing assistant has one hand on the patient's far shoulder and the other on the far hip.

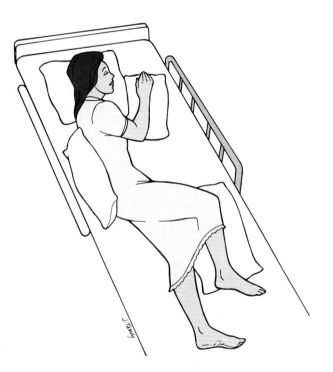

Fig. 10-17   The patient is positioned on the side in the middle of the bed. A pillow is in front of the bottom leg with the top leg on a pillow in the flexed position; a pillow is against the back; a small pillow supports the arm and hand; there is a pillow under the head and shoulder.

1 Follow steps 1 through 11 in *Turning the Patient Toward You* (see page 154.)
2 Stand with your feet about 12 inches apart. Flex your knees and keep your back straight.
3 Place one hand on the patient's shoulder and the other on the buttock near you.
4 Push the patient gently toward the other side of the bed (Fig. 10-18). Shift your weight from your rear leg to your front leg.

5 Make sure the patient is comfortable and in good body alignment. Use pillows to support the patient as in Figure 10-17. (See *Turning the Patient Toward You*, step 17).
6 Raise the side rail.
7 Place the signal light within the patient's reach.
8 Lower the bed to its lowest position.
9 Unscreen the patient.
10 Wash your hands.

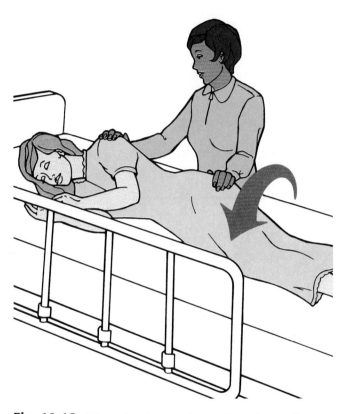

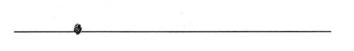

Fig. 10-18 The patient is turned away from the nursing assistant. The patient's arms and legs are crossed, and the nursing assistant has one hand on the patient's shoulder and the other on the patient's buttock.

Fig. 10-19 Logrolling. **A,** There is a pillow between the patient's legs, and the arms are crossed on the chest. The patient is on the far side of the bed. **B,** A turning sheet is used to logroll a patient.

Logrolling

Patients with spinal cord injuries or those recovering from spinal surgery must keep their spines straight at all times. The patient is rolled over in one motion. The back is kept in straight alignment when the patient is turned. *Logrolling* is turning the patient as a unit, in alignment, with one motion. Two workers are needed. Three are needed if a patient is tall or heavy. Sometimes a turning sheet is used for logrolling.

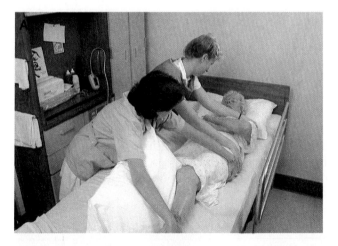

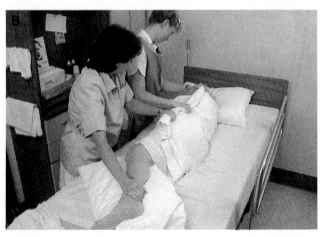

LOGROLLING A PATIENT

1 Ask a co-worker to help you.
2 Wash your hands.
3 Identify the patient. Check the ID bracelet and call the patient by name.
4 Explain the procedure to the patient.
5 Provide for privacy.
6 Make sure the bed wheels are locked.
7 Raise the bed to its highest level or to where you can use good body mechanics.
8 Make sure the bed is flat.
9 Make sure the side rail is up on the side to which the patient will be turned.
10 Stand on the other side. Lower the side rail.
11 Move the patient as a unit to the side of the bed near you. Use the turning sheet.
12 Place the patient's arms across the chest. Place a pillow between the knees (Fig. 10-19, *A*).
13 Raise the side rail. Go to the other side. Lower the side rail.
14 Position yourself near the shoulders and chest. Your helper should stand near the buttocks and thighs.

15 Stand with your feet about 12 inches apart. One foot should be in front of the other.
16 Ask the patient to hold his or her body rigid.
17 Roll the patient toward you as in Fig. 10-19, *A* or use a turning sheet as in Fig. 10-19, *B*. Make sure the patient is turned as a unit.
18 Make sure the patient is comfortable and in good body alignment:
   a Position a pillow against the back for support.
   b Put a pillow under the head and neck if allowed.
   c Place a pillow or folded bath blanket between the legs.
   d Support his or her arm and hand with a small pillow.
19 Place the signal light within reach.
20 Make sure both side rails are up.
21 Lower the bed to its lowest position.
22 Unscreen the patient.
23 Wash your hands.

SITTING ON THE SIDE OF THE BED

Patients are helped to sit on the side of the bed (*dangle*) for many reasons. Some gradually increase activity in stages. They progress from bed rest to sitting on the side of the bed and then to sitting in a chair. Walking in the room and then in the hallway are the next steps. Surgical patients are dangled some time after surgery. While dangling, they cough, deep breathe, and move their legs back and forth and in circles to stimulate circulation. Other reasons for dangling include preparing the patient to walk or for transfer to a chair or wheelchair.

Two workers may be needed. If there is a problem with balance or coordination, the patient must be supported. The patient should lie down if a feeling of faintness occurs. You must make certain observations while the patient is dangling. The patient's pulse and respirations are taken. You should observe for difficulty in breathing and pallor or cyanosis. Also note complaints of dizziness or lightheadedness.

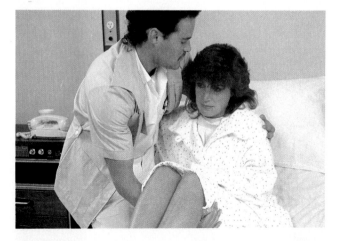

Fig. 10-20 A patient is prepared to sit on the side of the bed. The nursing assistant grasps the far shoulder and far knee.

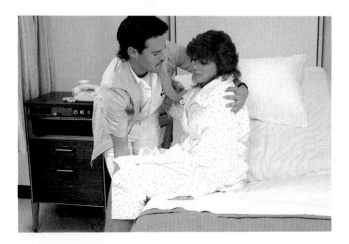

Fig. 10-21 The patient is upright with the legs over the edge of the mattress.

HELPING THE PATIENT TO SIT ON THE SIDE OF THE BED (DANGLE)

1 Explain the procedure to the patient.
2 Collect the following equipment:
  a Robe and slippers or shoes
  b Paper or sheet
3 Wash your hands.
4 Identify the patient. Check the ID bracelet and call the patient by name.
5 Determine which side of the bed to use.
6 Move furniture if necessary to provide moving space for you and the patient.
7 Provide for privacy.
8 Make sure the patient is supine and the bed wheels are locked.
9 Raise the bed to its highest level or to where you can use good body mechanics.
10 Assist the patient in moving up in bed.
11 Prepare the patient to get out of bed:
  a Fanfold top linens to the foot of the bed.
  b Place the paper or sheet under the patient's feet to protect the bottom linen from slippers or shoes.
  c Put the slippers or shoes on the patient.
12 Ask the patient to move to the side of the bed. Assist if necessary.
13 Raise the side rail if the bed is manually operated. Stand near the patient's waist if the bed is electric. This protects the patient from falling out of bed.
14 Raise the head of the bed so that the patient is in a sitting position.
15 Lower the side rail.
16 Slide one arm under the patient's neck and shoulders. Grasp the far shoulder. Place your other hand under the far knee (Fig. 10-20).

17 Turn the patient a quarter of a turn. As the legs go over the edge of the mattress, the trunk will be upright (Fig. 10-21).
18 Ask the patient to push both fists into the mattress (Fig. 10-22). This supports the patient in the sitting position.
19 Do not leave the patient alone. Provide support if necessary.
20 Ask how the patient feels. Check pulse and respirations. Help the patient lie down if necessary.
21 Help the patient put on a robe.
22 Lower the bed to its lowest position if the patient will be getting out of bed.
23 Reverse the procedure to return the patient to bed.
24 Lower the head of the bed after the patient has returned to bed. Help him or her move to the center of the bed.
25 Remove the slippers and the paper or sheet protecting the bottom linen.
26 Make sure the patient is comfortable and in good body alignment. Cover the patient.
27 Place the signal light within reach.
28 Lower the bed to its lowest position.
30 Return the robe and slippers to their proper place.
31 Return furniture to its proper location.
32 Unscreen the patient.
33 Wash your hands.
34 Report the following to the nurse:
  a How the patient tolerated the activity
  b The length of time he or she dangled
  c Pulse and respiratory rates
  d The amount of assistance required
  e Other observations or patient complaints

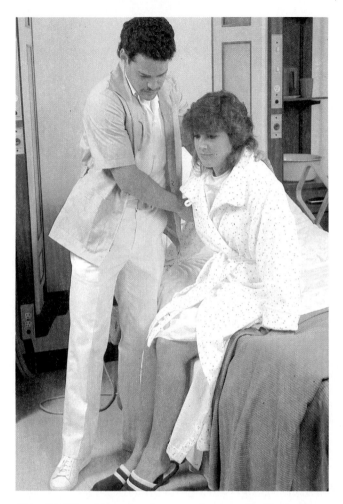

Fig. 10-22 The patient is supporting herself with the fists pushed into the mattress.

TRANSFERRING PATIENTS

Patients are often moved from beds to chairs, wheelchairs, or stretchers. Some need little help in transferring. Semi-helpless patients need the assistance of at least one person. A helpless patient is transferred by 2 or 3 people. The rules of body mechanics and the safety and comfort considerations described for lifting and moving patients also apply when transferring patients. The room should be arranged to allow enough space for a safe transfer. The chair, wheelchair, or stretcher must be placed correctly for a safe and efficient transfer.

A *transfer belt*, or safety belt, is useful when transferring semi-helpless or helpless patients. The belt goes around the patient's waist. You can grasp the belt to support the patient during the transfer. The belt is also called a *gait belt* and is used when walking with a patient.

Transferring a Patient to a Chair or Wheelchair

Safety is very important when transferring a patient to a chair or wheelchair. The patient must be protected from falling. The patient wears street shoes to prevent sliding or slipping on the floor. The chair or wheelchair must be sturdy enough to support the patient's weight. The number of workers needed for a transfer depends on the patient's physical capabilities, condition, and size. Encourage the patient to help in the transfer whenever possible to help increase muscle strength.

Most wheelchairs and bedside chairs have vinyl seats and backs. Vinyl retains body heat, causing the patient to become warmer and perspire more. You can cover the back and seat with a folded bath blanket or put a pillow on the seat. This increases the patient's comfort when in the chair.

You should help the patient out of bed on his or her strong side. If the left side is weak and the right side strong, get the patient out of bed on the right side. When transferring, the strong side moves first and pulls the weaker side along. Transferring a patient from the weak side results in an awkward and unsafe transfer.

The nurse may ask you take the patient's pulse before and after the transfer. The patient may have been on bed rest or may tire with even a little exertion. The pulse rate gives some information about how the activity was tolerated. Also observe and report if the patient tires easily, complains of weakness or being lightheaded, has pain or discomfort, or has difficulty breathing (dyspnea). Also report the amount of help needed and how the patient helped in the transfer.

Mechanical Lifts

Mechanical lifts are used to transfer helpless patients. A patient may be transferred to a chair, stretcher, bathtub, toilet, whirlpool, or car. Before using a lift, make sure it is functioning. You need to compare the patient's weight and the lift's weight limit. The lift must not be used if a patient's weight exceeds its capacity. See the box on page 164.

Many facilities require at least two people to transfer a patient with a mechanical lift. Be sure you know the policy of your facility regarding mechanical lifts.

Moving the Patient to a Stretcher

Patients are transferred to stretchers for transport to other areas. Stretchers are used for patients who are helpless and cannot sit up, those who must remain in a lying position, and for seriously ill patients.

The stretcher is covered with a folded flat sheet or bath blanket. A pillow and extra blankets are available. To increase the patient's comfort, raise the head of the stretcher to a sitting or semi-sitting position.

Text continued on p. 167.

APPLYING A TRANSFER (GAIT) BELT

1. Wash your hands.
2. Identify the patient. Check the ID bracelet and call the patient by name.
3. Explain the procedure to the patient.
4. Provide for privacy.
5. Assist the patient to a sitting position.
6. Apply the belt around the patient's waist over clothing. Do not apply it over bare skin.
7. Tighten the belt so that it is snug. It should not be so tight that it causes discomfort or impairs breathing.
8. Make sure that a woman's breasts are not caught under the belt.
9. Place the buckle either in the front, off center, or in the back for the patient's comfort (Fig. 10-23).

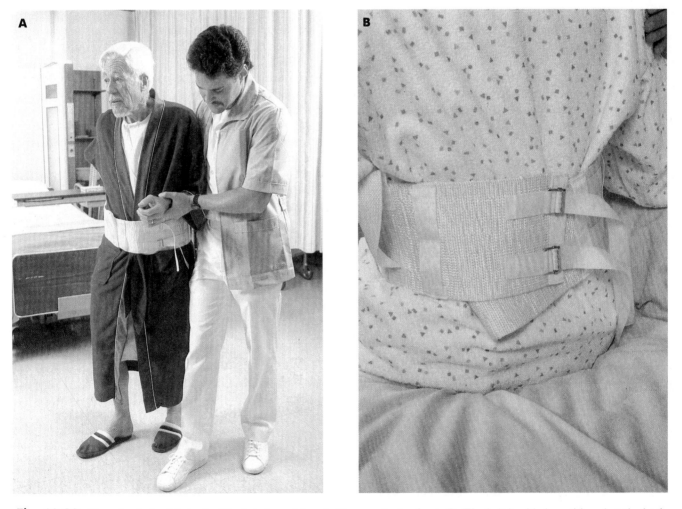

Fig. 10-23 Transfer (safety) belt. **A,** The belt is positioned off center in the front. **B,** The belt buckle is positioned at the back.

TRANSFERRING THE PATIENT TO A CHAIR OR WHEELCHAIR

1 Explain the procedure to the patient.
2 Collect the following equipment:
   a Wheelchair or arm chair
   b One or two bath blankets
   c Robe and shoes
   d Paper or sheet
   e Transfer (gait) belt if needed
   f Pillow
3 Wash your hands.
4 Identify the patient. Check the ID bracelet and call the patient by name.
5 Provide for privacy.
6 Determine which side of the bed to use. Move furniture to provide moving space.
7 Place the chair at the head of the bed. The chair back must be even with the headboard (Fig. 10-24).
8 Place the pillow or folded bath blanket on the seat. Lock the wheelchair wheels and raise the footrests.
9 Make sure the bed is in the lowest position and the bed wheels are locked.
10 Fan-fold top linens to the foot of the bed.
11 Place the paper or sheet under the patient's feet. Put the shoes on the patient.
12 Help the patient dangle. Make sure his or her feet touch the floor.
13 Help the patient put on a robe.
14 Apply the transfer belt if it will be used.
15 Assist the patient to a standing position.
   a Use this method if using a transfer belt:
      1 Stand in front of the patient.
      2 Ask the patient to place his or her hands on your shoulders.
      3 Grasp the transfer belt at each side.
      4 Brace your knees against the patient's knees and block his or her feet with your feet (Fig. 10-25).
      5 Pull the patient up into a standing position as you straighten your knees (Fig. 10-26).
   b Use this method if you are not using a transfer belt:
      1 Stand in front of the patient.
      2 Place your hands under his or her arms. Your hands should be around the shoulder blades (Fig. 10-27).
      3 Ask the patient to push the fists into the mattress and lean forward on the count of "3."
      4 Brace your knees against the patient's knees and block his or her feet with your feet.
      5 Pull the patient up into a standing position on the count of "3." Straighten your knees as you pull the patient up.
16 Support the patient in the standing position. Hold the transfer belt or keep your hands around the patient's shoulder blades. Continue to block the patient's feet and knees with your feet and knees. This helps prevent him or her from falling.
17 Turn the patient so that he or she can grasp the far arm of the chair. His or her legs will touch the edge of the chair as in Figure 10-28.
18 Continue to turn the patient until the other armrest is grasped.
19 Lower him or her into the chair as you bend your hips and knees (Fig. 10-29). The patient assists by leaning forward and bending the elbows and knees.
20 Make sure the buttocks are to the back of the seat. Position the patient in good alignment.
21 Position the feet on the wheelchair footrests.
22 Cover the patient's lap and legs with a bath blanket. Make sure the blanket does not dangle on the floor or hang over the wheels.
23 Remove the transfer belt if used.
24 Position the chair as the patient prefers.
25 Make sure the signal light and other necessary items are within reach.
26 Unscreen the patient.
27 Wash your hands.
28 Report the following to the nurse:
   a The pulse rate if taken
   b How well the activity was tolerated
   c Complaints of lightheadedness, pain, discomfort, difficulty breathing, weakness, or fatigue
   d The amount of assistance required to transfer the patient
29 Reverse the procedure to return the patient to bed.

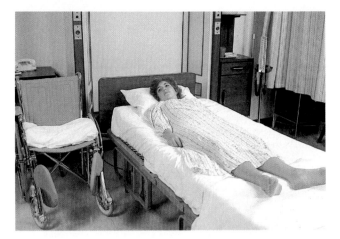

Fig. 10-24 The chair is positioned next to and even with the headboard.

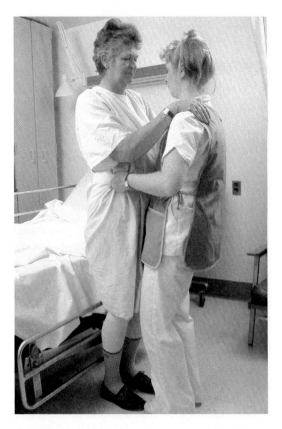

Fig. 10-26 The patient is pulled up to a standing position and supported by holding the transfer belt and blocking the patient's knees and feet.

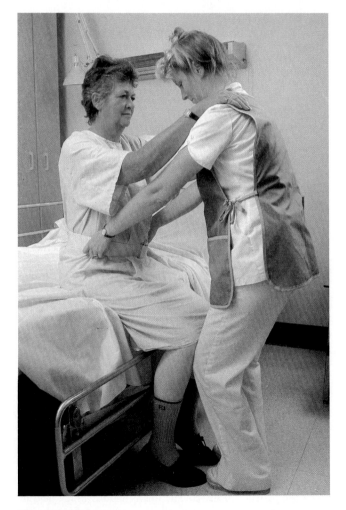

Fig. 10-25 Prevent the patient from sliding or falling by blocking the patient's knees and feet with your own knees and feet.

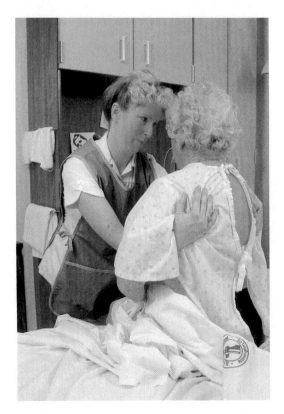

Fig. 10-27 A patient being prepared to stand. The hands are placed under the patient's arms and around to the shoulder blades.

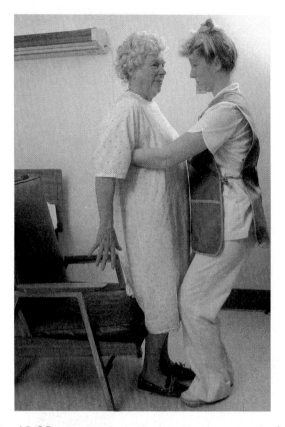

Fig. 10-28   The patient is supported as she grasps the far arm of the chair. The legs are against the chair.

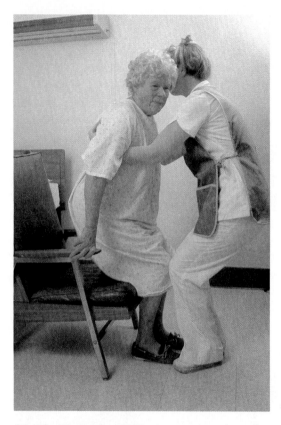

Fig. 10-29   The patient holds the arm rests, leans forward, and bends the elbows and knees while being lowered into the chair.

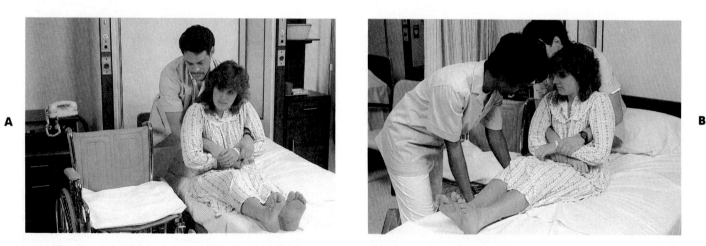

Fig. 10-30   A, Grasp the patient's forearms by putting your arms under the patient's arms. **B,** The thighs and calves are held to support the lower extremities during a transfer.

TRANSFERRING THE PATIENT TO A WHEELCHAIR (TWO WORKERS)

1 Ask a co-worker to help you.
2 Explain the procedure to the patient.
3 Collect the following equipment:
   a Wheelchair with removable armrests
   b Bath blankets
   c Shoes
   d Pillow
4 Wash your hands.
5 Identify the patient. Check the ID bracelet and call the patient by name.
6 Provide for privacy.
7 Determine which side of the bed to use. Move furniture to provide moving space.
8 Fanfold top linens to the foot of the bed.
9 Assist the patient to the side of the bed near you. Help him or her to a sitting position by raising the head of the bed.
10 Place the wheelchair by the bed so that the seat is even with the patient's hips.
11 Remove the armrest near the bed. Put the pillow or a folded bath blanket on the seat.
12 Lock the wheelchair wheels.
13 Stand behind the wheelchair at the head of the bed. Put your arms under the patient's arms and grasp the forearms (Fig. 10-30, *A*).
14 Have your assistant grasp the patient's thighs and calves (Fig. 10-30, *B*).

15 Bring the patient toward the chair on the count of "3." Lower him or her into the chair as in Figure 10-31.
16 Make sure the buttocks are to the back of the seat. Position the patient in good alignment.
17 Put the armrest back on the wheelchair.
18 Put the shoes on the patient. Position the feet on the footrests.
19 Cover the patient's lap and legs with a bath blanket. Make sure the blanket is not dangling on the floor or over the wheels.
20 Position the chair as the patient prefers.
21 Make sure the signal light and other necessary items are within reach.
22 Unscreen the patient.
23 Wash your hands.
24 Report the following to the nurse:
   a The pulse rate if taken
   b Complaints of lightheadedness, pain, discomfort, difficulty breathing, weakness, or fatigue
   c How well the activity was tolerated
25 Reverse the procedure to return the patient to bed.

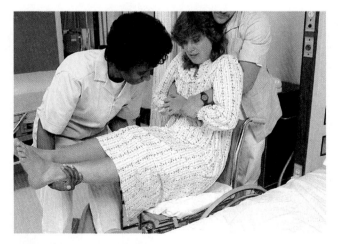

Fig. 10-31 The patient is supported while being lowered into the chair.

USING A MECHANICAL LIFT

1 Ask a co-worker to help you.
2 Explain the procedure to the patient.
3 Collect the following equipment:
   a Mechanical lift
   b Arm chair or wheelchair
   c Slippers
4 Wash your hands.
5 Identify the patient. Check the ID bracelet and call the patient by name.
6 Provide for privacy.
7 Center the sling under the patient. Turn him or her from side to side as if making an occupied bed to position the sling (see Chapter 12). The lower edge of the sling should be behind the knees (Fig. 10-32).
8 Place the chair at the head of the bed. It should be even with the headboard and about 1 foot away from the bed. Place a folded bath blanket in the chair.
9 Make sure the bed wheels are locked and the bed is in its lowest position.
10 Raise the head of the bed so that the patient is sitting.
11 Tighten the release valve so that it is closed (Fig. 10-33).
12 Raise the lift so that it can be positioned over the patient.
13 Widen the base by spreading the legs of the lift. Lock the legs in position.
14 Position the lift over the patient (Fig. 10-34).
15 Attach the sling to the straps or chains. Fasten hooks away from the patient (Fig. 10-35).

16 Attach the sling to the swivel bar (Fig. 10-36).
17 Cross the patient's arms over the chest. Let him or her hold onto the straps or chains, but not the swivel bar.
18 Pump the lift high enough until the patient and sling are free of the bed (Fig. 10-37).
19 Ask your co-worker to support the legs as you move the lift and patient away from the bed (Fig. 10-38).
20 Position the lift so that the patient's back is toward the chair.
21 Open the release valve slowly to gently lower the patient into the chair. Guide him or her into the chair as in Figure 10-39.
22 Lower the bar to unhook the sling. Leave the sling under the patient unless otherwise indicated.
23 Put the slippers on the patient. Position the feet on the footrests if a wheelchair is used.
24 Cover the patient's lap and legs with a bath blanket. Make sure the blanket is not dangling on the floor or over the wheels.
25 Position the chair as the patient prefers.
26 Make sure the signal light and other necessary items are within reach.
27 Wash your hands.
28 Report the following to the nurse:
   a The pulse rate if taken
   b Complaints of lightheadedness, pain, discomfort, difficulty breathing, weakness, or fatigue
   c How well the activity was tolerated
29 Reverse the procedure to return the patient to bed.

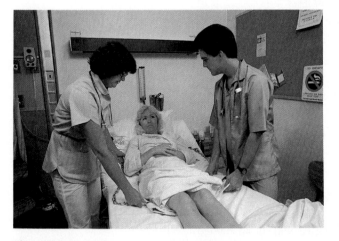

Fig. 10-32 The sling of the mechanical lift is positioned under the patient. The lower edge of the sling is behind the patient's knees.

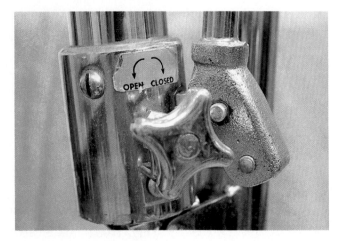

Fig. 10-33 Release valve.

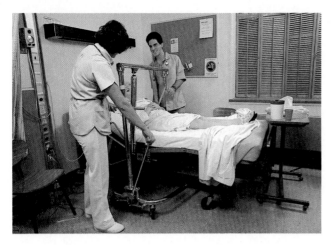

Fig. 10-34 The lift is positioned over the patient and the legs of the lift are spread to widen the base of support.

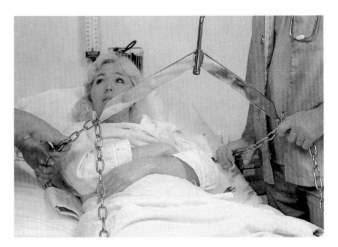

Fig. 10-35 The sling is attached so that the hooks are turned away from the patient's body.

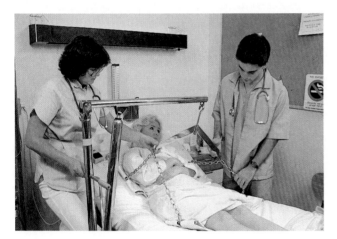

Fig. 10-36 The sling is attached to a swivel bar.

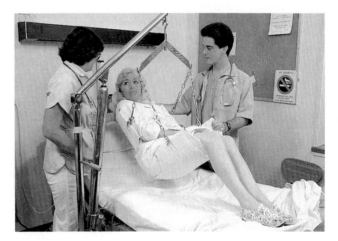

Fig. 10-37 The lift is raised until the sling and patient are off of the bed.

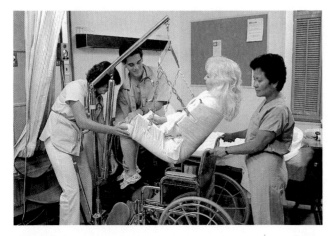

Fig. 10-38 The patient's legs are supported as the patient and lift are moved away from the bed.

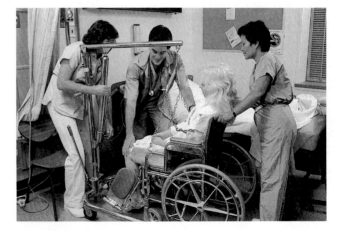

Fig. 10-39 The patient is guided into a chair.

MOVING THE PATIENT ONTO A STRETCHER WITH A DRAWSHEET
(3 ASSISTANTS)

1 Ask two co-workers to help you.
2 Explain the procedure to the patient.
3 Collect the following equipment:
   a Stretcher covered with a sheet or bath blanket
   b Bath blanket
   c Sheet or drawsheet
   d Pillow(s) if needed
4 Wash your hands.
5 Identify the patient. Check the ID bracelet and call the patient by name.
6 Provide for privacy.
7 Raise the bed to its highest level.
8 Cover the patient with a bath blanket. Fanfold top linens to the foot of the bed.
9 Loosen the cotton drawsheet on each side.
10 Lower the head of the bed so that it is as flat as possible.
11 Lower the side rail on the side to which the patient will be moved.
12 Ask your co-workers to help move the patient to the side of the bed with the drawsheet.
13 Go to the other side of the bed. Lower the side rail. Protect the patient from falling by holding the far arm and leg.
14 Have the co-workers position the stretcher next to the bed and stand behind the stretcher (Fig. 10-40).

15 Make sure the bed and stretcher wheels are locked.
16 Lay the clean sheet (or drawsheet) over the bottom sheet on the empty side of the bed.
17 Kneel on the bed at the patient's waist.
18 Roll up and grasp the drawsheet at the hip and mid-chest levels.
19 Ask your helpers to roll up and grasp the drawsheet. This supports the entire length of the patient's body.
20 Transfer the patient to the stretcher on the count of "3" by lifting and pulling him or her (Fig. 10-41). Make sure the patient is centered on the stretcher.
21 Place a pillow or pillows under the patient's head and shoulders if allowed.
22 Make sure the patient is covered and comfortable.
23 Fasten safety straps and raise the side rails.
24 Unlock the stretcher's wheels. Transport the patient.
25 Wash your hands.
26 Report the following to the nurse:
   a The time of the transport
   b Where the patient was transported to
   c Who accompanied him or her
   d How he or she tolerated the transfer
27 Reverse the procedure to return the patient to bed.

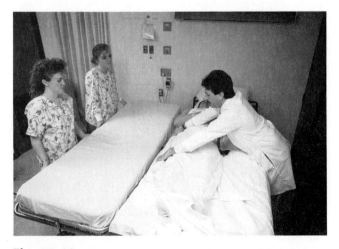

Fig. 10-40 The textrcher is against the bed and is held in place by two nursing assistants.

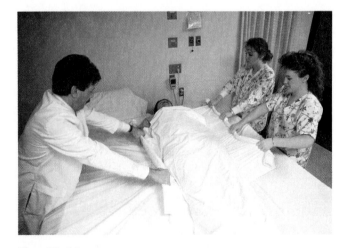

Fig. 10-41 The patient is transferred from the bed to a stretcher with workers using a drawsheet.

Safety straps are applied after the patient is transferred to the stretcher. The stretcher's side rails are kept up when transporting the patient. Move the patient's feet first so that the helper at the head of the stretcher can watch the patient's breathing and color during the transport. A patient on a stretcher must never be left unattended.

Using a drawsheet A drawsheet can be used to transfer a patient from the bed to a stretcher. At least 3 workers are needed for a safe transfer. Remember to keep the patient in good body alignment and to use good body mechanics.

POSITIONING

The patient must be properly positioned whether in bed or sitting in a chair. Physical comfort and well-being are promoted with regular position changes and good alignment. Breathing is easier and circulation is promoted. Proper positioning also helps prevent many complications. These include pressure areas on bony parts (see Chapter 13) and deformities (see Chapter 18). Some patients must be repositioned every hour or every 2 hours.

The doctor may order a particular position for a patient. A doctor may also restrict a patient from a certain position. You need to consult with the nurse and check the patient's care plan about position changes. You need to know how often to turn a patient and to what position. Other safety considerations include using good body mechanics and getting help if it is needed. Also be sure to explain the procedure to the patient. Be gentle when moving the patient and provide for privacy. The signal light must be within reach after repositioning.

Basic Positions for the Patient in Bed

Good body alignment and position changes are essential for patients confined to bed. Some patients can change positions without help, and others need some assistance. Others depend entirely on nursing personnel for position changes.

Fowler's position *Fowler's position* involves raising the head of the bed to a semi-sitting position. The head of the bed is raised 45 to 60 degrees. Good alignment for Fowler's position involves keeping the spine straight, supporting the head with a small pillow, and supporting the arms with pillows (Fig. 10-42). Patients with heart and respiratory disorders usually breathe more easily in Fowler's position. Eating, watching television, visiting, and reading are easier in Fowler's position.

Supine position The *supine* or *dorsal recumbent* position is the back-lying position. Good alignment involves having the bed flat, supporting the head and shoulders on a pillow, and placing the arms and hands at the patient's sides. The arms may be supported with regular-size pillows. The hands may be supported on small pillows with the palms down as in Figure 10-43.

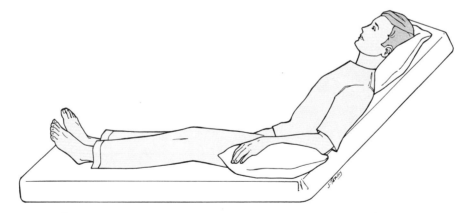

Fig. 10-42 Fowler's position. Pillows are used to maintain alignment.

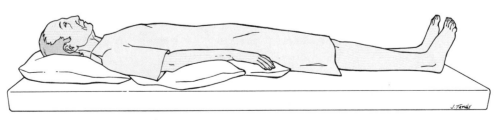

Fig. 10-43 Patient in supine position.

The nurse may ask you to place a folded or rolled towel under the small of the patient's back. A small pillow may be placed under the patient's thighs if requested by the nurse.

Prone position Patients in the *prone position* lie on their abdomens with their heads turned to one side.

Position the patient in good alignment by placing a small pillow under the head, one under the abdomen, and one under the lower legs (Fig. 10-44). The arms are flexed at the elbows with the hands near the head. Patients can also be positioned so that their feet hang over the end of the mattress (Fig. 10-45). If feet hang over the mattress, a pillow is not used under the lower legs.

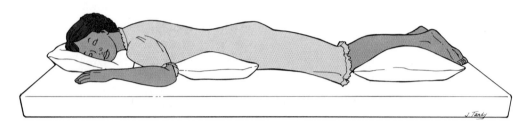

Fig. 10-44   Patient in prone position.

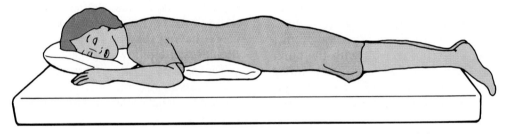

Fig. 10-45   Patient in prone position with the feet hanging over the edge of the mattress.

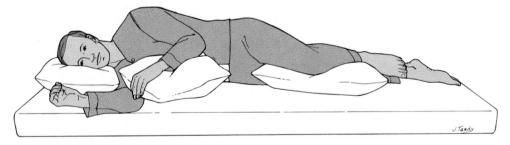

Fig. 10-46   Patient in lateral position with pillows used for support.

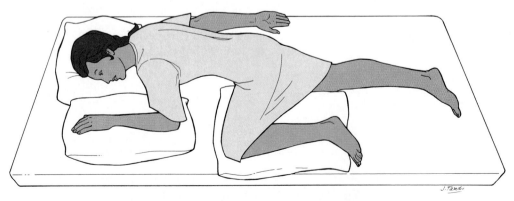

Fig. 10-47   Patient supported with pillows in Sims' position.

Lateral position A patient in the *lateral* or *side-lying position* lies on one side or the other (Fig. 10-46). Good alignment includes placing a pillow under the head and shoulders and supporting the upper leg and thigh with pillows. A small pillow is placed under the upper hand and arm, and a pillow is positioned against the patient's back.

Sims' position The *Sims' position* is a side-lying position. The upper leg is sharply flexed so that it is not on the lower leg, and the lower arm is behind the patient (Fig. 10-47). Good alignment involves placing a pillow under the patient's head and shoulder, supporting the upper leg with a pillow, and placing a pillow under the upper arm and hand.

Positioning in a Chair

Patients who sit in chairs must be able to hold their upper bodies and heads erect. Poor alignment results if the patient cannot stay in an erect position. The patient's back and buttocks should be against the back of the chair. Feet should be flat on the floor or on the wheelchair footrests. Backs of the knees and calves should be slightly away from the edge of the seat (Fig. 10-48). With the nurse's permission, you may put a small pillow between the patient's lower back and the chair. This gives support to the lower back. Paralyzed arms are positioned on pillows. Wrists are positioned at a slight upward angle (Fig. 10-49).

Patients may need postural supports if they cannot keep their upper bodies erect. Postural supports help keep patients in good body alignment. The jacket restraint (see Chapter 8) is sometimes used to support posture. The jacket restraint is used for this purpose only with the nurse's approval. The patient and family must clearly understand the purpose of the device. The safety rules described in Chapter 8 apply when the jacket restraint is used as a postural support.

SUMMARY

Good body mechanics must be used whenever lifting, moving, and transferring patients to protect yourself and them from injury. You need to keep yourself and

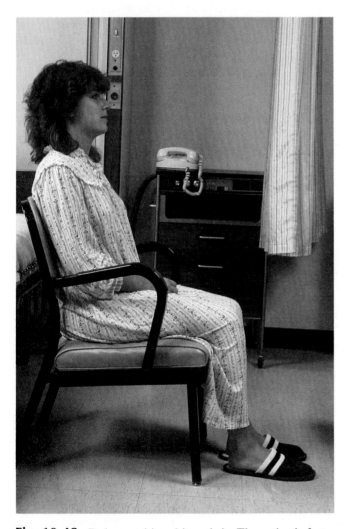

Fig. 10-48 Patient positioned in a chair. The patient's feet are flat on the floor, the calves do not touch the chair, and the back is straight and against the back of the chair.

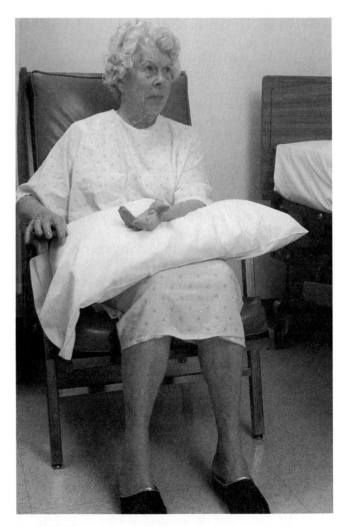

Fig. 10-49 A pillow is used to support the paralyzed arm. Note that the wrist is at a slight upward angle.

the patient in good alignment to promote comfort and well-being.

You have learned several ways to move, lift, transfer, and position patients. Their comfort and safety must always be considered during these activities. Be sure you know of any position restrictions ordered for a patient. Also be sure to provide for privacy and to protect the patient from falling. Encourage the patient to help with repositioning or transfers to the extent possible.

You may need to change some life-long habits in relation to your posture and the way you move your body. As you use good body mechanics, you will feel better and work with greater efficiency. Remember to follow the rules of body mechanics in all activities.

REVIEW QUESTIONS

Circle T *if the answer is true and* F *if the answer is false.*

T F **1** Body mechanics is the way body segments are aligned with one another.

T F **2** Good body mechanics helps protect you and your patients from injury.

T F **3** Base of support is the area on which an object rests.

T F **4** Objects are kept away from the body when lifting, moving, or carrying them.

T F **5** Face the direction in which you are working to prevent unnecessary twisting.

T F **6** Push, slide, or pull heavy objects rather than lift them.

T F **7** Consult with the nurse for any limitations or restrictions in positioning or moving a patient.

T F **8** The right to privacy must be protected when moving, lifting, or transferring patients.

T F **9** If help is needed to move a patient, ask a co-worker to help before you begin the procedure.

T F **10** A turning sheet should extend from the patient's shoulders to above the knees.

T F **11** A patient is moved to the side of the bed before being turned to the side-lying position.

T F **12** Logrolling is rolling the patient in segments.

T F **13** Patients with spinal cord injuries are logrolled.

T F **14** A patient may dangle to gradually increase activity.

T F **15** A transfer belt is part of a mechanical lift.

T F **16** A patient should be moved from the direction of the weak side of the body.

T F **17** Safety straps are applied only if the patient will be left unattended on a stretcher.

T F **18** Repositioning is essential to prevent deformities and pressure on body parts.

T F **19** The head of the bed is elevated 45 to 60 degrees for the supine position.

T F **20** The Sims' position is a side-lying position.

Circle the best *answer.*

21 Body mechanics involves the following *except*
  a Good posture
  b Balance
  c The small muscles of the body
  d The large muscles of the body

22 The small muscles of the body are located in the
  a Back
  b Shoulders
  c Upper arms
  d Hips and thighs

23 Which will *not* reduce friction?
  a Sliding the patient
  b Lifting the patient
  c Rolling the patient
  d Using a turning sheet

24 A patient is to be transferred from the bed to a chair. The patient should
  a Be barefoot
  b Wear socks
  c Wear slippers
  d Wear street shoes

25 A patient is positioned in a chair. Which is *false?*
  a The patient's back and buttocks should be against the back of the chair.
  b The patient's feet should be flat on the floor or wheelchair footrests.
  c A paralyzed arm should rest on the patient's lap.
  d The backs of the knees and calves should be away from the chair.

Answers

25	c	**17**	False	**9**	True
24	d	**16**	False	**8**	True
23	a	**15**	False	**7**	True
22	a	**14**	True	**6**	True
21	c	**13**	True	**5**	True
20	True	**12**	False	**4**	False
19	False	**11**	True	**3**	True
18	True	**10**	True	**2**	True
				1	False

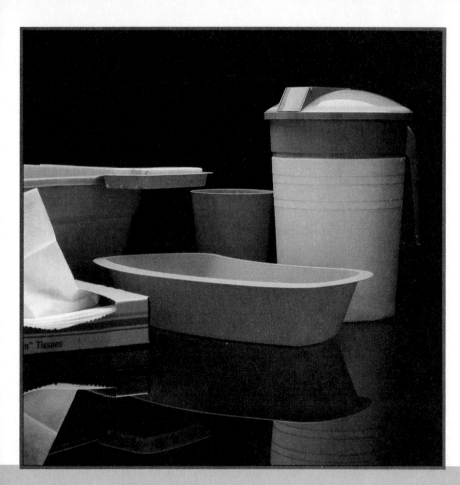

The Patient Unit

OBJECTIVES

- Define the key terms listed in this chapter
- Identify the temperature range that is comfortable for most people
- Describe how to protect patients from drafts
- List ways to prevent or reduce odors in patient rooms
- Identify the common causes of noise in health care facilities and how noise can be controlled
- Explain how lighting can affect the patient's comfort
- Know the basic bed positions
- Describe the use of furniture and equipment found in a patient unit
- Describe how a bathroom is equipped for the patient's use
- Explain how to maintain the patient's unit

caster A small wheel made of rubber or plastic

patient pack Personal care equipment provided by the health care facility (wash basin, emesis or kidney basin, bedpan, urinal, water pitcher and glass, soap, and soap dish)

patient unit The furniture and equipment provided for the individual by the health care facility

reverse Trendelenburg's position The head of the bed is raised, and the foot of the bed is lowered

semi-Fowler's position The head of the bed is raised 45 degrees, and the knee portion is raised 15 degrees; or the head of the bed is raised 30 degrees

Trendelenburg's position The head of the bed is lowered, and the foot of the bed is raised

Patients in hospitals and residents of long-term care facilities spend a lot of time in their rooms. Rooms may be private, for one person, or semiprivate, furnished for two people. Rooms should be comfortable and safe. There should be enough space for the individual to perform activities of daily living. This chapter describes the furnishings in a patient unit and the conditions that influence comfort. A *patient unit* is the furniture and equipment provided for the individual by the health care facility (Fig. 11-1).

COMFORT

Age, illness, and activity affect comfort. Comfort is also influenced by temperature, ventilation, noise, and odors. These conditions can usually be controlled to meet the person's needs.

Temperature and Ventilation

Health care facilities have heating, air conditioning, and ventilation systems. These systems maintain a comfortable temperature and provide fresh air in the rooms. A temperature range of 68° F to 74° F is usually comfortable for most healthy people. A comfortable temperature for one person may be too hot or too cold for another. Infants, the elderly, and ill persons generally need higher room temperatures to be comfortable. Therefore higher temperatures are usually needed in hospitals and nursing facilities. Physically active people are usually more comfortable where it is cooler.

Stale room air and lingering odors may cause a person to be uncomfortable and unable to rest. A good ventilation system provides fresh air and moves air in the room. Drafts can occur as air moves. In-fants, the elderly, and ill persons are sensitive to drafts. You can protect them from drafts by having them wear enough clothing. You should also make sure they are adequately covered with blankets. Move them from drafty areas whenever possible.

Odors

Many odors occur in health facilities. Some are pleasant, like food aromas and the scents of fresh flowers. Others are unpleasant. Draining wounds, vomitus, and bowel movements create unpleasant smells and can embarrass the patient. Body, breath, and smoking odors may be offensive to patients, visitors, and personnel. Ill people are usually very sensitive to odors and can become nauseated. Good ventilation helps eliminate odors. Nursing personnel can reduce odors by emptying and washing bedpans and emesis basins promptly and using room deodorizers when necessary. Good personal hygiene prevents body and breath odors.

Smoking presents special problems. Patients may be assigned to rooms on the basis of whether they smoke. If you smoke, do so only in designated areas. Wash your hands after handling smoking materials and before giving patient care. Careful attention must be given to uniforms, hair, and breath because of clinging smoke odors.

Many facilities ban smoking. Patients, staff, and visitors are not allowed to smoke anywhere in the building.

Noise

Ill people are sensitive to the noises and sounds around them. Patients and residents may be easily disturbed by common health care sounds. The clanging of metal equipment, such as bedpans, urinals, and wash basins, and the clatter of dishes and trays may be annoying. Loud talking and laughter in hallways and at the nurses' station, loud televisions and radios, ringing telephones, and the buzzing of an intercom system can be irritating. Noise from equipment in need of repair or oil is also disturbing. Wheels on stretchers, wheelchairs, utility carts, and other equipment must be oiled properly.

When in a strange place, people try to figure out the cause and meaning of strange sounds. This relates to the basic need to feel safe and secure. Patients may find sounds dangerous, frightening, or irritating. As a result, they may be upset, anxious, and uncomfortable. You must remember that what is noise to one person may not be noise to another. For example, a teenager's loud stereo music may be quite irritating to parents.

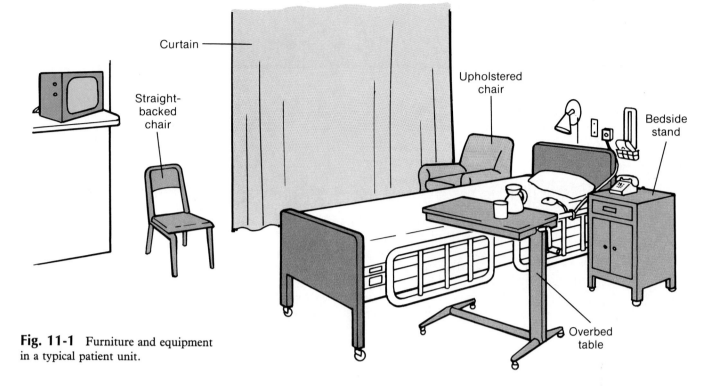

Fig. 11-1 Furniture and equipment in a typical patient unit.

Health care facilities are designed to reduce noise. Drapes, carpeting, and acoustical tiles all help absorb noise. Plastic equipment has replaced some metal equipment (bedpans, urinals, and wash basins). Workers can reduce noise by controlling the loudness of their voices and by handling equipment carefully. Making sure equipment is working properly and answering telephones and intercoms promptly also decrease noise.

Lighting

Good lighting is necessary for the safety and comfort of patients and staff. Glares, shadows, and dull lighting can cause falls, headaches, and eyestrain. People usually relax and rest better when lighting is dim. However, a bright room is more cheerful and stimulating.

Lighting can be adjusted to meet the changing needs of the patient. Shades can be pulled or drapes drawn to control natural light. The light above the bed usually can be adjusted to provide soft, medium, and bright lighting. Some facilities have ceiling lights over the beds. These provide lighting that may be very low to extremely bright. Bright lighting is helpful when health workers are performing procedures. Light controls should be within the patient's reach.

ROOM FURNITURE AND EQUIPMENT

Patient or resident rooms are furnished and equipped for the person's basic needs. There is furniture and equipment for comfort, sleep, elimination, nutrition, personal hygiene, and activity. There is also equipment for communicating with the nursing team, relatives, and friends. The right to privacy is considered when equipping the room.

The Bed

Hospital beds are adjusted electrically or manually. They can be raised horizontally so that care can be given without unnecessary bending or reaching. The lowest horizontal position lets the patient get out of bed with ease. The head of the bed can be kept flat or raised to varying degrees.

Electric beds are the most common. Bed positions are easily changed by use of hand controls. The location of the controls varies with the manufacturer. They may be on a side panel, attached to the bed by a cable, or on a panel at the foot of the bed (Fig. 11-2). Patients and residents need to know how to use the controls. They should be warned not to raise the bed to the high position and not to adjust the bed to harmful positions. They should be told if they are limited or restricted to certain positions.

Hand cranks are used to change the position of manually operated beds. The cranks are at the foot of the bed (Fig. 11-3). The left crank raises or lowers the head of the bed. The right crank adjusts the knee portion. The center crank raises or lowers the entire bed. The cranks are pulled up for use and kept down at all other times. Cranks kept in the "up" position are safety hazards because anyone walking past may bump into them.

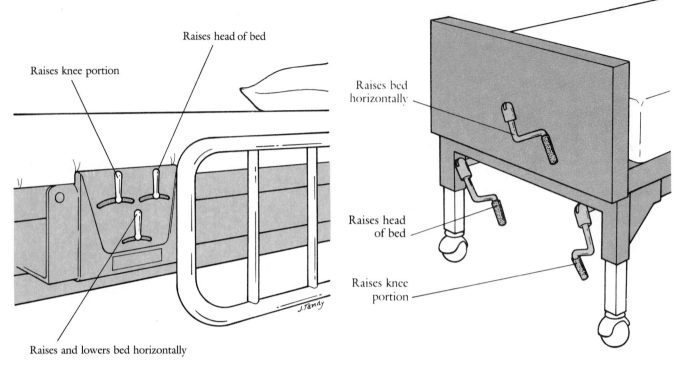

Raises head of bed

Raises knee portion

Raises and lowers bed horizontally

Fig. 11-2 Controls for an electric bed.

Raises bed horizontally

Raises head of bed

Raises knee portion

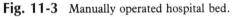

Fig. 11-3 Manually operated hospital bed.

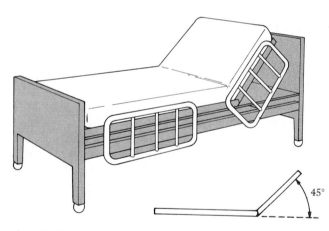

45°

Fig. 11-4 Fowler's position.

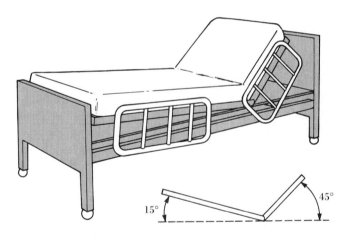

15° 45°

Fig. 11-5 Semi-Fowler's position.

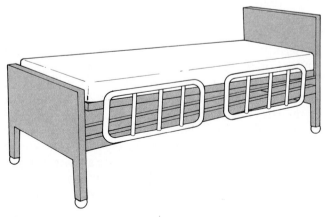

Fig. 11-6 Trendelenburg's position.

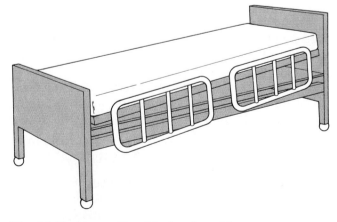

Fig. 11-7 Reverse Trendelenburg's position.

Bed positions There are four basic bed positions: Fowler's, semi-Fowler's, Trendelenburg's, and reverse Trendelenburg's.

Fowler's position is a semisitting position. The head of the bed is elevated 45 to 60 degrees (Fig. 11-4). The reasons for positioning a patient in Fowler's position are described in Chapter 10.

In *semi-Fowler's position* the head of the bed is raised 45 degrees and the knee portion is raised 15 degrees (Fig. 11-5). This position is comfortable and prevents patients from sliding down in bed. However, raising the knee portion can interfere with circulation. Consult with the nurse before positioning a patient in the semi-Fowler's position. Many facilities define semi-Fowler's position as when the head of the bed is elevated 30 degrees and the knee portion is *not* raised. You must know which definition your employer uses so that the patient is cared for safely.

Trendelenburg's position involves lowering the head of the bed and raising the foot of the bed (Fig. 11-6). This position is used only when ordered by a doctor or nurse. Blocks are placed under the lower legs of the bed. Some beds are made so that the entire bedframe can be tilted into Trendelenburg's position.

Reverse Trendelenburg's position is the opposite of Trendelenburg's position. The head of the bed is elevated and the foot of the bed lowered (Fig. 11-7). Blocks are put under the legs at the head of the bed, or the bedframe is tilted. This position also requires a doctor's order.

Safety Considerations

Bed legs usually have wheels or casters. A *caster* is a small wheel made of rubber or plastic that allows the bed to move easily. Each wheel or caster has a lock to prevent the bed from moving (Fig. 11-8). You must make sure the bed wheels are locked when giving bedside care. They should also be locked when you are transferring a patient to and from the bed. The patient can be injured if the bed moves.

The importance of side rails on hospital beds is discussed in Chapter 8.

The Overbed Table

The overbed table (see Fig. 11-1) can be positioned over the bed by sliding the base under the bed. You can raise or lower the table by turning the side handle. The height can be adjusted for the patient in bed or in a chair. The overbed table is used for meal trays and for eating, writing, reading, and other activities.

Many overbed tables have movable tops with a storage area underneath. The storage area is often used for makeup, hair care articles, or shaving items. Many also have a flip-up mirror.

The nursing team can use the overbed table as a working area. Only clean and sterile items are placed on the table. Be sure to clean the table after using it as a working surface.

The Bedside Stand

The bedside stand is located next to the bed. The stand is a storage area for the patient's personal belongings and personal care equipment. It has a drawer at the top and a lower cabinet with a shelf (Fig. 11-9). The drawer can be used for money, eyeglasses, books, and other personal possessions. The first shelf is used for the wash basin, which can hold personal

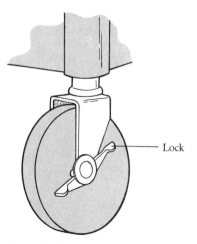

Fig. 11-8 Lock on a bed wheel.

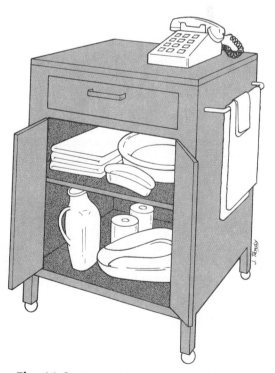

Fig. 11-9 The bedside stand is used to store the patient's personal care equipment.

care items. These include soap and soap dish, powder, lotion, deodorant, towels, washcloth, bath blanket, and a clean gown or pajamas. An emesis or kidney basin is often used to hold oral hygiene equipment. The kidney basin can be stored on the top shelf or in the drawer. The bedpan and its cover, the urinal, and toilet paper are on the lower shelf.

The top of the stand is often used for tissues and the telephone. The top may also be used for a radio, flowers, gifts, cards, and other items that are important to the patient. Some stands have a rod at the side or back for towels and washcloths.

Chairs

The patient unit usually has at least two chairs. One is a straight-back chair with no arms, and the other is an upholstered chair with arms. The upholstered chair is used most frequently by the patient and visitors. It is placed near the bed.

Curtains or Screens

Semiprivate rooms have a curtain between the two patient units. The curtain can be pulled around either bed to provide privacy for the patient. The curtain is always pulled while care is being given. If a portable screen is used (Fig. 11-10), it is placed between the two beds. Curtains and screens protect the patient from being seen by others. However, they do not block sound or prevent conversations from being overheard.

Personal Care Equipment

Personal care equipment refers to the items needed for hygiene and elimination. A *patient pack* is provided by the facility. It usually includes a wash basin, emesis or kidney basin, bedpan, urinal, water pitcher

and glass, and soap and soap dish. Powder, lotion, toothbrush, toothpaste, mouthwash, tissues, and a comb may also be provided. Usually patients bring their own oral hygiene equipment, hair care supplies, and deodorant. Some choose to use their own soap, lotion, and powder.

Call System

The call system lets the patient signal when help is needed. A signal light at the bedside is connected to a light above the room door and to a light panel or intercom system at the nurses' station. The signal light is at the end of a long cord. It can be attached to the bed or chair so that it is always within the patient's reach. The patient presses a button at the end of the signal light when assistance is needed (Fig. 11-11). The nurse or nursing assistant shuts off the light at the bedside when the patient is given the help needed.

An intercom system lets a member of the nursing team talk with the patient from the nurses' station. It also allows the light to be turned off from the station. Sometimes a tap bell is used in place of the signal light (Fig. 11-12). The signal light or tap bell must always be on the patient's good side. Patients are shown how to use the call system when admitted to the facility.

The Bathroom

Many health care facilities have a bathroom in each room. Some have a bathroom between two patient rooms. A toilet, sink, call system, and mirror are standard equipment. Some bathrooms are equipped with a shower or a tub and shower (Fig. 11-13). Hand rails, which the patient can use for support, are installed by the toilet. Toilets in some facilities are

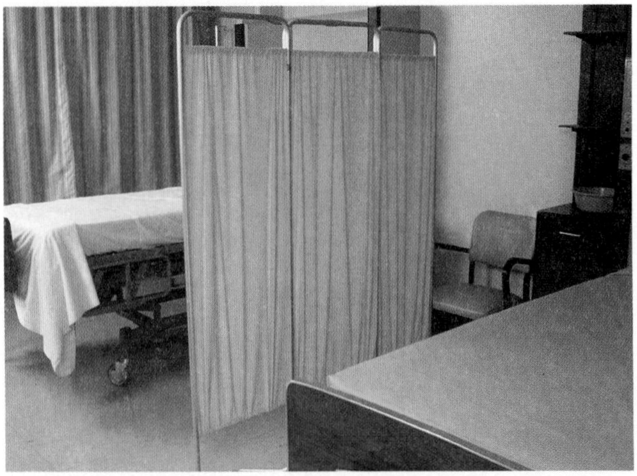

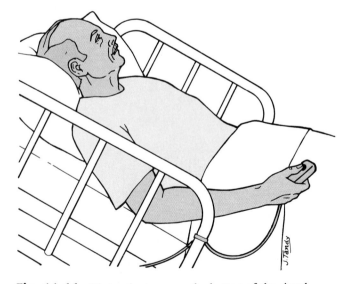

Fig. 11-11 The patient presses the button of the signal light when assistance is needed.

Fig. 11-10 Portable screen between two patient units.

higher than the standard toilet. The higher toilets make transfers to and from wheelchairs easier and are helpful for patients with joint problems.

Towel racks, toilet paper, soap, a paper towel dispenser, and the call system are found in the bathroom. They are placed within easy reach of the patient.

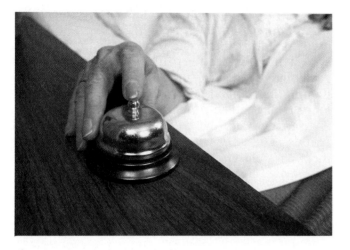

Fig. 11-12 Tap bell.

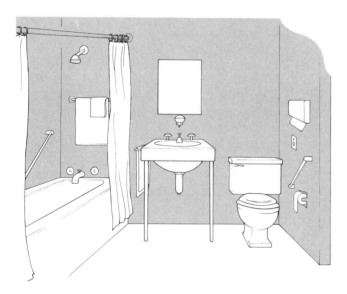

Fig. 11-13 Patient's bathroom in a health care facility.

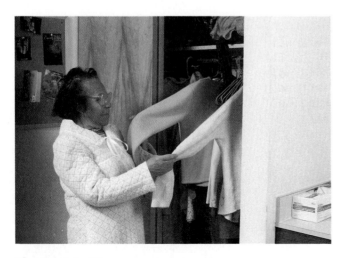

Fig. 11-14 The resident can access items in her closet.

Closet and Drawer Space

Most hospitals provide closet and extra drawer space for the patient's clothing. OBRA (see Chapter 7) requires nursing facilities to provide each resident with closet space. Such closet space must have shelves and a clothes rack (Fig. 11-14). The resident must have free access to the closet and its contents.

Items in the closet or drawers are the person's private property. You must not search the closet or drawers without the person's permission.

Sometimes people hoard items like napkins, straws, sugar, salt and pepper, and food in their drawers. Such hoarding can cause safety or health risks. Facility representatives can inspect a person's closet or drawers if hoarding is suspected. The person must be informed of the inspection and must be in the room when it takes place.

Other Equipment

Many facilities furnish patient units with additional equipment. A television and radio are often included for comfort and relaxation, along with a telephone for talking to family and friends. A wastebasket is placed by the bed.

Blood pressure equipment is often mounted on walls. There are also wall outlets for oxygen and suction (see Fig. 11-1). An IV pole (IV standard) is used to hang an intravenous infusion bottle or bag. Some hospital beds have an IV pole stored in the bedframe. The IV pole may be a separate piece of equipment that is brought to the patient's unit when needed.

General Rules

The patient's unit must be kept clean, neat, and safe. This is a responsibility of everyone involved in the person's care. The following rules will help guide you in maintaining the patient's unit:

1. Make sure the patient can reach the overbed table and the bedside stand.
2. Arrange personal belongings as the patient prefers. Make sure they are easily reached.
3. Keep the signal light within the patient's reach at all times.
4. Make sure the patient can reach the telephone, television, and light controls.
5. Provide the patient with enough tissues and toilet paper.

6. Adjust lighting, temperature, and ventilation for the patient's comfort.
7. Handle equipment carefully to prevent unnecessary noise.
8. Explain the causes of strange noises to the patient.
9. Use room deodorizers if necessary.
10. Empty the patient's wastebasket as often as needed.

SUMMARY

The patient's unit is designed and equipped to meet basic needs. Equipment is provided for comfort, hygiene, elimination, and activity. The overbed table is used for meals. Side rails, hand rails, and the call system are provided for patient safety. Safety is also promoted by controlling temperature, ventilation, lighting, noise, and odors. Curtains or screens provide privacy and help the patient feel safe and secure. A telephone lets the patient talk with family and friends. The television and radio provide entertainment and relaxation.

REVIEW QUESTIONS

Circle the best answer.

1 Which is a comfortable temperature range for most people?
   a 60° F to 66° F
   b 68° F to 74° F
   c 74° F to 80° F
   d 80° F to 86° F
2 A patient can be protected from drafts by
   a Wearing enough clothing
   b Being covered with adequate blankets
   c Being moved out of a drafty area
   d All of the above
3 Which does *not* prevent or reduce odors?
   a Placing fresh flowers in the room
   b Emptying bedpans promptly
   c Using room deodorizers
   d Practicing good personal hygiene
4 Which will *not* control noise?
   a Using equipment made of plastic
   b Handling dishes with care
   c Speaking softly
   d Talking with others in the hallway
5 Which is Fowler's position?
   a The head of the bed is raised 45 degrees.
   b The head of the bed is raised 45 degrees and the knee portion is raised 15 degrees.
   c The head of the bed is lowered and the foot of the bed is raised.
   d The head of the bed is raised and the foot of the bed is lowered.

6 The overbed table is *not* used
   a For eating
   b As a working surface
   c To store the urinal
   d To store shaving articles

Circle T if the answer is true and F if the answer is false.

T F 7 Soft, dim lighting is usually more relaxing and comfortable.
T F 8 The curtain is pulled around the patient's bed to provide privacy during conversations.
T F 9 The call system is used by the patient to signal when assistance is needed.
T F 10 The signal light must always be within the patient's reach except when the patient is in the bathroom.
T F 11 The overbed table and bedside stand should be within the patient's reach.
T F 12 You should explain the cause of strange noises to the patient.

Answers

12	True	6	c
11	True	5	a
10	False	4	d
9	True	3	a
8	False	2	d
7	True	1	b

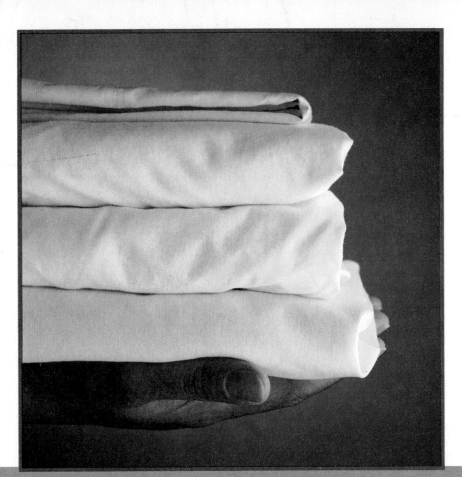

Bedmaking

OBJECTIVES

- Define the key terms listed in this chapter
- Describe the differences between open, closed, occupied, and surgical beds
- Identify when bed linens should be changed
- Explain the purposes of a plastic drawsheet and a cotton drawsheet
- Identify the type of bed that should be made in certain situations
- Handle linens according to the rules of medical asepsis
- Perform the procedures in this chapter

bath blanket   A thin, lightweight cotton blanket used to cover the patient during a bath or other procedures; it absorbs water and provides warmth

drawsheet   A small sheet placed over the middle of the bottom sheet; it helps keep the mattress and bottom linens clean and dry, and it can be used to turn and move patients in bed; the "cotton drawsheet"

mitered corner   A way of tucking linens under the mattress to help keep them straight and smooth

plastic drawsheet   A drawsheet made of plastic; it is placed between the bottom sheet and the cotton drawsheet to keep the mattress and bottom linens clean and dry

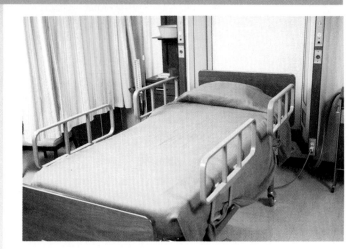

Fig. 12-1   Closed bed.

Patients spend a lot of time in bed. Some are out of bed part of the day; others must be in bed all the time. Meals are eaten in bed, and some patients are bathed in bed. Some cannot get out of bed to use the bathroom. Many procedures are done with the patient in bed.

Bedmaking is an important part of your job. A clean, neat bed helps make your patient more comfortable. Think of how nice it is to get into a freshly made bed at home. How does it feel getting into an unmade bed that does not have the sheets and blankets tucked in?

Beds are usually made in the morning after baths. The bed can also be made while the patient is in the shower or tub, or when the patient is out of the room. Patients like to have their beds made and rooms cleaned before visitors arrive.

Linens are straightened if they become loose and wrinkled during the day. Check linens for crumbs after meals and properly remove them. Be sure to straighten linens at bedtime. You must change linens if they become wet, soiled, or damp.

Beds are made in the following ways:

1. A *closed bed* is not being used. Top linens are not folded back, and the bed is ready for a new patient (Fig. 12-1).
2. An *open bed* is being used by a patient. Top linens are folded back so that the patient can get into bed. A closed bed becomes an open bed when the top linens are folded back (Fig. 12-2).
3. An *occupied bed* is made with the patient in it (Fig. 12-3).
4. A *surgical bed* is made so that the patient can be moved from a stretcher to the bed. It may be called a postoperative bed, recovery bed, or anesthetic bed (Fig. 12-4).

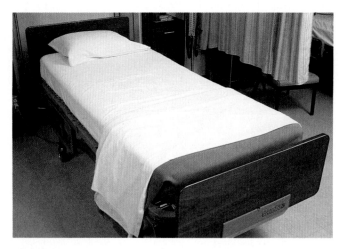

Fig. 12-2   Open bed. Top linens are folded to the foot of the bed.

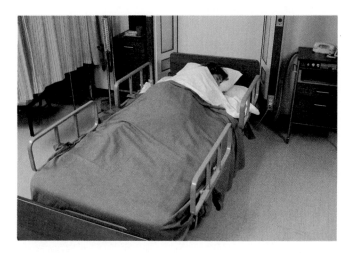

Fig. 12-3   Occupied bed.

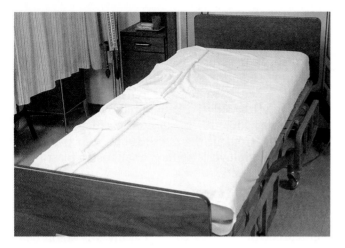

Fig. 12-4 Surgical bed.

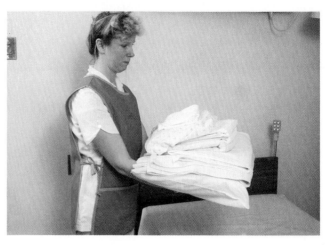

Fig. 12-5 Linens are held away from the body and uniform.

LINENS

Special attention is given to the care and use of linens. The rules of medical asepsis are followed when handling linens and making beds. Your uniform is considered dirty, so you must always hold linens away from your body and uniform (Fig. 12-5). Never shake linens in the air. Shaking them causes the spread of microorganisms. Clean linens are placed on a clean surface. Never put dirty linens on the floor.

Clean linens are collected in the order in which they will be used. Linens for the patient's personal care are also collected. Be sure to collect enough linens. If your patient has 2 pillows, get 2 pillowcases. Extra blankets may be needed for the patient's warmth. Do not bring unneeded linens to a patient's room. Extra linen in a patient's room is considered contaminated and cannot be used for another patient.

You should collect linens in the following order:
1. Mattress pad
2. Bottom sheet (flat sheet or contour sheet)
3. Plastic drawsheet
4. Cotton drawsheet
5. Top sheet (flat sheet)
6. Blanket
7. Bedspread
8. Pillowcase(s)
9. Bath towel(s)
10. Hand towel
11. Washcloth
12. Hospital gown
13. Bath blanket

Use one arm to hold the linens and the other hand to pick them up. The item to be used first is at the bottom of your stack. (You picked up the mattress pad first, therefore it is at the bottom. The bath blanket is on top.) You need the mattress pad first. To get it on top, simply place your arm over the bath blanket. Then turn the stack over to the arm on the

A

B

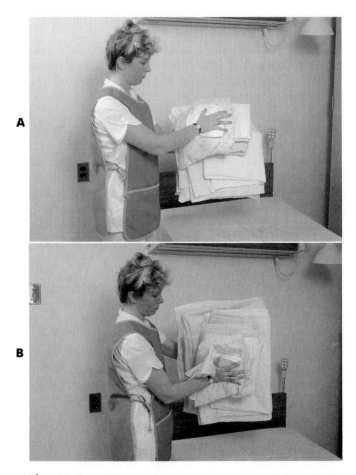

Fig. 12-6 **A,** The arm is placed over the top of the stack of linens. **B,** The stack of linens is turned over onto the arm.

bath blanket (Fig. 12-6). The arm that had been holding the linens will be free. Place the clean linens on a clean surface.

Linens are pressed and folded to prevent the spread of microbes and to make bedmaking easy. They are

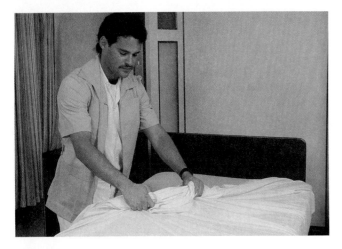

Fig. 12-7 Roll linens away from you when removing them from the bed.

pressed with a center crease, which is placed in the center of the bed from the head to the foot. The linens unfold easily.

To remove dirty linen from the bed, roll the linens up away from you. The side that touched the patient is inside the roll. The side that has not touched the patient is outside (Fig. 12-7).

Not all linens are changed every time the bed is made. Some are reused for an open bed. The mattress pad, plastic drawsheet, blanket, and bedspread may be reused for the same patient. They can be reused if not soiled, wet, or very wrinkled. Some facilities use only flat sheets. The flat top sheet can be reused as the bottom sheet. If a patient has been discharged, all linens are removed and a closed bed is made. Check the facility's policy about linen changes. *Remember, linens that are wet, damp, or soiled must be changed right away.*

A standard hospital bed may include a plastic drawsheet and a cotton drawsheet. A *drawsheet* is a small sheet placed over the middle of the bottom sheet. It helps keep the mattress and bottom linens clean and dry. A *plastic drawsheet* protects the mattress and bottom linens from becoming damp or soiled. It is placed between the bottom sheet and cotton drawsheet. The cotton drawsheet is needed to protect the patient from contact with the plastic and to absorb moisture. Although the bottom linen and mattress are protected, patient discomfort and skin breakdown may occur. This is because of heat retention and the difficulty in keeping the drawsheets tight and wrinkle free.

Most mattresses made for clinical use are covered with plastic. Plastic mattress covers may be used. Disposable waterproof bed protectors can be used. Plastic and cotton drawsheets may be used only for certain patients. They include those with bowel or bladder control problems or those who have excessive wound drainage.

A cotton drawsheet may be used without a plastic

drawsheet. Plasticized mattresses cause some patients to perspire heavily and can increase their discomfort. A cotton drawsheet helps to reduce heat retention and absorbs moisture. Cotton drawsheets are often used to move and position patients in bed (see Chapter 10). When used for this purpose, they are not tucked in at the sides. The bedmaking procedures in this chapter include the use of plastic and cotton drawsheets. Consult the nurse about their use. Also, know your employer's policies about using plastic and cotton drawsheets.

GENERAL RULES

Remember these rules when making a hospital bed.
1. Use good body mechanics at all times.
2. Follow the rules of medical asepsis.
3. Always wash your hands before handling clean linen and after handling dirty linen.
4. Bring enough linen to the patient's room.
5. Never shake linens. Shaking linens causes the spread of microorganisms.
6. Extra linen in a patient's room is considered contaminated. Do not use it for other patients. Put it in the dirty laundry so that it is not used for other patients.
7. Hold linens away from your uniform. Dirty and clean linen should never touch your uniform.
8. Never put dirty linens on the floor or on clean linens. Follow facility policy about dirty linen.
9. Linens the patient lies on (bottom linens) must be tightly tucked in without wrinkles.
10. A cotton drawsheet must completely cover the plastic drawsheet. A plastic drawsheet should never touch the patient's body.
11. Straighten and tighten loose sheets, blankets, and bedspreads whenever necessary.
12. Make as much of one side of the bed as possible before going to the other side. This saves time and energy.

THE CLOSED BED

A closed bed is made after a patient has been discharged so that it is ready for a new patient. The bed is made after the bed frame and mattress have been cleaned according to the facility's policy.

THE OPEN BED

The open bed is an unoccupied bed. Linens are folded back so that the patient can get into bed with ease. Open beds are made when patients are admitted to the facility. The are also made for patients who can be out of bed when their bed is being made. A closed bed becomes an open bed when the top linens are folded back.

1 Wash your hands.
2 Collect clean linen:
   a Mattress pad
   b Bottom sheet
   c Plastic drawsheet
   d Cotton drawsheet
   e Top sheet
   f Blanket
   g Bedspread
   h Two pillowcases
   i Bath towel(s)
   j Hand towel
   k Washcloth
   l Hospital gown
   m Bath blanket
3 Place linen on a clean surface.
4 Raise the bed to an appropriate level for good body mechanics.
5 Move the mattress to the head of the bed.
6 Put the mattress pad on the mattress. It should be even with the top of the mattress.
7 Place the bottom sheet on the mattress pad (Fig. 12-8):
   a Unfold it lengthwise.
   b Place the center crease in the middle of the bed.
   c Position the lower edge of the sheet even with the bottom of the mattress.
   d Place the large hem at the top and the small hem at the bottom.
   e Face the hem stitching downward.
8 Pick the sheet up from the side to open it. Fanfold it toward the other side of the bed as in Figure 12-9.
9 Go to the head of the bed. Tuck the top of the sheet under the mattress. You will have to lift the mattress slightly. Make sure the sheet is tight and smooth.
10 Make a mitered corner as in Figure 12-10.
11 Place the plastic drawsheet on the bed about 14 inches from the top of the mattress.
12 Open the plastic drawsheet and fanfold it toward the other side of the bed.
13 Place a cotton drawsheet over the plastic drawsheet. It must cover the entire plastic drawsheet (Fig. 12-11).
14 Open the cotton drawsheet and fanfold it toward the other side of the bed.
15 Tuck both drawsheets under the mattress. You may also tuck each in separately.
16 Go to the other side of the bed.
17 Miter the top corner of the bottom sheet.
18 Pull the bottom sheet tight so that there are no wrinkles. Tuck in the sheet.
19 Pull the drawsheets tight so that there are no wrinkles. Tuck both in together or pull each tight and tuck them in separately (Fig. 12-12).

20 Go to the other side of the bed.
21 Put the top sheet on the bed:
   a Unfold it lengthwise.
   b Place the center crease in the middle.
   c Place the large hem at the top, even with the top of the mattress.
   d Open the sheet and fanfold the extra part toward the other side.
   e Face the hem stitching outward.
   f Do not tuck the bottom in yet.
   g Never tuck top linens in on the sides.
22 Place the blanket on the bed:
   a Unfold it so that the center crease is in the middle.
   b Put the upper hem about 6 to 8 inches from the top of the mattress.
   c Open the blanket and fanfold the extra part toward the other side.
23 Place the bedspread on the bed:
   a Unfold it so that the center crease is in the middle.
   b Place the upper hem even with the top of the mattress.
   c Open the bedspread and fanfold the extra part toward the other side.
   d Make sure the bedspread facing the door is even and covers all top linens.
24 Tuck in top linens together at the foot of the bed. They should be smooth and tight. Make a mitered corner.
25 Go to the other side.
26 Straighten all top linen, working from the head of the bed to the foot.
27 Tuck in the top linens together. Make a mitered corner.
28 Turn the top hem of the bedspread under the blanket to make a cuff (Fig. 12-13).
29 Turn the top sheet down over the spread. Hem stitching is down. (Steps 28 and 29 are not done in some facilities.)
30 Place the pillow on the bed.
31 Open the pillowcase so that it is flat on the bed.
32 Put the pillowcase on the pillow as in Figure 12-14. Fold extra pillowcase material under the pillow at the seam end of the pillowcase.
33 Place the pillow on the bed so that the open end is away from the door. The seam of the pillowcase is toward the head of the bed.
34 Attach the signal light to the bed.
35 Lower the bed to its lowest position.
36 Put towels, washcloth, gown, and bath blanket in the bedside stand.
37 Wash your hands.

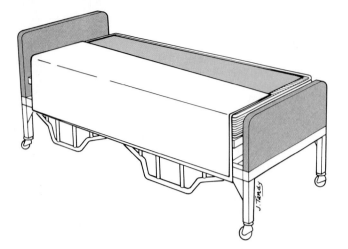

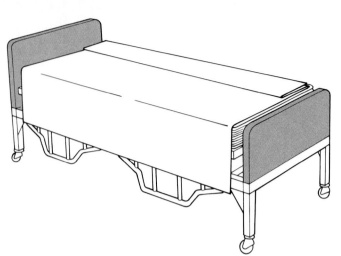

Fig. 12-8 The bottom sheet is on the bed with the center crease in the middle. The lower edge of the sheet is even with the bottom of the mattress.

Fig. 12-9 The bottom sheet is fanfolded to the other side of the bed.

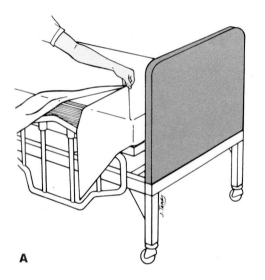

A

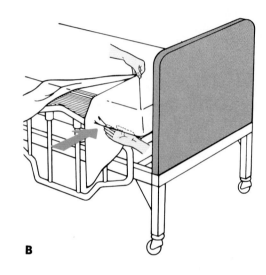

B

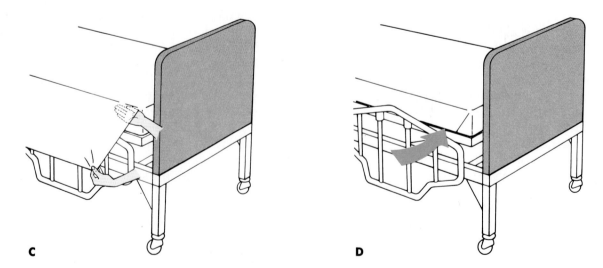

C

D

Fig. 12-10 Making a mitered corner. **A,** Bottom sheet is tucked under the mattress and the side of the sheet is raised onto the mattress. **B,** The remaining portion of the sheet is tucked under the mattress. **C,** The raised portion of the sheet is brought off the mattress. **D,** The entire side of the sheet is tucked under the mattress.

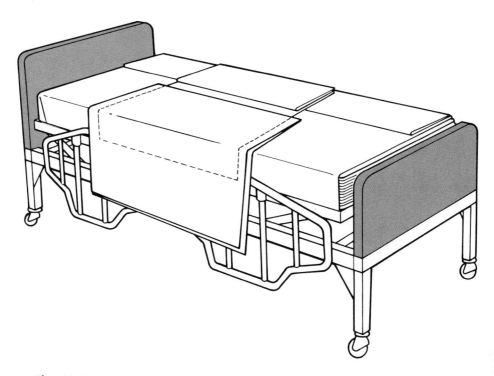

Fig. 12-11 A cotton drawsheet over the plastic drawsheet. The cotton drawsheet completely covers the plastic drawsheet.

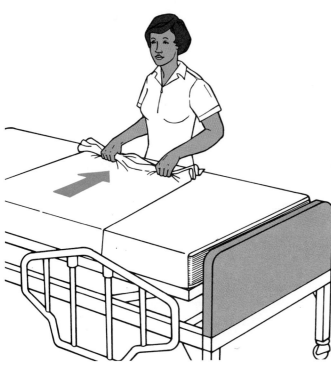

Fig. 12-12 The drawsheet is pulled tight to remove wrinkles.

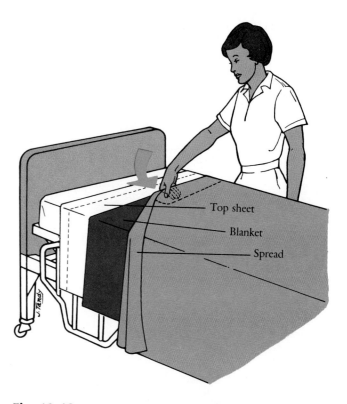

Top sheet

Blanket

Spread

Fig. 12-13 The top hem of the bedspread is turned under the top hem of the blanket to make a cuff.

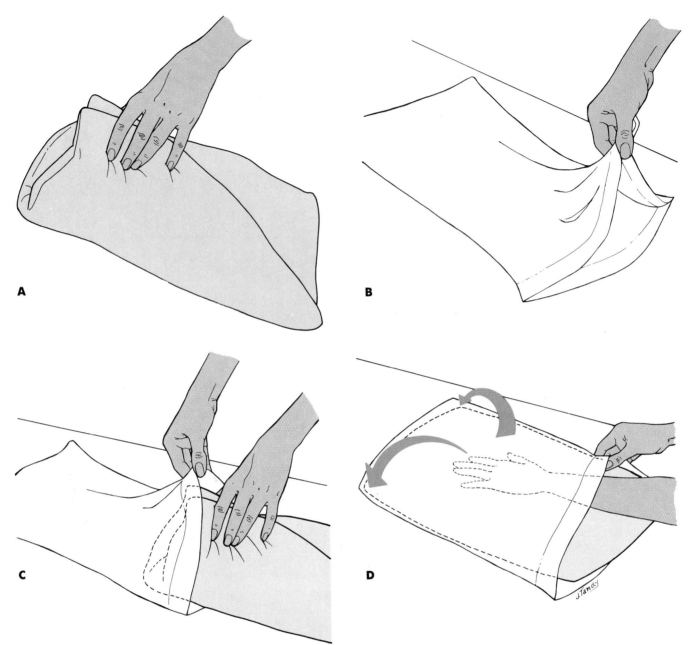

Fig. 12-14 Putting a pillowcase on a pillow. **A,** Grasp the corners of the pillow at the seam end and form a "V" with the pillow. **B,** The pillowcase is flat on the bed; the pillowcase is opened with the free hand. **C,** The "V" end of the pillow is guided into the pillowcase. **D,** The "V" end of the pillow falls into the corners of the pillowcase.

MAKING AN OPEN BED

1 Wash your hands.
2 Collect linen for a closed bed.
3 Make a closed bed.
4 Fanfold top linens to the foot of the bed (see Fig. 12-2).
5 Attach the signal light to the bed.

6 Lower the bed to its lowest position.
7 Put towels, washcloth, gown, and bath blanket in the bedside stand.
8 Place the dirty linen in the linen hamper.
9 Wash your hands.

THE OCCUPIED BED

An occupied bed is made when a patient cannot get out of bed because of illness or injury. When making an occupied bed, you must keep the patient in good body alignment. You must also be aware of restrictions or limitations in the patient's movement or positioning. Be sure to explain each step of the procedure to the patient before it is done.

THE SURGICAL BED

The surgical bed (recovery bed, postoperative bed, or anesthetic bed) is a form of the open bed. Top linens are folded in such a way that the patient can be transferred from a stretcher to the bed. The term *surgical bed* and its other names imply that the patient has had surgery. However, this type of bed is also needed for patients who arrive on a stretcher. If the bed is made for a postoperative (surgical) patient, a complete linen change is indicated. See the box on page 191.

MAKING AN OCCUPIED BED

1 Explain the procedure to the patient.
2 Wash your hands.
3 Collect clean linen (see *Making a Closed Bed*, page 183).
4 Place linen on a clean surface.
5 Provide for privacy.
6 Remove the signal light.
7 Raise the bed to an appropriate level for good body mechanics.
8 Lower the head of the bed to a level appropriate for the patient. It should be as flat as possible.
9 Lower the side rail near you. Make sure the opposite one is up and secure.
10 Loosen top linens at the foot of the bed.
11 Remove the bedspread and blanket separately. Fold them as in Figure 12-15 if they are to be reused.
12 Cover the patient with a bath blanket to provide warmth and privacy:
   a Unfold a bath blanket over the top sheet.
   b Ask the patient to hold onto the bath blanket. If he or she cannot, tuck the top part under the patient's shoulders.
   c Grasp the top sheet under the bath blanket at the shoulders. Bring the sheet down to the foot of the bed. Remove the sheet from under the blanket (Fig. 12-16).
13 Move the mattress to the head of the bed.
14 Position the patient on the side of the bed away from you. Adjust the pillow for the patient's comfort. It should be on the far side of the bed.
15 Loosen bottom linens from the head to the foot of the bed.
16 Fanfold bottom linens one at a time toward the patient: cotton drawsheet, plastic drawsheet, bottom sheet, and mattress pad (Fig. 12-17). Do not fanfold the mattress pad if it will be reused.

17 Place a clean mattress pad on the bed. Unfold it lengthwise so that the center crease is in the middle. Fanfold the top part toward the patient. If reusing the mattress pad, straighten and smooth any wrinkles.
18 Place the bottom sheet on the mattress pad so that the hem stitching is away from the patient. Unfold the sheet so that the crease is in the middle. The small hem should be even with the bottom of the mattress. Fanfold the top part toward the patient.
19 Make a mitered corner at the head of the bed. Tuck the sheet under the mattress from the head to the foot.
20 Pull the fanfolded plastic drawsheet toward you over the bottom sheet. Tuck excess material under the mattress. Do the following if you are using a clean plastic drawsheet (Fig. 12-18):
   a Place the plastic drawsheet on the bed about 14 inches from the mattress top.
   b Fanfold the top part toward the patient.
   c Tuck in the excess material.
21 Place the cotton drawsheet over the plastic drawsheet. It must cover the entire plastic drawsheet. Fanfold the top part toward the patient. Tuck in excess material.
22 Raise the side rail. Go to the other side and lower the side rail.
23 Position the patient on the side of the bed away from you. Adjust the pillow for the patient's comfort.
24 Loosen bottom linens. Remove the soiled linen one piece at a time.
25 Straighten and smooth the mattress pad.
26 Pull the clean bottom sheet toward you. Make a mitered corner at the top. Tuck the sheet under the mattress from the head to the foot of the bed.

Continued.

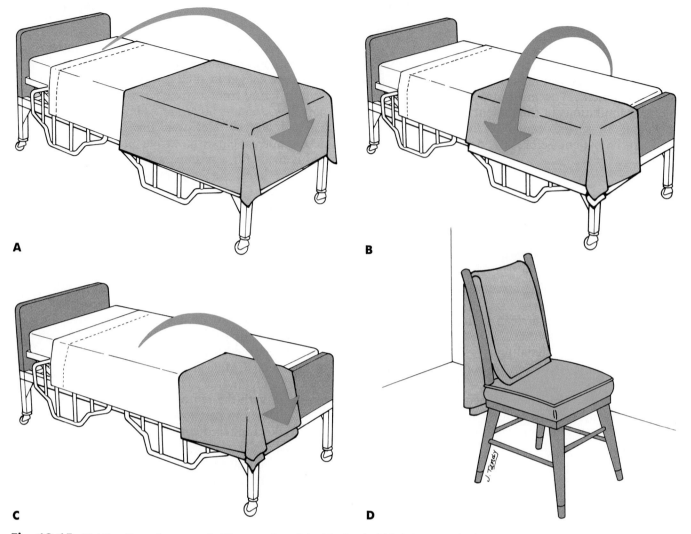

Fig. 12-15 Folding linen for reuse. **A,** The top edge of the blanket is folded down to the bottom edge. **B,** The blanket is folded from the far side of the bed to the near side. **C,** The top edge of the blanket is folded down to the bottom edge again. **D,** The folded blanket is placed over the back of a straight chair.

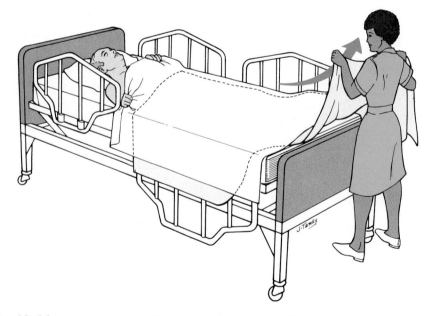

Fig. 12-16 The patient is holding onto the bath blanket. The nursing assistant at the foot of the bed is removing the top sheet from under the bath blanket.

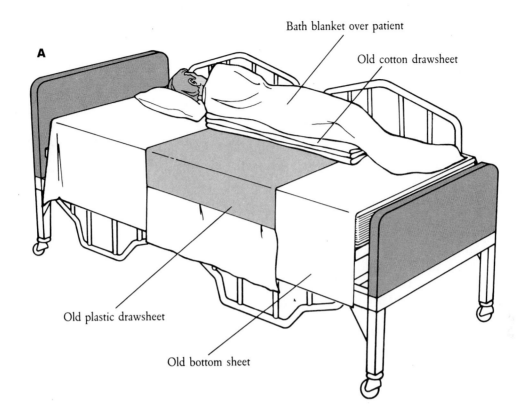

Bath blanket over patient

Old cotton drawsheet

Old plastic drawsheet

Old bottom sheet

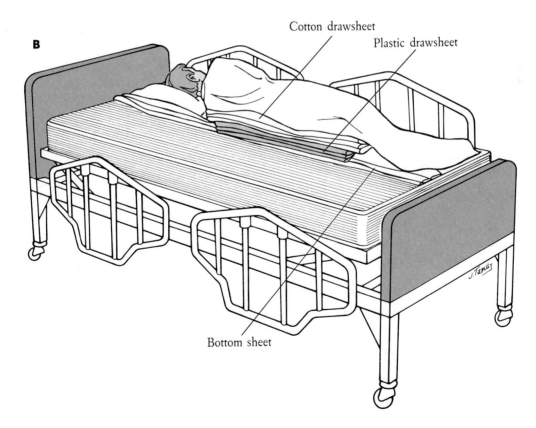

Cotton drawsheet

Plastic drawsheet

Bottom sheet

Fig. 12-17 Occupied bed. **A,** The cotton drawsheet is fanfolded and tucked under the patient. **B,** All bottom linens are tucked under the patient.

MAKING AN OCCUPIED BED—cont'd

27 Pull the drawsheets tightly toward you. Tuck both under together or tuck each in separately.

28 Position the patient supine in the center of the bed. Adjust the pillow for comfort.

29 Put the top sheet on the bed. Unfold it lengthwise. Make sure the crease is in the middle, the large hem is even with the top of the mattress, and hem stitching is on the outside.

30 Ask the patient to hold onto the top sheet so that you can remove the bath blanket. You may have to tuck the top sheet under the patient's shoulders. Remove the bath blanket.

31 Place the blanket on the bed. Unfold it so that the crease is in the middle. Unfold the blanket so that it covers the patient. The upper hem should be 6 to 8 inches from the top of the mattress.

32 Place the bedspread on the bed, unfolding it so that the center crease is in the middle. Unfold it so that it covers the patient. The top hem is even with the mattress top.

33 Turn the top hem of the bedspread under the blanket to make a cuff.

34 Bring the top sheet down over the bedspread to form a cuff.

35 Go to the foot of the bed.

36 Lift the mattress corner with one arm. Tuck all top linens under the mattress together. Be sure the linens are loose enough to allow movement of the patient's feet. Make a mitered corner.

37 Raise the side rail. Go to the other side and lower the side rail.

38 Straighten and smooth top linens.

39 Tuck the top linens under the mattress as in step 36. Make a mitered corner.

40 Change the pillowcase(s).

41 Place the signal light within reach.

42 Raise the side rail.

43 Raise the head of the bed to a level appropriate for the patient. Make sure the patient is comfortable.

44 Lower the bed to its lowest position.

45 Put towels, washcloth, gown, and bath blanket in the bedside stand.

46 Unscreen the patient. Thank him or her for cooperating.

47 Place the dirty linen in the linen hamper.

48 Wash your hands.

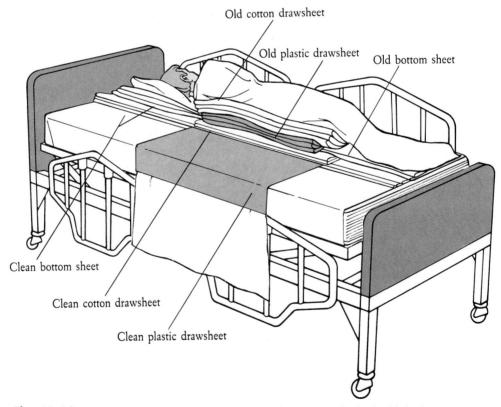

Fig. 12-18 A clean bottom sheet and plastic drawsheet are on the bed with both fanfolded and tucked under the patient. The clean cotton drawsheet is put in place in step 22.

MAKING A SURGICAL BED

1 Wash your hands.
2 Collect the following equipment:
    a Clean linen (see *Making a Closed Bed*, page 183)
    b IV pole
    c Tissues
    d Emesis basin
    e Other equipment as requested by the nurse
3 Place linen on a clean surface.
4 Remove the signal light.
5 Raise the bed to a level appropriate for good body mechanics.
6 Remove all linen from the bed.
7 Make a closed bed (see *Making a Closed Bed*, page 183). Do not tuck the top linens under the mattress.
8 Fold all top linen at the foot of the bed back onto the bed. The fold should be even with the edge of the mattress (Fig. 12-19).
9 Use one of these methods to fold top linen:
    a Fanfold linen lengthwise to the side of the bed farthest from the door (Fig. 12-20).
    b Fanfold linens from the head of the bed to the foot (Fig. 12-21).
10 Put the pillowcase(s) on the pillow(s).
11 Place the pillow(s) on a clean surface.
12 Leave the bed in its highest position.
13 Make sure both side rails are down.
14 Put the towels, washcloth, gown, and bath blanket in the bedside stand.
15 Place the tissues and emesis basin on the bedside stand. Place the IV pole near the head of the bed.
16 Move all furniture away from the bed. Make sure there is room for the stretcher and for the staff to move about.
17 Do not attach the signal light to the bed.
18 Place soiled linens in the linen hamper.
19 Wash your hands.

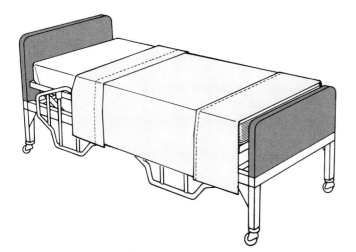

Fig. 12-19 Surgical bed. The bottom of the top linens is folded back onto the bed. The fold is even with the edge of the mattress.

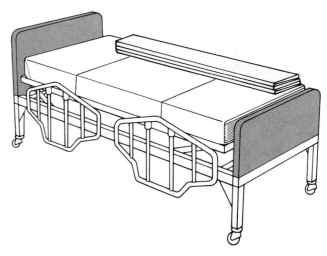

Fig. 12-20 A surgical bed with the top linens fanfolded lengthwise to the opposite side of the bed.

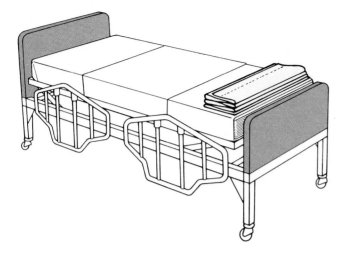

Fig. 12-21 A surgical bed with top linens fanfolded from the head of the bed to the foot.

SUMMARY

You have learned several ways to make hospital beds. You have also learned the principles of bedmaking and of handling linens. The facility's policies and procedures or a patient's condition may require changes in these procedures. However, the principles must be followed. The patient's comfort and safety are the focus of bedmaking. Remember that the patient spends a lot of time in bed. Therefore the bed must be neat, clean, and free of wrinkles. A well-made bed helps make your patient more comfortable.

Be sure to handle linens properly so that you do not spread microorganisms. Also follow the rules of medical asepsis, bedmaking, and good body mechanics.

REVIEW QUESTIONS

Circle T *if the statement is true and* F *if the statement is false.*

T F **1** Linens are changed whenever they become soiled, wet, or damp.

T F **2** An open bed is made after a patient is discharged.

T F **3** A surgical bed is only for patients who have had surgery.

T F **4** A postoperative bed is made with the patient in bed.

T F **5** Linens are held away from your body and uniform.

T F **6** Dirty linens can be put on the floor.

T F **7** Extra linen in a patient's room can be used for another patient.

T F **8** Complete linen changes are required for closed beds and surgical beds.

T F **9** A cotton drawsheet is always used when a plastic drawsheet is used.

T F **10** To remove crumbs from the bed, the linens are loosened and shaken in the air.

T F **11** The hem stitching of the bottom sheet should be downward so that it is away from the patient.

T F **12** The plastic drawsheet is placed 6 to 8 inches from the top of the mattress.

T F **13** A cotton drawsheet should completely cover the plastic drawsheet.

T F **14** The upper hem of the bedspread should be even with the top of the mattress.

T F **15** A closed bed becomes an open bed when top linens are fanfolded to the foot of the bed.

T F **16** An occupied bed is made for an ambulatory patient.

T F **17** A patient is screened when an occupied bed is made.

T F **18** When making an occupied bed, the far side rail should be up at all times.

T F **19** After a surgical bed is made, it is left in its lowest position.

T F **20** A cotton drawsheet is used only with a plastic drawsheet.

Answers

20 False	**10** False
19 False	**9** True
18 True	**8** True
17 True	**7** False
16 False	**6** False
15 True	**5** True
14 True	**4** False
13 True	**3** False
12 False	**2** False
11 True	**1** True

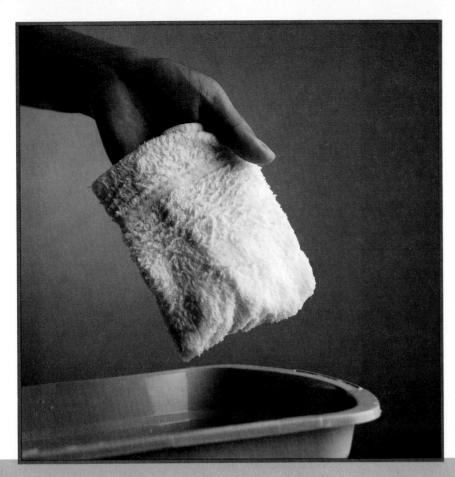

Cleanliness and Skin Care

OBJECTIVES

- Define the key terms listed in this chapter
- Explain the importance of cleanliness and skin care
- Describe the routine patient care performed before and after breakfast, after lunch, and in the evening
- Explain the importance of oral hygiene and list the observations to report
- Describe the general rules related to bathing patients and the observations to make
- Identify the safety precautions for patients taking tub baths or showers
- Identify the purposes of a back massage
- Identify the purposes of perineal care
- Explain the importance of hair care and shaving
- Explain the importance of nail and foot care
- Describe the signs, symptoms, and causes of decubiti
- Identify the pressure points of the body in the prone, supine, lateral, Fowler's, and sitting positions
- Describe how to prevent decubitus ulcers
- Perform the procedures described in this chapter

13

AM care   Routine care performed before breakfast; early morning care

antiperspirant   A skin care product that reduces the amount of perspiration

aspiration   Breathing fluid or an object into the lungs

bedsore   A decubitus ulcer; a pressure sore

decubitus ulcer   An area where the skin and underlying tissues are eroded because of a lack of blood flow; a bedsore or pressure sore

deodorant   A skin preparation that masks and controls body odors

hs care   Care given in the evening at bedtime

morning care   Care given after breakfast; cleanliness and skin care measures are more thorough at this time

oral hygiene   Measures performed to keep the mouth and teeth clean; mouth care

pericare   Perineal care

perineal care   Cleansing the genital and anal areas

pressure sore   A decubitus ulcer; a bedsore

Cleanliness and skin care are necessary for comfort, safety, and health. The skin is the body's first line of defense against disease. Intact skin prevents microorganisms from entering the body and causing an infection. Likewise, mucous membranes of the mouth, genital area, and anus must be kept clean and intact. Besides cleansing, hygiene practices prevent body and breath odors, promote relaxation, and increase circulation.

Culture and personal choice influence hygiene. Some people like to shower. Others like tub baths. One person may bathe at bedtime. Another may bathe in the morning. The frequency of bathing also varies among individuals. Some people do not have water for bathing. Others cannot afford such things as soap, deodorant, shampoo, or toothpaste.

Patients and residents usually need some help with personal hygiene. Weakness caused by illness and body changes from aging affect the ability to practice hygiene. The need for cleanliness and skin care is affected by perspiration, vomiting, urinary and bowel elimination, drainage from wounds or body openings, bed rest, and activity. The nurse decides the amount and type of personal hygiene you need to provide for an individual.

DAILY CARE OF THE PATIENT

Personal hygiene is performed as often as necessary to stay clean and comfortable. People who can take care of themselves practice hygiene routinely and out of habit. Teeth are brushed and the face and hands are washed after rising in the morning. These and other hygiene measures may be done routinely before and after meals and at bedtime.

Infants, young children, and some adults who are weak or disabled need help with hygiene. Routine care is given at certain times of the day. However, remember to assist a patient with personal hygiene whenever necessary.

Before Breakfast

Routine care before breakfast is often called *early morning care* or AM *care*. The night shift or day shift staff may be responsible for AM care. They get patients ready for breakfast or tests to be done early in the day. Personal hygiene measures performed at this time include:

1. Offering bedpans or urinals
2. Helping patients wash their faces and hands
3. Assisting patients with oral hygiene
4. Positioning patients in Fowler's position or in bedside chairs for breakfast
5. Straightening bed linens
6. Straightening patient units

After Breakfast

Morning care is given after breakfast. Cleanliness and skin care measures are more thorough at this time. Routine morning care usually involves:

1. Offering bedpans or urinals
2. Helping patients wash their faces and hands
3. Assisting patients with oral hygiene
4. Shaving male patients
5. Providing showers, tub baths, or bed baths
6. Giving perineal care
7. Giving back massages
8. Changing gowns or pajamas or dressing patients
9. Brushing and combing hair
10. Changing bed linens
11. Straightening patient units

Afternoon Care

Routine hygiene is performed after lunch and supper. If care is provided before visiting hours, patients will feel more refreshed. They can also visit with family and friends without interruption. Afternoon care consists of:

1. Offering bedpans or urinals
2. Helping patients wash their faces and hands
3. Assisting patients with oral hygiene
4. Changing gowns or pajamas if needed

5. Brushing or combing hair if needed
6. Changing damp or soiled bed linens
7. Straightening patient units

Evening Care

Care given at bedtime is called *hs care*. Hygiene measures are performed right before the patient is ready for sleep. They help promote comfort and relaxation. Hs care involves:
1. Offering bedpans or urinals
2. Helping patients wash their faces and hands
3. Assisting patients with oral hygiene
4. Changing damp or soiled linens and straightening all other linens
5. Changing gowns or pajamas if needed
6. Helping patients in street clothes to undress and put on gowns or pajamas
7. Giving back massages
8. Straightening patient units

ORAL HYGIENE

Oral hygiene, or mouth care, is done to keep the mouth and teeth clean. A clean mouth and clean teeth prevent mouth odors and infections, increase comfort, and make food taste better. Illness and disease may cause the patient to have a bad taste in the mouth. Some drugs and diseases cause the mouth and tongue to be coated with a whitish material. Other drugs and diseases cause redness and swelling of the mouth and tongue.

The nurse decides the type of mouth care and amount of assistance an individual needs. Oral hygiene is provided on awakening, after each meal, and at bedtime. Many people also practice oral hygiene before meals.

Equipment

A toothbrush, toothpaste, dental floss, and mouthwash are needed. The toothbrush should have soft or medium bristles. Patients with dentures need a denture cleaner, a denture cup, and a denture brush or a regular toothbrush. Toothettes are used for patients with sore, tender mouths and for unconscious patients. A *toothette* is a piece of spongy foam attached to a stick. Other needed items include an emesis basin, water glass, straw, tissues, and towels.

The equipment may be in the patient pack. Supply carts on nursing units usually have oral hygiene equipment. Most facility gift shops stock items for oral hygiene. However, many people bring oral hygiene equipment from home.

Universal precautions are necessary when giving oral hygiene. You will have contact with the person's mucous membranes. Gums may bleed during oral care. Also, many pathogens are in the mouth. Pathogens that are spread through sexual contact may be in the mouth of some individuals.

Brushing Teeth

The amount of assistance needed for toothbrushing varies. Many people perform oral hygiene themselves. Others need help in gathering and setting up

ASSISTING THE PATIENT TO BRUSH THE TEETH

1 Explain the procedure to the patient.
2 Wash your hands.
3 Collect the following equipment:
   a Toothbrush
   b Toothpaste or dentifrice
   c Mouthwash
   d Dental floss
   e Water glass with cool water
   f Straw
   g Emesis basin
   h Face towel
   i Paper towels
4 Place the paper towels on the overbed table. Arrange items on top of them.
5 Identify the patient. Check the ID bracelet and call the patient by name.
6 Provide for privacy.
7 Raise the head of the bed to a level where the patient can brush with ease.
8 Place the towel over the patient's chest to protect the gown and linens from spills.
9 Lower the side rail.
10 Move the overbed table in front of the patient. Adjust the table height so that the patient can work with ease.
11 Allow the patient to brush the teeth.
12 Move the overbed table next to the bed when the patient is finished. Lower it to a level appropriate for the patient.
13 Make sure the patient is comfortable.
14 Place the signal light within reach.
15 Raise the side rail.
16 Clean and return equipment to its proper place.
17 Wipe off the overbed table with the paper towels and discard them.
18 Unscreen the patient.
19 Place soiled linen in the linen hamper.
20 Wash your hands.
21 Report your observations to the nurse.

BRUSHING THE PATIENT'S TEETH

1 Explain the procedure to the patient.
2 Wash your hands.
3 Collect equipment. (See *Assisting the Patient to Brush the Teeth*, page 195.) Also get disposable gloves.
4 Place the paper towels on the overbed table. Arrange items on top of them.
5 Identify the patient. Check the ID bracelet and call the patient by name.
6 Provide for privacy.
7 Raise the bed to an appropriate level for good body mechanics.
8 Raise the head of the bed so that the patient can sit comfortably. Position the patient on the side near you if he or she cannot sit up.
9 Lower the side rail.
10 Place the towel over the patient's chest to protect the gown and linens from spills.
11 Position the overbed table so that you can reach it with ease. Adjust the height as needed.
12 Put on the gloves.
13 Apply toothpaste to the toothbrush.
14 Hold the toothbrush over the emesis basin. Pour some water over the brush.
15 Brush the patient's teeth gently as shown in Figure 13-1.
16 Let the patient have some water to rinse the mouth. Hold the emesis basin under the patient's chin (Fig. 13-2). Have the patient repeat rinsing as necessary.
17 Floss the patient's teeth (see *Flossing the Patient's Teeth*, page below).
18 Let the patient use mouthwash. Hold the emesis basin under the chin.
19 Remove and discard the gloves.
20 Make sure the patient is comfortable.
21 Place the signal light within reach.
22 Raise the side rail.
23 Lower the bed to its lowest position.
24 Clean and return equipment to its proper place.
25 Wipe off the overbed table with the paper towels and discard them.
26 Lower the overbed table to a level appropriate for the patient.
27 Unscreen the patient.
28 Place soiled linen in the linen hamper.
29 Wash your hands.
30 Report your observations to the nurse.

FLOSSING THE PATIENT'S TEETH

1 Explain to the patient what you are going to do.
2 Wash your hands.
3 Collect the following equipment:
  a Emesis basin
  b Water glass with cool water
  c Dental floss
  d Face towel
  e Paper towels
  f Disposable gloves
4 Place the paper towels on the overbed table. Arrange items on top of them.
5 Identify the patient. Check the ID bracelet and call the patient by name.
6 Provide for privacy.
7 Raise the bed to an appropriate level for good body mechanics.
8 Raise the head of the bed so that the patient can sit comfortably. Position the individual on the side near you if he or she cannot sit up.
9 Place the towel over the patient's chest to protect the gown and linens from spills.
10 Position the overbed table so that you can reach it with ease. Adjust the height as needed.
11 Wash your hands.
12 Lower the side rail.
13 Put on the gloves.
14 Break off an 18-inch piece of floss from the dispenser.
15 Hold the floss between the middle fingers of each hand (Fig. 13-3).
16 Stretch the floss with your thumbs.
17 Start at the upper back tooth on the right side and work around to the left side.
18 Move the floss gently up and down between the teeth (Fig. 13-4).
19 Move to a new section of floss after every second tooth.
20 Floss the lower teeth. Hold the floss with your index fingers (Fig. 13-5). Use back and forth motions and go under the gums as you did for the upper teeth. Start on the right side and work around to the left side.
21 Let the patient rinse his or her mouth. Hold the emesis basin under the chin. Repeat rinsing as necessary.
22 Follow steps 19 through 30 for *Brushing the Patient's Teeth*, above.

A

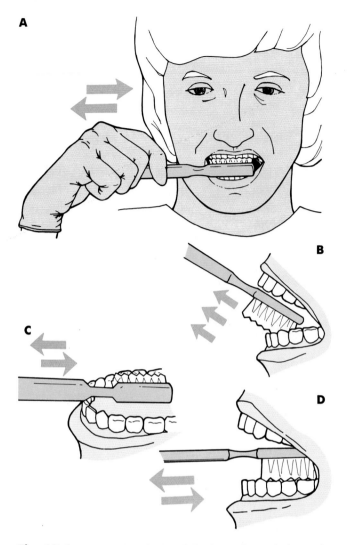

B

C

D

Fig. 13-1 **A,** Position the brush horizontally as shown and brush back and forth with short strokes. **B,** Position the brush at a 45 degree angle against the inside of the front teeth. Brush from the gum to the crown of the tooth with short strokes. Reposition the brush until all of the front teeth have been brushed. **C,** Hold the brush horizontally against the inner surfaces of the teeth and brush back and forth. **D,** Position the brush on the biting surfaces of the teeth as shown and brush back and forth.

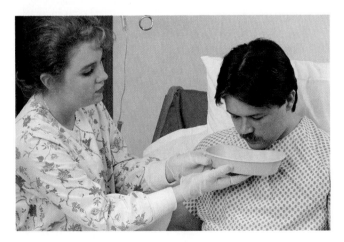

Fig. 13-2 The emesis basin is held under the patient's chin.

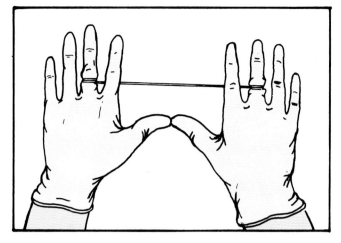

Fig. 13-3 Dental floss is held between the middle fingers to floss the upper teeth.

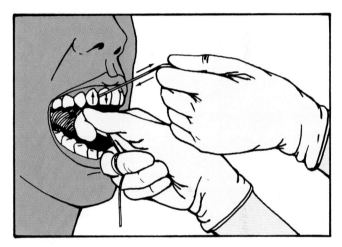

Fig. 13-4 Floss is moved in up and down motions between the teeth.

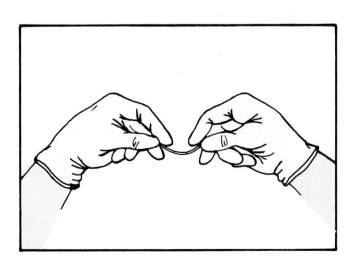

Fig. 13-5 Floss is held with the index fingers to floss the lower teeth.

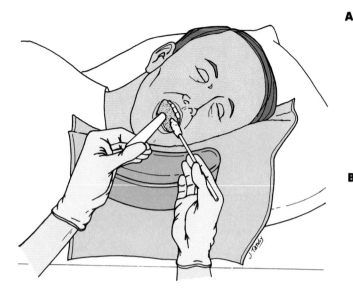

Fig. 13-6 The head of the unconscious patient is turned well to the side to prevent aspiration. A padded tongue blade is used to keep the mouth open while cleaning the mouth with applicators.

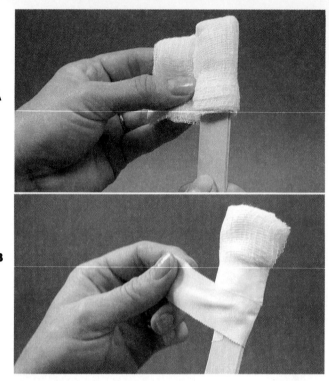

Fig. 13-7 Padded tongue blade. **A,** Place two wooden tongue blades together and wrap gauze around the top half. **B,** Tape the gauze in place.

PROVIDING MOUTH CARE FOR AN UNCONSCIOUS PATIENT

1 Wash your hands.
2 Collect the following equipment:
   a Lemon glycerine swabs
   b Antiseptic mouthwash or other solution
   c Toothettes or other applicators
   d Padded tongue blade
   e Water glass with cool water
   f Face towel
   g Emesis basin
   h Petrolatum
   i Paper towels
   j Disposable gloves
3 Place the paper towels on the overbed table. Arrange items on top of them.
4 Identify the patient. Check the ID bracelet and call the patient by name.
5 Explain the procedure to the patient.
6 Provide for privacy.
7 Raise the bed to an appropriate level for good body mechanics.
8 Lower the side rail near you.
9 Put on the gloves.
10 Position the patient on the side toward you. Turn his or her head well to the side.
11 Place the towel under the patient's face.
12 Place the emesis basin under his or her chin.
13 Position the overbed table so that you can reach it. Adjust the height as needed.
14 Separate the upper and lower teeth with the padded tongue blade.

15 Clean the mouth using the toothettes or applicators moistened with mouthwash or other solution (see Fig. 13-6).
   a Clean the chewing and inner surfaces of the teeth.
   b Swab the roof of the mouth, inside of the cheeks, and the lips.
   c Swab the tongue.
   d Moisten a clean applicator with water and swab the mouth to rinse.
   e Place used applicators in the emesis basin.
16 Repeat step 14 using lemon glycerine swabs.
17 Apply petrolatum to the patient's lips.
18 Remove and discard the gloves.
19 Explain that the procedure is done and that you will reposition him or her.
20 Reposition the patient.
21 Raise the side rail.
22 Lower the bed to its lowest position.
23 Clean and return equipment to its proper place. Discard disposable equipment.
24 Unscreen the patient.
25 Tell the patient that you are leaving the room.
26 Place soiled linen in the linen hamper.
27 Wash your hands.
28 Report your observations to the nurse.

the equipment. You may have to brush the teeth of patients who are very weak or are unable to use or move their arms. The following are reported to the nurse if observed when teeth are brushed:

1. Dry, cracked, swollen, or blistered lips
2. Redness, swelling, irritation, sores, or white patches in the mouth or on the tongue
3. Bleeding, swelling, or redness of the gums

Flossing

Flossing removes plaque and tartar from the teeth. These substances can cause serious gum disease, which can result in loosening and loss of teeth. Therefore dental flossing is a preventive measure. Flossing is also done to remove food from between the teeth. Flossing is usually done after brushing, but it can be done at other times. Some people floss after meals. If it is done only once a day, bedtime is the best time to floss.

Dental floss may be waxed or unwaxed. Waxed floss does not fray as easily as the unwaxed type. Some people find waxed floss easier to use because it slides between the teeth. However, particles on tooth surfaces are more likely to attach to unwaxed floss. Many dentists recommend unwaxed floss, which is thinner than waxed floss.

You need to floss for the patient if he or she cannot tend to oral hygiene. See the box on page 197.

Mouth Care for the Unconscious Patient

Unconscious patients need special mouth care. They cannot eat and drink, they breathe with their mouths open, and they are usually receiving supplemental oxygen. These factors cause the mouth to become dry and crusts to form on the tongue and mucous membranes. Good mouth care helps keep the mouth clean and moist and helps prevent infection.

Lemon glycerine swabs are often used to give mouth care to these patients. However, they have a drying effect and should not be the only method of mouth care used. Toothettes dipped in a small amount of mouthwash, hydrogen peroxide, or a salt solution can be used to clean the mouth. Petrolatum or other lubricant is applied to the lips after cleaning to prevent cracking.

Unconscious patients usually cannot swallow and must be protected from choking and aspiration. *Aspiration* is the breathing of fluid or an object into the lungs. To prevent aspiration, position the patient on one side with the head turned well to the side (Fig. 13-6). This position allows excess fluid to run out of the mouth, reducing the risk of aspiration. Using only a small amount of fluid also helps reduce the possibility of aspiration.

The patient's mouth must be kept open for mouth care. A padded tongue blade can be used for this purpose. (Figure 13-7 shows how to make a padded tongue blade.) Do not hold the mouth open with your fingers because the patient can bite down on them. Microorganisms can enter your body through the broken skin and cause an infection.

Unconscious patients cannot speak or respond to what is happening. However, they may be able to hear. Always assume that unconscious patients can hear. Explain what you are doing step by step. Also tell the patient when you are finished and when you are leaving the room.

Mouth care may be needed every 2 hours. Check with the nurse and the nursing care plan to see how often it is to be done and what solution is to be used. Unconscious patients should also be repositioned every 2 hours. Combining mouth care, skin care, and other comfort measures increases their comfort and safety. The possibility of forgetting to give mouth care is reduced if it is a part of the routine care given every 2 hours.

Denture Care

Dentures are cleaned for persons who cannot do this for themselves. Mouth care is provided and dentures are cleaned as often as natural teeth. Remember that dentures are the person's property and that they are expensive. Losing or damaging dentures is negligent conduct.

Dentures are slippery when they are wet. They are held firmly over a basin of water lined with a towel when being cleaned. They can easily break or chip if they are dropped onto a hard surface. Hot water causes them to warp. Do not use hot water to clean or store dentures. Some patients do not wear their

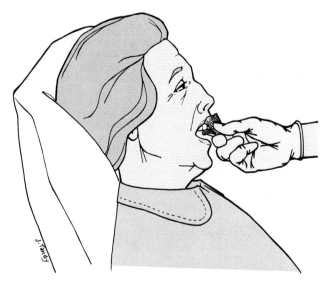

Fig. 13-8 Remove the upper denture by grasping it with the thumb and index finger of one hand. Use a piece of gauze to grasp the slippery denture.

DENTURE CARE

1 Explain the procedure to the patient.
2 Wash your hands.
3 Collect the following equipment:
   a Denture brush or toothbrush
   b Denture cup labeled with the patient's name and room number
   c Denture cleaner or toothpaste
   d Water glass with cool water
   e Straw
   f Mouthwash
   g Two face towels
   h Gauze squares
   i Disposable gloves
4 Identify the patient. Check the ID bracelet and call the patient by name.
5 Provide for privacy.
6 Lower the side rail.
7 Place a towel over the patient's chest.
8 Ask the patient to remove the dentures. Carefully place them in the emesis basin.
9 Put on gloves and remove the dentures using gauze squares if the patient cannot do so. (The gauze lets you get a good grip on the slippery dentures.)
   a Grasp the upper denture with your thumb and index finger (Fig. 13-8). You may need to break the seal that is holding it in place. Move the denture up and down slightly to break the seal. Gently remove the denture once the seal is broken. Place it in the emesis basin.
   b Remove the lower denture by grasping it with your thumb and index finger. Turn it slightly and lift it out of the patient's mouth. Place it in the emesis basin.
10 Raise the side rail.
11 Take the emesis basin, denture cup, brush, and denture cleaner or toothpaste to the sink.
12 Put on the gloves.
13 Rinse each denture under warm running water. Return them to the denture cup.
14 Line sink with a towel and fill it with water.

15 Apply denture cleaner or toothpaste to the brush.
16 Brush the dentures as in Figure 13-9.
17 Rinse the dentures under warm running water. Handle them carefully; do not drop them.
18 Place the dentures in the denture cup. Fill it with cool water until the dentures are covered.
19 Clean the emesis basin.
20 Bring the denture cup and emesis basin to the bedside table.
21 Lower the side rail.
22 Position the patient for oral hygiene.
23 Assist the patient to rinse out his or her mouth with mouthwash. Hold the emesis basin under the chin.
24 Ask the patient to insert the dentures. You must insert them if the patient cannot.
   a Grasp the upper denture firmly with your thumb and index finger. Raise the upper lip with the other hand and insert the denture. Use your index fingers to gently press on the denture to make sure that it is securely in place.
   b Grasp the lower denture securely with your thumb and index finger. Pull down slightly on the lower lip and insert the denture. Gently press down on it to make sure it is in place.
25 Remove the gloves.
26 Put the denture cup in the top drawer of the bedside stand if the dentures are not reinserted.
27 Make sure the patient is comfortable.
28 Make sure the signal light is within reach.
29 Raise the side rail.
30 Unscreen the patient.
31 Clean and return equipment to its proper place. Discard disposable equipment.
32 Place soiled linen in the linen hamper.
33 Wash your hands.
34 Report your observations to the nurse.

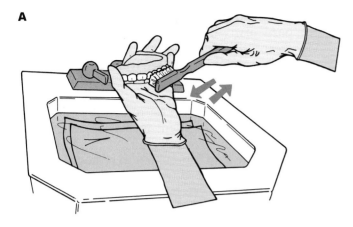

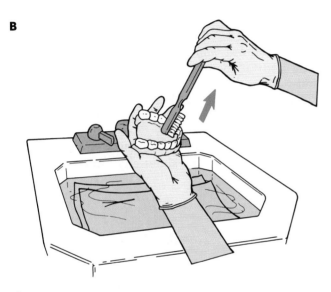

Fig. 13-9 A, Outer surfaces of the upper denture are brushed with back and forth motions. Note that the denture is held over the sink, which is filled halfway with water and lined with a towel. **B,** Position the brush vertically to clean the inner surfaces of the denture. Use upward strokes.

dentures. If dentures are not worn, they are stored in a container of cool water. Dentures can dry out and warp if they are not stored in water.

BATHING

Bathing has other purposes besides cleansing. A bath is refreshing and relaxing. Circulation is stimulated, and body parts are exercised. Observations can be made during the bath. The bath also gives you time to talk with and get to know the patient.

A patient may get a complete or partial bed bath, a tub bath, or a shower. The method depends on the patient's condition, ability to provide self-care, and personal choice. In health facilities, bathing usually occurs daily after breakfast. Again, personal choice should be considered regarding time of day and fre-

quency. A person who bathes at bedtime should be allowed to continue the practice if possible.

The frequency of bathing is an individual matter. Some people bathe at least once a day. Others take a complete bath only once or twice a week. Personal choice, the weather, physical activity, and illness influence how often a person bathes. Illness usually increases the need for bathing because of fever and increased perspiration. Other illnesses and dry skin may require bathing every 2 or 3 days.

Skin Care Products

There are many kinds of skin care products. Some are used for cleansing. Others protect the skin from drying or friction. The products used depend on personal choice and cost.

Soaps cleanse the skin. They remove dirt, dead skin, skin oil, some mircoorganisms, and perspiration. However, they tend to dry and irritate the skin. Dry skin is easily injured and causes itching and discomfort. Skin must be rinsed well to remove all soap.

Soap is not needed for every bath. Plain water can clean the skin. Plain water is often used for the elderly because of their dry skin. People with dry skin may prefer soaps containing bath oils. Soap should not be used if a person has very dry skin.

Bath oils keep the skin soft and prevent drying. Some soaps contain bath oils, or liquid bath oil can be added to bath water. Showers and tubs become slippery from bath oils. Safety precautions are necessary to prevent falls.

Creams and lotions protect the skin from the drying effect of air and evaporation. They do not feel greasy but leave an oily film on the skin. Most are scented.

Powders absorb moisture and prevent friction when two skin surfaces rub together. They are usually applied under the breasts, under the arms, and in the groin area. Sometimes powders are applied between the toes. Powder is applied to dry skin in a thin, even layer. Excessive amounts of powder cause caking and crusts that can irritate skin.

Deodorants and antiperspirants are applied to the axillae (underarms) after bathing. *Deodorants* mask and control body odors. *Antiperspirants* reduce the amount of perspiration. Deodorants and antiperspirants are not applied to irritated skin. They do not take the place of bathing.

Observations

When bathing a patient or assisting a patient to bathe, you should observe the skin. The following observations are reported to the nurse:

1. The color of the skin, lips, nail beds, and sclera (whites of the eyes)
2. The location and description of rashes
3. Dry skin

4. Bruises or open areas of the skin
5. Pale or reddened areas, particularly over bony parts
6. Drainage or bleeding from wounds or body openings
7. Skin temperature
8. Patient complaints of pain or discomfort

General Rules

Certain rules must be followed for bed baths, showers, or tub baths.

1. Ask the nurse what type of bath a patient is to have. Find out which skin care products to use. The person's personal choice should be allowed when possible.
2. Collect necessary equipment before beginning the procedure.
3. Protect the patient's privacy. Properly screen the patient and close doors.
4. Make sure the patient is adequately covered for warmth and privacy.
5. Reduce drafts by closing doors and windows.
6. Protect the patient from falling.
7. Use good body mechanics at all times.
8. Make sure water temperature is not too hot, particularly if the patient is elderly.
9. Keep soap in the soap dish between latherings. This prevents the water from becoming very soapy. If a tub bath is taken, the patient will not slip on the soap.
10. Wash from the cleanest to the dirtiest areas.
11. Encourage the patient to help as much as is safely possible.
12. Rinse the skin thoroughly to remove all soap.
13. Pat the skin dry to avoid irritating or breaking the skin.
14. Bathe the skin whenever fecal material or urine is on the skin.

The Complete Bed Bath

The *complete bed bath* involves washing the patient's entire body in bed. Patients who are unconscious, paralyzed, in a cast or traction, or are weak from illness or surgery generally require bed baths. Complete bed baths are given to patients who cannot bathe themselves.

Ask the nurse about the patient's ability to assist with the bath. Also ask about any limitations in ac-

GIVING A COMPLETE BED BATH

1   Identify the patient. Check the ID bracelet and call the patient by name.
2   Explain the procedure to the patient.
3   Offer the bedpan or urinal. Screen the patient if the bedpan or urinal is used.
4   Wash your hands.
5   Collect clean linen for a closed bed. Place the linen on a clean surface.
6   Collect the following equipment:
   a   Wash basin
   b   Soap dish with soap
   c   Bath thermometer
   d   Orange stick or nail file
   e   Washcloth
   f   Two bath towels and two face towels
   g   Bath blanket
   h   Gown or pajamas
   i   Equipment for oral hygiene
   j   Body lotion
   k   Talcum powder
   l   Deodorant or antiperspirant
   m   Brush and comb
   n   Other toilet articles if requested
   o   Paper towels
   p   Disposable gloves (for universal precautions)

7   Arrange equipment on the overbed table. Adjust the height as necessary. Use the bedside stand if necessary.
8   Close doors and windows to prevent drafts.
9   Provide for privacy.
10 Raise the bed to a level appropriate for good body mechanics.
11 Remove the signal light.
12 Provide oral hygiene.
13 Remove top linens and cover the patient with a bath blanket (see *Making an Occupied Bed*, pages 187-190).
14 Lower the head of the bed to a level appropriate for the patient. Keep it as flat as possible. Let the patient have at least one pillow.
15 Place the paper towels on the overbed table.
16 Fill the wash basin ⅔ full with water. Water temperature should be 110° to 115° F (43° to 46° C).
17 Place the basin on the overbed table on top of the paper towels.
18 Lower the side rail.
19 Place a face towel over the patient's chest.
20 Make a mitt with the washcloth (Fig. 13-10). Use a mitt throughout the procedure.

GIVING A COMPLETE BED BATH—cont'd

21 Wash the patient's eyes with water only. Do not use soap. Gently wipe from the inner aspect with a corner of the mitt (Fig. 13-11). Clean the eye farthest from you first. Repeat this step for the near eye.

22 Ask the patient if you should use soap to wash the face.

23 Wash his or her face, ears, and neck. Rinse and dry the skin well using the towel on the chest.

24 Help the patient move to the side of the bed near you.

25 Remove the gown. Do not expose the patient.

26 Place a bath towel lengthwise under the far arm.

27 Support the arm with the palm of your hand under the patient's elbow. His or her forearm should rest on your forearm.

28 Wash the arm, shoulder, and armpit with long, firm strokes (Fig. 13-12). Rinse and pat dry.

29 Place the basin on the towel. Put the patient's hand into the water (Fig. 13-13). Wash the hand well. Clean underneath the fingernails with an orange stick or nail file.

30 Encourage the patient to exercise the hand and fingers.

31 Remove the wash basin and dry the hand well. Cover the arm with the bath blanket.

32 Repeat steps 26-31 for the near arm.

33 Place a bath towel over the chest crosswise. Hold the towel in place and pull the bath blanket from under the towel to the waist.

34 Lift the towel slightly and wash the patient's chest (Fig. 13-14). Do not expose the patient. Rinse and pat dry.

35 Place the towel lengthwise over the chest and abdomen. Do not expose the patient. Pull the bath blanket down to the pubic area.

36 Lift the towel slightly and wash the abdomen (Fig. 13-15). Rinse and pat dry.

37 Pull the bath blanket up to the shoulders, covering both arms. Remove the towel.

38 Change the water if it is soapy or cool. Raise the side rail before you leave the bedside. Lower it when you return.

39 Uncover the far leg. Do not expose the genital area. Place a towel lengthwise under the foot and leg.

40 Bend the knee and support the leg with your arm. Wash the leg with long, firm strokes. Rinse and pat dry.

41 Place the basin on the towel near the foot.

42 Lift the leg slightly. Slide the basin under the foot.

43 Place the foot in the basin (Fig. 13-16). Use an orange stick or nail file to clean under the toenails if necessary.

44 Remove the basin and dry the leg. Cover the leg with the bath blanket. Remove the towel.

45 Repeat steps 39-44 for the near leg.

46 Change the water. Raise the side rail before leaving the bedside. Lower it when you return.

47 Turn the patient onto the side away from you. Keep him or her properly covered with the bath blanket.

48 Uncover the back and buttocks. Do not expose the patient. Place a towel lengthwise on the bed along the patient's back.

49 Wash the back, working from the back of the neck to the buttocks. Use long, firm, continuous strokes (Fig. 13-17). Rinse and dry the area well.

50 Give a back massage. (The patient may prefer to have the back massage after the bath.)

51 Turn the patient onto the back.

52 Change the water for perineal care. Raise the side rail before you leave the bedside. Lower it when you return.

53 Let the patient wash the genital area. Adjust the overbed table so that he or she can reach the wash basin, soap, and towels with ease. Place the signal light within reach. Ask him or her to signal when finished. Make sure the patient understands what to do. Answer the signal light promptly. Provide perineal care if the patient cannot do so (see *Perineal Care*, page 211).

54 Give a back massage if you have not already done so.

55 Apply deodorant or antiperspirant.

56 Put a clean gown or pajamas on the patient.

57 Comb and brush the hair.

58 Make the bed. Attach the signal light.

59 Make sure the patient is comfortable.

60 Make sure the side rails are up.

61 Lower the bed to its lowest position.

62 Empty and clean the wash basin.

63 Return the basin and supplies to their proper place.

64 Wipe off the overbed table with the paper towels and discard them.

65 Unscreen the patient.

66 Place soiled linen in the linen hamper.

67 Wash your hands.

68 Report your observations to the nurse.

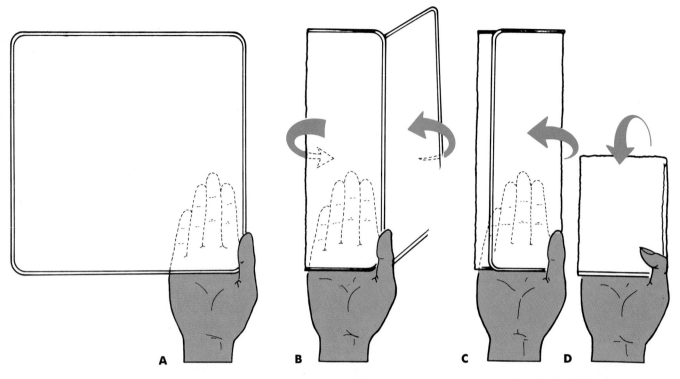

Fig. 13-10 **A,** Make a mitt with a washcloth by grasping the near side of the washcloth with your thumb. **B,** Bring the washcloth around and behind your hand. **C,** Fold the side of the washcloth over your palm as you grasp it with your thumb. **D,** Fold the top of the washcloth down and tuck it under next to your palm.

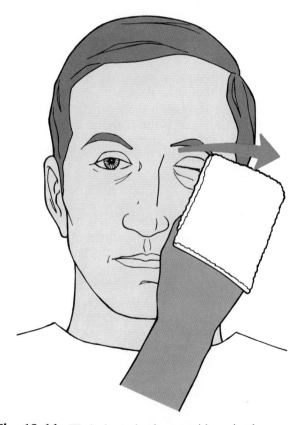

Fig. 13-11 Wash the patient's eyes with a mitted washcloth. Wipe from the inner to the outer aspect of the eye.

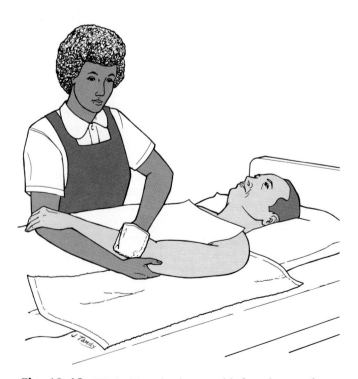

Fig. 13-12 Wash the patient's arm with firm, long strokes using a mitted washcloth.

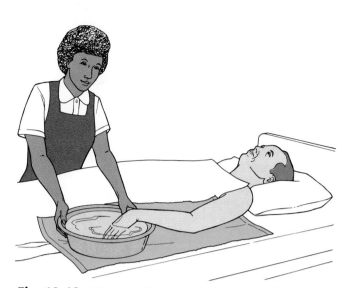

Fig. 13-13 The patient's hands are washed by placing the wash basin on the bed.

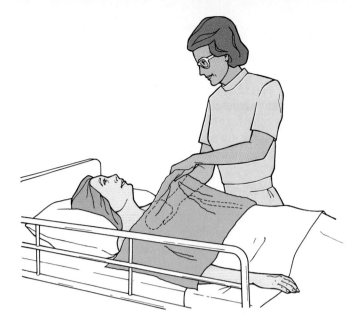

Fig. 13-14 The patient's breasts are not exposed during the bath. A bath towel is placed horizontally over the chest area. The towel is lifted slightly to reach under to wash the breasts and chest.

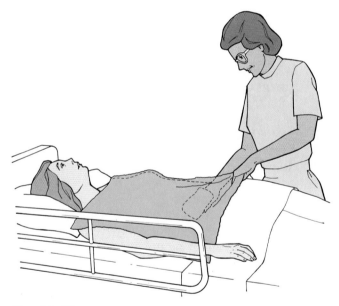

Fig. 13-15 The bath towel is turned so that it is vertical to cover the breasts and abdomen. The towel is lifted slightly to bathe the abdomen. The bath blanket covers the pubic area.

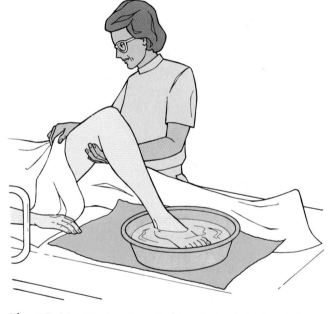

Fig. 13-16 The foot is washed by placing it in the wash basin on the bed.

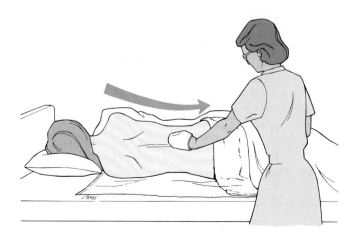

Fig. 13-17 The back is washed with long, firm, continuous strokes. Note that the patient is in a side-lying position. A towel is placed lengthwise on the bed to protect the linens from water.

tivity or position. Consult with the nurse about the need for universal precautions.

Many patients have never had a bed bath. They may be embarrassed to have another person see their body and may fear being exposed. Every patient must get an explanation about how a bed bath is given and how the body is covered to protect privacy.

The Partial Bath

The partial bath involves bathing the face, hands, axillae, genital area, back, and buttocks. These body areas may develop odors or cause discomfort if not clean. Partial bed baths are given to patients who cannot bathe themselves. Patients who are able may bathe themselves in bed or at the bathroom sink. Nursing personnel assist as needed, especially with washing the back.

The general rules for bathing apply for partial bed baths. The considerations involved in giving a complete bed bath also apply.

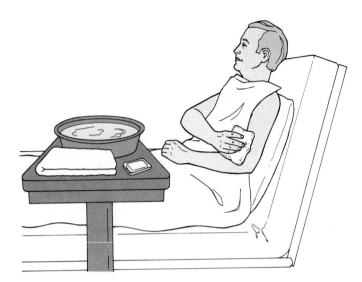

Fig. 13-18 The patient is bathing himself in bed. Necessary equipment is within his reach.

GIVING A PARTIAL BATH

1 Follow steps 1 through 9 in *Giving a Complete Bed Bath*, pages 202-203.
2 Make sure the bed is in the lowest position.
3 Assist the patient with oral hygiene. Adjust the height of the overbed table to an appropriate level.
4 Remove top linen. Cover the patient with a bath blanket.
5 Place the paper towels on the overbed table.
6 Fill the wash basin with water. Water temperature should be 110° to 115° F (43° to 46° C).
7 Place the basin on the overbed table on top of the paper towels.
8 Raise the head of the bed so that the patient can bathe comfortably. Assist him or her to sit at the bedside if allowed in this position.
9 Position the overbed table so that the patient can easily reach the basin and supplies.
10 Assist the patient with removing the gown.
11 Ask the patient to wash the parts of the body that can be reached with ease (Fig. 13-18). Explain that you will wash the back and those areas that cannot be reached.
12 Place the signal light within reach. Ask him or her to signal if help is needed or when bathing is complete.
13 Leave the room after washing your hands.
14 Return when the signal light is on. Knock before entering the room.
15 Change the bath water.

16 Ask what was washed. Wash the areas the patient could not reach. The face, hands, axillae, genital area, back, and buttocks are washed for the partial bath.
17 Give a back massage.
18 Apply deodorant or antiperspirant.
19 Help the patient put on a clean gown or pajamas.
20 Assist with hair care.
21 Assist him or her to a bedside chair. Turn the patient onto the side away from you if the patient cannot be up.
22 Make the bed.
23 Lower the bed to its lowest position.
24 Assist the patient to return to bed.
25 Make sure the patient is comfortable.
26 Place the signal light within reach.
27 Make sure the side rails are up.
28 Empty and clean the wash basin.
29 Return the basin and supplies to their proper place.
30 Wipe off the overbed table with the paper towels and discard them.
31 Unscreen the patient.
32 Place soiled linen in the linen hamper.
33 Wash your hands.
34 Report your observations to the nurse:
   a The condition of the patient's skin
   b The amount of assistance needed
   c How well the procedure was tolerated

The Tub Bath

Many people like tub baths. Patients may find them relaxing. Patients must be protected from falling when getting in and out of tubs and from burns caused by hot water temperatures. A tub bath can cause a person to feel faint, weak, or tired. This is more likely to occur if the person has been on bed rest. A bath should not last longer than 20 minutes.

Do not let a patient take a tub bath unless the nurse gives approval. Some patients have private baths. If not, you need to reserve the tub room. The tub should be cleaned before use. There must be a bath mat on the bottom of the tub to help prevent falls.

For safety, you may want to drain the tub before the person gets out of the tub. If the tub is drained first, keep the patient covered and protected from exposure and chilling. Changes in the procedure may be necessary for some patients. Consult with the nurse before assisting a patient with a tub bath.

Some facilities have portable tubs. The sides are lowered so that the patient can be transferred from the bed to the tub (Fig. 13-19). After the transfer, the sides are raised into position. The patient is then transported to the tub room. The portable tub is filled, and the patient is bathed in the usual manner. Nursing facilities, burn units, and rehabilitation units usually have portable tubs.

ASSISTING THE PATIENT WITH A TUB BATH

1. Reserve use of the bathtub if necessary.
2. Identify the patient. Check the ID bracelet and call the patient by name.
3. Explain the procedure to the patient.
4. Wash your hands.
5. Collect the following equipment:
   a. Washcloth
   b. Two bath towels
   c. Soap
   d. Bath thermometer
   e. Gown or pajamas
   f. Deodorant or antiperspirant
   g. Other toilet articles as requested
6. Place equipment in the bathroom in the space provided or on a chair.
7. Clean the tub if indicated.
8. Place a rubber bath mat in the tub.
9. Place a disposable bath mat or towel on the floor in front of the tub.
10. Place the "occupied" sign on the bathroom door.
11. Return to the patient's room. Provide for privacy.
12. Help the patient sit on the side of the bed.
13. Help the patient put on a robe and slippers.
14. Assist the patient to the bathroom. Use a wheelchair if necessary.
15. Have the patient sit on the chair by the tub.
16. Fill the tub halfway with water. Water temperature should be 105° F (41° C).
17. Help the patient remove slippers, robe, and gown.
18. Assist the patient into the tub (Fig. 13-20).
19. Explain how to use the signal light. Ask the patient to signal when finished bathing or when assistance is needed.
20. Remind him or her not to remain in the tub longer than 20 minutes.
21. Place a towel across the chair.
22. Leave the room and wash your hands.
23. Check the patient every 5 minutes.
24. Return when he or she has signaled for you. Knock before entering.
25. Help the patient out of the tub and onto the chair.
26. Help the patient dry off; pat gently.
27. Help the patient put on a clean gown or pajamas, a bathrobe, and slippers.
28. Assist the patient in returning to the room and to bed.
29. Provide a back massage.
30. Make sure the patient is comfortable.
31. Make sure the side rails are up.
32. Clean the tub. Remove soiled linen and discard disposable equipment. Put the "unoccupied" sign on the door. Return supplies to their proper place.
33. Place soiled linen in the linen hamper.
34. Wash your hands.
35. Report your observations to the nurse:
    a. The condition of the patient's skin
    b. The amount of assistance needed
    c. How well the procedure was tolerated

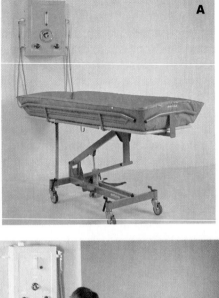

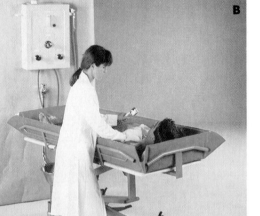

Fig. 13-19 **A,** Portable tub. **B,** The sides are lowered so that the patient can be transferred from the bed to the tub.

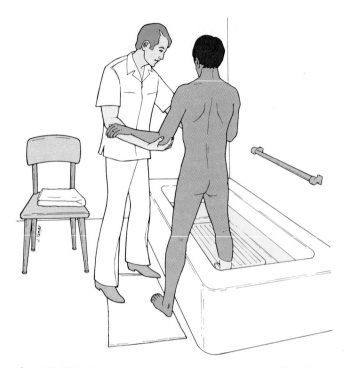

Fig. 13-20 The nursing assistant helps the patient into the tub to protect the patient from falling. A bath mat is in the tub, the tub is filled halfway with water, and a floor mat is in front of the tub.

The Shower

A shower may be part of the bathtub or a separate stall. A shower stall has advantages. The person can walk into the stall rather than having to step over the side of the tub. Weak and paralyzed patients can use a shower chair, which is wheeled into the shower stall. Shower chairs are made of plastic, with wheels on the legs. A round open area in the seat lets water drain (Fig. 13-21). The chair can be used to transport the person to and from the shower room. The wheels must be locked during the shower to prevent the chair from moving. A straight-backed chair or a stool can be used if a shower chair is not available. Lawn chairs have been used as shower chairs in private homes.

Patients must be protected from falling and chilling. Their privacy must also be protected. Weak or unsteady patients are not allowed to stand in the shower. They are not left unattended. Encourage patients to use the hand rails for support when getting in and out of the shower. Hand rails are especially important if the shower is in a tub. As with the tub

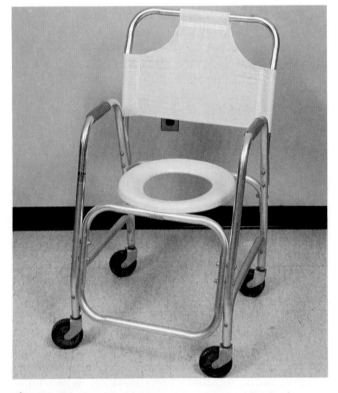

Fig. 13-21 A shower chair has a round opening in the center of the seat. The legs have wheels with locks to allow the chair to be used for transfers.

ASSISTING THE PATIENT TO SHOWER

1   Reserve the shower if necessary.
2   Identify the patient. Check the ID bracelet and call the patient by name.
3   Explain the procedure to the patient.
4   Wash your hands.
5   Collect the following equipment:
   a   Washcloth
   b   Two bath towels
   c   Soap
   d   Shower cap
   e   Gown or pajamas
   f   Deodorant or antiperspirant
   g   Other toilet articles as requested
6   Place the equipment on a chair or in the space provided near the shower.
7   Clean the shower if indicated.
8   Place a rubber bath mat on the floor of the shower. Do not block the drain.
9   Place a disposable bath mat or towel on the floor in front of the shower.
10   Place the "occupied" sign on the shower door.
11   Return to the patient's room. Provide for privacy.
12   Help the patient sit on the side of the bed.
13   Help the patient put on a robe and slippers.
14   Assist the patient to the shower room. Use a wheelchair or shower chair if necessary.
15   Explain how to use the signal light. Ask the patient to signal when finished showering or when assistance is needed.
16   Turn the shower on. Adjust the water temperature and pressure.
17   Help the patient remove slippers, gown, and robe.

18   Help him or her into the shower. If using a shower chair, place it in position and lock the wheels.
19   Assist the patient with washing if necessary.
20   Place a towel across the chair that is outside of the shower.
21   Wash your hands and leave the room only if the patient can stand without help. Stay outside of the stall if the patient is weak.
22   Return to the shower room when the patient has signaled. Knock before entering.
23   Turn the shower off.
24   Assist the patient out of the shower and onto the chair.
25   Help the patient dry off; pat gently.
26   Help him or her put on a clean gown or pajamas, a robe, and slippers.
27   Assist the patient in returning to the room and to bed.
28   Provide a back massage.
29   Make sure the patient is comfortable.
30   Make sure the side rails are up.
31   Place the signal light within reach.
32   Clean the shower. Remove soiled linen and discard disposable equipment. Put the "unoccupied" sign on the door. Return supplies to their proper place.
33   Place soiled linen in the linen hamper.
34   Wash your hands.
35   Report your observations to the nurse:
   a   The condition of the patient's skin
   b   The amount of assistance needed
   c   How well the procedure was tolerated

---

bath, patients may shower only with a nurse's approval.

THE BACK MASSAGE

The back massage, or back rub, relaxes muscles and stimulates circulation. The massage is normally given after the bath and as a part of hs care. It should last about 4 to 6 minutes. Observe the skin for abnormalities before beginning the procedure.

Lotion is used to reduce friction when giving the massage. It should be warmed before being applied. Place the lotion bottle in the bath water or hold it under warm running water to warm. You can also rub some between your hands.

The prone position is best for a massage. The side-lying position is often used. Firm strokes are used, and your hands should always be in contact with the patient's skin.

Some patients should not have back massages as described in this procedure. They may be dangerous for those with certain heart diseases, back injuries, back surgeries, skin diseases, and some lung disorders. Check with the nurse before giving back massages to patients with these conditions.

GIVING A BACK MASSAGE

1. Identify the patient. Check the ID bracelet and call the patient by name.
2. Explain the procedure to the patient.
3. Wash your hands.
4. Collect the following equipment:
   a. Bath blanket
   b. Bath towel
   c. Lotion
5. Provide for privacy.
6. Raise the bed to an appropriate level for good body mechanics.
7. Lower the side rail.
8. Position the patient in the prone or side-lying position with his or her back toward you.
9. Expose the back, shoulders, upper arms, and buttocks. Cover the rest of the body with the bath blanket.
10. Lay the towel on the bed along the back.
11. Warm the lotion bottle under running water or rub some lotion between your hands.
12. Explain that the lotion may feel cool and wet.
13. Apply lotion to the lower back area.
14. Stroke up from the buttocks to the shoulders. Then stroke down over the upper arms. Stroke up the upper arms, across the shoulders, and down the back to the buttocks (Fig. 13-22). Use firm strokes. Keep your hands in contact with the patient's skin.
15. Repeat step 14 for at least 3 minutes.
16. Knead by grasping tissue between your thumb and fingers (Fig. 13-23). Knead half of the back starting at the buttocks and moving up to the shoulder. Then knead down from the shoulder to the buttocks. Repeat on the other half of the back.
17. Massage bony areas. Use circular motions with the tips of your index and middle fingers.
18. Use fast movements to stimulate and slow movements to relax the patient.
19. Stroke with long, firm movements to end the massage. Tell the patient you are finishing.
20. Cover the patient. Remove the towel and bath blanket.

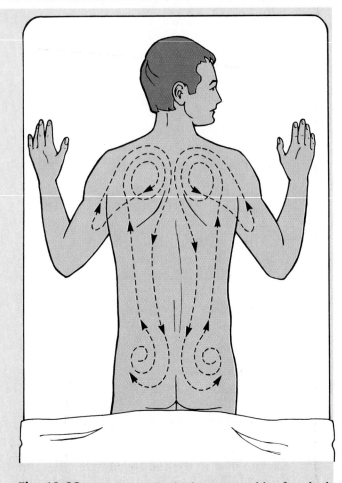

Fig. 13-22 The patient lies in the prone position for a back massage. Stroke upward from the buttocks to the shoulders, down over the upper arms, back up the upper arms, across the shoulders, and down the back to the buttocks.

21. Make sure the patient is comfortable.
22. Raise the side rail. Place the signal light within reach.
23. Lower the bed to its lowest position.
24. Return the lotion to its proper place.
25. Unscreen the patient.
26. Place soiled linen in the linen hamper.
27. Wash your hands.
28. Report your observations to the nurse.

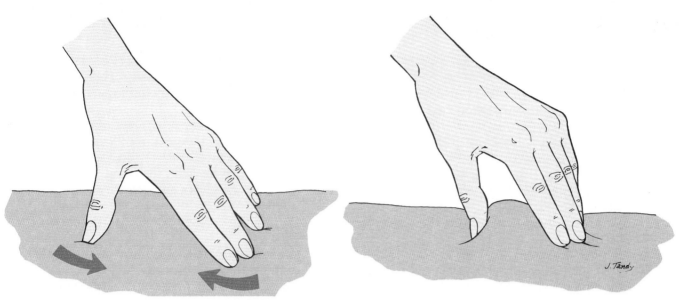

Fig. 13-23 Kneading is done by picking up tissue between the thumb and fingers.

PERINEAL CARE

Perineal care (pericare) involves cleaning the genital and anal areas. These areas are warm, moist, and dark. They provide a place for microorganisms to grow. The genital and anal areas are cleaned to prevent infection and odors and to promote comfort.

Perineal care is done at least once a day as part of the bath. The procedure is also done whenever the area is contaminated with urine or feces. Patients with certain disorders need more frequent perineal care. Perineal care is given before and after some surgeries and after childbirth.

Patients should do their own perineal care if able. Otherwise it is given by nursing personnel. Many patients and nursing personnel find the procedure embarrassing, especially when given to the opposite sex. Patients may not know the terms *perineum* and *perineal*. Most people understand one or more of the following terms: "privates," "private parts," "crotch," "genitals," or "the area between your legs." Be sure to use a term that the patient understands. The term should also be in good taste professionally.

Universal precautions and the rules of medical asepsis are followed. You will work from the cleanest area to the dirtiest. The urethral area is the cleanest and the anal area the dirtiest. Therefore clean from the urethra to the anal area. The perineal area is very delicate and is easily injured. Warm water, not hot water, is used. The area must be rinsed thoroughly. The perineum is patted dry after rinsing to reduce moisture and promote comfort.

GIVING FEMALE PERINEAL CARE

1 Explain the procedure to the patient.
2 Wash your hands.
3 Collect the following equipment:
  a Soap dish with soap
  b Three to ten disposable washcloths or a small package of cotton balls
  c Bath towel
  d Bath blanket
  e Bath thermometer
  f Waterproof pad
  g Disposable gloves
  h Paper towels
  i Disposable bag

4 Arrange the equipment on the overbed table.
5 Identify the patient. Check the ID bracelet and call her by name.
6 Provide for privacy.
7 Raise the bed to a level appropriate for good body mechanics.
8 Lower the side rail.
9 Cover the patient with a bath blanket. Move top linens to the foot of the bed.
10 Position the patient on her back.
11 Position the waterproof pad under her buttocks.

Continued.

GIVING FEMALE PERINEAL CARE—cont'd

12 Drape the patient as in Figure 13-24.
13 Raise the side rail.
14 Fill the wash basin. Water temperature should be approximately 105° to 109.4° F (41° to 43° C).
15 Place the basin on the overbed table on top of the paper towels.
16 Put the washcloths in the basin. Squeeze out excess water before using them.
17 Lower the side rail.
18 Help the patient flex her knees and spread her legs.
19 Put on the gloves.
20 Fold the corner of the bath blanket between the patient's legs onto her abdomen.
21 Apply soap to a washcloth.
22 Separate the labia. Clean downward from front to back with one stroke (Fig. 13-25). Discard the washcloth into the disposable bag.
23 Repeat steps 21 and 22 until the area is clean.
24 Rinse the perineum with a washcloth. Separate the labia. Stroke downward from front to back. Discard the washcloth and repeat the step as necessary.
25 Pat the area dry with the towel.
26 Fold the blanket back between her legs.
27 Help the patient lower her legs and turn onto her side away from you.
28 Apply soap to a washcloth.
29 Clean the rectal area. Clean from the vagina to the anus with one stroke (Fig. 13-26). Discard the washcloth.
30 Repeat steps 28 and 29 until the area is clean.
31 Rinse the rectal area with a washcloth. Stroke from the vagina to the anus. Discard the washcloth. Repeat the step as necessary.
32 Pat the area dry with the towel.
33 Remove the gloves and discard them into the bag.
34 Position the patient so that she is comfortable.
35 Return linens to their proper position and remove the bath blanket.
36 Raise the side rail. Place the signal light within reach.
37 Lower the bed to its lowest position.
38 Empty and clean the wash basin.
39 Return the basin and supplies to their proper place.
40 Wipe off the overbed table with the paper towels and discard them.
41 Unscreen the patient.
42 Take soiled linen and the disposable bag to the "dirty" utility room.
43 Wash your hands.
44 Report your observations to the nurse:
  a Any odors
  b Redness, swelling, discharge, or irritation
  c Patient complaints of pain, burning, or other discomfort

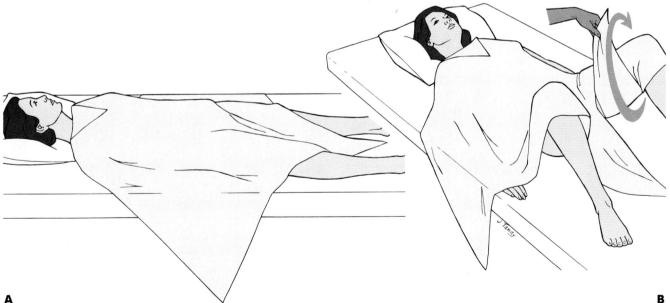

A   **B**

Fig. 13-24 A, Drape the patient for perineal care by positioning the bath blanket like a diamond: one corner is at the neck, there is a corner at each side, and one corner is between the patient's legs. **B,** Wrap the blanket around the leg by bringing the corner around under the leg and over the top. Tuck the corner under the hip.

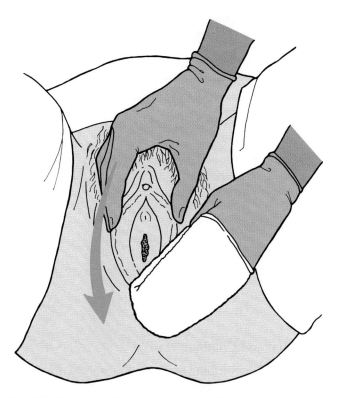

Fig. 13-25 Perineal care is given to the female by separating the labia with one hand. The nursing assistant uses a mitted washcloth to cleanse between the labia with downward strokes.

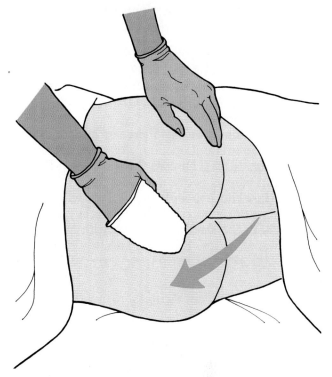

Fig. 13-26 The rectal area is cleaned by wiping from the vagina to the anus. The side-lying position allows the anal area to be cleaned more thoroughly.

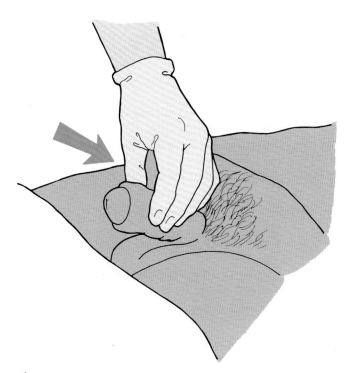

Fig. 13-27 The foreskin of the uncircumcised male is pulled back for perineal care. It is returned to the normal position immediately after cleaning.

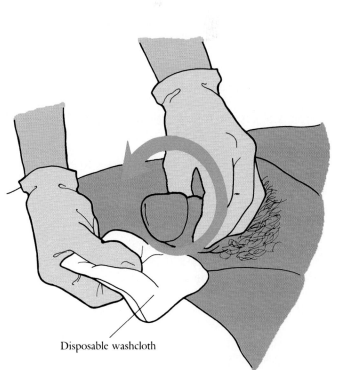

Disposable washcloth

Fig. 13-28 The penis is cleaned with circular motions starting at the urethra.

GIVING MALE PERINEAL CARE

1 Follow steps 1 through 21 in *Female Perineal Care*, pages 211-212.
2 Retract the foreskin if the patient is uncircumcised (Fig. 13-27).
3 Grasp the penis.
4 Clean the tip using a circular motion. Start at the urethral opening and work outward (Fig. 13-28). Discard the washcloth. Repeat this step as necessary.
5 Rinse the area with another washcloth.
6 Return the foreskin to its natural position.
7 Clean the shaft of the penis with firm downward strokes. Rinse the area.
8 Help the patient to flex his knees and spread his legs.
9 Clean the scrotum and rinse well.
10 Pat dry the penis and scrotum.
11 Fold the bath blanket back between his legs.
12 Help him lower his legs and turn onto his side away from you.
13 Clean the rectal area (see *Female Perineal Care*). Rinse and dry well.
14 Follow steps 33 through 44 in *Female Perineal Care*.

HAIR CARE

Appearance and mental well-being are affected by how the hair looks and feels. Illness and disability may prevent people from performing hair care. Patients and residents are assisted with hair care whenever necessary. Some facilities have barbers and beauticians for cutting, shampooing, and styling hair.

Brushing and Combing Hair

Brushing and combing are part of morning care. They are also done at other times of day if needed. Many people like to have their hair styled before visitors arrive. Encourage patients to do their own hair care. However, you should provide assistance as needed. Hair care is performed for those who cannot do so. Let the patient choose how hair is to be brushed, combed, and styled.

BRUSHING AND COMBING THE PATIENT'S HAIR

1 Identify the patient. Check the ID bracelet and call the patient by name.
2 Explain the procedure to the patient.
3 Collect the following equipment:
   a Comb and brush
   b Bath towel
   c Toilet articles as requested
4 Arrange equipment on the bedside stand.
5 Wash your hands.
6 Provide for privacy.
7 Lower the side rail.
8 Help the patient to a chair or to semi-Fowler's position if possible. The patient puts on a robe and slippers if he or she is to be up.
9 Place a towel across the shoulders. Place a towel across the pillow if the patient is in bed.
10 Ask the patient to remove eyeglasses. Put them in the glass case. Put the case inside the bedside stand.
11 Part the hair and divide it into 2 main sections (Fig. 13-29, A). Divide one side into 2 sections (Fig. 13-29, B).
12 Brush the hair. Start at the scalp and brush toward the hair ends (Fig. 13-30).
13 Style the hair as the patient prefers.
14 Remove the towel.
15 Let the patient put on the eyeglasses.
16 Assist him or her to assume a comfortable position.
17 Raise the side rail.
18 Place the signal light within reach.
19 Unscreen the patient.
20 Clean and return equipment to its proper place. Place soiled linen in the linen hamper.
21 Wash your hands.

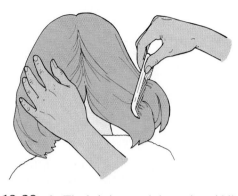

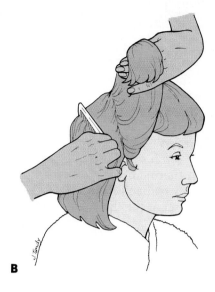

Fig. 13-29 A, The hair is parted down the middle and divided into two main sections. **B,** A main section is then parted into two smaller sections.

Long hair is easily matted and tangled during bed rest. Daily brushing and combing helps prevent this problem. Braiding also prevents matting and tangling. Hair is not braided unless the patient gives permission. Never cut hair to remove mats or tangles.

When giving hair care, protect the patient's gown or clothing by placing a towel across the shoulders. If hair care is provided when the patient is in bed, it is done before changing the pillowcase. If done after a linen change, place a towel across the pillow to collect falling hair.

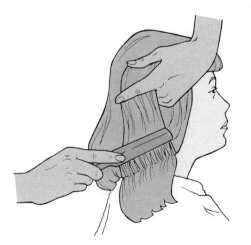

Fig. 13-30 The hair is brushed by starting at the scalp and brushing down to the hair ends.

Shampooing

Most people wash their hair at least once a week. Some shampoo 2 or 3 times a week. Others shampoo every day. Many factors influence the frequency of shampooing. These include the condition of the hair and scalp, hairstyle, and personal choice. Shampoo and hair conditioner also depend on personal choice.

Patients and residents probably need help shampooing. Personal choice is followed whenever possible. However, safety is necessary, and the nurse's approval is needed. If a shampoo is requested, inform the nurse of the request. Do not wash a person's hair unless a nurse directs you to do so.

There are several ways to shampoo hair. The method used depends on the person's condition, safety factors, and personal choice if possible. The nurse decides which method to use. Hair is dried and styled as quickly as possible after shampooing. Women may want their hair curled or rolled up before drying. Consult with the nurse before curling or rolling up a patient's hair.

Shampooing during the shower or tub bath Patients who can shower will probably be able to shampoo at the same time. Shampooing can also be done for those using shower chairs. A hand-held shower nozzle is used. It can also be used during a tub bath. A spray of water is directed to the hair. The person shampooing during a tub bath will probably need some help. An extra towel, shampoo, and hair conditioner (if requested) should be within the person's reach.

SHAMPOOING THE PATIENT'S HAIR

1 Explain the procedure to the patient.
2 Wash your hands.
3 Collect the following equipment:
  a Two bath towels
  b Face towel or washcloth folded lengthwise
  c Shampoo
  d Hair conditioner if requested
  e Bath thermometer
  f Pitcher or hand-held nozzle
  g Equipment for the shampoo in bed (if needed)
    1 Trough
    2 Basin or pail
    3 Bath blanket
    4 Waterproof bed protector
  h Comb and brush
  i Hair dryer
4 Arrange equipment in a convenient place.
5 Identify the patient. Check the ID bracelet and call the patient by name.
6 Provide for privacy.
7 Position the patient for the method you are going to use.
8 Place a bath towel across the shoulders or across the pillow under the patient's head.
9 Brush and comb the hair to remove snarls and tangles.
10 Obtain water. Water temperature should be about 110° F (43° to 44° C).
11 Ask the patient to hold the face towel or washcloth over the eyes.
12 Apply water until the hair is completely wet. Use the pitcher or nozzle.
13 Apply a small amount of shampoo.
14 Work up a lather with both hands. Start at the hairline and work toward the back.
15 Massage the scalp with your fingertips.
16 Rinse the hair with water.
17 Repeat steps 13 through 15.
18 Rinse the hair thoroughly.
19 Apply conditioner and rinse as directed on the container.
20 Wrap the patient's head with a bath towel.
21 Dry his or her face with the towel or washcloth used to protect the eyes.
22 Help the patient raise the head if appropriate.
23 Rub the hair and scalp with the towel. Use the second towel if the first is wet.
24 Comb the hair to remove snarls and tangles. A woman may want hair curled or rolled up.
25 Dry the hair as quickly as possible.
26 Make sure the patient is comfortable.
27 Place the signal light within reach.
28 Clean and return equipment to its proper place. Discard disposable items. Place soiled linen in the linen hamper.
29 Wash your hands.

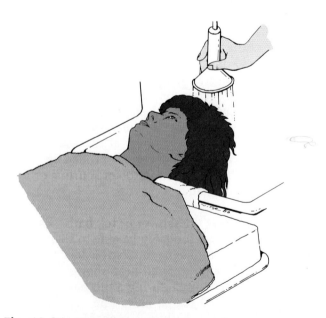

Fig. 13-31 Shampooing while on a stretcher. The stretcher is in front of the sink.

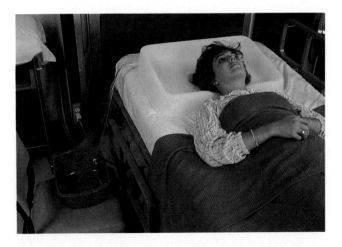

Fig. 13-32 A trough is used when shampooing a patient in bed. The trough is directed to the side of the bed so that water drains into a collecting basin.

Shampooing at the sink Individuals who can sit in a chair can usually be shampooed at a sink. The chair is placed so that the person faces away from the sink. The person's head is tilted back over the edge of the sink. A folded towel is placed over the sink edge to protect the neck. A water pitcher or hand-held nozzle is used to wet and rinse the hair.

Shampooing a patient on a stretcher Hair can be washed with the person lying on a stretcher. The stretcher is positioned in front of a sink. A pillow is placed under the head and neck, and the head is tilted over the edge of the sink (Fig. 13-31). A water pitcher or hand-held nozzle is used to wet and rinse the hair. Be sure to lock the wheels of the stretcher and to use the safety straps. Make sure the far side rail is raised.

Shampooing a patient in bed A shampoo can be given to a patient in bed. This method is used for those who cannot sit in a chair or be transferred to a stretcher. The patient's head and shoulders are moved to the edge of the bed if the position is allowed. A rubber or plastic trough is placed under the head to protect the linens and mattress from water. The trough also drains water into a basin placed on a chair by the bed (Fig. 13-32). A water pitcher is used to wet and rinse the hair.

SHAVING

A clean-shaven face is important for the comfort and well-being of many men. Likewise, most women shave their legs and underarms. Patients may prefer

---

SHAVING THE MALE PATIENT

1 Explain the procedure to the patient.
2 Wash your hands.
3 Collect the following equipment:
  a Wash basin
  b Bath towel
  c Face towel
  d Washcloth
  e Bath thermometer
  f Razor or shaver
  g Mirror
  h Shaving cream or soap
  i Shaving brush
  j After-shave lotion
  k Tissues
  l Paper towel
  m Disposable gloves
4 Arrange equipment on the overbed table.
5 Identify the patient. Check the ID bracelet and call the patient by name.
6 Provide for privacy.
7 Raise the bed to a level appropriate for good body mechanics.
8 Fill the wash basin. Water temperature should be approximately 115° F (46° C).
9 Place the basin on the overbed table on top of the paper towels.
10 Lower the side rail.
11 Position the patient in semi-Fowler's position if allowed or on his back.
12 Adjust lighting so that you can clearly see the patient's face.
13 Place the bath towel over the chest.
14 Position the overbed table within easy reach and at a comfortable working height.
15 Put on the gloves.
16 Wash the patient's face. Do not dry.
17 Place a washcloth or face towel in the water and wet it thoroughly. Wring it out.
18 Apply the washcloth or towel to the patient's face to soften the beard. Remove it after 3 to 5 minutes.
19 Apply shaving cream to the face with your hands. If apply lather, use a shaving brush.
20 Tighten the razor blade to the razor.
21 Hold the skin taut with your non-dominant hand.
22 Shave in the direction of hair growth. Use shorter strokes around the chin and lips (Fig. 13-33).
23 Rinse the razor often and wipe with tissues.
24 Apply direct pressure to any bleeding areas.
25 Wash off any remaining shaving cream or soap. Dry with a towel.
26 Apply after-shave lotion if requested.
27 Remove the gloves.
28 Move the overbed table to the side of the bed.
29 Make sure the patient is comfortable.
30 Place the signal light within reach.
31 Raise the side rail.
32 Lower the bed to its lowest position.
33 Clean and return equipment and supplies to their proper place. Discard disposable items.
34 Wipe off the overbed table with the paper towels. Discard the paper towels.
35 Position the table as appropriate for the patient.
36 Unscreen the patient.
37 Place soiled linen in the linen hamper.
38 Wash your hands.
39 Report any nicks or bleeding to the nurse.

electric shavers or razor blades. When using an electric shaver, practice safety precautions for using electrical equipment. Razor blades can cause nicks or cuts. Universal precautions may be necessary to prevent contact with the patient's blood.

The beard and skin are softened before shaving with a razor blade. The skin is softened by applying a warm washcloth or face towel to the face for a few minutes. Then the face is lathered with soap and water or a shaving cream. Be careful not to cut or irritate the skin while shaving. Women's legs and underarms can be shaved after the bath when the skin is soft. Soap and water or a shaving cream can also provide a lather for shaving the legs and underarms.

Many men have beards and mustaches, which need daily care. Ask the patient how he wants his beard or mustache groomed.

CARE OF NAILS AND FEET

Nails and feet need special attention to prevent infection, injury, and odors. Hangnails, ingrown nails (nails that grow in at the side), and nails torn away from the skin cause breaks in the skin. These breaks let microorganisms enter the body. Long or broken nails can scratch the skin or snag clothing. Dirty feet, socks, or stockings can harbor microorganisms and cause offensive odors.

Cleaning and trimming nails is easier after they have been soaked. Scissors are not used to cut fingernails. Extreme caution must be taken when clipping and trimming fingernails to prevent damage to surrounding tissues. Nursing assistants do not cut or trim toenails.

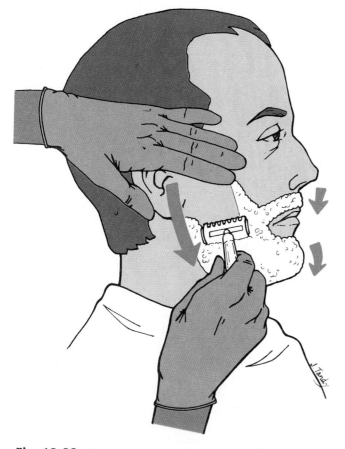

Fig. 13-33 Shaving is done in the direction of hair growth. Longer strokes are used on the larger areas of the face. Short strokes are used around the chin and lips.

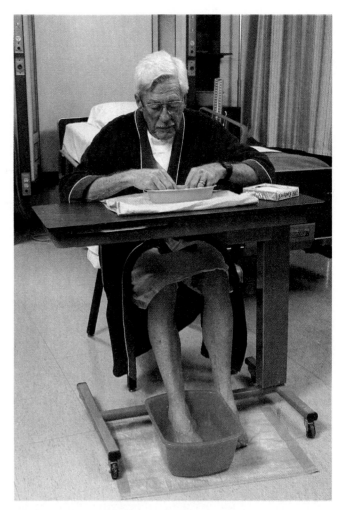

Fig. 13-34 Nail and foot care. The feet soak in a foot basin, and the fingers soak in the emesis basin.

GIVING NAIL AND FOOT CARE

1 Explain the procedure to the patient.
2 Wash your hands.
3 Collect the following equipment:
   a Wash basin
   b Bath thermometer
   c Bath towel
   d Face towel
   e Washcloth
   f Emesis basin
   g Nail clippers
   h Orange stick
   i Emery board or nail file
   j Lotion or petrolatum
   k Paper towels
   l Disposable bath mat
4 Arrange the equipment on the overbed table.
5 Identify the patient. Check the ID bracelet and call the patient by name.
6 Provide for privacy.
7 Help the patient to a bedside chair. Place the signal light within reach.
8 Place the bath mat under the patient's feet.
9 Fill the wash basin. Water temperature should be 109° to 111° F (43 to 44° C).
10 Place the basin on the bath mat. Help the patient put the feet into the basin.
11 Position the overbed table in front of the patient. It should be low and close to him or her.
12 Fill the emesis basin. Water temperature should be 109° to 111° F (43° to 44° C).
13 Place the basin on the overbed table on top of the paper towels.
14 Place the patient's fingers into the basin. Position the arms so that he or she is comfortable (Fig. 13-34).
15 Let the feet and fingernails soak for 20 to 30 minutes. Rewarm the water in 10 to 15 minutes.
16 Clean under the fingernails with the orange stick.
17 Remove the emesis basin and dry the fingers thoroughly.
18 Clip fingernails straight across with the nail clippers (Fig. 13-35).
19 Shape nails with an emery board or nail file.
20 Push cuticles back with the orange stick or a washcloth (Fig. 13-36).
21 Move the overbed table to the side.
22 Scrub callused areas of the feet with a washcloth.
23 Remove the feet from the basin. Dry thoroughly.
24 Apply lotion or petrolatum to the feet.
25 Assist the patient back to bed and to a comfortable position. Place the signal light within reach.
26 Raise the side rail.
27 Clean and return equipment and supplies to their proper place. Discard disposable supplies.
28 Unscreen the patient.
29 Take soiled linen to the "dirty" utility room.
30 Wash your hands.
31 Report your observations to the nurse:
   a Reddened, irritated, or callused areas
   b Breaks in the skin

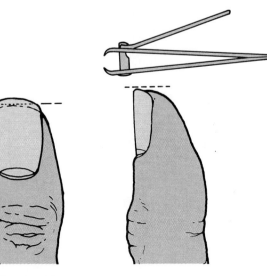

Fig. 13-35 Fingernails are clipped straight across. A nail clipper is used.

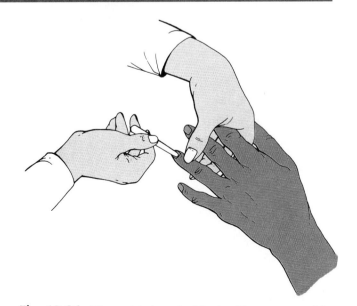

Fig. 13-36 The cuticle is pushed back with an orange stick.

CHANGING THE GOWN OF A PATIENT WITH AN IV

1 Explain the procedure to the patient.
2 Wash your hands.
3 Get a clean gown.
4 Identify the patient. Check the ID bracelet and call the patient by name.
5 Provide for privacy.
6 Untie the back of the gown. Free parts of the gown that the patient is lying on.
7 Remove the gown from the arm with no IV.
8 Gather up the sleeve of the arm with the IV. Slide it over the IV site and tubing. Remove the arm and hand from the sleeve (Fig. 13-37, *A*).
9 Keep the sleeve gathered. Slide your arm along the tubing to the bottle (Fig. 13-37, *B*).
10 Remove the bottle from the pole. Slide the bottle and tubing through the sleeve (Fig. 13-37, *C*). Do not pull on the tubing. Keep the bottle above the patient's arm.
11 Hang the IV bottle on the pole.
12 Gather the sleeve of the clean gown that will go on the arm with the IV infusion.
13 Remove the bottle from the pole. Quickly slip the gathered sleeve over the bottle at the shoulder part of the gown (Fig. 13-37, *D*). Hang the bottle on the pole.
14 Slide the gathered sleeve over the tubing, hand, arm, and IV site. Then slide the sleeve onto the patient's shoulder.
15 Put the other side of the gown on the patient.
16 Fasten the back of the gown.
17 Make sure the patient is comfortable.
18 Place the signal light within reach.
19 Raise the side rail. Lower the bed to its lowest position.
20 Unscreen the patient.
21 Take soiled linen to the "dirty" utility room.
22 Wash your hands.
23 Ask the nurse to check the IV flow rate.

CHANGING HOSPITAL GOWNS

The patient's gown is changed after the bath and when wet or soiled. Special measures are needed when there is an arm injury, paralysis, or an IV infusion. If there is injury or paralysis, the gown is removed from the unaffected arm first. The affected arm is supported while the gown is removed. The clean gown is put on the affected arm first and then on the unaffected arm.

Some facilities have special gowns for patients receiving IV infusions. The gowns open along the entire sleeve and are closed with ties or snaps. Traditional hospital gowns may be used for patients with IV infusions. You need to know how to change the gown of a patient with an IV.

A

B

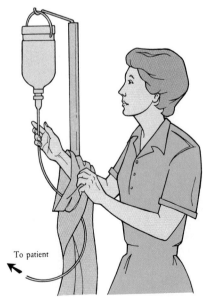

To patient

Fig. 13-37 A, The gown is removed from the uninvolved arm. The sleeve on the arm with the IV is gathered up, slipped over the IV site and tubing, and removed from the arm and hand.

C

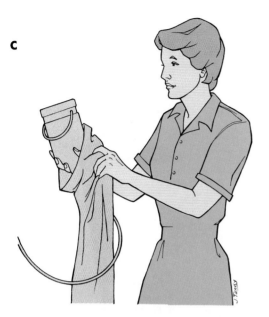

D

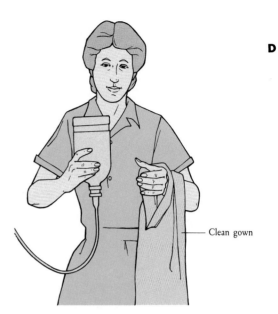

Clean gown

Fig. 13-37—cont'd B, The gathered sleeve is slipped along the IV tubing to the bottle. **C,** The IV bottle is removed from the pole and passed through the sleeve. **D,** The gathered sleeve of the clean gown is slipped over the IV bottle at the shoulder part of the gown.

DECUBITUS ULCERS

Decubitus ulcers (decubiti) are areas where skin and underlying tissues are eroded because of lack of blood flow (Fig. 13-38). They are also called *bedsores* and *pressure sores*. Decubiti occur most often in elderly, paralyzed, obese, or very thin and malnourished patients. The first sign of a decubitus ulcer is pale or white skin or a reddened area. The patient may complain of pain, burning, or tingling in the area. Some patients do not feel any abnormal sensations.

Sites

Decubitus ulcers usually occur over bony areas. The bony areas are called pressure points because they bear the weight of the body in a particular position. Pressure from body weight can reduce the blood supply to the area. Figure 13-39 shows the pressure points for the bed positions and the sitting position. In obese people, decubiti can develop in areas where skin is in contact with skin. Friction results when this occurs. Decubiti can develop between abdominal folds, the legs, and the buttocks, and underneath the breasts.

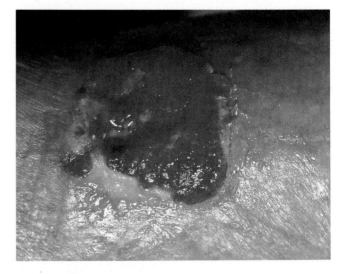

Fig. 13-38 A decubitus ulcer.

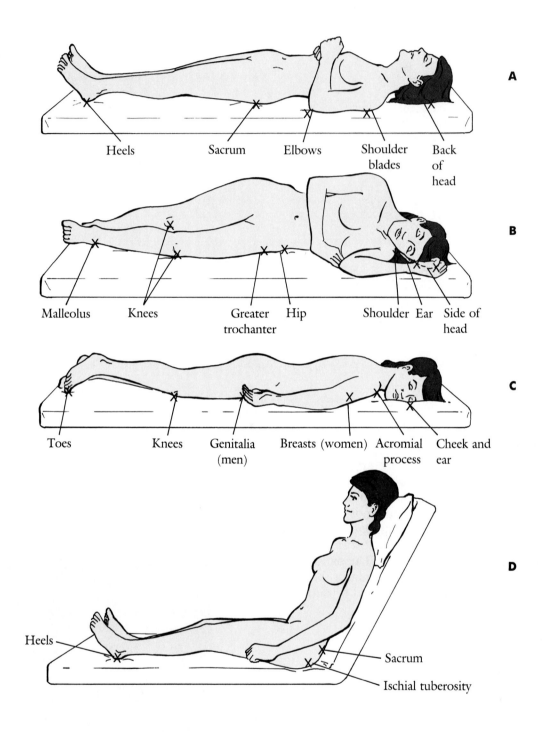

Fig. 13-39 Pressure points. **A,** The supine position. **B,** The lateral position. **C,** The prone position. **D,** Fowler's position.

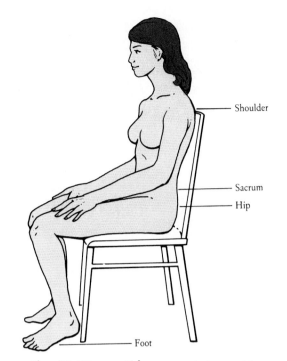

E

- Shoulder
- Sacrum
- Hip
- Foot

Fig. 13-39, cont'd **E**, The sitting position.

Causes

Pressure and friction are common causes of skin breakdown and decubiti. Other contributing factors include breaks in the skin, poor circulation to an area, moisture, dry skin, and irritation by urine and feces. Individuals who are inactive or cannot move or change positions are at risk for decubiti.

Prevention

Preventing decubitus ulcers is much easier than trying to heal them. Good nursing care, cleanliness, and skin care are essential. The following measures help prevent skin breakdown and decubiti:

1. Reposition the patient every 2 hours. Use pillows for support.
2. Provide good skin care. The skin must be clean and dry after bathing. Make sure the skin is free of urine, feces, and perspiration.
3. Apply lotion to dry areas such as the hands, elbows, legs, ankles, and heels.
4. Give a back massage when repositioning the patient.
5. Keep linens clean, dry, and free of wrinkles.
6. Apply powder where skin touches skin.
7. Do not irritate the skin. Avoid scrubbing or vigorous rubbing when bathing or drying the patient.
8. Massage reddened or pale pressure points. Use lotion and massage in a circular motion.
9. Use pillows and blankets to prevent skin from being in contact with skin and to reduce moisture and friction.
10. Report any signs of skin breakdown or decubiti immediately to the nurse.

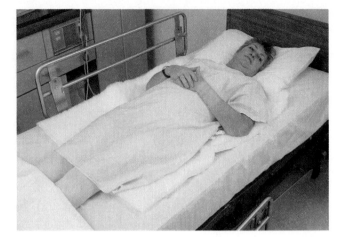

Fig. 13-40 Sheepskin.

Treatment

Treatment of decubitus ulcers is directed by the doctor. Drugs, treatments, and special equipment may be ordered to promote healing. The nurse and nursing care plan will tell you about a patient's treatment. Equipment used to treat and prevent decubiti are described in this section.

Sheepskin Sheepskin (lamb's wool) is placed on the bottom sheet (Fig. 13-40) to protect the skin from the irritating bed linens. Friction is reduced between the skin and the bottom sheet. Air circulates between the tufts to help keep the skin dry. Sheepskin comes in many sizes for use under the shoulders, buttocks, or heels.

Bed cradle A bed cradle is a metal frame placed on the bed and over the patient. Top linens are brought over the cradle to prevent pressure on the legs and feet (Fig. 13-41). Top linens are tucked in at the bottom of the mattress and mitered. They are also tucked under both sides of the mattress to protect the patient from air drafts and chilling. The bed cradle is also called an *Anderson frame.*

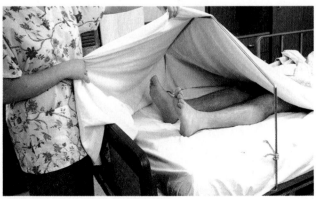

Fig. 13-41 A bed cradle is placed on top of the bed. Linens are brought over the top of the cradle.

A

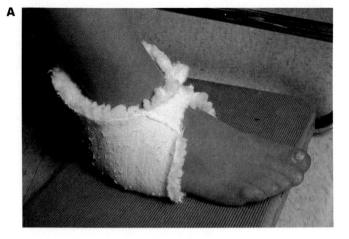

B

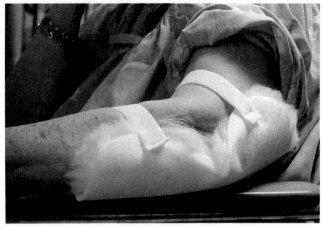

Fig. 13-42 A, Heel protector. **B,** Elbow protectors.

Heel and elbow protectors Heel and elbow protectors are made of foam rubber or sheepskin. They fit the shape of the heel or elbow (Fig. 13-42) and are secured in place with straps. Friction is prevented between the bed and the heel or elbow.

Flotation pad Flotation pads or cushions (Fig. 13-43) are similar to water beds. They are made of a gel-like substance. The outer case is heavy plastic. They are used for chairs and wheelchairs. The pad is put into a pillowcase to prevent contact between the plastic and the skin.

Egg crate mattress The egg crate mattress is a foam pad that looks like an egg carton (Fig. 13-44). Peaks in the mattress distribute the patient's weight more evenly. The egg crate mattress is placed on top of the regular mattress. Only a bottom sheet covers the egg crate mattress.

Water bed Water beds are used in many facilities. The patient "floats" on top of the mattress. Body weight is distributed along the entire length of the body. Therefore pressure on bony points is avoided.

Alternating pressure mattress An alternating pressure mattress is electrically operated. It has vertical tube-like sections (Fig. 13-45). Every other section is inflated with air. The other sections are deflated. Every 3 to 5 minutes the sections deflate or inflate automatically. With this mattress, constant pressure on any area is avoided.

Only a bottom sheet is used with an alternating pressure mattress. Drawsheets and waterproof bed protectors are avoided. They add layers of material between the patient and the air tubes. The air tubes should not be kinked. Pins are not used.

Clinitron bed The Clinitron bed has a specially designed mattress. Air that is kept at controlled tem-

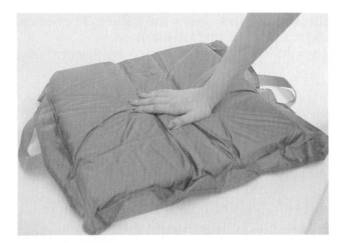

Fig. 13-43 Flotation pad.

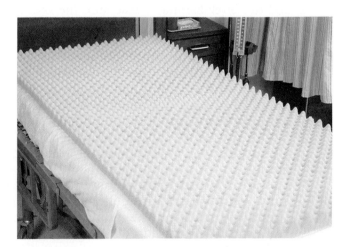

Fig. 13-44 Egg crate mattress on the bed.

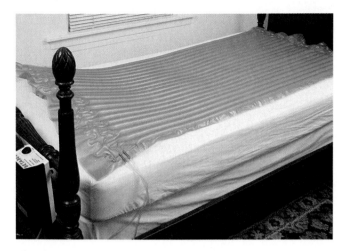

Fig. 13-45 Alternating pressure mattress.

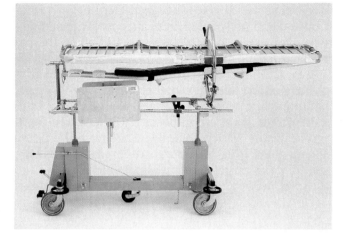

Fig. 13-46 The Stryker frame. (Courtesy The Stryker Corporation, Kalamazoo, Michigan.)

peratures flows through the mattress. The patient "floats" on the mattress. Body weight is distributed evenly, and pressure on body parts is minimal.

The Stryker frame   Two canvas frames are attached to a metal frame (Fig. 13-46). One is anterior (top) and the other is posterior (bottom). The patient is turned to the prone or supine position without moving. Body alignment is not changed during repositioning. Friction is reduced or eliminated completely during position changes. The *Foster frame* is like the Stryker frame, but it is larger and heavier.

The CircOlectric bed   The CircOlectric bed has a circular frame and anterior and posterior frames (Fig. 13-47). The bed is operated electrically to move the patient into various positions. The patient can be prone, supine, upright, or tilted to various degrees. Pressure points change as the patient's position changes. Friction is minimal during turning.

Guttman bed   The Guttman bed is used for position changes. The patient is rotated from right to left and to the supine position. The bed is useful for patients with spinal cord injuries.

Roto Rest treatment table   The Roto Rest treatment table is a bed that constantly moves from side to side (Fig. 13-48). The patient is continuously rotated from the left side-lying to the right side-lying position every 3 minutes. This device is also useful for patients with spinal cord injuries.

Other equipment   Trochanter rolls and footboards are also used to prevent and treat decubiti. These are described in Chapter 18.

SUMMARY

Promoting cleanliness and providing skin care are important responsibilities. Physical and psychological

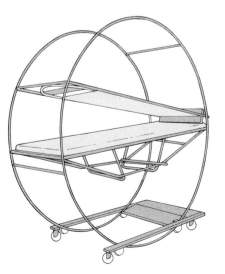

Fig. 13-47 The CircOlectric bed.

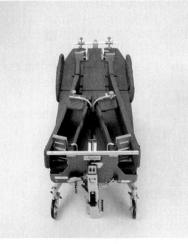

Fig. 13-48 Roto Rest treatment table. (Courtesy Kenetics Concepts Inc.)

well-being are affected by good personal hygiene. Cultural and personal choice influence hygiene practices. Whenever possible, you should allow the patient's choice.

The skin must be kept clean and intact. This promotes comfort and prevents infection. Oral hygiene, bathing, back massages, perineal care, hair care, and nail and foot care are important to the patient both physically and psychologically. Shaving and wearing a clean gown or pajamas are also appreciated. Patients should do as much self-care as possible. You need to assist as necessary. Giving personal care provides a good time to get to know the person and to observe the skin.

Decubitus ulcers result from poor nursing and skin care. They are very difficult to heal. The ulcers can have a serious effect on the patient and can cause death. The patient faces prolonged nursing and medical care. The bills from such care can be a great financial burden. You must practice the measures that prevent decubiti. Should decubiti occur, follow the nurse's directions for treating them. Remember, it is easier to prevent decubiti than to treat and heal them.

REVIEW QUESTIONS

Circle T *if the answer is true or* F *if the answer is false.*

T F **1** Cleanliness and skin care are necessary for comfort, safety, and health.

T F **2** A back massage is given only during morning care.

T F **3** A hard-bristled toothbrush is best.

T F **4** Unconscious patients are supine for mouth care.

T F **5** Use your fingers to keep the mouth of an unconscious patient open for mouth care.

T F **6** Dentures are washed in warm water over a hard surface.

T F **7** Bath oils cleanse and soften the skin.

T F **8** Powders absorb moisture and prevent friction.

T F **9** Deodorants reduce the amount of perspiration.

T F **10** A tub bath should not last longer than 20 minutes.

T F **11** You can give permission for tub baths or showers.

T F **12** Weak patients can be left alone in the shower if they are sitting in shower chairs.

T F **13** A back massage relaxes muscles and stimulates circulation.

T F **14** Perineal care helps prevent infection.

T F **15** Scissors are used to cut fingernails and toenails.

T F **16** A gown is removed from the unaffected side first.

T F **17** White or reddened skin is the first sign of a decubitus ulcer.

T F **18** Decubiti usually occur over bony areas.

T F **19** Pressure is a cause of decubiti.

Read each question carefully and circle the best *answer.*

20 Oral hygiene is part of
   a AM care tend hs care
   b Morning care
   c Care given after lunch
   d All of the above

21 You have brushed a patient's teeth. Which should be reported to the nurse?
   a Bleeding, swelling, or redness of the gums
   b Irritations, sores, or white patches in the mouth or on the tongue
   c Lips that are dry, cracked, swollen, or blistered
   d All of the above

22 Which is *not* a purpose of bathing?
   a Increasing circulation
   b Promoting drying of the skin
   c Exercising body parts
   d Refreshing and relaxing the patient

23 Soaps do the following *except*
   a Remove dirt and dead skin
   b Remove pathogens
   c Remove skin oil and perspiration
   d Dry the skin

24 Which action is *incorrect* when bathing an individual?
   a Cover the patient for warmth and privacy.
   b Rinse the skin thoroughly to remove all soaps.
   c Wash from the dirtiest to cleanest area.
   d Pat the skin dry.

25 Bath water for a complete bed bath should be
   a 100° F
   b 105° F
   c 110° F
   d 120° F

26 You are to give a back massage. Which is *false?*
   a The massage should last about 4 to 6 minutes.
   b Lotion is warmed before being applied.
   c The hands are always in contact with the skin.
   d The side-lying position is best.

27 A patient's hair can be washed
   a In the tub or shower
   b In bed

c On a stretcher or in a chair

d All of the above

28 Before shaving a man's face, you should

a Dry his face thoroughly

b Apply a cold washcloth to his face

c Soften his skin

d Apply after-shave lotion

29 Which will *not* prevent decubiti?

a Repositioning the patient every 2 hours

b Applying lotion to dry areas

c Scrubbing and rubbing the skin vigorously

d Keeping bed linens clean, dry, and free of wrinkles

30 Which are *not* used to treat decubiti?

a Stryker frame and CircOlectric bed

b Water bed and flotation pad

c Plastic drawsheet and sheepskin

d Heel and elbow protectors and bed cradle

Answers

10 True	**20** d	**30** c
9 False	**19** True	**29** c
8 True	**18** True	**28** c
7 False	**17** True	**27** d
6 False	**16** True	**26** d
5 False	**15** False	**25** c
4 False	**14** True	**24** c
3 False	**13** True	**23** b
2 False	**12** False	**22** b
1 True	**11** False	**21** d

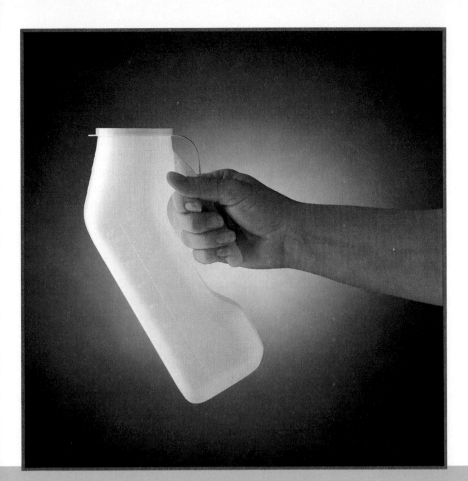

Urinary
Elimination

- Define the key terms listed in this chapter
- Identify the characteristics of normal urine
- Identify the usual times for urination
- Describe the general rules for maintaining normal urinary elimination
- List the observations to be made about urine
- Describe urinary incontinence and the care required
- Explain why catheters are used
- Describe the rules for caring for patients with catheters
- Describe two methods of bladder training
- Describe the rules for collecting urine specimens
- Perform the procedures described in this chapter

14

acetone Ketone bodies that appear in the urine because of the rapid breakdown of fat for energy

catheter A tube used to drain or inject fluid through a body opening

catheterization The process of inserting a catheter

diabetes mellitus A chronic disease in which the pancreas fails to secrete enough insulin; the body is prevented from using sugar for energy

dysuria Painful or difficult (dys) urination (uria)

Foley catheter A catheter that is left in the urinary bladder so that urine drains continuously into a collection bag; an indwelling or retention catheter

glucosuria Sugar (glucos) in the urine (uria)

indwelling catheter A retention or Foley catheter

ketone body Acetone

micturition The process of emptying the bladder; urination or voiding

retention catheter A Foley or indwelling catheter

urinary incontinence The inability to control the passage of urine from the bladder

urination The process of emptying the bladder; micturition or voiding

voiding Urination or micturition

The urinary system removes much of the waste from the body and regulates the amount of water in the body. The kidneys, ureters, urinary bladder, and urethra are the major urinary tract structures (see Chapter 5). Blood passes through the two kidneys, where urine is formed. Urine consists of the wastes and excess fluids that are filtered out of the blood. Urine flows through the two ureters to the urinary bladder, where it is stored until urination. The urethra is the tube that connects the urinary bladder to the outside of the body. Urine is eliminated from the body through the urethra. *Urination, micturition,* and *voiding* all mean the process of emptying the bladder.

NORMAL URINATION

The healthy adult excretes about 1000 to 1500 ml (milliliters) (2 to 3 pints) of urine a day. Many factors affect the amount of urine produced. These include age, illnesses, the amount and kinds of fluid ingested, the amount of salt in the diet, and medications being taken. Certain substances increase urine production. Examples are coffee, tea, alcohol, and some drugs. A diet high in salt causes the body to retain water. When water is retained, less urine is produced. Urine production is also influenced by body temperature, the amount of perspiration, and the external temperature.

Urinary frequency also depends on many factors. The amount of fluid ingested, personal habits, and available toilet facilities affect frequency, as do activity, work, and illness. People usually urinate at bedtime and after getting up. Some people urinate every 2 to 3 hours. Others void every 8 to 12 hours. Sleep may be disturbed if large amounts of urine are being produced.

MAINTAINING NORMAL URINATION

Patients or residents may need help maintaining normal elimination. Some need help getting to the bathroom. Others use bedpans, urinals, or commodes.

General Rules

You need to follow these rules to help individuals maintain normal urinary elimination. The rules of medical asepsis and universal precautions are also practiced.

1. Provide the bedpan, urinal, or commode, or help the person to the bathroom as soon as the request is made. The need to void may be urgent.
2. Help the person assume a normal position for voiding if possible. Women use the sitting or squatting position. Men stand to urinate.
3. Make sure the bedpan or urinal is warm.
4. Cover the person for warmth and privacy.
5. Provide for privacy. Pull the curtain around the bed, close doors to the room and bathroom, and pull drapes or window shades. Leave the room if the person is strong enough to be alone.
6. Remain nearby if the person is weak or unsteady.
7. Place the signal light and toilet paper within reach.
8. Allow the individual enough time to void.
9. Run water in a nearby sink if the person has difficulty starting the stream. You may need to place the person's fingers in some water.
10. Provide perineal care as needed.
11. Provide a wash basin, soap, washcloth, and towel after urination. Assist as necessary.
12. Offer the bedpan or urinal at regular intervals. Some people are embarrassed or are too weak to ask.

What to Report to the Nurse

Before urine is disposed of, it is carefully observed. Urine is observed for color, clarity, odor, amount, and the presence of particles. Urine that looks abnormal is saved for the nurse to observe. Complaints of urgency, burning on urination, or dysuria are also reported. *Dysuria* means painful or difficult (dys) urination (uria).

Bedpans

Bedpans are used by persons who cannot be out of bed. Women use bedpans for urination and bowel movements. Men use them for bowel movements only. Bedpans are made of plastic or stainless steel. Stainless steel bedpans tend to be cold and are warmed before being given to patients.

Fracture pans are also available (Fig. 14-1). A *fracture pan* has a thinner rim and is only about ½ inch deep at one end. The smaller end is placed under the buttocks (Fig. 14-2). Fracture pans are used for patients with casts or those in traction.

The bedpan is covered after being used and is taken to the toilet or "dirty" utility room. After being emptied and rinsed, it is cleaned with a disinfectant. The bedpan is returned to the bedside stand with a clean cover.

GIVING THE BEDPAN

1 Provide for privacy.
2 Collect the following equipment:
 a Bedpan
 b Bedpan cover
 c Toilet tissue
 d Disposable gloves
3 Arrange the equipment on the chair or bed.
4 Explain the procedure to the patient.
5 Raise the bed to a level appropriate for good body mechanics.
6 Make sure the side rails are up.
7 Warm and dry the bedpan if necessary.
8 Lower the side rail.
9 Position the patient supine. The head of the bed should be slightly elevated.
10 Fold the top linens and gown out of the way. Keep the lower body covered.
11 Ask the patient to flex the knees and raise the buttocks by pushing against the mattress with his or her feet.
12 Slide your hand under the lower back and help him or her raise the buttocks.
13 Slide the bedpan under the patient (Fig. 14-3).
14 Do the following if the patient cannot assist in getting on the bedpan:
 a Turn the patient onto the side away from you.
 b Place the bedpan firmly against the buttocks (Fig. 14-4, A).
 c Push the bedpan down and toward the patient (Fig. 14-4, B).
 d Hold the bedpan securely. Turn the patient onto the back. Make sure the bedpan is centered under the patient.
15 Return top linens to their proper position.
16 Raise the head of the bed so that the patient is in a sitting position.
17 Make sure he or she is correctly positioned on the bedpan (Fig. 14-5).
18 Raise the side rail.
19 Place the toilet tissue and signal light within reach.
20 Ask him or her to signal when finished or when assistance is needed.
21 Leave the room and close the door. Wash your hands.
22 Return when the patient signals. Knock before entering.
23 Lower the side rail and the head of the bed.
24 Put on the gloves.
25 Ask the patient to raise the buttocks. Slide the bedpan out. You may also hold the bedpan securely and turn him or her onto the side away from you.
26 Clean the genital area if the patient cannot do so. Clean from front to back with toilet tissue. Provide perineal care if necessary.
27 Cover the bedpan. Take it to the bathroom or "dirty" utility room. Raise the side rail before leaving the bedside.
28 Measure urine if the patient is on intake and output (I&O) (see Chapter 16). Collect a urine specimen if needed. Note the color, amount, and character of the urine or feces.
29 Empty and rinse the bedpan. Clean it with a disinfectant.
30 Remove the gloves.
31 Return the bedpan and clean cover to the bedside stand.
32 Help the patient wash the hands.
33 Make sure he or she is comfortable and the side rails are up.
34 Place the signal light within reach.
35 Lower the bed to its lowest position.
36 Unscreen the patient.
37 Place soiled linen in the linen hamper.
38 Wash your hands.
39 Report your observations to the nurse.

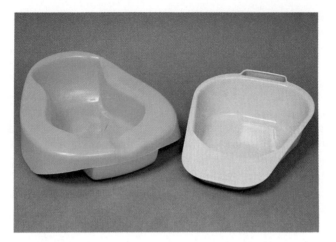

Fig. 14-1 The regular bedpan and the fracture pan.

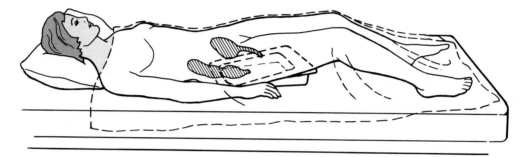

Fig. 14-2 A patient positioned on a fracture pan. The smaller end is placed under the buttocks.

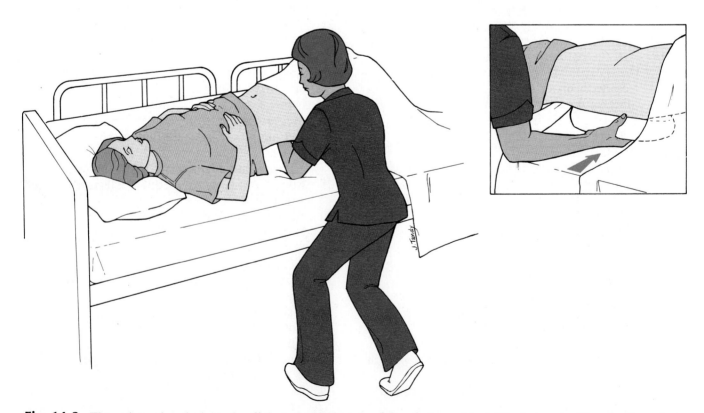

Fig. 14-3 The patient raises the buttocks off the bed with the help of the nursing assistant. The bedpan is slid under the patient.

A **B**

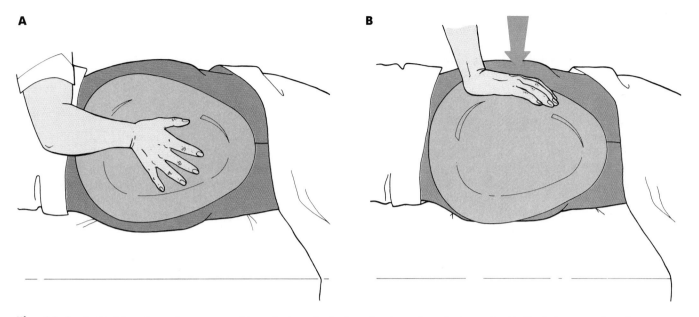

Fig. 14-4 A, Position the patient on one side and place the bedpan firmly against the buttocks. **B,** Push downward on the bedpan and toward the patient.

Urinals

Urinals (Fig. 14-6, *A*) are used by men for urination. They are made of the same materials as bedpans. Plastic urinals have caps at the top and hook-type handles. The hook allows the urinal to hang from the side rail within the man's reach (Fig. 14-6, *B*). The urinal is used while lying in bed, sitting on the edge of the bed, or standing at the bedside. If possible, the man should stand. Some men need to be supported in the standing position by 1 or 2 workers. You may have to place and hold the urinal for some men.

Urinals are emptied promptly to prevent odors and the spread of microorganisms. A filled urinal can easily spill and cause safety hazards. Urinals are cleaned like bedpans.

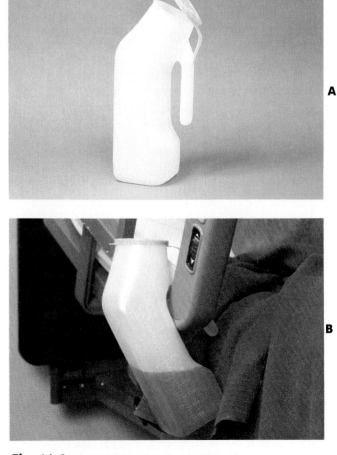

A

B

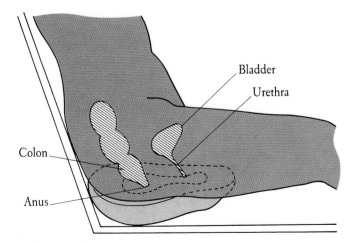

Bladder

Urethra

Colon

Anus

Fig. 14-5 The patient is positioned on the bedpan so that the urethra and anus are directly over the opening.

Fig. 14-6 A, Urinal for a male. **B,** The urinal hangs from the side rail within the patient's reach.

GIVING THE URINAL

1 Provide for privacy.
2 Determine if the man will stay in bed or stand.
3 Give him the urinal if he will stay in bed. Remind him to tilt the bottom down to prevent spills.
4 Do the following if he is going to stand:
   a Help him sit on the side of the bed.
   b Put slippers on him.
   c Assist him to a standing position.
   d Provide support if he is unsteady.
   e Give him the urinal.
5 Position the urinal between his legs if necessary. Position his penis in the urinal if he cannot hold the urinal. (Wear gloves for this step.)
6 Cover him to provide for privacy.
7 Place the signal light within reach. Ask him to signal when finished or when he needs assistance.
8 Leave the room and close the door. Wash your hands.
9 Return when he signals for you. Knock before entering.
10 Put on gloves.
11 Cover the urinal. Take it to the bathroom or "dirty" utility room.
12 Measure urine if he is on I&O. Collect a urine specimen if needed. Note the color, amount, and character of the urine.
13 Empty the urinal and rinse it with cold water. Clean it with a disinfectant.
14 Remove the gloves.
15 Return the urinal to the bedside stand.
16 Help the patient wash his hands.
17 Make sure he is comfortable and the side rails are up.
18 Place the signal light within reach.
19 Unscreen him.
20 Wash your hands.
21 Report your observations to the nurse.

HELPING THE PATIENT TO THE COMMODE

1 Explain the procedure to the patient.
2 Provide for privacy.
3 Collect the following equipment:
   a Commode
   b Toilet tissue
   c Bath blanket
   d Disposable gloves
4 Bring the commode next to the bed. Remove the seat and lid from the container.
5 Help the patient sit on the side of the bed.
6 Help him or her put on a robe and slippers.
7 Assist him or her to the commode.
8 Place a bath blanket over his or her lap for warmth.
9 Place the toilet tissue and signal light within reach.
10 Ask him or her to signal when finished or when assistance is needed.
11 Leave the room and close the door. Wash your hands.
12 Return when the patient signals. Knock before entering.
13 Put on the gloves.
14 Help the person clean the genital area if indicated. Remove the gloves.
15 Help him or her back to bed. Remove the robe and slippers. Raise the side rail.
16 Put on another pair of gloves. Cover and remove the container from the commode. Clean the commode if necessary.
17 Take the container to the bathroom or "dirty" utility room.
18 Check urine and feces for color, amount, and character. Measure urine if the patient is on I&O. Collect a specimen if one is needed.
19 Clean and disinfect the container. Remove the gloves.
20 Return the container to the commode. Return other supplies to their proper place.
21 Return the commode to its proper place.
22 Help the patient wash the hands.
23 Make sure he or she is comfortable and the signal light is within reach. Raise the side rail.
24 Unscreen the patient.
25 Place soiled linen in the linen hamper.
26 Wash your hands.
27 Report your observations to the nurse.

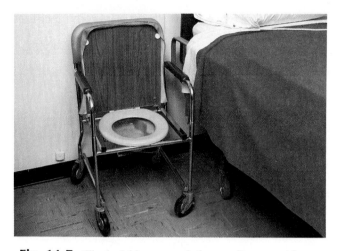

Fig. 14-7 The bedside commode has a toilet seat with a container. The container slides out from under the toilet seat for emptying.

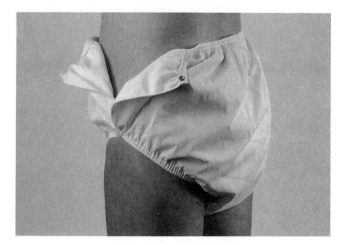

Fig. 14-8 Garment protector (incontinence pad).

After using urinals, many men hang them on side rails or place them on nearby tables until someone empties them. This practice is to be discouraged. They should be reminded to signal when urinals need to be emptied.

Commodes

A bedside commode is a portable chair or wheelchair with an opening for a bedpan or similar receptacle (Fig. 14-7). Patients unable to walk to the bathroom may be allowed to use the commode. The commode lets the patient assume a normal position for elimination. The bedpan or receptacle is cleaned after use like the regular bedpan.

URINARY INCONTINENCE

Urinary incontinence is the inability to control the passage of urine from the bladder. Some people dribble only when laughing, sneezing, coughing, lifting, or straining. Others dribble constantly. Some people have no control over urination. The many causes of incontinence include spinal cord injuries, central nervous system disorders, aging, and confusion. Certain medications, weak pelvic muscles, reproductive system surgeries, childbirth, and urinary tract infections are also causes. Sometimes it occurs because the person cannot use the toilet, bedpan, urinal, or commode in time. Difficulty removing clothes may delay urination. Incontinence may be temporary or permanent.

Incontinence is embarrassing to the person. Clothing becomes wet, odors develop, and the person is uncomfortable. Irritation, infection, and decubiti can also occur. Good skin care is essential.

Following the rules for maintaining normal urinary elimination will prevent incontinence in some people.

Others need bladder training programs (see pages 239-240). Sometimes catheters are ordered (see below). Some people wear garment protectors or incontinence pads (Fig. 14-8).

CATHETERS

A *catheter* is a rubber or plastic tube used to drain or inject fluid through a body opening. A urinary catheter is inserted through the urethra into the bladder to drain urine. An *indwelling catheter* is left in the bladder so that urine drains continuously into a drainage bag. The indwelling catheter is also called a *retention* or *Foley catheter*. A balloon near the tip is inflated after the catheter is inserted. The balloon prevents the catheter from slipping out of the bladder (Fig. 14-9). Tubing connects the catheter to the collection bag. Catheter insertion (*catheterization*) is done by a nurse or doctor.

Catheters may be used preoperatively and postoperatively to keep the bladder empty. A full bladder can be accidentally injured during surgery. After surgery a full bladder can cause pressure on nearby organs. A catheter may be used for urinary incontinence.

General Rules

You may care for patients with indwelling catheters. The following rules will promote their comfort and safety:

1. Make sure urine flows freely through the catheter or tubing. The tubing should not have kinks.
2. Keep the drainage bag below the level of the bladder. This prevents urine from flowing backward into the bladder. Attach the drainage bag to the bed frame.

3. Coil the drainage tubing on the bed and pin it to the bottom linen (Fig. 14-10).
4. Tape the catheter to the inner thigh as in Figure 14-10, or tape the catheter to the man's abdomen. This prevents excessive movement of the catheter and reduces friction at the insertion site.
5. Provide catheter care in addition to perineal care. Catheter care is done daily (q.d.) and may be done twice a day (b.i.d.) in some facilities (see *Catheter Care,* page 237).
6. Empty the drainage bag at the end of the shift or at time intervals as directed by the nurse. Measure and record the amount of urine (see *Emptying a Urinary Drainage Bag,* page 238).
7. Report patient complaints to the nurse immediately. These include complaints of pain, burning, the need to urinate, or irritation. Also report the color, clarity, and odor of urine.
8. Follow the rules of medical asepsis and universal precautions at all times.

A

B

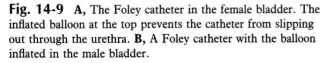

Fig. 14-9 A, The Foley catheter in the female bladder. The inflated balloon at the top prevents the catheter from slipping out through the urethra. **B,** A Foley catheter with the balloon inflated in the male bladder.

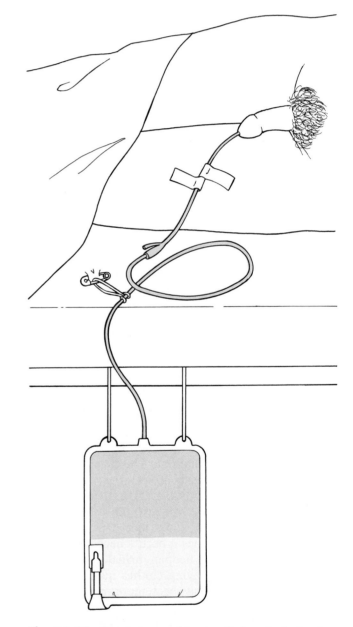

Fig. 14-10 The drainage tubing is coiled on the bed and pinned to the bottom linens so urine flows freely. A rubber band is placed around the tubing with a clove hitch. The safety pin is passed through the loops and pinned to the linens. The catheter is taped to the inner thigh. Enough slack is left on the catheter to prevent friction at the urethra.

CATHETER CARE

1 Explain the procedure to the patient.
2 Wash your hands.
3 Collect the following equipment:
   a Equipment for perineal care
   b Catheter care kit (if used in your facility)
   c Disposable gloves
   d Disposable bed protector
   e Disposable bag
4 Identify the patient. Check the ID bracelet with the treatment card.
5 Provide for privacy.
6 Raise the bed to a level appropriate for good body mechanics.
7 Lower the side rail.
8 Cover the patient with a bath blanket. Fanfold top linens to the foot of the bed.
9 Drape the patient for perineal care (see Fig. 13-24).
10 Put on gloves. Perform perineal care (see *Female Perineal Care* or *Male Perineal Care*, pages 211-214).
11 Place the bed protector under the buttocks. Ask the patient to flex the knees and raise the buttocks off the bed by pushing against the mattress with the feet.
12 Fold back the bath blanket between the legs to expose the genital area.
13 Open the catheter care kit (if used in your facility).
14 Put on the gloves.
15 Apply antiseptic solution to the applicators. You may also use soap and a washcloth.

16 Separate the labia (female) or retract the foreskin (uncircumcised male) as in Figure 14-11. Check for crusts, abnormal drainage, or secretions.
17 Apply antiseptic solution to the labia or to the head of the penis. Apply the solution from front to back with an applicator. Discard the applicator after one stroke. Repeat this step as necessary. Use soap and a washcloth if that is your facility's policy.
18 Clean the catheter from the meatus down the catheter about 4 inches (Fig. 14-12). Use one applicator per stroke. Avoid tugging or pulling on the catheter.
19 Make sure the catheter is taped properly. Coil and secure tubing as in Figure 14-10.
20 Remove the bed protector.
21 Remove the gloves and discard them into the bag.
22 Make sure the patient is comfortable.
23 Cover the patient and remove the bath blanket.
24 Raise the side rail.
25 Lower the bed to its lowest position.
26 Clean and return equipment to its proper place. Discard disposable equipment.
27 Unscreen the patient.
28 Take soiled linen and the disposable bag to the "dirty" utility room.
29 Wash your hands.
30 Report your observations to the nurse.

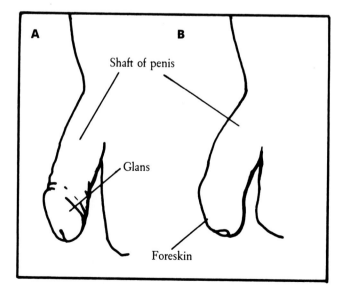

Fig. 14-11 **A,** Circumcised male. **B,** Uncircumcised male.

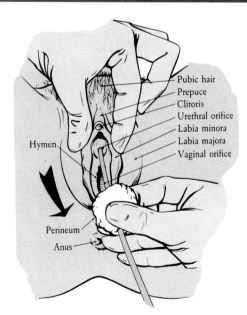

Fig. 14-12 The catheter is cleaned beginning at the meatus. About 4 inches of the catheter is cleaned.

EMPTYING A URINARY DRAINAGE BAG

1 Collect equipment:
   a Graduate
   b Disposable gloves
2 Wash your hands.
3 Explain the procedure to the patient.
4 Identify the patient. Check the ID bracelet and call the patient by name.
5 Provide for privacy.
6 Put on the gloves.
7 Place the graduate so that urine can be collected when the drain is opened.
8 Open the clamp on the bottom of the drainage bag.
9 Let all urine drain into the graduate. Do not let the drain touch the graduate (Fig. 14-13).
10 Close the clamp. Replace the clamped drain in the holder on the bag (see Fig. 14-10).
11 Measure the urinary output.
12 Rinse the graduate and return it to its proper place.
13 Remove the gloves and wash your hands.
14 Record the time and amount on the I&O record.
15 Unscreen the patient.
16 Report the amount and other observations.

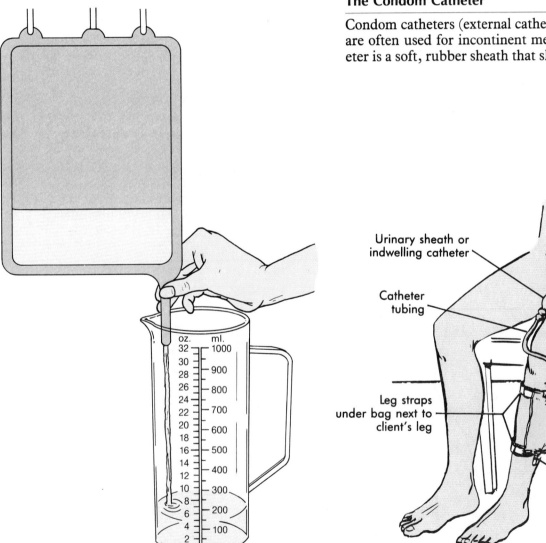

Fig. 14-13 The clamp on the drainage bag is opened and the drain is directed into the graduate. The drain must not touch the inside of the graduate.

The Condom Catheter

Condom catheters (external catheter, Texas catheter) are often used for incontinent men. A condom catheter is a soft, rubber sheath that slides over the penis.

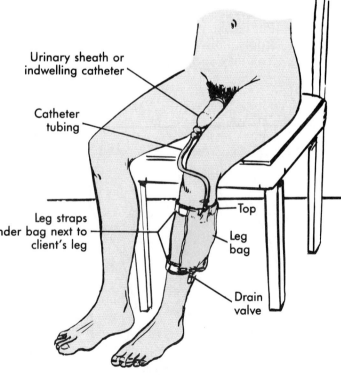

Fig. 14-14 A condom catheter attached to a leg bag. (From Hoeman SP: *Rehabilitation/Restorative Care in the Community*, St Louis, 1990, Mosby–Year Book.)

APPLYING A CONDOM CATHETER

1 Explain the procedure to the man.
2 Wash your hands.
3 Collect the following equipment:
   a Condom catheter
   b Elastic tape
   c Drainage bag or leg bag
   d Basin of warm water
   e Soap
   f Towel
   g Washcloths
   h Bath blanket
   i Disposable gloves
   j Disposable bed protector
   k Bag for disposable supplies
   l Paper towels
4 Arrange paper towels and equipment on the overbed table.
5 Provide for privacy.
6 Raise the bed to an appropriate level for good body mechanics.
7 Lower the side rail.
8 Cover the patient with a bath blanket. Bring top linens to the foot of the bed.
9 Ask the patient to raise his buttocks off the bed. You may need to turn the patient onto his side away from you.
10 Slide the bed protector under his buttocks.
11 Have the patient lower his buttocks or turn him onto his back.
12 Bring top linens up to cover his knees and lower legs.
13 Secure the drainage bag to the bed frame. Have the leg bag ready if one will be used. Make sure the drain is closed.
14 Raise the bath blanket to expose the genital area.
15 Put on the gloves.

16 Remove the condom catheter.
   a Remove the tape and roll the sheath toward the penis.
   b Disconnect the drainage tubing from the condom.
   c Place the tape and condom in the bag.
17 Provide perineal care (see *Male Perineal Care*, page 214). Observe the penis for skin breakdown or irritation.
18 Remove the protective backing from the condom. This exposes the adhesive strip.
19 Hold the penis firmly. Roll the condom onto the penis. Leave a 1-inch space between the penis and the end of the catheter (Fig. 14-15).
20 Secure the condom with tape. Apply tape in a spiral (Fig. 14-16). Tape must not go completely around the penis.
21 Connect the condom to the drainage tubing. Coil excess tubing on the bed as in Figure 14-10, or attach the leg bag.
22 Remove the bed protector.
23 Remove the gloves.
24 Return top linens and remove the bath blanket.
25 Make sure the patient is comfortable. Place the signal light within reach. Raise the side rail.
26 Clean and return the wash basin and other equipment to their proper place.
27 Unscreen the patient.
28 Take the bag, used collection bag, and disposable supplies to the "dirty" utility room. Measure and record the amount of urine in the bag. Make sure you use universal precautions.
29 Wash your hands.
30 Report your observations.

Tubing connects the condom catheter and the drainage bag. Residents and home care patients may prefer leg bags during the day (Fig. 14-14).

A new condom catheter is applied daily. The penis is thoroughly washed with soap and water and dried before a new catheter is applied. Universal precautions are followed when removing or applying condom catheters.

BLADDER TRAINING

Bladder training programs may be developed for patients with urinary incontinence. Voluntary control of urination is the goal. With the doctor's approval, the nurse develops a plan to bladder train an individual. The bladder training program is part of the nursing care plan. You will assist in the bladder training program as directed by the nurse.

There are two basic methods for bladder training. With one, the person uses the toilet, commode, bedpan, or urinal at scheduled intervals. The person is given 15 or 20 minutes to start voiding. The rules for helping to maintain normal urination are followed during bladder training. The normal position for urination should be assumed if possible. Privacy is important.

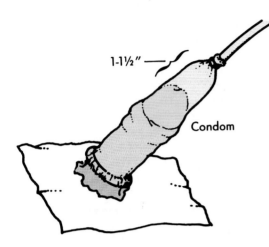

Fig. 14-15 A condom catheter applied to the penis. There is a 1-inch space between the penis and the end of the catheter. (From Hoeman SP: *Rehabilitation/Restorative Care in the Community*, St Louis, 1990, Mosby–Year Book.)

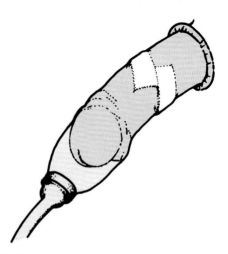

Fig. 14-16 Tape is applied in spiral fashion to secure the condom catheter to the penis. (From Hoeman SP: *Rehabilitation/Restorative Care in the Community*, St Louis, 1990, Mosby–Year Book.)

The second method is used for those with catheters. The catheter is clamped (Fig. 14-17) to prevent urine from draining out of the bladder. Usually the catheter is clamped for 1 hour at first. Eventually it is clamped for 3 to 4 hours at a time. When the catheter is removed, the toilet, commode, bedpan, or urinal is used every 3 to 4 hours.

COLLECTING AND TESTING URINE SPECIMENS

Urine specimens (samples) are collected for laboratory study. Urine is examined to help the doctor diagnose a problem or evaluate the effectiveness of treatment. There are many types of specimens. A

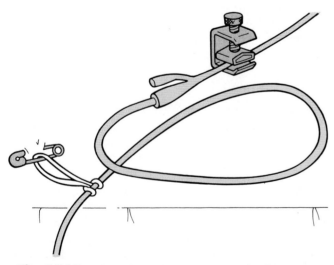

Fig. 14-17 The catheter clamp prevents urine from draining out of the bladder. The clamp is applied directly to the catheter—not to the drainage tubing.

laboratory requisition slip is completed for each specimen to be sent to the laboratory. The nurse is responsible for accurately completing the requisition. It has the patient's identifying information and the laboratory test to be done. Nursing assistants are often asked to collect specimens.

General Rules

The following rules are practiced when collecting urine specimens:

1. Wash your hands before and after collecting the specimen.
2. Use universal precautions.
3. Use a clean container for each specimen.
4. Use a container appropriate for the specimen.
5. Label the container accurately with the requested information. Most request the patient's full name, room and bed number, date, and time the specimen was collected.
6. Do not touch the inside of the container or lid.
7. Collect the specimen at the time specified.
8. Ask the patient not to have a bowel movement while the specimen is being collected. The specimen must be free of fecal material.
9. Ask the patient to put toilet tissue in the toilet or wastebasket. The specimen should not contain tissue.
10. Take the specimen and requisition slip to the laboratory or designated storage place.

The Routine Urine Specimen

The routine urine specimen is also called the random urine sample or routine urinalysis. The test is done for all patients admitted to hospitals. The test is also done before surgery and for physical examinations. Many patients can collect the specimen themselves. Weak and very ill patients need assistance.

The Clean-Catch Urine Specimen

The clean-catch urine specimen is also called a mid-stream specimen or clean-voided specimen. The perineal area is cleaned before collecting the specimen. Perineal care reduces the number of microbes in the urethral area at the time the specimen is collected. The patient begins to void into the toilet, bedpan, urinal, or commode. Then the stream is stopped and the specimen container is positioned. The patient then voids into the container until the specimen is obtained.

Many people find it hard to stop the stream of urine. You may need to position and hold the specimen container in place after the patient has started to void. Be sure to wear gloves when collecting a clean-catch urine specimen. Clean-catch specimen kits are obtained from the central supply area. See the box on page 242.

The 24-Hour Urine Specimen

All urine voided during a 24-hour period is collected for a 24-hour urine specimen. Urine is chilled on ice or refrigerated during the collection period to prevent the growth of microorganisms. A preservative is added to the collection container for some tests.

The patient voids to begin the test; this voiding is discarded. *All* voidings during the next 24 hours are collected. The procedure and test period must be clearly understood by the patient and everyone involved in the patient's care. The rules for collecting urine specimens are also followed. See the box on page 243.

The Fresh-Fractional Urine Specimen

A "double-voided specimen" is another term for a fresh-fractional urine specimen. This is because the patient voids twice. The patient voids to empty the bladder, which contains "stale" urine. In 30 minutes, the patient voids again. "Fresh" urine has collected in the bladder since the first voiding. The second voiding is usually a very small or "fractional" amount of urine. See the box on page 243.

Fresh-fractional specimens are used to test urine for sugar. The tests are described later in this chapter.

Collecting a Specimen From an Infant or Child

Specimens may be needed from infants and children who have not been toilet trained. They need to have a collection bag applied over the urethra. Two workers may be needed to apply the bag if the baby or child is agitated.

COLLECTING A ROUTINE URINE SPECIMEN

1 Explain the procedure to the patient.
2 Wash your hands.
3 Collect the following equipment:
  a Bedpan and cover, urinal, or disposable specimen pan
  b Specimen container and lid
  c Label
  d Disposable gloves
4 Fill out the label. Put it on the container.
5 Put the container and lid in the bathroom or "dirty" utility room.
6 Identify the patient. Check the ID bracelet against the laboratory requisition slip.
7 Provide for privacy.
8 Ask the patient to urinate in the appropriate receptacle. Remind him or her to put toilet tissue into the wastebasket or toilet. Caution the patient not to put toilet tissue into the bedpan or specimen pan.
9 Put on the gloves.
10 Take the bedpan or urinal to the bathroom or "dirty" utility room.

11 Measure urine if the patient is on I&O.
12 Pour urine into the specimen container until it is about ¾ full. Dispose of excess urine.
13 Place the lid on the specimen container.
14 Clean the bedpan or urinal. Remove the gloves.
15 Return the bedpan or urinal to its proper place.
16 Help the patient to wash the hands.
17 Make sure he or she is comfortable. Raise the side rail.
18 Place the signal light within reach.
19 Unscreen the patient.
20 Take the specimen to the nurses' station or laboratory. Be sure you have the laboratory requisition slip if you are taking the specimen to the laboratory.
21 Wash your hands.
22 Report your observations to the nurse.

COLLECTING A CLEAN-CATCH URINE SPECIMEN

1 Explain the procedure to the patient.
2 Wash your hands.
3 Collect the following equipment:
   a Clean-catch specimen kit
   b Disposable gloves
   c Bedpan, urinal, or commode if the patient cannot use the bathroom
4 Label the container with the requested information.
5 Identify the patient. Check the ID bracelet with the laboratory requisition slip.
6 Provide for privacy.
7 Let the patient complete the procedure if able. Place the signal light within reach.
8 Assist the patient if necessary.
9 Offer the bedpan or assist him or her to the bathroom or commode. Be sure the patient has on a robe and slippers if he or she is to be up.
10 Open the kit. Remove the specimen container and towelettes. Put on the gloves.
11 Clean the penis or perineal area with towelettes or other specified solution (see *Male Perineal Care* or *Female Perineal Care*, pages 211-214).
12 Keep the woman's labia separated until the specimen is collected. If the patient is an uncircumcised male, keep the foreskin retracted until the specimen is collected.

13 Collect the specimen:
   a Ask the patient to urinate into the receptacle.
   b Ask him or her to stop the stream.
   c Hold the specimen container under the patient.
   d Ask him or her to start urinating again.
   e Ask the patient to stop the stream when urine has been collected.
   f Let him or her finish urinating.
14 Put the lid on the container immediately. Do not touch the inside of the lid.
15 Help the patient clean the perineal area. Return the foreskin to its natural position.
16 Clean the bedpan or commode. Remove the gloves.
17 Return equipment to its proper place. Discard disposable items.
18 Help the patient wash the hands.
19 Make sure the patient is comfortable. Raise the side rails and place the signal light within reach.
20 Unscreen the patient.
21 Take the specimen to the nurses' station or laboratory. Be sure you have the laboratory requisition slip if you are taking the specimen to the laboratory.
22 Wash your hands.
23 Report your observations to the nurse.

Testing Urine

You may be responsible for testing the urine of patients with diabetes mellitus. *Diabetes mellitus* is a chronic disease in which the pancreas fails to secrete enough insulin. The insufficient amount of insulin prevents the body from using sugar for energy. Sugar builds up in the blood if it cannot be used. Some of the sugar appears in the urine. *Glucosuria* is the medical term for sugar (glucos) in the urine (uria).

The diabetic patient may also have *acetone (ketone bodies, ketones)* in the urine. These appear in urine because of the rapid breakdown of fat for energy. Fat is used for energy if the body cannot use sugar because of the lack of insulin.

The doctor orders the type and frequency of urine tests. They are usually done four times a day: 30 minutes before each meal (a.c.) and at bedtime (h.s.). The doctor uses the test results to regulate the amount of medication given. They are also used to regulate the patient's diet. You must be accurate when testing urine, and promptly report the results to the nurse. Fresh-fractional urine specimens are best for testing urine for sugar and ketones.

Testape Testape is used to test urine for sugar. A strip of tape is removed from the Testape dispenser and dipped into the specimen. Then the strip is compared to the color chart on the dispenser. See the box on page 245.

Clinitest The Clinitest tests urine for sugar. A Clinitest tablet is added to a test tube with urine and water. The solution turns various colors depending on the amount of sugar in the urine. The Clinitest kit contains the instructions and color chart for the test. The kit is labeled with the person's name and room number. See the box on page 245.

Acetest The Acetest determines if acetone or ketone bodies are in the urine. An Acetest tablet is added to urine. The urine changes color depending on how much acetone is in the urine. See the box on page 247.

COLLECTING A 24-HOUR URINE SPECIMEN

1 Review the procedure with the nurse. Ask if a preservative is to be used and if the urine is to be preserved on ice.
2 Explain the procedure to the patient.
3 Wash your hands.
4 Collect the following equipment:
   a Urine container for a 24-hour collection
   b Preservative from the laboratory
   c Bucket with ice
   d Two labels stating a 24-hour urine specimen is being collected
   e Funnel
   f Bedpan, urinal, commode, or specimen pan
   g Disposable gloves
5 Write the requested information on the specimen container.
6 Identify the patient. Check the ID bracelet with the laboratory requisition slip.
7 Arrange the equipment in the patient's bathroom or "dirty" utility room.
8 Place one label (stating a 24-hour urine specimen is being collected) in the appropriate place in the bathroom or "dirty" utility room. Place the other near the bed.
9 Offer the bedpan or urinal, or assist the patient to the bathroom or bedside commode. Be sure the patient has on a robe and slippers when up.
10 Ask the patient to void. Discard the specimen (wear gloves for this step) and note the time. This begins the 24-hour collection period.
11 Mark the time the test began and the time it will end on the labels in the room and bathroom. Also mark the specimen container.
12 Ask the patient to use the bedpan, urinal, commode, or specimen pan when urinating during the next 24 hours. Have the patient signal when urine should be emptied. Remind him or her not to have a bowel movement at the same time and not to put toilet tissue in the receptacle.
13 Measure all urine if the patient is on I&O.
14 Pour urine into the specimen container using the funnel. Be careful not to spill any urine. The test is restarted if urine is spilled or discarded.
15 Add ice to the bucket as necessary.
16 Ask the patient to void at the end of the 24-hour period. Pour the urine into the specimen container.
17 Take the specimen and requisition slip to the laboratory.
18 Remove the labels from the room and bathroom. Clean and return equipment to its proper place. Discard disposable items.
19 Thank the patient for cooperating.
20 Make sure he or she is comfortable, the signal light is within reach, and the side rails are up.
21 Wash your hands.
22 Report your observations to the nurse.

COLLECTING A FRESH-FRACTIONAL URINE SPECIMEN

1 Explain the procedure to the patient.
2 Wash your hands.
3 Collect the following equipment:
   a Bedpan, urinal, commode, or disposable specimen pan
   b Two specimen containers
   c Urine testing equipment
   d Disposable gloves
4 Identify the patient. Check the ID bracelet with the treatment card.
5 Provide for privacy.
6 Offer the bedpan or urinal, or assist the patient to the bathroom or commode. Be sure he or she has on a robe and slippers when up.
7 Ask the patient to urinate.
8 Put on the gloves.
9 Take the receptacle to the bathroom or "dirty" utility room.
10 Measure urine if the patient is on I&O. Pour some urine into the specimen container.
11 Test the specimen in case a second one cannot be obtained. Discard the urine.
12 Clean the receptacle. Remove the gloves.
13 Return the receptacle to its proper place.
14 Help the patient wash the hands.
15 Make sure the patient is comfortable, the side rails are up, and the signal light is within reach. Unscreen the patient.
16 Remove the gloves and wash your hands.
17 Return to the room in 20 to 30 minutes.
18 Repeat steps 5 through 16.
19 Report the results of the second test and any other observations to the nurse.

COLLECTING A URINE SPECIMEN FROM AN INFANT OR CHILD

1 Explain the procedure to the child.
2 Wash your hands.
3 Collect the following equipment:
   a Disposable collection bag
   b Wash basin
   c Sterile cotton balls
   d Bath towel
   e Two diapers
   f Specimen container
   g Disposable gloves
4 Identify the child. Check the ID bracelet with the laboratory requisition slip.
5 Provide for privacy.
6 Put on the gloves.
7 Remove the diaper and dispose of it properly.
8 Clean the perineal area. Use a sterile cotton ball for each stroke. Rinse and dry the area.
9 Position the child on the back. Flex the child's knees and separate the legs.
10 Remove the adhesive backing from the collection bag.
11 Apply the bag to the perineum. Do not cover the anus (Fig. 14-18).
12 Diaper the child. Remove the gloves.
13 Raise the head of the crib if allowed. This helps the urine to collect in the bottom of the bag.
14 Unscreen the child.
15 Return to the room periodically. Open the diaper to see if the child has urinated. Provide for privacy if the child has urinated.
16 Put on gloves and remove the diaper.
17 Remove the collection bag gently.
18 Press the adhesive surfaces of the bag together. You may also transfer urine to the specimen container through the drainage tab.
19 Clean the perineal area, rinse, and dry well.
20 Diaper the child and remove the gloves.
21 Make sure the child is comfortable. Raise the side rail.
22 Unscreen the child.
23 Write the requested information on the specimen container.
24 Clean and return equipment to its proper place. Discard disposable items.
25 Take the specimen to the nurses' station or laboratory. Make sure you have the laboratory requisition slip if you are taking the specimen to the laboratory.
26 Wash your hands.
27 Report your observations to the nurse.

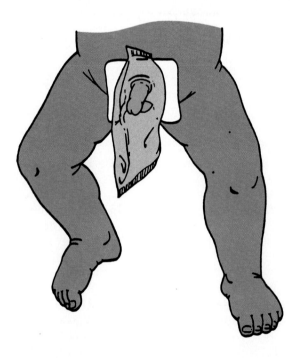

Fig. 14-18 A disposable collection bag is applied to the perineal area of the infant. Urine collects in the bag for a specimen.

TESTING URINE—TESTAPE

1 Explain the procedure to the patient.
2 Wash your hands.
3 Identify the patient. Check the ID bracelet with the treatment card.
4 Collect the following:
   a Fresh-fractional urine specimen (see *Collecting a Fresh-Fractional Urine Specimen*, page 243)
   b Testape
   c Wristwatch
   d Disposable gloves
5 Put on the gloves.
6 Open the dispenser. Withdraw about 1½ inches of Testape.
7 Tear the strip off the dispenser.
8 Dip about ¼ inch of the Testape into the specimen. Remove it immediately.
9 Hold the Testape downward (Fig. 14-19, *A*). Do not set the Testape down.
10 Wait 60 seconds.
11 Compare the darkest area of the Testape with the color chart on the dispenser (Fig. 14-19, *B*).
12 Read the number corresponding with the color that matches the Testape.
13 Discard the used Testape and urine.
14 Clean the equipment. Remove the gloves.
15 Return equipment to its proper place.
16 Wash your hands.
17 Report the results and other observations.

TESTING URINE—CLINITEST

1 Explain the procedure to the patient.
2 Wash your hands.
3 Identify the patient. Check the ID bracelet with the treatment card.
4 Collect the following:
   a Fresh-fractional urine specimen (see *Collecting a Fresh-Fractional Urine Specimen*, page 243)
   b Wristwatch
   c Clinitest kit (test tube, tablets, medicine dropper, test tube holder, and color chart)
   d Disposable gloves
   e Paper towels
   f Two medicine cups with water
5 Put on the gloves.
6 Place the paper towels over the working area.
7 Arrange the specimen, Clinitest equipment, and medicine cups on the paper towels.
8 Place the clean test tube in the test tube holder.
9 Rinse the medicine dropper with water from one of the medicine cups.
10 Draw urine into the medicine dropper. Keep the medicine dropper upright.
11 Place 5 drops of urine in the test tube (Fig. 14-20).
12 Rinse the medicine dropper. Use the medicine cup previously used for rinsing. Discard the medicine cup.
13 Draw water into the medicine dropper. Use the other medicine cup for the water.
14 Add 10 drops of water to the test tube.
15 Drop one tablet into the test tube:
   a Open the bottle.
   b Hold the bottle in one hand. Hold the bottle cap in the other.
   c Tap the bottle gently so that a tablet falls into the bottle cap (Fig. 14-21).
   d Drop the tablet in the cap into the test tube.
   e Put the cap tightly on the bottle.
   f Do not let the tablet touch your skin, eyes, mucous membranes, or clothing. It can cause burns and other damage.
16 Watch the boiling reaction. Do not shake or touch the test tube. Keep it away from your eyes.
17 Wait 15 seconds after the boiling has stopped. Then shake the tube gently.
18 Compare the liquid in the test tube with the color chart.
19 Match the color of the liquid in the test tube with the color chart. Read the matching number.
20 Discard the contents of the test tube and the urine specimen.
21 Clean the test tube and medicine dropper. Place them in the kit. Place the test tube upside down in the kit.
22 Clean other equipment. Discard disposable equipment.
23 Remove the gloves.
24 Return equipment to its proper place.
25 Wipe off the working area with paper towels.
26 Wash your hands.
27 Report the results and your observations.

A

B

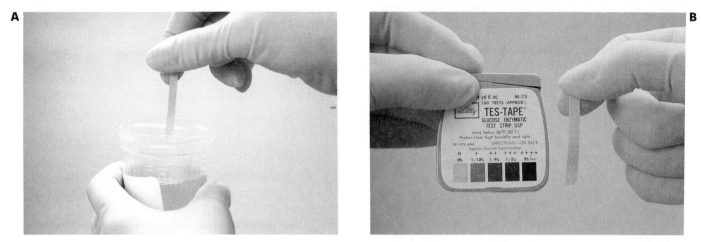

Fig. 14-19 **A,** The 1½ inch strip of Testape is held downward after being dipped into the urine. **B,** The Testape is compared to the color chart on the dispenser to determine the amount of sugar in the urine.

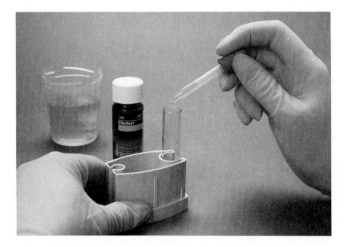

Fig. 14-20 A medicine dropper is used to place five drops of urine in the test tube during the Clinitest.

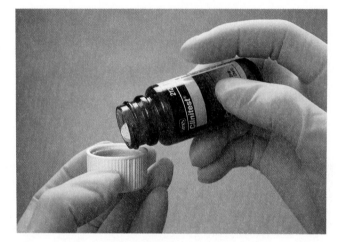

Fig. 14-21 A Clinitest tablet is transferred from the bottle to the bottle cap by tapping the bottle gently. The tablet is then dropped from the cap into the test tube.

Keto-Diastix The Keto-Diastix (Fig. 14-22) determines if sugar and ketones (acetone) are in the urine. The plastic strip has two test areas at the bottom. The strip is dipped into a urine specimen. The test areas change color if sugar or ketones are present. The strip is compared to a color chart.

Straining Urine

Stones (calculi) can develop in the urinary system. They may be in the kidneys, ureters, or bladder. Stones may be as small as a pin head or as large as an orange. Stones that cause severe pain and damage to the urinary system may be removed by special surgical procedures. A stone may exit the body with the urine. All of the patient's urine must be strained. If a stone is passed, it is sent to the laboratory to be examined. See the box on page 248.

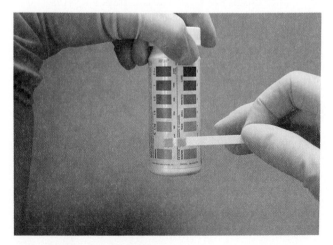

Fig. 14-22 Keto-Diastix.

TESTING URINE—ACETEST

1 Explain the procedure to the patient.
2 Wash your hands.
3 Identify the patient. Check the ID bracelet with the treatment card.
4 Collect the following:
  a Fresh-fractional urine specimen (see *Collecting a Fresh-Fractional Urine Specimen,* page 243)
  b Acetest tablets
  c Medicine dropper
  d Color chart
  e Medicine cup with water
  f Paper towels
  g Disposable gloves
  h Wristwatch
5 Put on the gloves.
6 Place the paper towels over the working area.
7 Place the Acetest tablet on the paper towel:
  a Open the bottle.
  b Hold the bottle in one hand. Hold the cap in the other.
  c Tap the bottle so that a tablet falls into the cap.
  d Drop the tablet onto the paper towel.
  e Put the cap tightly on the bottle.
  f Do not let the tablet touch your skin, eyes, mucous membranes, or clothing.
8 Rinse the medicine dropper with water from the medicine cup.
9 Draw some urine into the medicine dropper.
10 Drop 1 drop of urine onto the tablet.
11 Wait 30 seconds.
12 Compare the tablet with the color chart.
13 Read the result that matches the color chart.
14 Discard the paper towel, Acetest tablet, urine, and other disposable equipment.
15 Clean the medicine dropper and other equipment. Remove the gloves.
16 Return equipment to its proper place.
17 Wash your hands.
18 Report the results and your other observations.

TESTING URINE—KETO-DIASTIX

1 Explain the procedure to the patient.
2 Wash your hands.
3 Identify the patient. Check the ID bracelet with the treatment card.
4 Collect the following:
  a Fresh-fractional urine specimen (see *Collecting a Fresh-Fractional Urine Specimen,* page 243)
  b Keto-Diastix
  c Wristwatch
  d Disposable gloves
5 Put on the gloves.
6 Remove a strip from the bottle. Put the cap on the bottle immediately. Make sure it is tight.
7 Dip the 2 test areas of the strip into the specimen for 2 seconds.
8 Remove the strip after 2 seconds.
9 Tap the strip gently against the container to remove excess urine.
10 Wait 15 seconds. Compare the strip with the color chart on the bottle for ketones. The color is buff before testing. Read the results.
11 Compare the strip with the color chart for glucose after 30 seconds. The color is light blue before testing. Read the results.
12 Discard disposable equipment and the specimen.
13 Clean equipment. Remove the gloves.
14 Return equipment to its proper place.
15 Wash your hands.
16 Report the results and your other observations.

STRAINING URINE

1 Explain the procedure to the patient. Also explain that the urinal, bedpan, commode, or specimen pan should be used for voiding.
2 Wash your hands.
3 Collect the following:
  a Disposable strainer or 4 × 4 gauze
  b Specimen container
  c Urinal, bedpan, commode, or specimen pan
  d Labels for the room and bathroom (labels state that all urine is strained)
  e Disposable gloves
4 Identify the patient. Check the ID bracelet with the treatment card.
5 Arrange equipment in the patient's bathroom.
6 Place one label in the bathroom. Place the other near the bed.
7 Offer the bedpan or urinal, or assist the patient to the bedside commode or bathroom. Be sure the patient has on a robe and slippers when up. Provide for privacy.
8 Ask the patient to signal after voiding.
9 Put on the gloves.
10 Place the strainer or gauze into the specimen container.
11 Pour the urine into the specimen container. The urine will pass through the strainer or gauze (Fig. 14-23).
12 Place the strainer or gauze in the container if any crystals, stones, or particles appear.
13 Discard the urine.
14 Help the patient clean the perineal area if necessary.
15 Help the patient wash the hands.
16 Remove the gloves.
17 Make sure the patient is comfortable, the side rails are up, and the signal light is within reach. Unscreen the patient.
18 Label the specimen container with the requested information.
19 Clean and return equipment to its proper place.
20 Take the specimen to the nurses' station or laboratory. Make sure you have a requisition slip if you are taking the specimen to the laboratory.
21 Wash your hands.
22 Report your observations to the nurse.

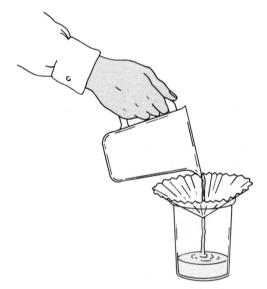

Fig. 14-23 A disposable strainer is placed in a specimen container. Urine is poured through the strainer into the specimen container.

SUMMARY

You are responsible for helping patients and residents maintain normal urination. You also assist with bladder training, collect specimens, and test urine for sugar and acetone. You must follow the rules of medical asepsis, universal precautions, cleanliness, and skin care. Your observations of the person's urine are valuable to doctors and nurses. They use your observations to plan and evaluate the person's treatment and progress.

Position and privacy are important for urinary elimination. Urination is considered a private function. Voiding is easier and more comfortable if the person can urinate in a normal position and in private.

REVIEW QUESTIONS

Circle the best *answer.*

1 Which mean urination?
   a Glucosuria and dysuria
   b Acetone and ketone bodies
   c Micturition and voiding
   d Catheter and urinal

2 Which statement is *false*?
   a Urine is normally clear and yellow or amber in color.
   b Urine normally has an ammonia odor.
   c People normally urinate before going to bed and on rising.
   d A person normally urinates about 1000 ml to 1500 ml a day.

3 Which is *not* a rule for maintaining normal elimination?
   a Help the person assume a normal position for urination.
   b Provide for privacy.
   c Help the person to the bathroom or commode, or provide the bedpan or urinal as soon as requested.
   d Always stay with the person who is on a bedpan.

4 The best position for using a bedpan is
   a Fowler's position
   b The supine position
   c The prone position
   d The side-lying position

5 After a man uses the urinal, you should ask him to
   a Cover the urinal
   b Put the signal light on
   c Put the urinal on the overbed table
   d Empty the urinal

6 Urinary incontinence
   a Is always permanent
   b Requires good skin care
   c Is treated with a catheter
   d All of the above

7 A patient has a catheter. Which is *incorrect?*
   a Keep the drainage bag above the level of the bladder.
   b Make sure the drainage tubing is free of kinks.
   c Coil the drainage tubing on the bed.
   d Tape the catheter to the inner thigh.

8 A patient has a catheter. Which is *false?*
   a Daily perineal care is sufficient.
   b The rules of medical asepsis are followed.
   c The drainage bag is emptied at the end of each shift.
   d Complaints of pain, burning, the need to urinate, or irritation are reported immediately.

9 A man has a condom catheter. Tape is applied
   a Completely around the penis
   b To the inner thigh
   c To the abdomen
   d In a spiral fashion

10 The goal of bladder training is to
   a Remove the catheter
   b Allow the person to walk to the bathroom
   c Gain voluntary control of urination
   d All of the above

11 When collecting a urine specimen, you should
   a Label the container with the requested information
   b Use the appropriate container
   c Collect the specimen at the time specified
   d All of the above

12 The perineal area is cleaned immediately before collecting a
   a Routine urine specimen
   b Clean-catch urine specimen
   c 24-hour urine specimen
   d Fresh-fractional urine specimen

13 A 24-hour urine specimen involves
   a Collecting all of the urine voided by a patient during a 24-hour period
   b Collecting a routine urine specimen every hour for 24 hours
   c A catheterization
   d Testing the urine for sugar and acetone

14 Urine is tested for sugar and acetone
   a At bedtime
   b 30 minutes after meals and at bedtime
   c 30 minutes before meals and at bedtime
   d Before breakfast

15 Which specimen is best for sugar and acetone testing?
   a A routine urine specimen
   b A clean-catch urine specimen
   c A 24-hour urine specimen
   d A fresh-fractional urine specimen

16 Which measures sugar and acetone in the urine?
   a Testape
   b Clinitest
   c Acetest
   d Keto-Diastix

Answers

				9	b
16	d	11	d	5	b
15	d	10	c	4	a
14	c	9	d	3	d
13	a	8	a	2	b
12	b	7	a	1	c

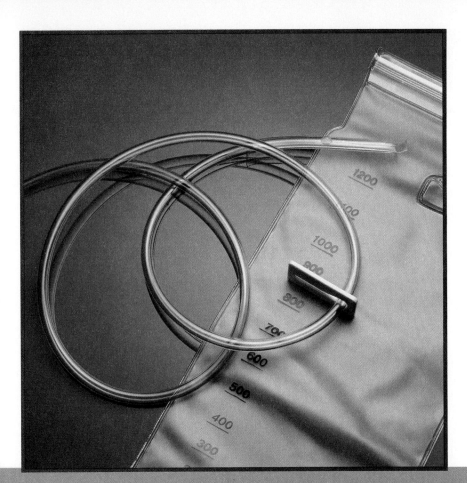

Bowel Elimination

OBJECTIVES

- Define the key terms listed in this chapter
- Describe a normal stool and the normal pattern and frequency of bowel movements
- List the observations about defecation that are reported to the nurse
- Identify the factors that affect bowel elimination
- Describe common problems relating to defecation
- Describe the measures that promote comfort and safety during defecation
- Describe bowel training
- Explain why enemas are given
- Know the common enema solutions
- Describe the rules for administering enemas
- Explain the purpose of rectal tubes
- Insert a rectal tube
- Describe how to care for a patient with a colostomy or ileostomy
- Perform the procedures described in this chapter

anal incontinence   The inability to control the passage of feces and gas through the anus

chyme   Partially digested food and fluid that pass from the stomach into the small intestine

colostomy   An artificial opening between the colon and abdomen

constipation   The passage of a hard, dry stool

defecation   The process of excreting feces from the rectum through the anus; a bowel movement

diarrhea   The frequent passage of liquid stools

enema   The introduction of fluid into the rectum and lower colon

fecal impaction   The prolonged retention and accumulation of feces in the rectum

feces   The semisolid mass of waste products in the colon

flatulence   The excessive formation of gas in the stomach and intestines

flatus   Gas or air in the stomach or intestines

ileostomy   An artificial opening between the ileum (small intestine) and the abdomen

ostomy   The surgical creation of an artificial opening

peristalsis   The alternating contraction and relaxation of intestinal muscles

stoma   An opening; see colostomy and ileostomy

stool   Feces that have been excreted

suppository   A cone-shaped solid medication that is inserted into a body opening; it melts at body temperature

NORMAL BOWEL MOVEMENTS

The frequency of bowel movements is highly individualized. Some people have a bowel movement every day. Others have a bowel movement every 2 to 3 days. Some people have 2 or 3 bowel movements a day. The pattern of elimination also involves the time of day. Many people defecate after breakfast; others do so in the evening.

Stools are normally brown in color. Bleeding in the stomach, intestines, or colon affects the color of stools. Color is also affected by certain diseases and foods. A diet high in beets causes red-colored feces. A diet high in green vegetables can cause green stools.

Feces are normally soft, formed, and shaped like the rectum. Feces that move rapidly through the intestine are watery and unformed. This is called *diarrhea*. Stools that move slowly through the intestines are harder than normal. *Constipation* is the excretion of a hard, dry stool.

Feces have a characteristic odor. The odor is due to bacterial action in the intestines. Certain foods and drugs can affect the odor of stools.

What to Report to the Nurse

Stools are carefully observed before disposal. Note the color, amount, consistency, and odor. The shape and size of feces and frequency of defecation are reported. Also report any complaints of pain. Abnormal stools should be observed by the nurse.

Bowel elimination is the excretion of wastes from the gastrointestinal system. Foods and fluids are normally taken in through the mouth and are partially digested in the stomach. The partially digested foods and fluids are called *chyme*. Chyme passes from the stomach into the small intestine. Further digestion and absorption of nutrients occur as the chyme passes through the small bowel. The chyme eventually enters the large intestine (large bowel or colon), where fluid is absorbed. There the chyme becomes less fluid and more solid in consistency. *Feces* refers to the semisolid mass of waste products in the colon.

Feces move through the intestines by *peristalsis*, the alternating contraction and relaxation of intestinal muscles. The feces move through the large intestine to the rectum. Feces are stored in the rectum until excreted from the body (Fig. 15-1). *Defecation (bowel movement)* is the process of excreting feces from the rectum through the anus. The term *stool* refers to feces that have been excreted.

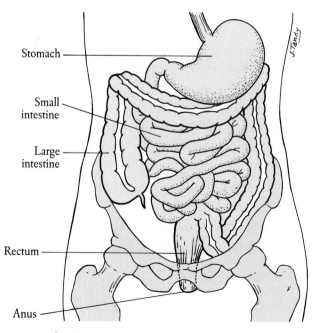

Stomach

Small intestine

Large intestine

Rectum

Anus

Fig. 15-1   The gastrointestinal system.

FACTORS AFFECTING BOWEL ELIMINATION

Normal defecation is affected by many factors. Regularity, frequency, consistency, color, and odor of stools can be affected by psychological and physical factors.

Privacy

Like urination, bowel elimination is a private act. Lack of privacy may prevent a person from defecating even though the urge is felt. The odors and sounds from a bowel movement can be embarrassing. Imagine what it is like using a bedpan or commode for bowel elimination in a semiprivate room. Individuals may ignore the urge to defecate to avoid having a bowel movement in the presence of others.

Age

Infants and toddlers do not have voluntary control of bowel movements. Defecation occurs whenever feces enter the rectum. Bowel training is learned between 2 and 3 years of age. The elderly may lose control over defecation because of changes in the body caused by aging. Aging can also cause the passage of feces through the intestine to slow down. This results in constipation.

Diet

A well-balanced diet is important for normal bowel elimination. A certain amount of bulk is needed. Foods high in fiber are not completely digested and leave a residue that provides needed bulk. A diet low in fiber reduces the frequency of defecation, resulting in constipation. Fruits and vegetables are high in fiber.

Individual reaction to certain foods can cause diarrhea or constipation. Milk may cause constipation in some people and diarrhea in others. Chocolate and other foods can cause similar reactions.

Gas-forming foods can stimulate peristalsis. Increased peristalsis results in defecation. Gas-forming foods include onions, beans, cabbage, cauliflower, radishes, and cucumbers.

Fluids

Fecal material contains a certain amount of water. Water is absorbed from feces as they move through the large intestine. Stool consistency depends on how much water is absorbed. The amount of fluid ingested and the amount of urine both affect the amount of water absorbed by the large intestine.

Activity

Exercise and activity maintain muscle tone and stimulate peristalsis. Irregular elimination and constipation are often due to inactivity and bed rest. Inactivity may result from disease, surgery, injury, and aging.

Medications

Medications can prevent constipation or control diarrhea. Other medications that are unrelated to bowel elimination may cause the side effects of diarrhea or constipation. Drugs for pain relief often cause constipation. Antibiotics, used to fight or prevent infection, often cause diarrhea. Diarrhea results because the antibiotics kill the normal bacteria in the large intestine. Normal bacteria are necessary for the formation of stool.

COMMON PROBLEMS

Many factors can affect normal bowel elimination. Common problems include constipation, fecal impaction, diarrhea, anal incontinence, and flatulence.

Constipation

Constipation is the passage of a hard, dry stool. The person usually strains to have a bowel movement. The stool may be large or marble-sized. Large stools cause pain as they pass through the anus. Constipation occurs when feces move through the intestine slowly, allowing more time for the absorption of water. Common causes of constipation include diet, ignoring the urge to defecate, decreased fluid intake, inactivity, medications, aging, and certain diseases.

Fecal Impaction

A *fecal impaction* is the prolonged retention and accumulation of feces in the rectum. Fecal material is hard or putty-like in consistency. A fecal impaction results if constipation is not relieved. The person cannot defecate, and more water is absorbed from the already hardened feces. Liquid seeping from the anus is a sign of fecal impaction. Liquid feces pass around the hardened fecal mass in the rectum.

The person with a fecal impaction may try several times to have a bowel movement. Abdominal discomfort and rectal pain may be reported. The doctor may order medications and enemas to remove the impaction. The nurse may have to remove the fecal mass with a gloved finger.

Diarrhea

Diarrhea is the frequent passage of liquid stools. Feces move through the intestines rapidly, reducing the time for fluid absorption. There is an urgent need to defecate. Some people have difficulty maintaining control of elimination. Abdominal cramping, nausea, and vomiting may also occur.

Causes include infections, certain medications, irritating foods, and microorganisms in food and water. Medical treatment involves reducing peristalsis by diet or medications. You must provide the bedpan or commode promptly for the person with diarrhea. Prompt disposal of the stool is necessary to reduce odors and prevent the spread of microorganisms. Good skin care is essential. Liquid feces are very irritating to the skin. Frequent wiping of the anal area with toilet tissue is also irritating. Decubiti may develop if cleanliness and good skin care are not practiced.

Anal Incontinence

Anal incontinence (fecal incontinence) is the inability to control the passage of feces and gas through the anus. Infants and toddlers normally have anal incontinence until they are toilet trained. Diseases or injuries to the nervous system may cause anal incontinence. Sometimes it results from an unanswered signal light when the person needs the bedpan or requires help getting to the commode or bathroom.

The person with anal incontinence needs good skin care. A bowel training program may be developed. Providing the bedpan or commode after meals or every 2 to 3 hours may be helpful. Consider the psychological impact of anal incontinence on the person. Frustration, embarrassment, anger, and humiliation are a few of the emotions experienced.

Flatulence

Gas or air in the stomach or intestines is called *flatus*. Swallowing air while eating and drinking and bacterial action in the intestines are common sources of flatus. Normally flatus is expelled through the mouth and anus.

Flatulence is the excessive formation of gas in the stomach and intestines. If the gas is not expelled, the intestines distend. In other words, they swell or enlarge from the pressure of the gases. The person may have abdominal cramping, shortness of breath, and a swollen abdomen. Flatulence may be caused by gasforming foods, constipation, medications, and abdominal surgery. In addition, tense or anxious people may swallow large amounts of air when drinking. Doctors may prescribe enemas, medications, or rectal tubes to relieve distention.

COMFORT AND SAFETY DURING ELIMINATION

Certain measures help promote normal bowel elimination. The nurse plans measures that involve diet, fluids, and exercise. The following actions should be routinely practiced to promote bowel elimination, comfort, and safety.

1. Provide the bedpan or help the patient to the toilet or commode as soon as requested.
2. Provide for privacy. Ask visitors to leave the room. Close doors, pull curtains around the bed, and pull window curtains or shades. Remember that defecation is a private act. Leave the room if the person can be alone.
3. Make sure the bedpan is warm.
4. Position the person in a normal sitting or squatting position.
5. Make sure the individual is adequately covered for warmth and privacy.
6. Allow enough time for defecation.
7. Place the signal light and toilet tissue within the person's reach.
8. Stay nearby if the person is weak or unsteady.
9. Provide perineal care.
10. Dispose of feces promptly. This reduces odors and prevents the spread of microorganisms.
11. Let the person wash the hands after defecating and wiping with toilet tissue.
12. Offer the bedpan after meals if the person has the problem of incontinence.
13. Use universal precautions if contact with feces is possible.

BOWEL TRAINING

Bowel training involves two aspects. One is gaining control of bowel movements. The other is developing a regular pattern of elimination. Fecal impaction, constipation, and anal incontinence are prevented.

The urge to defecate is usually felt after a meal, particularly breakfast. Therefore the use of the toilet, commode, or bedpan is encouraged at this time. Other factors that influence elimination are included in the nursing care plan and bowel training program. These include diet, fluids, activity, and privacy. The nurse will give you instructions about an individual's bowel training program.

The physician may order a suppository to stimulate defecation. A *suppository* is a cone-shaped solid medication that is inserted into a body opening. It melts at body temperature. The rectal suppository is inserted into the rectum by the nurse. It is inserted about 30 minutes before the time selected for the bowel movement. Enemas may also be ordered.

ENEMAS

An *enema* is the introduction of fluid into the rectum and lower colon. Enemas are ordered by doctors. They are given to remove feces and to relieve constipation or fecal impaction. They are also ordered to clean the bowel of feces before certain surgeries, x-ray procedures, or childbirth. Sometimes enemas are ordered to remove flatus and relieve intestinal distention. Bowel training programs can involve enemas.

Enema Solutions

The enema solution ordered by the doctor depends on the purpose of the enema. The solution may be *tap water* obtained from a faucet. A *soap suds* enema (SSE) is prepared by adding 5 ml of liquid soap to 1000 ml of water. A *saline* enema is a solution of salt and water. These solutions are generally used for cleansing enemas. Cleansing enemas involve the removal of feces from the rectum and colon.

Oil is used for oil-retention enemas. They are given for constipation or fecal impactions. The oil is retained in the rectum for 30 to 60 minutes to soften the feces and lubricate the rectum. This allows feces to pass with ease. Mineral oil, olive oil, or a commercial oil-retention enema may be used.

Commercial enemas are often ordered for constipated patients. They are also ordered when complete cleansing of the bowel is not indicated. The enema contains about 120 ml (4 ounces) of a solution. It causes defecation by irritating and distending the rectum.

Other enema solutions may be ordered. Consult with the nurse and use the procedure manual to safely prepare and give uncommon enemas.

Equipment

Disposable enema kits are available from the central supply area. The kit (Fig. 15-2) includes a plastic enema bag, tubing, a clamp for the tubing, and a waterproof bed protector. The enema bag holds the solution. Most kits have packets of castile soap for soap suds enemas. Lubricant is needed if the tubing end is not prelubricated. A bath thermometer is used to measure the temperature of the solution. Some solutions are obtained from central supply. If a commercial enema has been ordered, you need the enema and a waterproof bed protector. A bedpan is usually needed for an enema. Enema procedures also require gloves for universal precautions.

General Rules

The administration of an enema is generally a safe procedure. Many people give themselves enemas at home. However, enemas are dangerous for people with certain heart and kidney diseases. Give an enema only after receiving clear instructions and after reviewing the procedure with the nurse.

Comfort and safety measures are practiced when giving an enema. In addition, these rules must be followed.

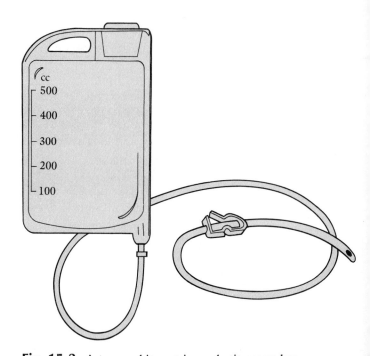

Fig. 15-2 An enema kit contains a plastic enema bag, tubing, and a clamp.

1. Solution temperature should be 105° F (40.5° C). Measure the temperature with a bath thermometer.
2. The amount of solution to be given depends on the enema's purpose and the person's age. Adults generally receive 750 to 1000 ml. Young children receive no more than 500 ml.
3. The left Sims' position is usually used (see Fig. 10-47). However, a comfortable left side-lying position may be allowed.
4. The enema bag is raised no more than 18 inches above the level of the mattress.
5. The lubricated enema tubing is inserted only 2 to 4 inches into the rectum. The intestine can be injured if the tube is inserted any deeper.
6. The solution is administered slowly. Usually it takes 10 to 15 minutes to give 750 to 1000 ml.
7. The solution should be retained in the bowel for a certain length of time. The length of time depends on the amount and type of solution.
8. The enema tube is held in place while the solution is being administered.
9. The bathroom must be vacant when the person has the urge to defecate. Make sure that the bathroom will not be used by another patient.
10. The nurse is asked to observe the results of the enema.
11. Universal precautions are used.

GIVING A CLEANSING ENEMA

1 Explain the procedure to the patient.
2 Wash your hands.
3 Collect the following equipment:
  a Bedpan or bedside commode
  b Disposable enema kit (enema bag, tubing, and clamp)
  c Bath thermometer
  d Waterproof bed protector
  e Water-soluble lubricant
  f Disposable gloves
  g Material for enema solution: 5 ml castile soap or 2 teaspoons of salt
  h Toilet tissue
  i Bath blanket
  j IV pole
  k Large measuring container
  l Robe and slippers
  m Specimen container if needed
  n Paper towels
4 Identify the patient. Check the ID bracelet with the treatment card.
5 Provide for privacy.
6 Raise the bed to an appropriate level for good body mechanics.
7 Lower the side rail.
8 Cover the patient with a bath blanket. Fanfold top linens to the foot of the bed.
9 Position the IV pole so that the enema bag will be 12 inches above the anus or 18 inches above the level of the mattress.
10 Raise the side rail.
11 Prepare the enema:
  a Close the clamp on the tubing.
  b Adjust water flow until it is lukewarm.
  c Fill the measuring container to the 1000 ml mark or as otherwise ordered.
  d Measure the temperature of the water. It should be 105° F (40.5° C).
  e Prepare the enema solution:
    1 Saline enema: add 2 teaspoons of salt
    2 Soap suds enema: add 5 ml of castile soap
    3 Tap water enema: add nothing to the water
  f Stir the solution with the bath thermometer. Scoop off any suds (SSE).
  g Pour the solution into the enema bag.
  h Seal the top of the bag.
  i Hang the bag on the IV pole.
12 Lower the side rail.
13 Position the patient in the left Sims' position or in a comfortable left side-lying position.

14 Place the waterproof pad under the buttocks.
15 Expose the anal area.
16 Put on the gloves.
17 Place the bedpan behind the patient.
18 Position the enema tubing in the bedpan. Open the clamp. Let solution flow through the tubing to remove air. Clamp the tubing.
19 Lubricate the tubing with the lubricant. Lubricate 2 to 4 inches from the tip.
20 Separate the buttocks to see the anus.
21 Ask the patient to take a deep breath through the mouth.
22 Insert the tubing gently 2 to 4 inches into the rectum when the patient is exhaling (Fig. 15-3). Stop if he or she complains of pain or if you feel resistance.
23 Check how much solution is in the enema bag.
24 Unclamp the tubing and administer the solution slowly (Fig. 15-4).
25 Ask the patient to take slow deep breaths. This helps the patient relax while the enema is being administered.
26 Clamp the tubing if the patient has a desire to defecate, complains of abdominal cramping, or begins to expel solution. Unclamp when the symptoms subside.
27 Give at least 750 ml or the desired amount. You may have to stop if the person cannot tolerate the procedure.
28 Clamp the tubing before it is empty. This prevents air from entering the bowel.
29 Hold several thicknesses of toilet tissue around the tubing and against the anus. Remove the tubing.
30 Discard the soiled toilet tissue into the bedpan.
31 Wrap the tubing tip with paper towels and place it inside the enema bag.
32 Help the patient onto the bedpan. Raise the head of the bed. Assist the patient to the bathroom or commode if appropriate. The patient wears a robe and slippers when up. The bed is in the lowest position.
33 Place the signal light and toilet tissue within reach. Remind the patient not to flush the toilet.
34 Leave the room if the patient can be alone. Discard disposable equipment. Remove the gloves. Wash your hands.
35 Return when the patient signals. Knock before entering.

GIVING A CLEANSING ENEMA—cont'd

36 Observe enema results for amount, color, consistency, and odor.
37 Put on gloves.
38 Obtain a stool specimen if ordered.
39 Help the patient clean the perineal area if indicated.
40 Remove the bed protector.
41 Empty, clean, and disinfect the bedpan or commode. Flush the toilet after the nurse observes the results. Return equipment to its proper place. Remove the gloves.

42 Help the patient wash the hands.
43 Return top linens and remove the bath blanket.
44 Make sure the patient is comfortable and the signal light is within reach.
45 Lower the bed to its lowest position.
46 Raise the side rail. Unscreen the patient.
47 Place soiled linen in the linen hamper.
48 Wash your hands.
49 Report your observations.

The Cleansing Enema

Cleansing enemas are often given to clean the bowel of feces and flatus. They are sometimes given before surgery, x-ray procedures, and childbirth. The doctor may order a soap suds, tap water, or saline enema. The doctor may order "enemas until clear." Enemas are given until the return solution is clear and free of fecal material. Check with the nurse to see how many enemas can be given. The facility may allow enemas to be repeated only 2 or 3 times.

Tap water enemas can be dangerous. The large intestine may absorb some of the water into the bloodstream. This creates a fluid imbalance in the body. Repeated enemas increase the risk of excessive fluid absorption. Soap suds enemas are very irritating to the bowel's mucous lining. Damage to the bowel can result with repeated enemas. Using more than 5 ml of castile soap and using stronger soaps can also damage the bowel. The saline enema solution is similar to body fluid. However, some people may absorb some of the salt in the solution.

The Commercial Enema

The commerical enema is ready to be given (Fig. 15-5). The solution is usually given at room temperature. However, the nurse may have you warm the enema in a basin of warm water. The left Sims' or a left side-lying position is often used. Some nursing theories suggest using the knee-chest position (see Fig. 20-2, *C*) The knee-chest position lets more so-

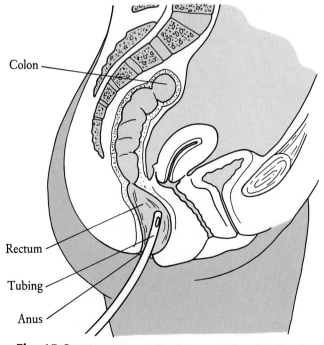

Fig. 15-3 The enema tubing is inserted 2 to 4 inches into the rectum.

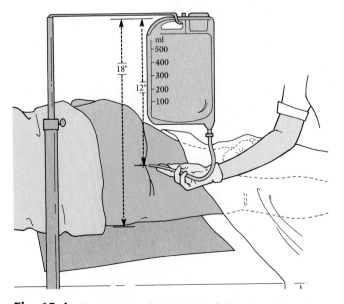

Fig. 15-4 An enema is given in the left Sims' position. The IV pole is positioned so that the enema bag is 12 inches above the anus and 18 inches above the mattress.

GIVING A COMMERCIAL ENEMA

1 Explain the procedure to the patient.
2 Wash your hands.
3 Collect the following equipment:
   a Commercial enema
   b Bedpan, commode, or specimen pan
   c Waterproof bed protector
   d Toilet tissue
   e Disposable gloves
   f Robe and slippers
   g Specimen container if needed
   h Bath blanket
4 Identify the patient. Check the ID bracelet with the treatment card.
5 Provide for privacy.
6 Raise the bed to a level appropriate for good body mechanics.
7 Lower the side rail.
8 Cover the patient with a bath blanket. Fan-fold top linens to the foot of the bed.
9 Position the patient in the left Sims' or a comfortable side-lying position.
10 Place the bed protector under the buttocks.
11 Expose the anal area.
12 Position the bedpan near the patient.
13 Put on the gloves.
14 Remove the cap from the enema.
15 Separate the buttocks to see the anus.
16 Ask the patient to take a deep breath through the mouth.
17 Insert the enema tip 2 inches into the rectum when the patient is exhaling (Fig. 15-6). Insert the tip gently.
18 Squeeze and roll the bottle gently. Do not release pressure on the bottle until all solution has been given.
19 Remove the tip from the rectum. Put the bottle into the box, tip first.

20 Remove and discard the gloves.
21 Help the patient onto the bedpan. Raise the head of the bed. Assist the patient to the bathroom or commode if appropriate. The patient wears a robe and slippers when up, and the bed is in the lowest position.
22 Place the signal light and toilet tissue within reach. Remind the patient not to flush the toilet.
23 Leave the room if the patient can be alone. Discard used disposable items. Wash your hands.
24 Return when the patient signals. Knock before entering.
25 Observe enema results for amount, color, consistency, and odor.
26 Put on gloves.
27 Obtain a stool specimen if ordered.
28 Help the patient clean the perineal area if indicated.
29 Remove the bed protector.
30 Empty, clean, and disinfect the bedpan or commode. Flush the toilet after the nurse observes the results. Return equipment. Remove the gloves.
31 Help the patient wash the hands.
32 Cover the patient. Remove the bath blanket.
33 Make sure the patient is comfortable and the signal light is within reach.
34 Lower the bed to its lowest position.
35 Raise the side rail.
36 Unscreen the patient.
37 Place soiled linen in the linen hamper.
38 Wash your hands.
39 Report your observations to the nurse.

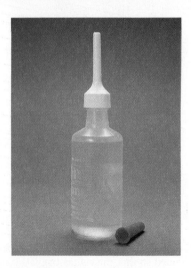

Fig. 15-5 A commercial enema.

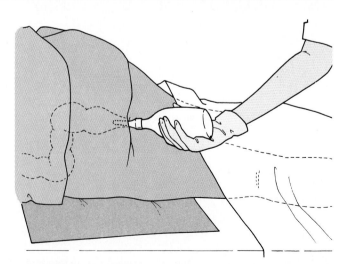

Fig. 15-6 The tip of the commercial enema is inserted 2 inches into the rectum.

GIVING AN OIL-RETENTION ENEMA

1 Explain the procedure to the patient.
2 Wash your hands.
3 Collect the following equipment:
   a Commercial oil-retention enema
   b Waterproof bed protector
   c Disposable gloves
   d Bath blanket
4 Identify the patient. Check the ID bracelet with the treatment card.
5 Provide for privacy.
6 Raise the bed to an appropriate level for good body mechanics.
7 Lower the side rail.
8 Cover the patient with a bath blanket. Fanfold top linens to the foot of the bed.
9 Position the patient in the left Sims' or side-lying position.
10 Place a bed protector under the buttocks.
11 Drape the patient to expose the anal area.
12 Put on the gloves.
13 Remove the cap from the enema.
14 Separate the buttocks to see the anus.
15 Ask the patient to take a deep breath through the mouth.
16 Insert the tip 2 inches into the rectum when the patient is exhaling. Insert the tip gently.
17 Squeeze the bottle slowly and gently until all solution has been given.
18 Remove the tip from the rectum. Put the bottle in the box, tip first.
19 Remove and discard the gloves.
20 Cover the patient. Leave him or her in the Sims' or side-lying position.
21 Encourage him or her to retain the enema for the time ordered.
22 Place additional waterproof protectors on the bed if indicated.
23 Raise the side rail.
24 Lower the bed to its lowest position.
25 Make sure the patient is comfortable and the signal light is within reach.
26 Unscreen the patient.
27 Discard used disposable equipment.
28 Wash your hands.
29 Check the patient frequently.
30 Report your observations to the nurse.

lution flow into the colon. The nurse will tell you how to position the patient.

The plastic bottle is squeezed and rolled up from the bottom to administer the solution. Squeezing and rolling are continued until all solution has been given. Do not release pressure on the bottle. If pressure is released, solution is withdrawn from the rectum back into the bottle. Encourage the patient to retain the solution until the urge to defecate is felt. Remaining in the Sims' or side-lying position will help the person retain the enema longer.

The Oil-Retention Enema

Commercial oil-retention enemas are administered like other commercial enemas. However, the solution is retained in the rectum so that the feces soften. The enema is retained for a specified length of time, usually for 30 to 60 minutes. Oil-retention enemas are ordered to relieve constipation or fecal impaction.

RECTAL TUBES

A rectal tube is inserted into the rectum to relieve flatulence and intestinal distention. Flatus passes from the body without effort or straining. The disposable kit contains a tube and flatus bag (Fig. 15-7). The bag collects feces that may be expelled

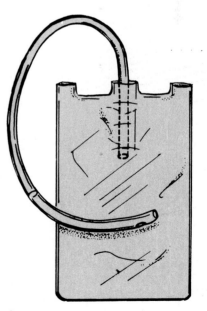

Fig. 15-7 A rectal tube and flatus bag.

USING A RECTAL TUBE

1 Explain the procedure to the patient.
2 Wash your hands.
3 Collect the following equipment:
  a Disposable rectal tube with flatus bag
  b Water-soluble lubricant
  c Adhesive tape
  d Disposable gloves
  e Waterproof bed protector if needed
4 Identify the patient. Check the ID bracelet with the treatment card.
5 Provide for privacy.
6 Raise the bed to a level appropriate for good body mechanics.
7 Lower the side rail.
8 Position the patient in the left Sims' or left side-lying position.
9 Expose the anal area.
10 Put on the gloves.
11 Lubricate 2 to 4 inches up from the tip of the tube.
12 Separate the buttocks to see the anus.
13 Ask the patient to take a deep breath through the mouth.
14 Insert the tube gently 2 to 4 inches into the rectum when the patient is exhaling. Stop if he or she complains of pain or if you feel resistance.

15 Tape the rectal tube to the buttocks.
16 Position the flatus bag so that it rests on the bed (Fig. 15-8). Remove the gloves.
17 Cover the patient.
18 Leave the tube in place for 20 minutes.
19 Lower the bed to its lowest position. Place the signal light within reach.
20 Leave the room and wash your hands.
21 Put on the gloves.
22 Remove the tube after 20 minutes. Wipe the rectal area.
23 Ask the patient about the amount of gas expelled.
24 Make sure he or she is comfortable. Place the signal light within reach.
25 Unscreen the patient.
26 Take used disposable equipment and soiled linen to the "dirty" utility room. Remove the gloves.
27 Wash your hands.
28 Report your observations to the nurse.

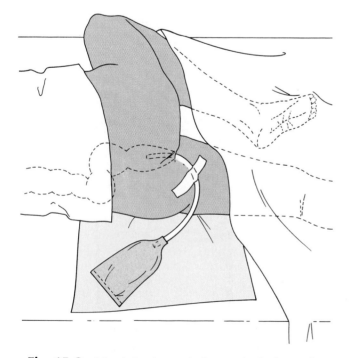

Fig. 15-8 After being inserted, the rectal tube is taped to the buttocks and the flatus bag rests on the bed. The tube is inserted 2 to 4 inches into the rectum.

along with flatus. If a flatus bag is not included, place the open end of the tube in a folded waterproof pad.

The rectal tube is removed after 20 to 30 minutes. This helps prevent rectal irritation. The nurse tells you when to insert the tube and how long to leave it in place.

THE PATIENT WITH AN OSTOMY

Sometimes it is necessary to surgically remove part of the intestines. Cancer, diseases of the bowel, and trauma (for example, stab wounds or bullet wounds) are common reasons for intestinal surgery. An ostomy may be necessary. An *ostomy* is the surgical creation of an artificial opening. The opening is called the *stoma*. The nurse may need your assistance in giving postoperative care. You may care for a person who has had an ostomy for a long time.

Colostomy

A *colostomy* is the surgical creation of an artificial opening between the colon and the abdomen. Part of the colon is brought out onto the abdominal wall, and a stoma is made. Feces and flatus pass through the

CARING FOR A PERSON WITH A COLOSTOMY

1. Explain the procedure to the patient.
2. Wash your hands.
3. Collect the following equipment:
   a. Bedpan with cover
   b. Waterproof bed protectors
   c. Bath blanket
   d. Toilet tissue
   e. Clean colostomy appliance
   f. Clean ostomy belt
   g. Wash basin
   h. Bath thermometer
   i. Prescribed soap or cleansing agent
   j. Karaya powder, karaya ring, or other skin barrier if ordered
   k. Deodorant for the appliance
   l. Disposable bag
   m. Paper towels
   n. Disposable gloves
4. Identify the patient. Check the ID bracelet and call the patient by name.
5. Provide for privacy.
6. Raise the bed to a level appropriate for good body mechanics.
7. Lower the side rail.
8. Cover the patient with a bath blanket. Fanfold linens to the foot of the bed.
9. Place the waterproof pad under the buttocks.
10. Put on the gloves.
11. Disconnect the appliance from the belt.
12. Remove the colostomy belt.
13. Remove the appliance gently. Place it in the bedpan.
14. Wipe around the stoma with toilet tissue to remove any mucus or feces. Place soiled tissue in the bedpan.
15. Cover the bedpan and take it to the bathroom.
16. Empty the appliance and bedpan into the toilet. Note the color, amount, consistency, and odor of feces. Put the appliance in the disposable bag.
17. Fill the wash basin. Water temperature should be 115° F (46.1° C). Place the basin on the overbed table on top of the paper towels.
18. Clean the skin around the stoma with water. Rinse and pat dry. Use soap or other cleansing agent if ordered.
19. Apply the karaya powder, karaya ring, or other skin barrier.
20. Put a clean colostomy belt on the patient.
21. Add deodorant to the new appliance.
22. Remove the adhesive backing on the appliance.
23. Center the appliance over the stoma. Make sure it is sealed to the skin. Apply gentle pressure to the adhesive surface from the stoma outward.
24. Connect the belt to the appliance.
25. Remove the bed protector. Remove the gloves.
26. Cover the patient. Remove the bath blanket.
27. Make sure the patient is comfortable.
28. Lower the bed to its lowest position.
29. Raise the side rail. Place the signal light within reach. Unscreen the patient.
30. Clean the bedpan, wash basin, and other equipment. Place used disposable equipment in the bag. (Wear gloves if necessary.)
31. Return equipment to its proper place.
32. Take the disposable bag and soiled linen to the "dirty" utility room.
33. Wash your hands.
34. Report your observations to the nurse.

stoma rather than the anus. Colostomies may be permanent or temporary. If permanent, the diseased part of the colon is removed. A temporary colostomy gives the diseased or injured bowel time to heal. After healing occurs, surgery is done to reconnect the bowel.

The colostomy location depends on the part of the colon that is diseased or injured. Figure 15-9 shows common colostomy sites. Stool consistency depends on the location of the colostomy. The stool can be liquid to formed. The more colon remaining to absorb water, the more solid and formed the stool. If the colostomy is near the beginning of the colon, stools will be liquid in consistency. A colostomy near the end of the large intestine results in formed stools.

The individual wears a colostomy appliance. The appliance is a disposable plastic bag applied over the stoma. It collects feces expelled through the stoma. When the appliance becomes soiled, it is removed and a new one is applied. Skin care is given to prevent skin breakdown around the stoma. The appliance has an adhesive backing that is applied to the skin. Many people also secure the appliance to an ostomy belt (Fig. 15-10). Many people manage their colostomies without assistance. If this is the case, they are allowed to do so in the health care facility.

Odors should be prevented. Good hygiene is essential. A new bag is applied whenever soiling occurs. Emptying the bag of feces and avoiding gas-forming

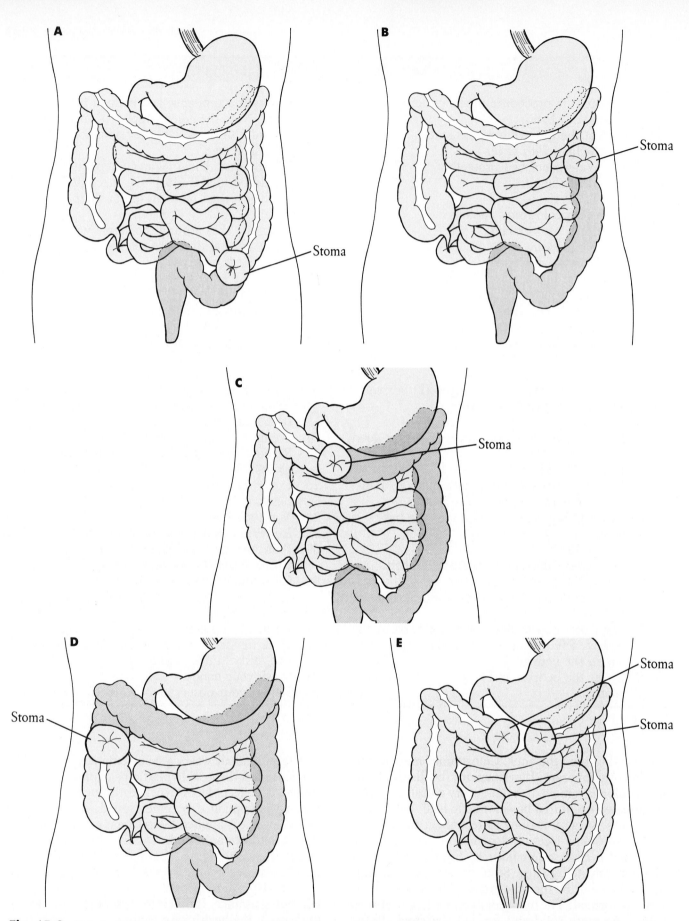

Fig. 15-9 Colostomy sites with the shaded area indicating the part of the bowel that has been surgically removed. **A,** Sigmoid colostomy. **B,** Descending colostomy. **C,** Transverse colostomy. **D,** Ascending colostomy. **E,** Double-barrel colostomy. Two stomas are created: one allows for the excretion of fecal material. The other allows medication to be introduced to help the bowel heal. This type of colostomy is usually temporary.

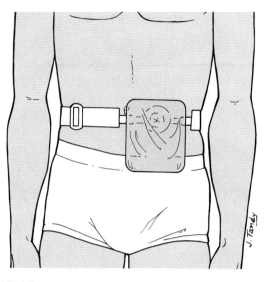

Fig. 15-10 A colostomy appliance is in place over the stoma and is secured with a colostomy belt.

foods also help to control odors. Special deodorants can be put into the appliance. The nurse will tell you which one to use.

Ileostomy

An *ileostomy* is the surgical creation of an artificial opening between the ileum (small intestine) and the abdomen. Part of the ileum is brought out onto the abdominal wall, and a stoma is made. The entire large intestine is removed (Fig. 15-11). Liquid feces drain constantly from an ileostomy. Water is not absorbed because the colon has been removed. Feces in the small intestine contain digestive juices and are very irritating to the skin. The ileostomy appliance must fit well so that feces do not touch the skin. The appliance is sealed to the skin and is removed every 2 to 4 days. Good skin care is essential.

There are disposable and reusable ileostomy ap-

CARING FOR A PERSON WITH AN ILEOSTOMY

1 Explain the procedure to the patient.
2 Wash your hands.
3 Collect the following equipment:
  a Prescribed solvent
  b Medicine dropper
  c Clean appliance
  d Clean belt
  e Clamp for the appliance
  f Gauze dressing
  g Disposable washcloth
  h Towels
  i Cotton balls
  j Prescribed soap or other cleansing agent
  k Karaya ring
  l Soft brush
  m Deodorant
  n Disposable gloves
  o Robe and slippers
4 Arrange equipment in the bathroom.
5 Identify the patient. Check the ID bracelet and call the patient by name.
6 Provide for privacy.
7 Help the patient put on a robe and slippers.
8 Assist the patient to the bathroom.
9 Help him or her sit on the toilet.
10 Put on the gloves.
11 Direct the appliance into the toilet. (See Fig. 15-12). Remove the clamp.
12 Let the appliance empty into the toilet. Wipe the end with toilet tissue. Discard tissue into the toilet. Observe feces for amount, color, odor.
13 Disconnect the appliance from the belt. Remove the belt.

14 Apply a few drops of solvent to the skin around the appliance. (Use the medicine dropper.) The appliance will loosen and can be gently removed.
15 Cover the stoma with a gauze dressing to absorb drainage.
16 Wet the skin around the stoma with a cotton ball soaked with solvent.
17 Clean the skin around the stoma with warm water. Rinse and pat dry. Use soap or cleansing agent only if ordered.
18 Moisten a karaya ring.
19 Remove the gauze dressing.
20 Apply the karaya ring (when sticky) around the stoma.
21 Add deodorant to the appliance.
22 Apply the appliance to the karaya ring. Be sure the bottom is clamped.
23 Put a clean belt on the patient. Connect the belt to the appliance. Remove the gloves.
24 Help the patient wash the hands.
25 Make sure he or she is comfortable. Place the signal light within reach. Unscreen the patient.
26 Discard disposable equipment. Clean the used appliance with soap and water using the soft brush. Wash the belt. Allow both items to dry. Clean equipment. (Wear gloves for this step.)
27 Return equipment to its proper place.
28 Wash your hands.
29 Report your observations to the nurse.

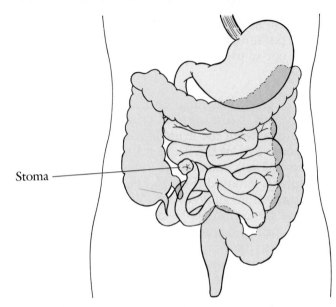

Stoma

Fig. 15-11 An ileostomy. The entire large intestine is surgically removed during the operation.

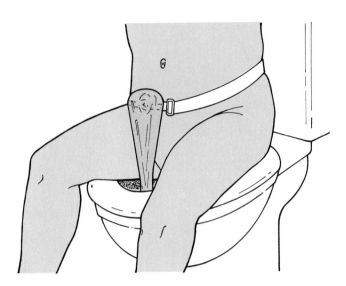

Fig. 15-12 An ileostomy appliance is emptied by directing it into the toilet and unclamping the end.

COLLECTING A STOOL SPECIMEN

1   Explain the procedure to the patient.
2   Wash your hands.
3   Collect the following equipment:
   a   Bedpan and cover (another bedpan may be needed if the patient needs to urinate) or bedside commode
   b   Urinal
   c   Specimen pan if the bathroom or commode will be used
   d   Specimen container and lid
   e   Tongue blade
   f   Disposable bag
   g   Disposable gloves
   h   Toilet tissue
   i   Laboratory requisition slip
4   Label the container with the requested information.
5   Identify the patient. Check the ID bracelet with the requisition slip.
6   Provide for privacy.
7   Offer the bedpan or urinal for urination.
8   Assist the person onto the bedpan or commode. Place the specimen pan under the toilet seat (Fig. 15-13). The patient wears a robe and slippers when up.
9   Ask the patient not to put toilet tissue in the bedpan, commode, or specimen pan. Provide a disposable bag for toilet tissue.
10   Place the signal light and toilet tissue within reach.
11   Leave the room and wash your hands.
12   Return when the patient signals. Knock before entering.
13   Put on the gloves. Provide perineal care if necessary.
14   Use a tongue blade to take about 2 tablespoons of feces from the bedpan to the specimen container (Fig. 15-14).
15   Put the lid on the container. Do not touch the inside of the lid or container.
16   Place the tongue blade in the bag.
17   Empty, clean, and disinfect the bedpan, commode container, or specimen pan. Remove the gloves.
18   Return equipment to its proper place.
19   Help the patient wash the hands.
20   Make sure the patient is comfortable. Place the signal light within reach.
21   Lower the bed to its lowest position. Raise the side rail.
22   Unscreen the patient.
23   Take the specimen and requisition slip to the laboratory.
24   Wash your hands.
25   Report your observations to the nurse.

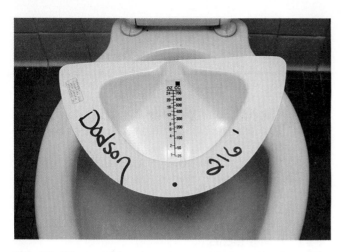

Fig. 15-13 A specimen pan is placed in the toilet for a stool specimen.

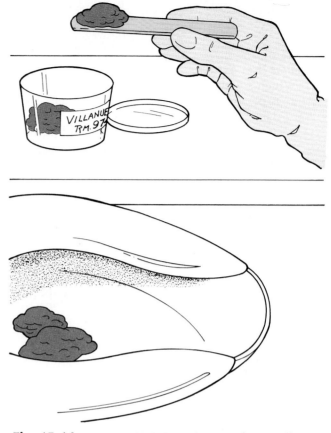

Fig. 15-14 A tongue blade is used to transfer a small amount of stool from the bedpan to the specimen container.

pliances. The appliance is clamped at the end so that feces collect in the bag. To empty the bag, direct it into the toilet and remove the clamp (Fig. 15-12). The appliance is emptied every 4 to 6 hours (q4h to q6h) or when the person urinates. Reusable bags are washed with soap and water and allowed to dry and air out. The care of an ileostomy patient is similar to that of a colostomy patient.

COLLECTING STOOL SPECIMENS

Stool specimens are sent to the laboratory. When internal bleeding is suspected, feces are checked for the presence of blood. Stools are also studied for fat, microorganisms, worms, and other abnormal contents. The rules for collecting urine specimens (see Chapter 14, page 240) apply when collecting stool specimens. Universal precautions are also necessary.

The stool specimen must not be contaminated with urine. Some tests require a warm stool. The specimen is taken to the laboratory immediately if a warm stool is needed.

SUMMARY

Your responsibilities in assisting individuals with bowel elimination are similar to those for urinary elimination. The act of defecation is private. Bowel control is important to people, as are the hygiene practices that follow bowel movements. Well-being is closely associated with maintaining normal bowel

function. The personal routines related to defecation also affect well-being.

Normal bowel elimination is not always possible. Constipation, fecal impaction, diarrhea, anal incontinence, and flatulence are common problems. The doctor may order enemas, rectal tubes, medications, or dietary changes to relieve the problem. The nurse may direct you to give an enema or insert a rectal tube. The instructions and procedure must be thoroughly understood. Sometimes ileostomies or colostomies are necessary to treat bowel problems.

When assisting the person with bowel elimination, always consider the person's need for privacy and bowel control. The person's dignity and psychological well-being are just as important as the physical act of defecation. In addition, the rules of medical asepsis, universal precautions, cleanliness, skin care, and safety must be followed.

REVIEW QUESTIONS

Circle the best *answer.*

1 Which statement is *false?*
a A person must have a bowel movement every day.
b Stools are normally brown, soft, and formed.
c Diarrhea occurs when feces move through the intestines rapidly.
d Constipation results when feces move through the large intestine slowly.

2 Bowel elimination is affected by
a Privacy and age
b Medications and diet
c Fluid intake and activity
d All of the above

3 The prolonged retention and accumulation of feces in the rectum is called
a Constipation
b Fecal impaction
c Flatulence
d Anal incontinence

4 Which will *not* promote comfort and safety in relation to bowel elimination?
a Asking visitors to leave the room
b Helping the patient to assume a sitting position
c Offering the bedpan after meals
d Telling the person that you will return very soon

5 Bowel training is aimed at
a Gaining control of bowel movements
b Developing a regular pattern of elimination
c Preventing fecal impaction, constipation, and anal incontinence
d All of the above

6 Which is *not* used for a cleansing enema?
a Soap suds
b Saline
c Oil
d Tap water

7 Which is *false?*
a Enema solutions should be 105° F (40.5° C).
b The left Sims' position is used for an enema.
c The enema bag is held 12 inches above the anus.
d The enema solution is administered rapidly.

8 The enema tube is inserted
a 1 to 2 inches
b 2 to 4 inches
c 4 to 6 inches
d 6 to 8 inches

9 The oil retention enema should be retained for
a 10 to 15 minutes
b 15 to 30 minutes
c 30 to 60 minutes
d 60 to 90 minutes

10 Rectal tubes are left in place no longer than
a 20 to 30 minutes
b 10 to 20 minutes
c 10 to 15 minutes
d 5 to 10 minutes

11 Which statement about colostomies and ileostomies is *false?*
a Good skin care around the stoma is essential.
b Odors can be controlled with deodorant.
c The individual will have to wear an appliance.
d Fecal material is always liquid in consistency.

12 The ileostomy appliance is usually emptied
a Every 4 to 6 hours
b Every morning
c Every 2 to 3 days
d When the doctor gives the order to do so

Answers

12 a	**8** b	**4** d
11 d	**7** d	**3** b
10 a	**6** c	**2** d
9 c	**5** d	**1** a

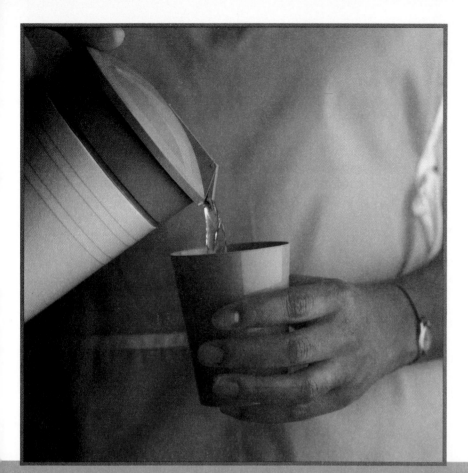

Foods and Fluids

16

OBJECTIVES

- Define the key terms listed in this chapter
- Identify the foods found in the four basic foods groups
- Explain the importance of protein, carbohydrates, and fats
- Identify major sources of proteins, carbohydrates, and fats
- Describe the functions of vitamins and minerals
- Identify the dietary sources of vitamins and minerals
- Describe six factors that affect eating and nutrition
- Describe the special diets
- Describe normal adult fluid requirements and the common causes of dehydration
- Explain your responsibilities when forced fluids, restricted fluids, or NPO is ordered
- Explain the purpose of intake and output records
- Identify foods that are counted as fluid intake
- Describe between-meal nourishments, tube feedings, intravenous therapy, and hyperalimentation
- Perform the procedures described in this chapter

anorexia Loss of appetite

calorie The amount of energy produced from the burning of food by the body

dehydration A decrease in the amount of water in body tissues

dysphagia Difficulty or discomfort (dys) in swallowing (phagia)

edema The swelling of body tissues with water

gastrostomy Surgically created opening in the stomach that allows feeding

gavage Tube feeding

graduate A calibrated container used to measure fluid

intravenous therapy Fluid administered through a needle within a vein; often referred to as "IV" and "IV infusion"

nutrient A substance that is ingested, digested, absorbed, and used by the body

nutrition The many processes involved in the ingestion, digestion, absorption, and use of foods and fluids by the body

The need for food and water is a basic physical need that is necessary for life and health. The amount and quality of foods and fluids in the diet are important. They influence a person's current and future physical and psychological well-being. A poor diet and poor eating habits make a person more susceptible to infection and chronic diseases. Healing problems and abnormalities in body functions are also related to poor diet and eating habits. Poor physical and mental functioning put an individual at risk for accidents and injuries. Besides being necessary for survival, eating and drinking provide pleasure. They are associated with social activities with family and friends.

Dietary practices are influenced by many factors, including culture, finances, and personal choice. These practices include the selection of food and the way it is prepared and served.

BASIC NUTRITION

Nutrition has been defined in many ways. Essentially, *nutrition* is the many processes involved in the ingestion, digestion, absorption, and use of foods and fluids by the body. Good nutrition is needed for growth, healing, and maintaining body functions. It begins with the proper selection of foods and fluids. They must provide a well-balanced diet and appropriate caloric intake. A diet that includes many foods high in calories will cause excessive weight gain or obesity. The inadequate intake of calories results in weight loss.

Foods and fluids contain nutrients. A *nutrient* is a substance that is ingested, digested, absorbed, and used by the body. At least 35 nutrients are considered essential for body functioning. They are grouped into the categories of fats, proteins, carbohydrates, vitamins, and minerals. The essential nutrients are found in the four basic food groups.

Fats, proteins, and carbohydrates provide the body with fuel for energy. The amount of energy provided by a nutrient is measured in calories. A *calorie* is the amount of energy produced from the burning of food by the body. Energy is needed for all body functions—even sitting in a chair. The amount of calories needed by a person depends on many factors. These factors include age, sex, activity, climate, state of health, and the amount of sleep obtained.

Food Groups

There are four basic food groups: milk and dairy products, meats and fish, fruits and vegetables, and breads and cereals (Fig. 16-1). The essential nutrients are found in varying amounts in each group. A well-balanced daily diet includes the recommended number of servings from each group and all of the essential nutrients. Usually the daily diet includes three regular meals.

Milk and dairy products The main nutrients found in milk and dairy products are protein, fat, carbohydrates, calcium, and riboflavin. Milk and foods and fluids made from whole or skim milk (cheese and ice cream) are in this group. Children younger than 11 years of age need at least 3 to 4 cups of milk a day (1 cup = 8 ounces). Teenagers need 4 or more cups. Adults need 2 or more cups. Pregnant women and breast-feeding mothers need 6 or more cups. This amount meets their own and the baby's nutritional needs.

Meats and fish Protein, fat, iron, and thiamin are the main nutrients found in meats and fish. An individual needs 2 or more servings daily from this group. The meat and fish group includes beef, veal, lamb, poultry, pork, fish, eggs, and cheese. Alternatives or substitutes for meat and fish are dry beans, peas, nuts, and peanut butter.

Serving size is important when planning a well-balanced diet. This is especially important for meat and fish because they contain many calories. Serving size is influenced by many factors, including culture, appetite, personal choice, and the recipe used. A

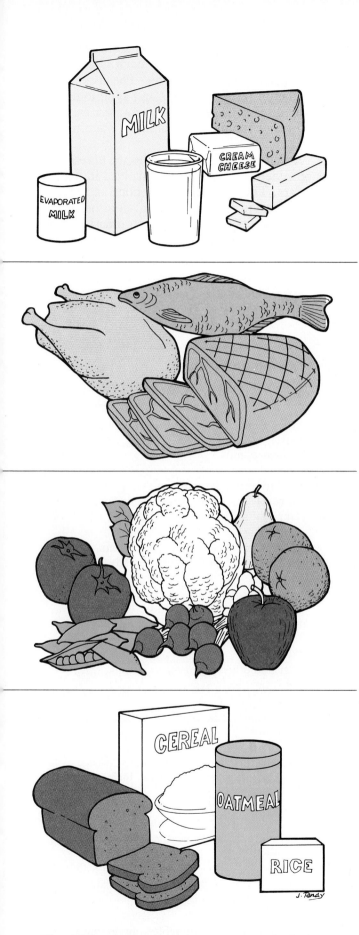

Fig. 16-1 The four basic food groups and the foods included in each group.

quarter-pound hamburger, a 12-ounce T-bone steak, a 10-ounce lobster tail, and a quarter of a chicken are a few examples of serving portions advertised by restaurants. Nutritionists consider 2 to 3 ounces of boned meat, fish, or poultry to be one serving. A 12-ounce steak is equal to 4 to 6 servings of the meat and fish group!

Fruits and vegetables Vitamins A and C, carbohydrates, and small amounts of other nutrients are found in fruits and vegetables. Four or more servings should be part of the daily diet. This group includes fruits, dark green and yellow vegetables, tomatoes, potatoes, and fruit and vegetable juices.

Breads and cereals Four or more servings of bread and cereal are needed daily for a well-balanced diet. Protein, carbohydrates, iron, thiamin, niacin, and riboflavin are the main nutrients in this group. Foods included in this group are bread, cereal, pasta, and crackers.

Nutrients

No one food or food group contains all the essential nutrients needed by the body. A well-balanced diet consists of servings from each food group. This ensures an adequate intake of the essential nutrients.

Protein Protein is the most important nutrient—it is needed for tissue growth and repair. One gram (g) of protein provides 4 calories. Sources of protein include meat, fish, poultry, eggs, milk and milk products, cereals, beans, peas, and nuts. Foods high in protein are usually expensive. Therefore protein is often lacking in the diets of people with low incomes.

Every body cell is made up of protein. Execessive protein intake causes some protein to be excreted in the urine. Some protein changes into body fat, and some changes into carbohydrates.

Carbohydrates Carbohydrates provide the body with energy. They also provide fiber for bowel elimination. Carbohydrates are found in fruits, vegetables, breads, cereals, and sugar. These foods are rather inexpensive. Rarely are carbohydrates lacking in the diet. One gram of carbohydrate provides 4 calories.

Carbohydrates are broken down into sugars during digestion. The sugars are then absorbed into the bloodstream. The fiber in foods that contain carbohydrates is not digested; it provides the bulky part of chyme in the elimination process. Excess carbohydrate intake results in some of the nutrient being stored in the liver. The rest changes into body fat.

Fats Fats also provide energy. One gram of fat provides 9 calories. Besides being a source of energy, fats serve many other functions. They add flavor to food and help the body use certain vitamins. Fats also conserve body heat and protect organs from injury. Sources of fat include the fat in meats, lard, butter, shortenings, salad and vegetable oils, milk, cheese, egg yolks, and nuts. These sources are more expensive than sources of carbohydrates. Dietary fat not needed by the body is stored as body fat (adipose tissue).

Vitamins   Although they do not provide calories, vitamins are essential nutrients. They are ingested through food and most cannot be produced by the body. Vitamins A, D, E, and K can be stored by the body. Vitamin C and the B complex vitamins are not stored and must be ingested daily. Each vitamin is needed for specific body functions. The lack of a particular vitamin results in signs and symptoms of a particular disease. Table 16-1 summarizes the sources and major functions of common vitamins.

Minerals   A well-balanced diet supplies the necessary amounts of minerals. Minerals are involved in many body processes. They are needed for bone and tooth formation, nerve and muscle function, fluid balance, and other body processes. Table 16-2 summarizes the major functions and dietary sources of common minerals.

TABLE 16-1   Major Functions and Sources of Common Vitamins

Vitamin	Major Functions	Sources
Vitamin A	Growth; vision; healthy hair, skin, and mucous membranes; resistance to infection	Liver, spinach, green leafy and yellow vegetables, fruits, fish liver oils, egg yolk, butter, cream, milk
Vitamin B_1 (thiamin)	Muscle tone; nerve function; digestion; appetite; normal elimination; utilization of carbohydrates	Pork, liver and other organ meats, breads and cereals, potatoes, peas, beans, and soybeans
Vitamin B_2 (riboflavin)	Growth; healthy eyes; protein and carbohydrate metabolism; healthy skin and mucous membranes	Milk and milk products, organ meats, green leafy vegetables, eggs, breads and cereals
Vitamin B_3 (niacin)	Protein, fat, and carbohydrate metabolism; functioning of the nervous system; appetite; functioning of the digestive system	Meat, poultry, fish, peanut butter, breads and cereals, peas and beans, eggs, liver
Vitamin B_{12}	Formation of red blood cells; protein metabolism; functioning of the nervous system	Liver and other organ meats, meats, fish, eggs, green leafy vegetables
Folic acid	Formation of red blood cells; functioning of the intestines; protein metabolism	Liver, meats, fish, yeast, green leafy vegetables, eggs, mushrooms
Vitamin C (ascorbic acid)	Formation of substances that hold tissues together; healthy blood vessels, skin, gums, bones, and teeth; wound healing; prevention of bleeding; resistance to infection	Citrus fruits, tomatoes, potatoes, cabbage, strawberries, green vegetables, melons
Vitamin D	Absorption and metabolism of calcium and phosphorus; healthy bones	Fish liver oils, milk, butter, liver, exposure to sunlight
Vitamin E	Normal reproduction; formation of red blood cells; muscle function	Vegetable oils, milk, eggs, meats, fish, cereals, green leafy vegetables
Vitamin K	Blood clotting	Liver, green leafy vegetables, margarine, soybean and vegetable oils, eggs

TABLE 16-2 **The Major Functions and Sources of Common Minerals**

Mineral	Major Function	Source
Calcium	Formation of teeth and bones; blood clotting; muscle contraction; heart function; nerve function	Milk and milk products, green leafy vegetables
Phosphorus	Formation of bones and teeth; utilization of proteins, fats, and carbohydrates; nerve and muscle function	Meat, fish, poultry, milk and milk products, nuts, eggs
Iron	Allows red blood cells to carry oxygen	Liver and other organ meats, egg yolks, green leafy vegetables, breads and cereals
Iodine	Thyroid gland function, growth, and metabolism	Iodized salt, seafood and shellfish, vegetables
Sodium	Fluid balance; nerve and muscle function	Almost all foods
Potassium	Nerve function; muscle contraction; heart function	Fruits, vegetables, cereals, coffee, meats

FACTORS THAT AFFECT EATING AND NUTRITION

Nutrition and eating habits are influenced by many factors. Some begin during infancy and continue throughout life. Others develop later.

Culture

Dietary practices are greatly influenced by culture. The types of foods available in the region of a particular ethnic group also influence diet. Rice and tea are common in the diets of Chinese, Japanese, Korean, and other peoples of the Far East. Hispanic people like tacos, tamales, and burritos. Italians are known for their spaghetti, lasagna, and other pastas. Scandinavians have a lot of fish in their diet. Americans enjoy foods from the meat group, fast foods, and processed foods (canned and frozen foods.)

Culture also influences food preparation. Frying, baking, smoking, or roasting food or eating raw food are influenced by culture. The use of sauces and spices is also related to culture.

Religion

Many religious beliefs involve dietary practices. The selection, preparation, and eating of food are often regulated by religious practices. Some religions require days of fasting. During a fast, all or certain foods are avoided. Members of a religious group may not follow each dietary practice of their faith. Others follow all dietary teachings. You need to respect the individual's religious dietary practices. Table 16-3 summarizes the dietary practices of the major religious groups.

Finances

The amount of money available is a major factor in food selection. People with limited incomes, like the elderly, usually buy the cheaper carbohydrate-containing foods. Therefore protein and certain vitamins and minerals are often lacking in their diets.

Appetite

Appetite relates to the desire for food. Hunger is an unpleasant feeling caused by the lack of food. Hunger causes a person to seek food and eat until the appetite is satisfied. Aromas and thoughts of food can also stimulate the appetite. Loss of appetite, *anorexia*, can also occur. The many causes of anorexia include illness, medications, unpleasant thoughts or sights, anxiety, and fear.

Personal Preference

The like or dislike of particular foods is an individual matter. Food preferences begin in childhood. They are influenced by the kinds of food served in the home. As a child grows older, new foods are introduced through school and social activities. Many people decide if they like or dislike a specific food by the

TABLE 16-3 **Religion and Dietary Practices**

Religion	Dietary Practice
Adventist (Seventh Day Adventist)	Coffee, tea, and alcohol are not allowed; beverages with caffeine (colas) are not allowed; some groups forbid the eating of meat
Baptist	Some groups forbid coffee, tea, and alcohol
Christian Scientist	Alcohol and coffee are not allowed
Church of Jesus Christ of Latter Day Saints (Mormon)	Alcohol and hot drinks, such as coffee and tea, are not allowed; meat is not forbidden, but members are encouraged to eat meat infrequently
Greek Orthodox Church	Wednesdays, Fridays, and Lent are days of fasting; meat and dairy products are usually avoided during days of fast
Islamic (Muslim or Moslem)	All pork and pork products are forbidden; alcohol is not allowed except for medical reasons
Judaism (Jewish faith)	Foods must be kosher (prepared according to Jewish law); meat of kosher animals (cows, goats, and sheep) can be eaten; chickens, ducks, and geese are kosher fowls; kosher fish have scales and fins, such as tuna, sardines, carp, and salmon; shellfish cannot be eaten; milk, milk products, and eggs from kosher animals and fowl are acceptable; milk and milk products cannot be eaten with or immediately after eating meat; milk and milk products can be eaten 6 hours after eating meat; milk and milk products can be a part of the same meal with meat—they are served separately and before the meat; kosher foods cannot be prepared in utensils used to prepare nonkosher foods; breads, cakes, cookies, noodles, and alcoholic beverages are not consumed during Passover
Roman Catholic	Fasting for 1 hour before receiving Holy Communion; fasting from meat on Ash Wednesday and Good Friday—some may continue to fast from meat on Fridays

way it looks, the way it is prepared, its smell, or the recipe ingredients. Usually individuals develop a wider variety of food preferences with age and with increased social experiences.

Food preferences are also influenced by body reactions. People usually avoid foods that cause allergic reactions, nausea, vomiting, diarrhea, indigestion, or headaches.

Illness

Appetite usually decreases during illness and recovery from injuries. However, nutritional needs are increased at these times. The body needs to fight infection, heal tissue, and replace lost blood cells. Nutrients lost through vomiting and diarrhea must also be replaced. Some diseases and medications cause a sore mouth, which makes eating painful. The loss of teeth also affects the ability to chew foods, especially those that provide protein.

SPECIAL DIETS

Doctors may prescribe special diets. A special diet may be ordered because of a nutritional deficiency or a disease, to eliminate or decrease certain substances in the diet, or for weight control. The doctor, nurses, and dietician all work together to meet the person's nutritional needs. They consider the need for dietary changes, personal preferences, religion, culture, and eating problems.

Many patients do not need special diets. *General diet, routine hospital diet,* and *house diet* are terms used in many facilities when there are no dietary restrictions or modifications. Special or therapeutic diets are ordered for preoperative and postoperative surgical patients and for those with diabetes. Patients with diseases of the heart, kidneys, gallbladder, liver, stomach, or intestines may receive special diets. Allergies, obesity, and other disorders also require ther-

TABLE 16-4 **Common Therapeutic Diets**

Diet	Description	Use	Foods Allowed
Clear-liquid	Clear liquids that do not leave a residue; nonirritating and nongasforming	Postoperatively; for acute illness and nausea and vomiting	Water, tea, and coffee (without milk or cream); carbonated beverages; gelatin; clear fruit juices (apple, grape, and cranberry); fat-free clear broth; hard candy, sugar, and popsicles
Full-liquid	Foods that are liquid at room temperature or that melt at body temperature	Advance from clear-liquid diet; postoperatively, for stomach irritation, fever, and nausea and vomiting	All foods allowed on a clear-liquid diet; custard; eggnog; strained soups; strained fruit and vegetable juices; milk; creamed cereals; ice cream and sherbet
Soft	Semisolid foods that are easily digested	Advance from full-liquid diet; for chewing difficulties, gastrointestinal disorders, and infections	All liquids; eggs (not fried); broiled, baked, or roasted meat, fish, or poultry; mild cheeses (American, Swiss, cheddar, cream, and cottage); strained fruit juices; refined bread and crackers; cooked or pureed vegetables; cooked or canned fruit without skin or seeds; pudding; plain cakes
Low-residue	Food that leaves a small amount of residue in the colon	For diseases of the colon and diarrhea	Coffee, tea, milk, carbonated beverages, strained fruit juices; refined bread and crackers; creamed and refined cereal; rice; cottage and cream cheese; eggs (not fried); plain puddings and cakes; gelatin; custard; sherbet and ice cream; strained vegetable juices; canned or cooked fruit without skin or seeds; potatoes (not fried); strained cooked vegetables; plain pasta
High-residue	Foods that increase the amount of residue in the colon to stimulate peristalsis	For constipation and colon disorders	All fruits and vegetables; whole wheat bread; whole grain cereals; fried foods; whole grain rice; milk, cream, butter, and cheese; meats
Bland	Foods that are mechanically and chemically nonirritating and low in roughage; foods served at moderate temperatures; strong spices and condiments are avoided	For ulcers, gallbladder disorders, and some intestinal disorders; postoperatively following abdominal surgery	Lean meats; white bread; creamed and refined cereals; cream or cottage cheese; gelatin, plain puddings, cakes, and cookies; eggs (not fried); butter and cream; canned fruits and vegetables without skin and seeds; strained fruit juices; potatoes (not fried); pastas and rice; strained or soft cooked carrots, peas, beets, spinach, squash, and asparagus tips; creamed soups from allowed vegetables; no fried foods are allowed
High-calorie	The number of calories is increased to approximately 4000; includes three full meals and between-meal snacks	For weight gain and some thyroid imbalances	Dietary increases in all foods

Continued.

TABLE 16-4   **Common Therapeutic Diets—cont'd**

Diet	Description	Use	Foods Allowed
Low-calorie	The number of calories is reduced below the minimum daily requirements	For weight reduction	Foods low in fats and carbohydrates and lean meats; avoid butter, cream, rice, gravies, salad oils, noodles, cakes, pastries, carbonated and alcoholic beverages, candy, potato chips, and similar foods
High-iron	Foods that are high in iron	For anemia; following blood loss; for women during the reproductive years	Liver and other organ meats; lean meats; egg yolks; shellfish; dried fruits; dried beans; green leafy vegetables; lima beans; peanut butter; enriched breads and cereals
Low-fat (low-cholesterol)	Protein and carbohydrates are increased with a limited amount of fat in the diet	For heart disease, gallbladder disease, disorders of fat digestion, and liver disease	Skim milk or buttermilk; cottage cheese (no other cheeses are allowed); gelatin; sherbet; fruit; lean meat, poultry, and fish (baked, broiled, or roasted); fat-free broth; soups made with skim milk; margarine; rice, pasta, breads and cereals; vegetables; potatoes
High-protein	Protein is increased to aid and promote tissue healing	For burns, high fever, infection, and some liver diseases	Meat, milk, eggs, cheese, fish, poultry; breads and cereals; green leafy vegetables
Sodium-restricted	A specific amount of sodium is allowed; there are five basic levels of sodium restriction ranging from mild to severe	For heart disease, fluid retention, and some kidney diseases	Fruits and vegetables and unsalted butter are allowed; adding salt at the table is not allowed; highly salted foods and foods high in sodium are not allowed; the use of salt during cooking may be restricted
Diabetic	The amount of carbohydrates and number of calories are regulated; protein and fat are also regulated	For diabetes mellitus	Determined by nutritional and energy requirements

apeutic diets. Table 16-4 summarizes the common therapeutic diets.

The sodium-restricted diet and diabetic diet are commonly ordered. Nursing assistants working in hospitals, nursing facilities, or private homes are likely to encounter these diets. They are described in greater detail.

The Sodium-Restricted Diet

The average amount of sodium in the daily diet is 3000 to 5000 mg. The body needs only half this amount daily. Healthy people excrete excess sodium in the urine. Heart and kidney diseases cause the body to retain the extra sodium.

Sodium-restricted diets are ordered for people with heart disease. They may also be ordered for those with liver diseases, kidney disease, certain complications of pregnancy, and when certain medications are being taken. Sodium causes the body to retain water. If there is too much sodium, the body retains more water. Body tissues swell with water, and there are excess amounts of fluid in the blood vessels. The increased fluid in the tissues and bloodstream forces the heart to work harder. In other words, the work load of the heart increases. With heart disease, the extra work load can cause serious complications or death. Restricting the amount of sodium in the diet decreases the amount of sodium in the body. The body retains less water. Less water in the tissues and blood vessels reduces the amount of work for the heart.

There are five levels of sodium-restricted diets. They range from mild to severe. The doctor orders the amount of restriction for the person. People on sodium-restricted diets need to learn how to calculate the amount of sodium in the diet. They also need to know which foods are high and which are low in sodium. A nurse or dietician teaches patients and families about the diet.

1. *2000-3000 mg. sodium diet.* This is called the low-salt diet. Sodium restriction is mild. A minimum amount of salt is used for cooking, and salt is not added to foods at the table. Highly salted foods and salty seasonings (catsup, celery salt, garlic salt, chili sauce, etc.) are omitted from the diet. Also omitted are canned and processed foods high in salt, ham, bacon, frankfurters, potato chips, olives, pickles, luncheon meats, and salted or smoked fish.
2. *1000 mg. sodium diet.* Sodium restriction is moderate. Food is cooked without salt. Foods high in sodium are omitted. Vegetables high in sodium are restricted in amount. Salt-free products, such as salt-free bread, are used. Diet planning is necessary.
3. *800 mg. sodium diet.* Restrictions for the low-salt diet and the 1000 mg. diet are followed. Diet planning is necessary to further reduce the amount of sodium in the diet.
4. *500 mg. sodium diet.* Sodium restriction is "strict." Restrictions for the less restricted diets are followed. In addition, vegetables high in sodium are omitted. Milk is limited to 2 cups per day, and only 1 egg per day is allowed. Meat is limited to 5 to 6 ounces per day. Diet planning is essential.
5. *250 mg. sodium diet.* This diet is described as "severe." The diet is similar to the 500 mg. sodium diet. However, milk is eliminated. Low-sodium milk can be substituted for regular whole or skim milk.

The Diabetic Diet

The diabetic diet is ordered for people with diabetes mellitus. Diabetes mellitus is a chronic disease in which there is a deficiency of insulin in the body. Insulin is produced and secreted by the pancreas and is needed for the body to use sugar. If there is not enough insulin, sugar builds up in the bloodstream rather than being used by cells for energy. Diabetes is usually treated with insulin therapy, diet, and exercise.

Carbohydrates are broken down into sugar during digestion. The amount of carbohydrates is controlled with the diabetic diet. By controlling carbohydrates, the person takes in the amount needed by the body. Unneeded carbohydrates are eliminated so that the body does not have to use or store the excess. Therefore the diabetic diet involves the correct amount and kind of food for the individual. The doctor determines the amount of carbohydrate, fat, protein, and calories an individual should have. The person's age, sex, activity, and weight are considered.

The calories and nutrients allowed are divided among 3 meals and between-meal nourishments. The person must eat only what is allowed and all that is allowed. This is important so that the person does not get too many or too few carbohydrates. The American Diabetes Association provides food lists that have equal value in terms of nutrients and calories. The foods are grouped into 6 categories: milk, vegetables, fruits, bread, meat foods, and fat. The 6 groups are called "exchange lists" or "exchanges." The exchanges allow variety in menu planning. For example, a person may not want grapefruit. The exchange list is checked for other fruits. The person notes that one small orange equals one-half grapefruit. Therefore the person knows how much to eat. The nurse and dietician help the individual and family learn how to use the exchange lists.

You must serve the person's tray on time. The diabetic must eat at regular intervals to maintain a certain blood sugar level. You need to check the tray to determine what has been eaten. If all food has not been eaten, a between-meal nourishment is needed. The nourishment makes up for what was not eaten at the regular meal. The amount of insulin given also depends on how much the person has eaten during the day.

FLUID BALANCE

After oxygen, water is the most important physical need for survival. Death can result from an inadequate water intake or from excessive fluid loss. Water enters the body through fluids and foods. Water is lost through the urine and feces, through the skin as perspiration, and through the lungs with expiration. Fluid balance must be maintained for health. There must be a balance between the amount of fluid taken in and the amount lost.

The amount of fluid taken in and the amount lost must be equal. If the fluid intake exceeds fluid output (the amount lost), body tissues swell with water. This is called *edema.* Edema is common in people with heart and kidney diseases. *Dehydration* is a decrease in the amount of water in the tissues. It results when fluid output exceeds intake. Inadequate fluid intake, vomiting, diarrhea, bleeding, excessive sweating, and increased urine production are common causes of dehydration.

Normal Requirements

An adult needs 1500 ml of water daily to survive. Approximately 2000 to 2500 ml of fluid per day is required to maintain a normal fluid balance. The water requirement increases with high weather temperatures, exercise, fever, and illness. Excessive fluid losses also increase the water requirement.

Minimum daily water requirements vary with age. Infants and young children have more body water. They need more fluids than adults do. Consequently, excessive fluid losses cannot be tolerated and will quickly cause death in an infant or child.

Special Orders

The doctor may order the amount of fluid that a person can have during a 24-hour period. This is done to maintain fluid balance. It may be necessary to *force fluids*. Force fluids involves having the individual consume an increased amount of fluid. The force fluids order may be general or for a specific amount. A "force fluids" sign is placed above the bed. Records are kept of the amount ingested. A variety of allowed fluids are provided. They must be within the person's reach and served at the appropriate temperature. You need to regularly offer fluids to patients who have force fluids orders but who cannot feed themselves.

The doctor may order *restrict fluids*. Fluids are restricted to a specific amount. Water is offered in small amounts and in small containers. The water pitcher is removed from the room or kept out of sight. Like with the force fluids order, a sign is posted above the bed and accurate intake records are kept. Patients with restricted fluid intake need frequent oral hygiene. Oral hygiene helps keep mucous membranes of the mouth moist.

Some patients can have *nothing by mouth*. The person cannot eat or drink anything. NPO is the abbreviation for the Latin term *nils per os*, which means nothing by mouth. Patients are usually NPO before and after surgery, before some laboratory tests and x-ray procedures, and in the treatment of certain illnesses. An NPO sign is posted above the bed, and the water pitcher and glass are removed. Frequent oral hygiene is allowed, but the patient cannot swallow any fluid. The patient is kept NPO starting at midnight before the scheduled surgery, laboratory tests, or x-ray procedures.

Intake and Output Records

The doctor or nurse may want a patient's fluid intake and output to be measured. This involves keeping intake and output (I&O) records. I&O records are used to evaluate fluid balance and kidney function, and to determine and evaluate medical treatment. I&O records are also necessary when forcing fluids or restricting fluid intake.

To measure fluid intake, all liquid ingested by the patient through the mouth is measured. Fluids given in IV therapy and tube feedings are also measured.

The obvious fluids are measured: water, milk, coffee, tea, juices, soups, and soft drinks. Soft and semi-solid foods such as ice cream, sherbet, custard, pudding, creamed cereals, gelatin, and popsicles are also measured. Output includes urinary output, vomitus, diarrhea, and wound drainage.

Measuring Intake and Output

Intake and output are measured in milliliters (ml) or in cubic centimeters (cc). These metric system measurements are equal in amount. One ounce equals 30 ml. A pint is about 500 ml. There are about 1000 ml in a quart. You need to know the fluid capacity of bowls, dishes, cups, pitchers, glasses, and other containers used to serve fluids. Most facilities have tables on the I&O record for use in measuring intake.

A container called a *graduate* is used to measure fluids. You will use a graduate to measure leftover fluids, urine, vomitus, and drainage from suction (see Chapter 22). The graduate is like a measuring cup; it shows calibrations for amounts. Some graduates are marked in ounces and in milliliters or cubic centimeters (Fig. 16-2). Plastic urinals and emesis basins are often calibrated.

An I&O record is kept at the bedside. Whenever fluid is ingested or output is measured, the amount is recorded in the appropriate column (Fig. 16-3). The amounts are totaled at the end of the shift. The nurse records the amount in the patient's record. The patient's I&O are also communicated to the next shift during the end-of-shift report. The nurse records any intake through IV therapy or tube feedings.

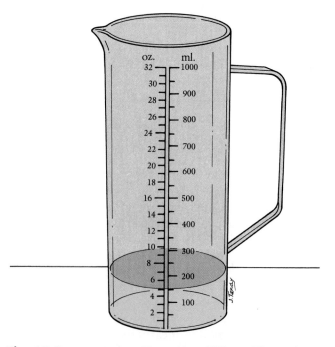

Fig. 16-2 A graduate calibrated in milliliters. The graduate shown is filled to 150 ml.

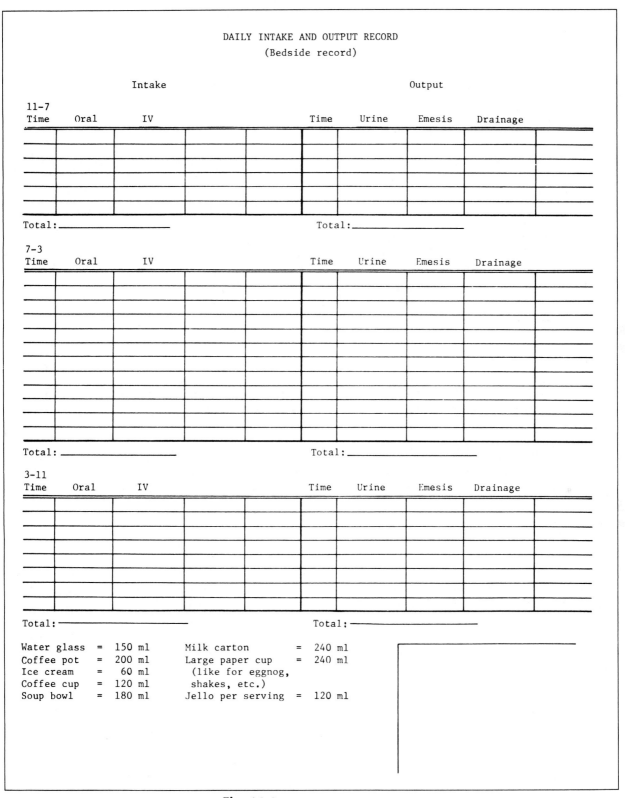

DAILY INTAKE AND OUTPUT RECORD
(Bedside record)

Intake   Output

11-7
Time   Oral   IV   Time   Urine   Emesis   Drainage

Total:_____   Total:_____

7-3
Time   Oral   IV   Time   Urine   Emesis   Drainage

Total:_____   Total:_____

3-11
Time   Oral   IV   Time   Urine   Emesis   Drainage

Total:_____   Total:_____

Water glass	=	150 ml	Milk carton	= 240 ml
Coffee pot	=	200 ml	Large paper cup	= 240 ml
Ice cream	=	60 ml	(like for eggnog,	
Coffee cup	=	120 ml	shakes, etc.)	
Soup bowl	=	180 ml	Jello per serving	= 120 ml

Fig. 16-3 An intake and output record.

MEASURING INTAKE AND OUTPUT

1 Explain the procedure to the patient.
2 Collect the following equipment:
   a Intake and output (I&O) record
   b Two I&O labels
   c Graduate
   d Disposable gloves
3 Place the I&O record at the bedside.
4 Place one label in the bathroom. Place the other in the appropriate place near the bed.
5 Measure intake as follows:
   a Pour liquid remaining in a container into the graduate.
   b Measure the amount at eye level.
   c Check the amount of the serving on the I&O record.
   d Subtract the remaining amount from the full serving amount.
   e Repeat steps 5a through 5d for each liquid.

f Add the amounts from 5e together. Record the time and amount on the I&O record.
6 Measure output as follows. (Wear gloves for this step.)
   a Pour the fluid into the graduate.
   b Measure the amount at eye level.
   c Record the time and amount on the I&O record.
   d Rinse and return the graduate to its proper place.
   e Clean and rinse the bedpan, urinal, emesis basin, or other drainage container. Return it to its proper place. Remove the gloves.
7 Wash your hands.
8 Report your observations to the nurse.

The patient should receive an explanation about the purpose of measuring intake and output and how to participate in the process. Some patients measure and record their own intake. Patients need to use the urinal, commode, bedpan, or specimen pan for urination. They need to be reminded not to put toilet tissue into the receptacle. Because urine will be measured, the patient should not urinate in the toilet.

ASSISTING THE INDIVIDUAL WITH FOODS AND FLUIDS

Weakness and illness can affect a patient's appetite and ability to eat. Odors, the sight of unpleasant equipment, an uncomfortable position, the need for oral hygiene, and the need to urinate are some factors that affect appetite. Nursing personnel can control these factors. You will often be responsible for preparing patients for meals.

GETTING THE PATIENT READY FOR MEALS

1 Explain the procedure to the patient.
2 Wash your hands.
3 Collect the following equipment:
   a Equipment for oral hygiene
   b Bedpan or urinal
   c Wash basin
   d Soap
   e Washcloth
   f Towel
   g Robe and slippers
4 Provide for privacy.
5 Assist the patient with oral hygiene.
6 Offer the bedpan or urinal. Assist the patient to the bathroom or bedside commode if he or she is able to be up. The patient wears a robe and slippers when up.

7 Help the patient wash the hands.
8 Raise the head of the bed to a comfortable sitting position. Position the overbed table in front of the patient. Make sure it is clean.
9 Help the patient to the chair if he or she is able to be up. Position the overbed table in front of the patient. Place the signal light within reach.
10 Clean and return equipment to its proper place. (Wear gloves if contact with body fluids or substances is possible.)
11 Straighten the room. Eliminate any unpleasant noise, odors, or equipment.
12 Unscreen the patient.
13 Wash your hands.

SERVING MEAL TRAYS

1 Wash your hands.
2 Check the items on the tray with the dietary card to make sure the tray is complete.
3 Identify the patient. Check the ID bracelet with the dietary card.
4 Have the patient in a sitting position if possible.
5 Place the tray on the overbed table within the patient's reach. Adjust table height as necessary.
6 Remove food covers. Open milk cartons and cereal boxes, cut meat, and butter bread if indicated (Fig. 16-4).
7 Place the napkin and silverware within reach.

8 Serve trays last to patients who must be fed.
9 Measure and record intake if ordered. Note the amount and type of foods eaten.
10 Remove the tray.
11 Assist the patient with oral hygiene.
12 Clean any spills and change soiled linen.
13 Help the patient return to bed if indicated.
14 Make sure the patient is comfortable, the signal light is within reach, and the side rails are up.
15 Wash your hands.
16 Report your observations to the nurse.

Serving Meal Trays

Food is usually served in the patient's room. However, some patients are allowed to eat in the cafeteria or lounge area. Residents of nursing facilities are served in dining rooms if they can be up. Food is served in containers that keep foods hot or cold as appropriate. You will help serve meal trays after preparing patients for the meals. Having patients already prepared for eating allows prompt serving of the trays. If trays are served promptly, the food will be at the desired temperature.

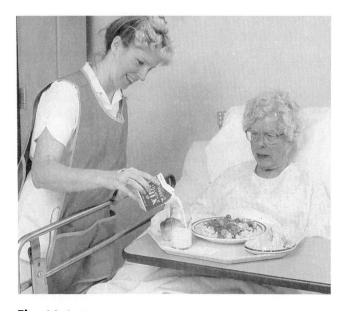

Fig. 16-4 The nursing assistant opens cartons and other containers for the patient.

Feeding the Patient

Some patients cannot feed themselves. Weakness, paralysis, casts, and other physical limitations may make self-feeding impossible. These patients must be fed. When feeding a patient, you should be in a comfortable position. You also need to provide a relaxed mood so that the patient does not feel rushed. Many people say a prayer before eating. Providing time and privacy for a prayer shows a great deal of care and respect for the patient. You also need to ask the patient about the order in which to offer foods and fluids. Spoons are used to feed patients. They are less likely to cause injury. The spoon should be only one third full. This provides a manageable portion of food to be chewed and swallowed.

Patients who are unable to feed themselves may feel anger, humiliation, and embarrassment at being dependent on others. Some may be depressed or resentful, or may refuse to eat. These patients should be allowed to feed themselves as much as possible. However, they should not exceed limitations ordered by the doctor. In addition, you should provide the patient with support and encouragement.

Many blind people are keenly aware of food aromas. However, they need to know what foods and fluids are on the tray. When feeding a blind patient, always tell the person what you are offering. If the blind person does not need to be fed, identify the foods and their location on the tray. Use the numbers on a clock to identify the location of foods (Fig. 16-5).

Mealtime provides social contact with others. You should engage the patient in pleasant conversation. However, be sure to allow the patient enough time to chew and swallow food.

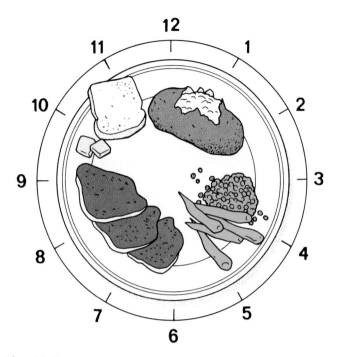

Fig. 16-5   The numbers on a clock are used to help the blind person locate food on the tray.

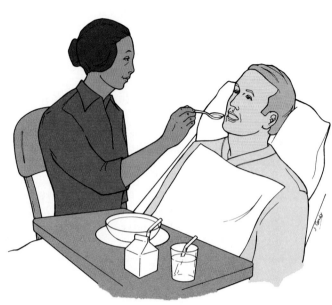

Fig. 16-6   A spoon is used to feed patients. The spoon should be no more than ⅓ full.

FEEDING THE PATIENT

1   Explain the procedure to the patient.
2   Wash your hands.
3   Position the patient in a comfortable sitting position.
4   Bring the tray into the room. Place it on the overbed table.
5   Identify the patient. Check the ID bracelet with the dietary card.
6   Drape a napkin across the patient's chest and underneath the chin.
7   Prepare the food for eating.
8   Tell the patient what foods are on the tray.
9   Serve foods in the order preferred by the patient. Alternate between solid and liquid foods. Use a spoon for safety as in Figure 16-6. Allow enough time for chewing. Do not rush the patient.
10 Use straws for liquids if the patient cannot drink out of a glass or cup. Have one straw for each liquid. Provide a short straw for weak patients.

11 Converse with the patient in a pleasant manner.
12 Encourage him or her to eat as much as possible.
13 Wipe the patient's mouth with a napkin.
14 Note how much and which foods were eaten.
15 Measure and record intake if applicable.
16 Remove the tray.
17 Provide oral hygiene.
18 Make sure the patient is comfortable, the signal light is within reach, and the side rails are up.
19 Wash your hands.
20 Report your observations to the nurse:
    a   The amount and kind of food eaten
    b   Complaints of nausea or *dysphagia*—difficulty or discomfort (dys) in swallowing (phagia)

PROVIDING FRESH DRINKING WATER

1 Get a list of patients who have special fluid orders (NPO, fluid restriction, or no ice). The list is obtained from the nurse.
2 Wash your hands.
3 Collect the following equipment:
   a Cart
   b Ice chest filled with ice cubes and a cover for the chest
   c Scoop
   d Disposable cups
   e Straws
   f Paper towels
   g Large water pitcher filled with cold water (optional, depending on facility procedure)
4 Arrange equipment on the cart on top of the paper towels.
5 Move the cart until you are just outside a patient's room. Check the list to see if the patient has special orders.
6 Check the ID bracelet and call the patient by name.
7 Take the water pitcher from the overbed table. Empty it into the sink in the bathroom.
8 Fill the pitcher half full with water. Get water from the tap or pitcher on the cart.
9 Fill the water pitcher with ice if it is allowed. Use the scoop for the ice (Fig. 16-7).
10 Place the pitcher, disposable cup, and straw on the overbed table. Make sure the patient can reach the articles with ease.
11 Fill the disposable cup with fresh water.
12 Repeat steps 5 through 11 for each patient.
13 Return the equipment to the "clean" utility room. Clean and return equipment to its proper place.
14 Wash your hands.

Between-Meal Nourishments

Many therapeutic diets involve between-meal nourishments. Commonly served nourishments are crackers, milk, juice, a milkshake, a piece of cake, wafers, a sandwich, gelatin, and custard. Nourishments are served as soon as they arrive on the nursing unit. The necessary eating utensils, a straw, and a napkin are provided. The same considerations and procedures described for serving meal trays and feeding patients are followed.

Providing Drinking Water

Patients need to have fresh drinking water at periodic intervals. Fresh water is usually provided during the day and evening and whenever the pitcher is empty. Before passing water you need to ask the nurse about any special orders. Some patients may be NPO, on restricted fluids, or not allowed ice. You need to practice the rules of medical asepsis when passing drinking water.

Other Methods of Maintaining Food and Fluid Needs

Many people cannot eat or drink because of illness, surgery, or injury. Other methods must be used to meet the basic need for foods and fluids. These methods are ordered by the doctor. The nurse is responsible for carrying out the order.

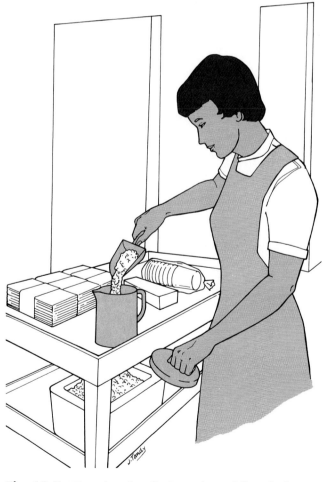

Fig. 16-7 The rules of medical asepsis are followed when passing drinking water. The scoop does not touch any part of the water pitcher when ice is being added.

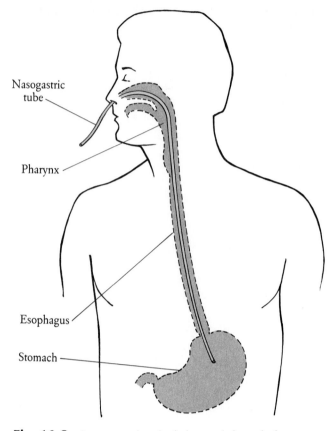

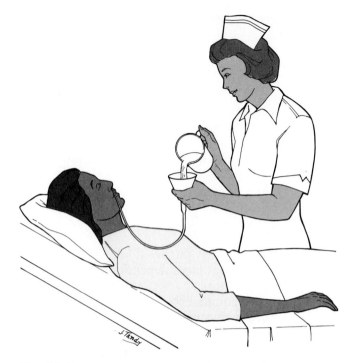

Fig. 16-9 The nurse gives a tube feeding. A funnel is attached to the end of the NG tube. The blended fluid is poured into the funnel.

Fig. 16-8 A nasogastric tube is inserted through the nose into the stomach.

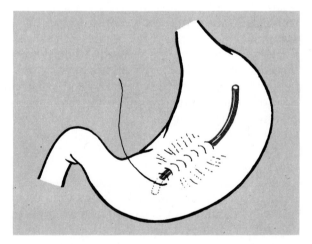

Fig. 16-10 A gastrostomy tube.

Tube feedings The doctor may order a nasogastric tube (NG tube, Levine tube) so that the patient can be fed through the tube. The nurse inserts the tube through the nose into the stomach (Fig. 16-8). Commercial or blended fluids are passed through the tube into the stomach. The feeding can be given at sched-uled intervals using a syringe or funnel (Fig. 16-9). The feeding may also be administered continuously by a special pump. *Gavage* is another term for a tube feeding.

A patient may have a gastrostomy. A *gastrostomy* is an opening (stomy) in the stomach (gastro). The opening is created surgically. A tube is inserted into the opening (Fig. 16-10). Commercial or blended foods are passed through the tube into the stomach.

A gastrostomy is indicated when food cannot pass normally from the mouth into the esophagus and then into the stomach. Cancer of the head, neck, or esophagus may require a gastrostomy. The patient with a gastrostomy cannot eat or drink fluids.

Intravenous therapy Many patients receive fluid through a needle that is inserted in a vein. Minerals and vitamins are often given in the same way. *IV* and *IV infusion* are often used in referring to *intravenous therapy*. The fluid is in a bottle or plastic bag. Clear IV tubing connects the container to the needle in a vein (Fig. 16-11). The amount of fluid given (infused) per hour is ordered by the doctor. The nurse is responsible for making sure this amount is given. This is done by controlling the number of drops (the flow rate) per minute. Nursing assistants are *never* responsible for IV therapy or for regulating the flow rate.

Hyperalimentation Hyperalimentation is the intravenous administration of a solution highly concentrated with proteins, carbohydrates, vitamins, and minerals. The solution is far more nutritious than a regular IV solution. Hyperalimentation is used for seriously ill and injured patients. Nursing assistants are *never* responsible for administering or regulating hyperalimentation solutions.

SUMMARY

The need for foods and fluids is basic for health and survival. A well-balanced diet contains foods from the four basic food groups. The diet provides the necessary amounts of proteins, carbohydrates, fats, vitamins, and minerals. Eating habits vary among individuals and are affected by many factors, including religion and culture. When assisting a patient in meeting nutritional needs, you must consider the factors that affect eating. Also try to make the meal as pleasant as possible for the individual.

Fluid balance is essential for health and life. The amount of fluid taken in must equal the amount lost. Fluid is lost through the urine, feces, skin, and lungs. You will assist doctors and nurses in evaluating a person's fluid balance by keeping accurate I&O records when directed to do so.

Patients and residents depend on nursing personnel to meet part or all of their food and fluid needs.

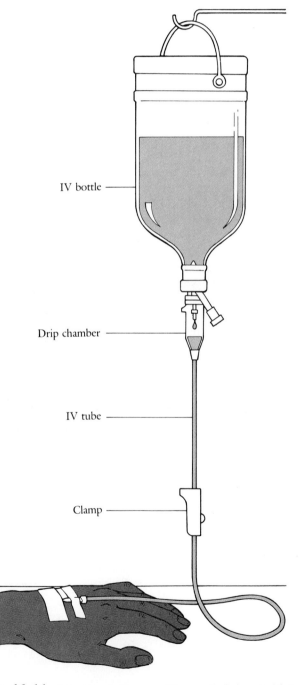

IV bottle

Drip chamber

IV tube

Clamp

Fig. 16-11 Intravenous therapy. The needle is inserted into a vein in the arm or hand. The needle is attached to the bottle by tubing.

Even patients who are up and about rely on the nursing team to serve meal trays. They also need nourishments and fresh drinking water. Some patients need to be fed. Remember that meals provide plea- sure and socialization. The person will enjoy the meal even more if he or she is refreshed and in a comfortable position.

REVIEW QUESTIONS

Circle the best answer.

1 Nutrition is
   a Fats, proteins, carbohydrates, vitamins, and minerals
   b The many processes involved in the ingestion, digestion, absorption, and use of food and fluids by the body
   c The four basic food groups
   d The balance between fluids taken in and lost by the body
2 Protein is needed for
   a Tissue growth and repair
   b Energy and the fiber for bowel elimination
   c Body heat and the protection of organs from injury
   d Improving the taste of food
3 Which foods provide the *most* protein?
   a Butter and cream
   b Tomatoes and potatoes
   c Meats and fish
   d Corn and lettuce
4 Eating and nutrition are affected by
   a A person's culture and religious practices
   b Personal preferences and how food is prepared
   c The amount of money available to buy food
   d All of the above
5 Sodium-restricted diets are usually ordered for all of the following patients *except* those with
   a Diabetes mellitus
   b Heart disease
   c Kidney disease
   d Liver disease
6 Mrs. Ronan is on a sodium-restricted diet. She asks you to bring some salt for her chicken. You should bring her the salt.
   a True
   b False
7 The diabetic diet controls the amount of
   a Water
   b Sodium
   c Carbohydrates
   d Nutrients
8 Diet planning for the diabetic diet involves

a Calculating the amount of sodium
b Exchange lists
c Measuring fluid intake
d Giving insulin with meals
9 Fluids are lost from the body through the
   a Urine and feces
   b Skin and lungs
   c Vomitus
   d All of the above
10 Fluid intake and the amount of fluid lost from the body must be equal.
   a True
   b False
11 Adult fluid requirements for normal fluid balance are about
   a 1000 to 1500 ml daily
   b 1500 to 2000 ml daily
   c 2000 to 2500 ml daily
   d 2500 to 3000 ml daily
12 A patient is NPO. You should
   a Provide a variety of fluids
   b Offer fluids in small amounts and small containers
   c Remove the water pitcher and glass
   d Prevent the patient from having oral hygiene
13 Which are *not* counted as liquid foods?
   a Coffee, tea, juices, and soft drinks
   b Butter, spaghetti sauce, and melted cheese
   c Ice cream, sherbet, custard, and pudding
   d Jello, popsicles, soup, and creamed cereals
14 Which statement about feeding a patient is *false?*
   a Ask if he or she wants to pray before eating.
   b A fork is used to feed a patient.
   c The patient should be asked the order in which foods should be served.
   d Engage the patient in a pleasant conversation.

Answers

		10 a	5 a	
14 b		9 d	4 d	
13 b		8 b	3 c	
12 c		7 c	2 a	
11 c		6 b	1 b	

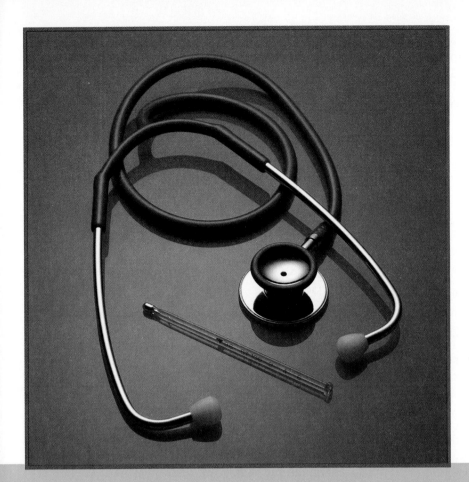

Measurement of Vital Signs

17

OBJECTIVES

- Define the key terms listed in this chapter
- Explain why vital signs are measured
- List ten factors that can affect vital signs
- Identify the normal ranges of oral, rectal, and axillary body temperatures
- Know when to take oral, rectal, and axillary temperatures
- Identify the sites for taking a pulse and know the normal pulse ranges of the different age-groups
- Describe normal respirations
- Know the normal ranges for adult blood pressures
- Describe the differences between mercury and aneroid sphygmomanometers
- Describe the practices you should follow when measuring blood pressure
- Perform the procedures described in this chapter

apical-radial pulse   Taking the apical and radial pulses at the same time

apnea   The lack or absence of (a) breathing (pnea)

blood pressure   The amount of force exerted against the walls of an artery by the blood

body temperature   The amount of heat in the body that is a balance between the amount of heat produced and the amount lost by the body

bradypnea   Slow (brady) breathing (pnea); the respiratory rate is less than 10 respirations per minute

Cheyne-Stokes   A pattern of breathing in which respirations gradually increase in rate and depth and then become shallow and slow; breathing may stop for 10 to 20 seconds

diastole   The period of heart muscle relaxation

diastolic pressure   The pressure in the arteries when the heart is at rest

dyspnea   Difficult, labored, or painful (dys) breathing (pnea)

hypertension   Persistent blood pressure measurements above the normal systolic (150 mm Hg) or diastolic (90 mm Hg) pressures

hyperventilation   Respirations that are rapid and deeper than normal

hypotension   A condition in which the systolic blood pressure is below 100 mm Hg and the diastolic pressure is below 60 mm Hg

hypoventilation   Respirations that are slow, shallow, and sometimes irregular

pulse   The beat of the heart felt at an artery as a wave of blood passes through the artery

pulse deficit   The difference between the apical and radial pulse rates

pulse rate   The number of heartbeats or pulses felt in 1 minute

respiration   The act of breathing air into (inhalation) and out of (exhalation) the lungs

sphygmomanometer   The instrument used to measure blood pressure

stethoscope   An instrument used to listen to the sounds produced by the heart, lungs, and other body organs

systole   The period of heart muscle contraction

systolic pressure   The amount of force it takes to pump blood out of the heart into the arterial circulation

tachypnea   Rapid (tachy) breathing (pnea); the respiratory rate is usually greater than 24 respirations per minute

vital signs   Temperature, pulse, respirations, and blood pressure

Vital signs reflect the function of three body processes essential for life: regulation of body temperature, breathing, and heart function. The four *vital signs* of body function are temperature, pulse, respirations, and blood pressure.

Nursing assistants frequently measure vital signs. Accuracy is absolutely essential. You must be accurate in measuring, reporting, and recording vital signs.

MEASURING AND REPORTING VITAL SIGNS

Vital signs are measured to detect changes in normal body function. They are also used to determine a person's response to treatment. Life-threatening situations can also be recognized. A person's temperature, pulse, and respirations (TPR) and blood pressure (BP) will vary within certain limits during any 24-hour period. Many factors affect vital signs. They include sleep, activity, eating, weather, noise, exercise, medications, fear, anxiety, and illness.

The vital signs are measured during routine physical examinations. They are also measured when a person is admitted to a health care facility. Hospitalized patients have vital signs measured several times a day. The doctor or nurse compares each measurement with previous ones. Residents of nursing facilities do not have their vital signs measured as often. The nurse will tell you when to obtain vital signs. Unless otherwise ordered, vital signs are taken with the person lying or sitting. The person should be at rest when vital signs are measured.

Vital signs reflect even minor changes in a person's condition. They must be measured accurately. If you are unsure of your measurements, promptly ask the nurse to take them again. Vital signs must also be accurately reported and recorded. Any vital sign that is changed from a previous measurement must be reported to the nurse immediately. Vital signs that are above or below the normal range must also be reported immediately.

Many facilities have a "temp board" or a "TPR book." These are divided into columns. The names of individuals are written down the left side of the page. Times of day (such as 8:00 AM, 12:00 PM, 4:00 PM, 8:00 PM) are at the top of the other columns. You will record vital signs on the line in the column appropriate for the patient and time. In some facilities, changed or abnormal vital signs are circled in red. Besides recording them, verbally report changed or abnormal vital signs to the nurse right away.

BODY TEMPERATURE

Body temperature is the amount of heat in the body. It is a balance between the amount of heat produced and the amount lost by the body. Heat is produced as food is used for energy. It is lost through the skin, breathing, urine, and feces. Body temperature remains fairly stable. It is lower in the morning and higher in the afternoon and evening. Factors affecting body temperature include age, weather, exercise, pregnancy, the menstrual cycle, emotions, and illness.

Normal Body Temperature

The Fahrenheit (F) and Centigrade or Celsius (C) scales are used to measure temperature. Common sites for measuring body temperature are the mouth, rectum, and axilla. Normal body temperature is 98.6° F (37° C) when measured orally. The normal rectal temperature is 1° higher, or 99.6° F (37.5° C). The average axillary temperature is 97.6° F (36.5° C). Body temperature usually stays within a normal range. Normal ranges of body temperature for adults are:

Oral—97.6° to 99.6° F (36.5° to 37.5° C)
Rectal—98.6° to 100.6° F (37.0° to 38.1° C)
Axillary—96.6° to 98.6° F (36.0° to 37.0° C)

Types of Thermometers

A thermometer is used to measure temperature. The glass thermometer is familiar to most people. There are other kinds of thermometers for measuring body temperature.

Glass thermometers The glass thermometer (clinical thermometer) is a hollow glass tube with a bulb filled with mercury. When heated by the body, the mercury expands and rises in the tube. The mercury contracts and moves down the tube when cooled.

There are three types of glass thermometers. Each has a different bulb or tip (Fig. 17-1). Long- or slender-tip thermometers are used for oral and axillary

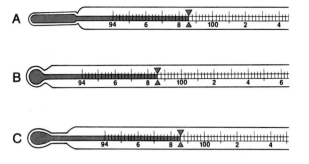

Fig. 17-1 Types of glass thermometers. **A,** The long or slender tip. **B,** The stubby tip (rectal thermometer). **C,** The pear-shaped tip.

temperatures, as are stubby- and pear-shaped-tip thermometers. Rectal thermometers have stubby tips that are color-coded in red. Glass thermometers are available in Fahrenheit and Centigrade scales. Some have both scales.

How to read a glass thermometer. Fahrenheit thermometers have long and short lines. Every other long line is marked in an even degree from 94° to 108° F. The short lines indicate 0.2 (two tenths) of a degree (Fig. 17-2, *A*). Centigrade thermometers also have long and short lines. Each long line represents one degree, from 34° to 42° C. Each short line represents 0.1 (one tenth) of a degree (Fig. 17-2, *B*). Table 17-1 shows equivalent values for Fahrenheit and Centigrade scales.

Using a glass thermometer. The thermometer is inserted into the mouth, rectum, or axilla. Each area has many microorganisms. There is one thermometer for each patient to prevent the spread of microbes and infection. Thermometers are disinfected after use. They are often stored in a disinfectant solution between uses. Before being used again, a thermometer is rinsed under cold running water and wiped with a tissue to remove the disinfectant.

Methods for cleaning thermometers vary among facilities. The thermometer is usually first wiped with a tissue to remove mucus or feces. Then it is washed in cold soapy water. Hot water is not used; it causes

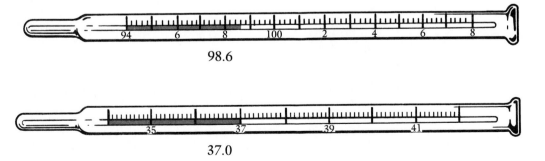

98.6

37.0

Fig. 17-2 **A,** Fahrenheit thermometer. The mercury level is at 98.6° F. **B,** Centigrade thermometer. The mercury level is at 37.0° C.

TABLE 17-1 **Fahrenheit and Centigrade Equivalents**

Fahrenheit	Centigrade
95.0	35.0
95.9	35.5
96.8	36.0
97.7	36.5
98.6	37.0
99.5	37.5
100.4	38.0
101.3	38.5
102.2	39.0
103.1	39.5
104.0	40.0
104.9	40.5
105.8	41.0
106.7	41.5
107.6	42.0
108.5	42.5
109.4	43.0
110.3	43.5

the mercury to expand so much that the thermometer could break. After cleaning, thermometers are rinsed under cold running water. They are stored in a case or a container filled with disinfectant solution.

Many facilities use plastic covers for thermometers (Fig. 17-3). A cover is used once and then discarded. The thermometer is inserted into a cover and the temperature is taken. The cover is removed to read the thermometer. The thermometer is then inserted into a clean cover and is ready for use. Disinfection and cleaning are not necessary because the thermometer never touches the patient.

Before taking a temperature, you must shake the thermometer down to move the mercury into the bulb. The thermometer is checked for breaks or chips, which could cause patient injury.

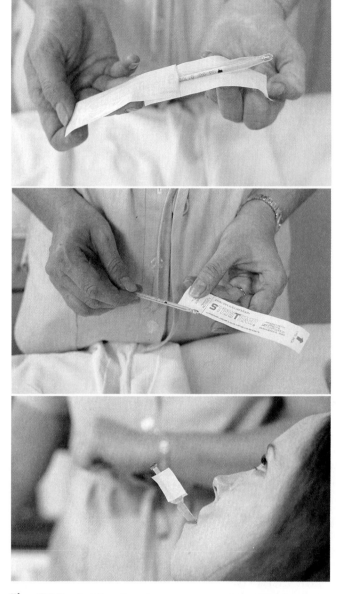

Fig. 17-3 A, The glass thermometer and plastic cover. **B,** The thermometer is inserted into a plastic cover. **C,** The patient's temperature is taken with the thermometer in the plastic cover.

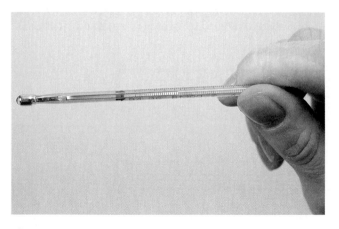

Fig. 17-4 The termometer is held at the stem with the thumb and fingertips.

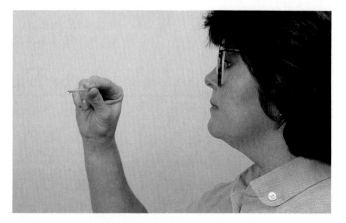

Fig. 17-5 The thermometer is read at eye level.

HOW TO READ A GLASS THERMOMETER

1 Make sure you have good lighting.
2 Hold the thermometer at the stem with your thumb and fingertips (Fig. 17-4).
3 Bring the thermometer to eye level (Fig. 17-5).
4 Rotate the thermometer until you can see both the numbers and the long and short lines.
5 Note that each long line measures 1° and each small line measures 0.1° on a Centigrade thermometer. Each small line on a Fahrenheit thermometer represents 0.2° (see Fig. 17-2).

6 Turn the thermometer back and forth slowly until the silver (or red) mercury line is seen.
7 Read the thermometer to the nearest degree (long line). Read the nearest tenth of a degree (short line)—an even number if you are using a Fahrenheit thermometer.
8 Record the patient's name and temperature.

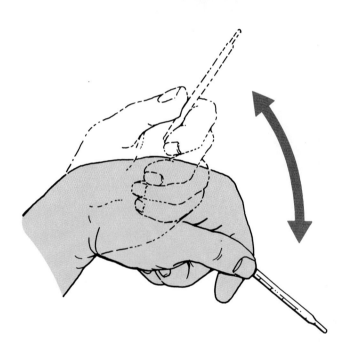

Fig. 17-6 The wrist is snapped to shake down the thermometer.

HOW TO USE A GLASS THERMOMETER

1 Collect the following equipment:
   a Thermometer
   b Tissues
2 Wash your hands.
3 Hold the thermometer at the stem.
4 Rinse the thermometer under cold running water if it was soaking in a disinfectant. Dry it from the stem to the bulb end with tissues.
5 Shake down the thermometer. The mercury must be below the lines and numbers.
   a Hold the thermometer at the stem.
   b Stand away from walls, tables, or other hard surfaces to avoid breaking the thermometer.

   c Flex and snap your wrist until the mercury is shaken down (Fig. 17-6).
6 Take the patient's temperature. Read the thermometer and record the temperature.
7 Shake down the thermometer after use.
8 Wipe the thermometer with tissues. Clean it if plastic covers are not used.
9 Place the thermometer in a disinfectant solution or in a plastic cover.

Electronic thermometers Electronic thermometers are portable and battery operated (Fig. 17-7). They measure temperatures in 2 to 60 seconds. The temperature is displayed on the front of the instrument. The hand-held unit is kept in a battery charger when not in use.

Oral and rectal probes are supplied with electronic thermometers. A disposable cover or sheath covers the probe. Disposable probe covers are used only once and then are discarded.

Electronic thermometers are expensive. However, they have several advantages. Disposable probe covers reduce the possibility of spreading infection. The temperature is measured rapidly, and the temperature display is easily read.

Disposable oral thermometers Disposable oral thermometers (Fig. 17-8) have small chemical dots. The dots change color when heated by the body. Each dot must be heated to a certain temperature before it

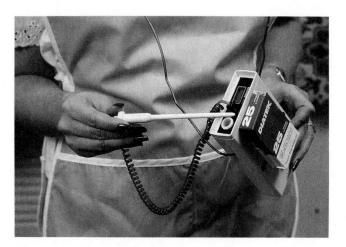

Fig. 17-7 An electronic thermometer.

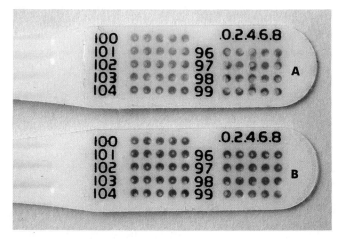

Fig. 17-8 **A,** Disposable oral thermometer with chemical dots. **B,** The dots change color when the temperature is taken.

TAKING AN ORAL TEMPERATURE WITH A GLASS THERMOMETER

1 Explain the procedure to the patient. Ask him or her not to eat, drink, smoke, or chew gum for 15 minutes.
2 Collect the following equipment:
    a Oral thermometer and holder
    b Tissues
    c Plastic covers if used
3 Wash your hands.
4 Identify the patient. Check the ID bracelet and call the patient by name.
5 Provide for privacy.
6 Rinse the thermometer in cold water if it was soaking in a disinfectant solution. Dry it with tissues.
7 Check the thermometer for breaks or chips.
8 Shake down the thermometer.
9 Place a plastic cover on the thermometer.
10 Ask the patient to moisten his or her lips.
11 Place the bulb end of the thermometer under the patient's tongue (Fig. 17-9).
12 Ask the patient to close his or her lips around the thermometer to hold it in place.

13 Leave the thermometer in place for 2 to 3 minutes.
14 Grasp the stem of the thermometer. Remove it from the patient's mouth.
15 Use tissues to remove the plastic cover. Wipe the thermometer with a tissue from the stem to the bulb end if no cover was used.
16 Read the thermometer.
17 Record the patient's name and temperature.
18 Shake down the thermometer.
19 Rinse and wash the thermometer.
20 Place the thermometer in the holder with disinfectant or in a plastic cover.
21 Make sure the patient is comfortable and the signal light is within reach.
22 Unscreen the patient.
23 Wash your hands.
24 Report any abnormal temperature to the nurse. Record the measurement in the proper place.

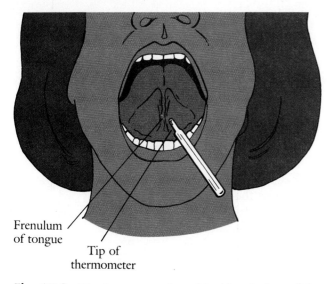

Frenulum
of tongue

Tip of
thermometer

Fig. 17-9 The thermometer is positioned at the base of the tongue next to the frenulum.

changes color. These thermometers are used only once. They measure the temperature in about 45 seconds.

Temperature-sensitive tape Temperature-sensitive tape changes color in response to body heat. The tape is applied to the forehead or abdomen. It indicates if the temperature is normal or above normal but does not measure exact body temperature. The color change takes about 15 seconds.

Taking Oral Temperatures

Oral temperatures are usually taken on older children and adults. Drinking and eating hot or cold foods or fluids, smoking, and chewing gum cause inaccurate measurements. If the patient has engaged in these activities, wait 15 minutes before taking an oral temperature. The glass thermometer must remain in place 2 to 3 minutes for an accurate measurement.

Temperatures are not taken orally if the patient:

1. Is an infant or a child younger than 4 or 5 years of age
2. Is unconscious
3. Has had surgery or an injury to the face, neck, nose, or mouth
4. Is receiving oxygen
5. Breathes through the mouth
6. Has a nasogastric tube in place
7. Is delerious, restless, confused, or disoriented
8. Is paralyzed on one side of the body
9. Has a sore mouth

Taking Rectal Temperatures

The rectal temperature is the most accurate and reliable measurement of body temperature. This route is used when oral temperatures cannot be taken (see above). Rectal temperatures are not taken if the patient has diarrhea, a rectal disorder or injury, heart disease, or has had rectal surgery.

The rectal thermometer is lubricated for easy insertion and to prevent tissue injury. The thermometer is held in place so that it is not lost into the rectum or broken. A glass thermometer must remain in the rectum for 2 minutes for an accurate measurement.

TAKING AN ORAL TEMPERATURE WITH A DISPOSABLE THERMOMETER

1 Explain the procedure to the patient. Ask him or her not to eat, drink, smoke, or chew gum for 15 minutes.
2 Get a disposable thermometer.
3 Wash your hands.
4 Identify the patient. Check the ID bracelet and call the patient by name.
5 Provide for privacy.
6 Remove the wrapper from the thermometer.
7 Ask the patient to open the mouth and raise the tongue.
8 Place the thermometer at the base of the tongue on either side.
9 Ask the patient to lower the tongue and close the mouth.
10 Leave the thermometer in place for 45 seconds.
11 Remove the thermometer and read the last colored dot.
12 Record the patient's name and temperature.
13 Make sure the patient is comfortable and the signal light is within reach.
14 Unscreen the patient.
15 Wash your hands.
16 Report any abnormal temperature to the nurse. Record the measurement in the proper place.

TAKING AN ORAL TEMPERATURE WITH AN ELECTRONIC THERMOMETER

1 Explain the procedure to the patient. Ask him or her not to eat, drink, smoke, or chew gum for 15 minutes.
2 Collect the following equipment:
   a Electronic thermometer
   b Oral probe (usually blue)
   c Disposable probe covers
3 Plug the oral probe into the thermometer.
4 Wash your hands.
5 Identify the patient. Check the ID bracelet and call the patient by name.
6 Provide for privacy.
7 Insert the probe into a probe cover.
8 Ask the patient to open the mouth and raise the tongue.
9 Place the covered probe at the base of the tongue on either side (Fig. 17-10). Ask the patient to lower the tongue and close the mouth.
10 Hold the probe in place.
11 Read the temperature on the display. A tone or a flashing or steady light means the temperature has been measured.
12 Remove the probe from the patient's mouth. Press the eject button to discard the cover.
13 Record the patient's name and temperature.
14 Return the probe to the holder.
15 Make sure the patient is comfortable and the signal light is within reach.
16 Unscreen the patient.
17 Return the thermometer to the charging unit.
18 Wash your hands.
19 Report any abnormal temperature to the nurse. Record the measurement in the proper place.

TAKING A RECTAL TEMPERATURE WITH A GLASS THERMOMETER

1 Explain the procedure to the patient.
2 Collect the following equipment:
   a Rectal thermometer and holder
   b Toilet tissue
   c Plastic covers if used
   d Disposable gloves
   e Water-soluble lubricant
3 Wash your hands.
4 Identify the patient. Check the ID bracelet and call the patient by name.
5 Provide for privacy.
6 Rinse the thermometer in cold water if it was soaking in a disinfectant solution. Dry it with tissues.
7 Check the thermometer for breaks or chips.
8 Shake down the thermometer.
9 Place a plastic cover on the thermometer.
10 Position the patient in Sims' position.
11 Put on the gloves.
12 Put a small amount of lubricant on a tissue. Lubricate the bulb end of the thermometer.
13 Fold back top linens to expose the anal area.
14 Raise the upper buttock to expose the anus (Fig. 17-11).
15 Insert the thermometer 1 inch into the rectum.
16 Hold it in place for 2 minutes (Fig. 17-12).
17 Remove the thermometer.
18 Remove the plastic cover. Wipe the thermometer with tissues from the stem to the bulb end if no cover was used.
19 Place the used toilet tissue on a paper towel or several thicknesses of toilet tissue. Place the thermometer on clean toilet tissue.
20 Wipe the anal area to remove excess lubricant and any feces. Cover the patient.
21 Discard soiled toilet tissue into the toilet.
22 Remove the gloves.
23 Read the thermometer. Record the patient's name and temperature. Write "R" to indicate a rectal temperature.
24 Make sure the patient is comfortable and the signal light is within reach.
25 Shake down the thermometer.
26 Rinse and wash the thermometer.
27 Place the thermometer in the holder with disinfectant or in a plastic cover.
28 Unscreen the patient.
29 Wash your hands.
30 Report any abnormal temperature. Record the measurement with an "R" in the proper place.

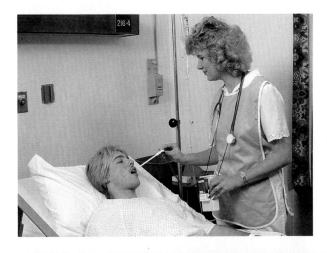

Fig. 17-10 The covered probe of the electronic thermometer is inserted under the tongue. The unit is carried in the hand with the carrying strap around the neck.

TAKING A RECTAL TEMPERATURE WITH AN ELECTRONIC THERMOMETER

1 Explain the procedure to the patient.
2 Collect the following equipment:
  a Electronic thermometer
  b Rectal probe (usually red)
  c Disposable probe covers
  d Toilet tissue
  e Water-soluble lubricant
  f Disposable gloves
3 Plug the rectal probe into the thermometer.
4 Wash your hands.
5 Identify the patient. Check the ID bracelet and call the patient by name.
6 Provide for privacy.
7 Position the patient in Sims' position.
8 Put on the gloves.
9 Put a small amount of lubricant on some toilet tissue.
10 Insert the probe into a probe cover.
11 Lubricate the end of the covered probe using the lubricant on the toilet tissue.
12 Fold back top linens to expose the anal area.
13 Raise the upper buttock to expose the anus.

14 Insert the probe ½ inch into the rectum.
15 Hold the probe in place until you hear a tone or see a flashing or steady light.
16 Read the temperature on the display.
17 Remove the probe from the rectum.
18 Press the eject button to discard the probe cover. Return the probe to the holder.
19 Wipe the anal area with toilet tissue to remove excess lubricant and any feces. Cover the patient.
20 Discard used toilet tissue into the toilet.
21 Remove the gloves.
22 Record the patient's name and temperature with an "R" (for rectal temperature).
23 Make sure the patient is comfortable and the signal light is within reach.
24 Unscreen the patient.
25 Return the thermometer to the charging unit.
26 Wash your hands.
27 Report any abnormal temperature. Record the measurement with an "R" in the proper place.

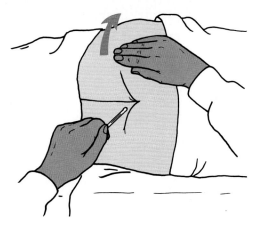

Fig. 17-11 The rectal temperature is taken with the patient in Sims' position. The buttock is raised to expose the anus.

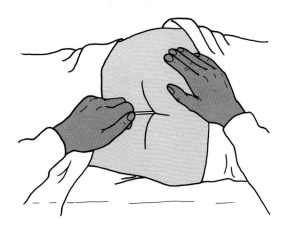

Fig. 17-12 The rectal thermometer is held in place during the measurement.

TAKING AN AXILLARY TEMPERATURE WITH A GLASS THERMOMETER

1 Explain the procedure to the patient.
2 Collect the following equipment:
   a Oral glass thermometer and holder
   b Plastic covers if used
   c Tissues
   d Towel
3 Wash your hands.
4 Identify the patient. Check the ID bracelet and call the patient by name.
5 Provide for privacy.
6 Rinse the thermometer in cold water if it was soaking in a disinfectant solution. Dry it with tissues.
7 Check the thermometer for breaks or chips.
8 Shake down the thermometer.
9 Place a plastic cover on the thermometer.
10 Help the patient remove an arm from the gown. Do not expose the patient.
11 Dry the axilla with the towel.
12 Place the bulb end of the thermometer in the center of the axilla.
13 Ask the patient to place the arm over the chest to hold the thermometer in place (Fig. 17-13). Hold it and the arm in place if he or she cannot help or if the patient is an infant or child (Fig. 17-14).
14 Leave the thermometer in place for 9 minutes.
15 Remove the thermometer from the plastic cover. Wipe it with tissues from the stem to the bulb end if no cover was used.
16 Read the thermometer.
17 Record the patient's name and temperature with an "A" (for axillary temperature).
18 Help the patient put the gown back on.
19 Make sure the patient is comfortable and the signal light is within reach.
20 Shake down the thermometer.
21 Rinse and wash the thermometer. Place it in the holder with disinfectant or in a plastic cover.
22 Unscreen the patient.
23 Place the towel in the linen hamper.
24 Wash your hands.
25 Report any abnormal temperature. Record the measurement with an "A" in the proper place.

TAKING AN AXILLARY TEMPERATURE WITH AN ELECTRONIC THERMOMETER

1 Explain the procedure to the patient.
2 Collect the following equipment:
   a Electronic thermometer
   b Oral probe (usually blue)
   c Disposable probe covers
   d Towel
3 Plug the oral probe into the thermometer.
4 Wash your hands.
5 Identify the patient. Check the ID bracelet and call the patient by name.
6 Provide for privacy.
7 Help the patient remove an arm from the gown. Do not expose the patient.
8 Dry the axilla with the towel.
9 Insert the probe into a probe cover.
10 Place the covered probe in the axilla. Place the patient's arm over the chest. Hold the probe in place until your hear a tone or see a steady or flashing light.
11 Remove the probe. Read the temperature on the display.
12 Record the patient's name and temperature with an "A" (for axillary temperature).
13 Press the eject button and discard the probe cover. Return the probe to the holder.
14 Help the patient put the gown back on.
15 Make sure the patient is comfortable and the signal light is within reach.
16 Unscreen the patient.
17 Place the towel in the linen hamper.
18 Return the thermometer to the charging unit.
19 Wash your hands.
20 Report any abnormal temperature. Record the measurement with an "A" in the proper place.

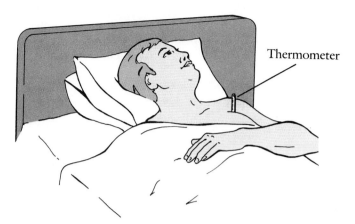

Fig. 17-13 The thermometer is held in place in the axilla by bringing the patient's arm over the chest.

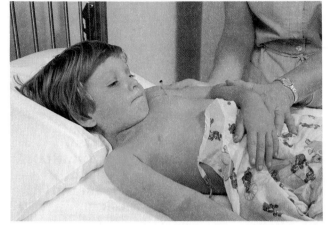

Fig. 17-14 Axillary temperature taken on a child. The nursing assistant holds the thermometer and the child's arm in place.

Taking Axillary Temperatures

Axillary temperatures are less reliable than oral or rectal temperatures. They are used when the temperature cannot be measured orally or rectally. This site should not be used right after the axilla has been bathed. The axilla should be dry for the measurement. The thermometer must be held in place to maintain proper position. A glass thermometer is held in place for 9 minutes for a reliable measurement.

PULSE

The *pulse* is defined as the beat of the heart felt at an artery as a wave of blood passes through the artery. A pulse can be felt every time the heart beats.

Sites for Taking a Pulse

The pulse can be taken at a number of sites (Fig. 17-15). Pulses are easy to feel at these sites. The arteries are close to the body's surface and lie over a bone. The radial site is used most often because it is easily accessible. The radial pulse can be taken without disturbing or exposing the patient.

The temporal, carotid, brachial, radial, femoral, popliteal, and dorsalis pedis (pedal) arteries are found on both sides of the body. The apical pulse is felt over the apex of the heart. It is taken with a stethoscope.

Using a Stethoscope

A *stethoscope* is an instrument used to listen to the sounds produced by the heart, lungs, and other body organs. The stethoscope amplifies the sounds so that they can be heard easily. The parts of a stethoscope

are shown in Figure 17-16. The earpieces should fit snugly to block out external noises. However, they should not cause pain or ear discomfort.

Stethoscopes are expensive and are shared by doctors and the nursing team. Care must be taken when using stethoscopes because they will be in contact with many patients and workers. The earpieces and diaphragm are cleaned before and after use. Cleaning prevents the spread of microorganisms.

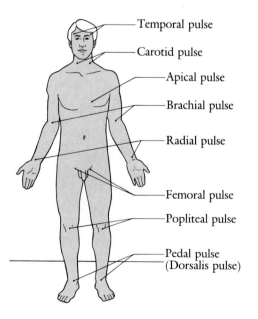

Fig. 17-15 The pulse sites.

HOW TO USE A STETHOSCOPE

1. Collect the following equipment:
   a. Stethoscope with diaphragm
   b. Alcohol wipes
2. Wash your hands.
3. Wipe the earpieces and diaphragm with alcohol wipes.
4. Warm the diaphragm in your hand.
5. Place the earpiece tips in your ears so that the bend of the tips points forward.
6. Place the diaphragm over the artery. Hold it in place with your two middle fingers (Fig. 17-17).
7. Do not let anything touch the tubing.
8. Ask the patient to be silent during the procedure.
9. Wipe the earpiece tips and diaphragm with alcohol wipes when the procedure is completed.
10. Return the stethoscope to its proper place.

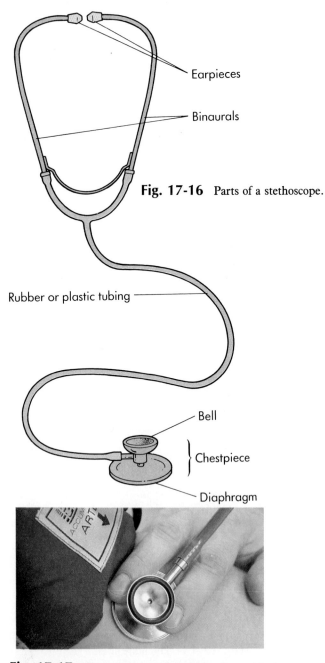

Fig. 17-16 Parts of a stethoscope.

Earpieces

Binaurals

Rubber or plastic tubing

Bell

Chestpiece

Diaphragm

Fig. 17-17 The stethoscope is held in place with the fingertips of the index and middle fingers.

Pulse Rate

The *pulse rate* is the number of heartbeats or pulses felt in 1 minute. The rate varies for different age-groups (Table 17-2). The pulse rate is influenced by many factors. They include elevated body temperature (fever), exercise, fear, anger, anxiety, excitement, heat, position, and pain. These and other factors cause the heart to beat faster. Some medications also increase the pulse rate. Other drugs slow down the pulse.

The adult pulse rate is between 60 and 100 beats per minute. A rate of less than 60 or greater than 100 is considered abnormal. Abnormal rates are reported to the nurse immediately.

TABLE 17-2 Pulse Ranges for the Different Age-Groups

Age-group	Pulse rates per minute
Newborns (Birth to 4 weeks)	70-170
Infants to 1 year (4 weeks to 1 year)	80-130
Toddlers and preschoolers (2 to 6 years)	80-120
School-age children (6 to 12 years)	70-110
Teenagers and adults (12 years and older)	70-80

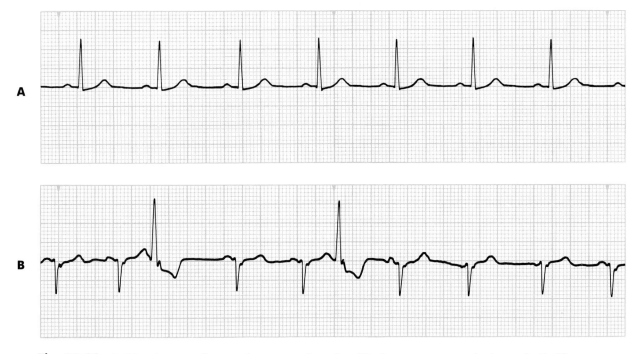

Fig. 17-18 **A,** The electrocardiogram shows a regular pulse. The beats occur at regular intervals. **B,** The beats in this electrocardiogram occur at irregular intervals. (From Huszar RJ: *Basic dysrhythmias: interpretation and management,* St Louis, 1988, Mosby–Year Book.)

Rhythm and Force of the Pulse

When taking a pulse, give attention to its rhythm and force. The rhythm should be regular. That is, a pulse should be felt in a pattern. The same time interval should occur between beats (Fig. 17-18, *A*). An irregular pulse occurs when the beats are unevenly spaced or beats are skipped (Fig. 17-18, *B*). The force of the pulse relates to its strength. A forceful pulse is easy to feel and is described as strong, full, or bounding. Pulses that are hard to feel are described as weak, thready, or feeble.

Electronic blood pressure equipment (see page 301) also counts pulses. The pulse rate is displayed along with the blood pressure. However, no information is given about the rhythm and force of the pulse. If electronic blood pressure equipment is used, you still need to feel the pulse to determine rhythm and force.

Taking a Radial Pulse

The radial pulse is used for routine vital signs. The pulse is felt by placing the first three fingers of one hand against the radial artery. The radial artery is on the thumb side of the wrist (Fig. 17-19). Do not use your thumb to take a pulse; the thumb has a pulse of its own. The pulse in your thumb could be mistaken for the patient's pulse. The pulse is counted for 30 seconds. The number is multiplied by 2 to obtain the number of beats per minute. If the pulse is irregular, it is counted for 1 full minute.

Taking an Apical Pulse

The apical pulse is taken with a stethoscope. This method is used on infants and children up to about 3 years of age. Apical pulses are also taken on adults who have heart diseases or who are taking medications that affect the heart. The apical pulse is on the left side of the chest slightly below the nipple (Fig. 17-20). The apical pulse is counted for 1 full minute.

The heartbeat normally sounds like a "lub-dub." Each "lub-dub" is counted as one beat. Do not count the "lub" as one beat and the "dub" as another.

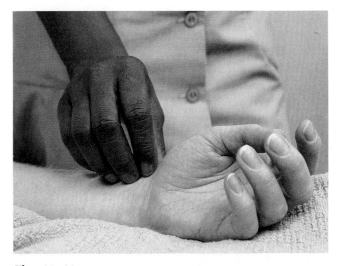

Fig. 17-19 The middle three fingers are used to locate the radial pulse on the thumb side of the wrist.

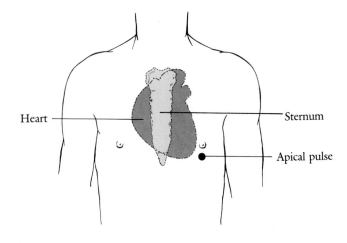

Fig. 17-20   The apical pulse is located 2 to 3 inches to the left of the sternum (breast bone) and below the left nipple.

TAKING A RADIAL PULSE

1 Wash your hands.
2 Identify the patient. Check the ID bracelet and call the patient by name.
3 Explain the procedure to the patient.
4 Provide for privacy.
5 Have the patient sit or lie down.
6 Locate the radial pulse with your 3 middle fingers (see Fig. 17-19).
7 Note if the pulse is strong or weak, and regular or irregular.
8 Count the pulse for 30 seconds. Multiply the number of beats by 2.
9 Count the pulse for 1 full minute if it is irregular.
10 Record the patient's name and pulse. Make a notation about the strength of the pulse and if it was regular or irregular.

11 Make sure the patient is comfortable and the signal light is within reach.
12 Unscreen the patient.
13 Wash your hands.
14 Report the following to the nurse:
   a A pulse rate of less than 60 or greater than 100 beats per minute should be reported immediately
   b Whether the pulse is regular or irregular
   c The pulse rate
   d The strength of the pulse (strong, full, or bounding; or weak, thready, or feeble)
15 Record the pulse rate in the proper place.

TAKING AN APICAL PULSE

1 Collect the following equipment:
   a Stethoscope with diaphragm
   b Alcohol wipes
2 Wash your hands.
3 Identify the patient. Check the ID bracelet and call the patient by name.
4 Explain the procedure to the patient.
5 Provide for privacy.
6 Wipe the earpieces and diaphragm with alcohol wipes.
7 Have the patient sit or lie down.
8 Expose the nipple area of the left chest.
9 Warm the diaphragm in your palm.
10 Place the earpieces in your ears.
11 Locate the apical pulse. Place the diaphragm 2 to 3 inches to the left of the breastbone and below the left nipple (see Fig. 17-20).
12 Count the pulse for 1 full minute. Note if it is regular or irregular.

13 Cover the patient. Remove the earpieces.
14 Record the patient's name and pulse. Note whether the pulse was regular or irregular.
15 Make sure the patient is comfortable and the signal light is within reach.
16 Unscreen the patient.
17 Clean the earpieces and diaphragm of the stethoscope with alcohol wipes.
18 Return the stethoscope to its proper place.
19 Wash your hands.
20 Report the following to the nurse:
   a A pulse rate of less than 60 or greater than 100 beats per minute should be reported immediately
   b Whether the pulse was regular or irregular
   c The pulse rate
   d Any unusual heart sounds
21 Record the pulse rate in the proper place with an "Ap" for an apical pulse.

Taking an Apical-Radial Pulse

The apical and radial pulse rates should be equal. Sometimes heart contractions are not strong enough to create pulses in the radial artery. This may occur in people with heart disease. The radial pulse may be less than the apical pulse. To see if there is a difference between the apical and radial rates, the pulses are taken at the same time by two workers. This is called an *apical-radial pulse*. The *pulse deficit* is the difference between the apical and radial pulse rates. To obtain the pulse deficit, subtract the radial rate from the apical rate. The apical pulse rate is never less than the radial pulse rate.

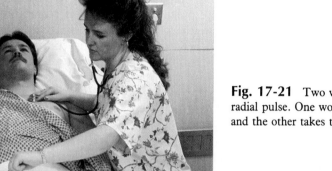

Fig. 17-21 Two workers take an apical-radial pulse. One worker takes the apical pulse, and the other takes the radial pulse.

TAKING AN APICAL-RADIAL PULSE

1 Ask a nurse or another nursing assistant to help you.
2 Collect the following equipment:
   a Stethoscope with diaphragm
   b Alcohol wipes
3 Wash your hands.
4 Identify the patient. Check the ID bracelet and call the patient by name.
5 Explain the procedure to the patient.
6 Provide for privacy.
7 Wipe the earpieces and diaphragm with the alcohol wipes.
8 Have the patient sit or lie down.
9 Expose the left nipple area of the chest.
10 Warm the diaphragm in your palm.
11 Place the earpieces in your ears.
12 Find the apical pulse. Have your helper find the radial pulse (Fig. 17-21).
13 Give the signal to begin counting.
14 Count the pulse for 1 full minute.
15 Give the signal to stop counting.
16 Cover the patient. Remove the earpieces.
17 Record the patient's name and the apical and radial pulses. Subtract the radial pulse from the apical pulse for the pulse deficit.

Note whether the pulse was regular or irregular.
18 Make sure the patient is comfortable and the signal light is within reach.
19 Unscreen the patient.
20 Clean the earpieces and diaphragm with alcohol wipes.
21 Return the stethoscope to its proper place.
22 Wash your hands.
23 Report the following to the nurse:
   a An apical pulse rate of less than 60 or greater than 100 beats per minute should be reported immediately
   b The apical and radial pulse rates
   c The pulse deficit
   d Whether the pulse was regular or irregular
   e Any unusual heart sounds
24 Record the pulses in the proper place. Indicate that an apical-radial pulse was taken.

RESPIRATIONS

Respiration is the act of breathing air into the lungs (inhalation) and out of the lungs (exhalation). Oxygen is taken into the lungs during inhalation. Carbon dioxide is moved out of the lungs during exhalation. Each respiration involves one inhalation and one exhalation. The chest rises during inhalation and falls during exhalation.

The healthy adult has 14 to 20 respirations per minute. Infants and children normally breathe faster than adults. The respiratory rate is affected by many of the factors that affect body temperature and pulse. Heart and respiratory diseases usually cause an increased number of respirations per minute.

Abnormal Respirations

Normal respirations occur between 14 and 20 times per minute in the adult. They are quiet, effortless, and regular. Both sides of the chest rise and fall equally. You should know the following abnormal respiratory patterns:

1. *Tachypnea*—rapid (tachy) breathing (pnea); the respiratory rate is usually greater than 24 respirations per minute
2. *Bradypnea*—slow (brady) breathing (pnea); the respiratory rate is less than 10 respirations per minute
3. *Apnea*—the lack or absence (a) of breathing (pnea)
4. *Hypoventilation*—respirations that are slow (hypo), shallow, and sometimes irregular
5. *Hyperventilation*—respirations that are rapid (hyper) and deeper than normal
6. *Dyspnea*—difficult, labored, or painful (dys) breathing (pnea)
7. *Cheyne-Stokes*—a breathing pattern in which respirations gradually increase in rate and depth and then become shallow and slow; breathing may stop (apnea) for 10 to 20 seconds

Counting Respirations

Respirations are counted when the patient is at rest. The patient should be positioned so that you can see the chest rise and fall. The depth and rate of breathing can be voluntarily controlled to a certain extent. People tend to change breathing patterns when they know their respirations are being counted. Therefore the patient should be unaware that the respirations are being counted.

Respirations are counted right after taking a pulse. The fingers or stethoscope stay over the pulse site. The patient assumes that the pulse is still being taken. Respirations are counted by watching the rise and fall of the chest. They are counted for 30 seconds. The number is multiplied by 2 for the total number of respirations in 1 minute. If an abnormal pattern is noted, the respirations are counted for 1 full minute.

BLOOD PRESSURE

Blood pressure is the amount of force exerted against the walls of an artery by the blood. Blood pressure is controlled by the force of heart contractions, the amount of blood pumped with each heartbeat, and how easily the blood flows through the blood vessels. The period of heart muscle contraction is called *systole*. The period of heart muscle relaxation is called *diastole*.

Both the systolic and diastolic pressures are measured. The *systolic pressure* is the higher pressure. It represents the amount of force needed to pump blood

COUNTING THE PATIENT'S RESPIRATIONS

1 Continue to hold the wrist after taking the radial pulse. Keep the stethoscope in place if you took an apical pulse.
2 Do not tell the patient you are counting respirations.
3 Begin counting when the chest rises. Count each rise and fall of the chest as 1 respiration.
4 Observe if respirations are regular and if both sides of the chest rise equally. Also note the depth of respirations and if the patient has any pain or difficulty in breathing.
5 Count respirations for 30 seconds. Multiply the number by 2. Count an infant's respirations for 1 minute.
6 Count an adult's respirations for 1 full minute if they are abnormal or irregular.
7 Record the patient's name, respiratory rate, and other observations.
8 Make sure the patient is comfortable and the signal light is within reach.
9 Wash your hands.
10 Report the following to the nurse:
   a The respiratory rate
   b Equality and depth of respirations
   c If the respirations were regular or irregular
   d If the patient experienced pain or difficulty in breathing
   e Any respiratory noises
   f Any abnormal respiratory patterns
11 Record the respiratory rate in the proper place.

out of the heart into the arterial circulation. The *diastolic pressure* is the lower pressure. It reflects the pressure in the arteries when the heart is at rest. Blood pressure is measured in millimeters (mm) of mercury (Hg). The systolic pressure is recorded over the diastolic pressure. The average adult has a systolic pressure of 120 mm Hg and a diastolic pressure of 80 mm Hg. This is written as 120/80 mm Hg.

Factors That Affect Blood Pressure

Blood pressure is affected by many factors and can change from minute to minute. Age, sex, the amount of blood in the system, and emotions affect blood pressure. Pain, exercise, body size, and medications also have an effect. Because it can vary so easily, blood pressure has normal ranges. Systolic pressures between 100 and 150 mm Hg are considered normal. Normal diastolic pressures are between 60 and 90 mm Hg.

Persistent measurements above the normal systolic and diastolic pressures are abnormal. This condition is known as *hypertension*. Report any systolic pressure above 150 mm Hg to the nurse immediately. A diastolic pressure above 90 mm Hg also must be reported immediately. Likewise, systolic pressures below 100 mm Hg and diastolic pressures below 60 mm Hg are

reported. This is called *hypotension*. Some people normally have low blood pressures. However, hypotension is a sign of a serious condition that can lead to death if it is not corrected.

Equipment

A stethoscope and a sphygmomanometer are used to measure blood pressure. The *sphygmomanometer* (blood pressure cuff) consists of a cuff and a measuring device. There are three types of sphygmomanometers: aneroid, mercury (Fig. 17-22), and electronic. The aneroid type has a round dial and a needle that points to the calibrations. The aneroid manometer is small and easy to carry. The mercury manometer is more accurate than the aneroid type. The mercury type has a column of mercury within a calibrated tube. Many facilities have wall-mounted mercury sphygmomanometers in patient rooms.

The blood pressure cuff is wrapped around the upper arm. Tubing connects the cuff to the manometer. Another tube connects the cuff to a small handheld bulb. A valve on the bulb is turned to allow inflation of the cuff as the bulb is squeezed. The inflated cuff causes pressure over the brachial artery. The valve is turned in the opposite direction for cuff deflation. Blood pressure is measured as the cuff is deflated.

Sounds are produced as blood flows through the arteries. The stethoscope is used to hear the sounds in the brachial artery as the cuff is deflated. Stethoscopes are not needed with electronic sphygmomanometers.

There are many types of electronic sphygmomanometers (Fig. 17-23). The systolic and diastolic blood pressures are displayed on the front of the instrument. The pulse is usually displayed also. The cuff automatically inflates and deflates on some models. Others have automatic deflation only. If elec-

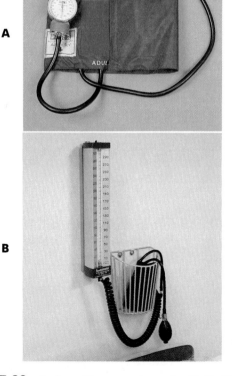

Fig. 17-22 **A,** Aneroid manometer and cuff. **B,** Mercury manometer and cuff.

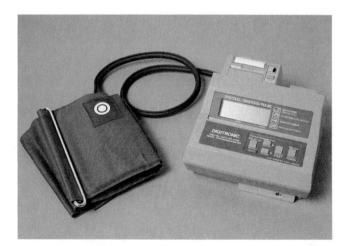

Fig. 17-23 Electronic sphygmomanometer.

tronic blood pressure equipment is used where you work, you need to learn how to use the equipment. Ask the nurse to show you what to do. The manufacturer's instructions are also helpful.

Measuring Blood Pressure

Blood pressure is normally measured in the brachial artery. You should practice the following guidelines when measuring blood pressure.

1. Blood pressure is not taken on an arm with an IV infusion or a cast, or on an injured arm. If a patient has had breast surgery, blood pressure is not taken on that side.
2. Let the patient rest for about 15 minutes before measuring the blood pressure.
3. The cuff is applied to the bare upper arm; it is not applied over clothing. Clothing can affect the measurement.
4. The diaphragm of the stethoscope is placed firmly over the artery. The entire diaphragm must be in contact with the skin.
5. The room should be quiet so that the blood

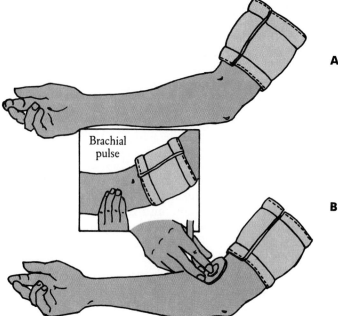

Fig. 17-24 A, The cuff is over the brachial artery. **B,** The diaphragm of the stethoscope is over the brachial artery.

MEASURING BLOOD PRESSURE

1 Collect the following equipment:
  a Sphygmomanometer (blood pressure cuff)
  b Stethoscope
  c Alcohol wipes
2 Wash your hands.
3 Identify the patient. Check the ID bracelet and call the patient by name.
4 Explain the procedure to the patient.
5 Provide for privacy.
6 Wipe the stethoscope earpieces and diaphragm with alcohol wipes.
7 Have the patient sit or lie down.
8 Position the patient's arm so that it is level with the heart. The palm should be up.
9 Stand no more than 3 feet away from the sphygmomanometer. A mercury model should be vertical, on a flat surface, and at eye level. The aneroid type should be directly in front of you.
10 Expose the upper arm.
11 Squeeze the cuff to expel any remaining air. Close the valve on the bulb.
12 Find the brachial artery at the inner aspect of the elbow.
13 Place the arrow on the cuff over the brachial artery (Fig. 17-24, *A*). Wrap the cuff around the upper arm at least 1 inch above the elbow. It should be even and snug.
14 Place the stethoscope earpieces in your ears.

15 Locate the radial artery. Inflate the cuff until you can no longer feel the pulse. Inflate the cuff 30 mm Hg beyond the point at which you last felt the pulse.
16 Position the diaphragm over the brachial artery (Fig. 17-24, *B*).
17 Deflate the cuff at an even rate of 2 to 4 millimeters per second. Turn the valve counterclockwise to deflate the cuff.
18 Note the point on the scale where you hear the first sound. This is the systolic reading. It should be near the point where the radial pulse disappeared.
19 Continue to deflate the cuff. Note the point where the sound disappears for the diastolic reading.
20 Deflate the cuff completely. Remove it from the patient's arm. Remove the stethoscope.
21 Record the patient's name and blood pressure.
22 Return the cuff to the case or wall holder.
23 Make sure the patient is comfortable and the signal light is within reach.
24 Unscreen the patient.
25 Clean the earpieces and diaphragm with alcohol wipes.
26 Return the equipment to its proper place.
27 Wash your hands.
28 Report the blood pressure. Record it in the proper place.

pressure can be heard. Talking, television, radio, and sounds from the hallway can interfere with an accurate measurement.

6. The sphygmomanometer must be clearly visible.
7. The radial artery is located, and the cuff is inflated. When the radial pulse is no longer felt, the cuff is inflated an additional 30 mm Hg. This prevents cuff inflation to an unnecessarily high pressure, which is painful to the patient.
8. The point at which the radial pulse is no longer felt is where you should expect to hear the first blood pressure sound. The first sound is the systolic pressure. The point where the sound disappears is the diastolic pressure.

SUMMARY

Temperature, pulse, respirations, and blood pressure give valuable information about a person's state of health or illness. Vital signs can vary within certain normal ranges. Changes above or below the normal range signal a disorder or serious illness. Vital signs can change in response to the slightest change in body functions. Therefore they are a part of routine physical examinations and are taken several times a day for hospitalized patients.

Measuring vital signs is a very important part of your job. Vital signs must be accurately measured. Any abnormal measurements are immediately reported to the nurse. They could signal serious threats to the patient's life. Clear and accurate recording of vital signs is equally important. Doctors and nurses use them to decide on treatment and to evaluate care.

REVIEW QUESTIONS

Circle the best *answer.*

1 Which statement is *false?*
   a The vital signs are temperature, pulse, respirations, and blood pressure.
   b Vital signs detect changes in body function.
   c Vital signs change only when a person is ill.
   d Sleep, exercise, medications, emotions, and noise affect vital signs.
2 Which temperature should you report immediately?
   a An oral temperature of 98.4° F
   b A rectal temperature of 101.6° F
   c An axillary temperature of 97.6° F
   d An oral temperature of 99.0° F
3 Electronic thermometers measure temperatures in
   a 2 to 60 seconds
   b 45 seconds
   c 2 to 3 minutes
   d 8 to 9 minutes
4 A rectal temperature is *not* taken when the patient
   a Is unconscious
   b Is an infant
   c Has a nasogastric tube
   d Has had rectal surgery
5 Which gives the most accurate measurement of body temperature?
   a Oral temperature
   b Rectal temperature
   c Axillary temperature
   d An electronic thermometer

6 Which is usually used to take a pulse?
   a The radial pulse
   b The apical-radial pulse
   c The apical pulse
   d The brachial pulse
7 Which is reported to the nurse immediately?
   a An adult has a pulse of 120 beats per minute
   b An infant has a pulse of 130 beats per minute
   c An adult has a pulse of 80 beats per minute
   d All of the above
8 Which statement about apical-radial pulses is *true?*
   a The pulse can be taken by one person.
   b The radial pulse can be greater than the apical pulse.
   c The apical pulse can be greater than the radial pulse.
   d The apical and radial pulses are always equal.
9 Normal respirations are
   a Between 14 and 20 per minute
   b Quiet and effortless
   c Regular with both sides of the chest rising and falling equally
   d All of the above
10 Difficult, painful, or labored breathing is known as
   a Tachypnea
   b Bradypnea
   c Apnea
   d Dyspnea
11 Respirations are usually counted
   a After taking the temperature

b After taking the pulse
c Before taking the pulse
d After taking the blood pressure
12 Which blood pressure is normal?
a 88/54 mm Hg
b 210/100 mm Hg
c 130/82 mm Hg
d 152/90 mm Hg
13 When taking a blood pressure, you should do the following *except*
a Take the blood pressure in the arm with an IV infusion
b Apply the cuff to a bare upper arm
c Turn off the television and radio
d Locate the brachial artery
14 Which is the systolic blood pressure?
a The point at which the pulse is no longer felt
b The point where the first sound is heard
c The point where the last sound is heard
d The point 30 mm Hg above where the pulse was felt

Answers

	10 d	5 b
14 b	9 d	4 d
13 a	8 c	3 a
12 c	7 a	2 b
11 b	6 a	1 c

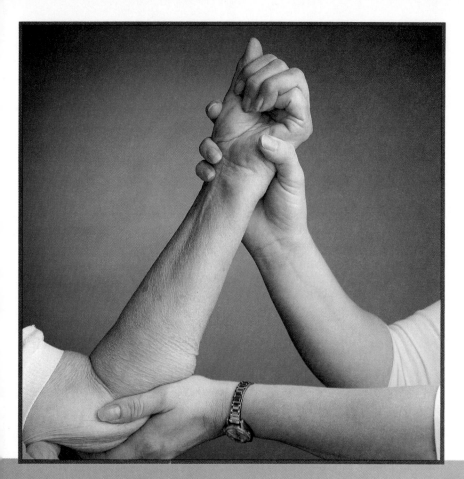

Exercise and Activity

18

abduction Moving a body part away from the body

adduction Moving a body part toward the body

atrophy A decrease in size or a wasting away of tissue

contracture The abnormal shortening of a muscle

dorsiflexion Bending backward

extension Straightening of a body part

external rotation Turning the joint outward

flexion Bending a body part

footdrop Plantar flexion

hyperextension Excessive straightening of a body part

internal rotation Turning the joint inward

plantar flexion The foot is bent; footdrop

pronation Turning downward

range of motion The movement of a joint to the extent possible without causing pain

supination Turning upward

Being active is important for physical and psychological well-being. Ideally, we can move about and function without help. However, illnesses, surgery, and injuries result in weakness and some degree of activity limitation. Some people are tired and weak. Others are confined to bed for a long time. Inactivity, whether minimal or severe, can affect the normal function of every body system.

Nursing personnel are responsible for promoting exercise and activity in all patients to the degree possible. The nurse will tell you about a patient's activity level and what exercises to perform. To effectively assist in promoting exercise and activity, you need to understand certain concepts. You need to understand bed rest and how to prevent the complications of bed rest. You also need to know how to help patients exercise.

BED REST

Bed rest has many meanings. The person on bed rest may be allowed to participate in activities of daily living (ADL). Bathing, oral hygiene, hair care, and feeding may be allowed. If "strict" or "absolute" bed rest is ordered, everything is done for the patient. The patient is not allowed to perform any activities of daily living.

Bed rest may be ordered by the doctor because of a person's health problem. It may also be a nursing measure because of a person's apparent helplessness. You must know the activities that are allowed for each person on bed rest. The nurse will provide this information.

The Complications of Bed Rest

Bed rest has many useful purposes. The person is allowed to rest and does not have to move about as usual. Pain is reduced, and healing is promoted. However, bed rest and the lack of exercise and activity can cause serious complications. Decubitus ulcers, constipation, and fecal impaction can result. Blood clots, urinary tract infections, and pneumonia (infection of the lung) can also occur. Contractures and muscle atrophy are other complications.

A *contracture* is the abnormal shortening of a muscle. The contracted muscle is fixed into position (Fig. 18-1), is permanently deformed, and cannot be stretched. The person is permanently deformed and disabled. Contractures must be prevented. *Atrophy* is the decrease in size or the wasting away of tissue. Muscle atrophy is a decrease in size or a wasting away of muscle (Fig. 18-2). These complications must be prevented so that normal body movement can occur.

Preventing the Complications of Bed Rest

The complications of bed rest can be prevented by good nursing care. You have an important role in preventing contractures and muscle atrophy. Positioning in good body alignment is essential. Performing range-of-motion exercises is another important preventive measure.

Positioning Body alignment and positioning were discussed in Chapter 10. Besides positioning the person in good body alignment, supportive devices may be necessary. They support and maintain the person in a particular position.

Bed boards. Bed boards are placed under the mattress. They keep the patient in better alignment by

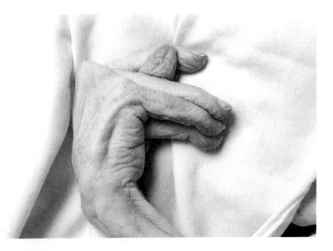

Fig. 18-1 A contracture.

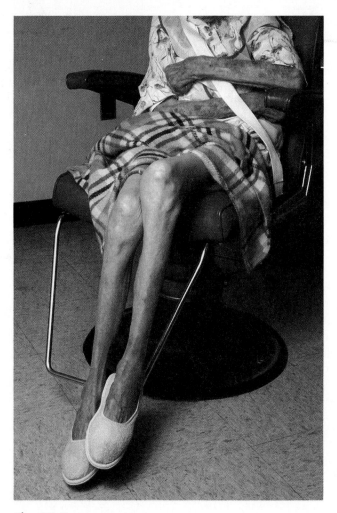

Fig. 18-2 Muscle atrophy.

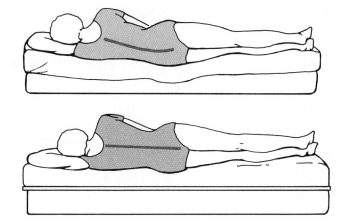

Fig. 18-3 **A**, Mattress sagging without bed boards. **B**, Bed boards are placed under the mattress. No sagging occurs.

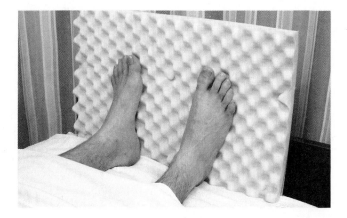

Fig. 18-4 Footboard. Feet are flush with the board to keep them in normal alignment.

preventing the mattress from sagging (Fig. 18-3). Bed boards are usually made of plywood and are covered with canvas or some other material. They are in two sections. One is for the head of the bed and the other for the foot. The two sections allow the head of the bed to be raised.

Footboards. A footboard (Fig. 18-4) is placed at the foot of the mattress to prevent *plantar flexion (footdrop)*. In plantar flexion the foot (plantar) is bent (flexion). The footboard is positioned so that the soles of the feet are flush against the footboard. The feet are in good body alignment as in the standing position. The footboard can be used as a bed cradle to keep top linens off of the feet.

Trochanter rolls. Trochanter rolls (Fig. 18-5) prevent the hips and legs from turning outward (external rotation). Bath blankets are used for trochanter rolls. The blanket is folded to the desired length and rolled up. The loose end is placed under the person from the hip to the knee. Then the roll is tucked alongside the body. Pillows or sandbags can also be used to keep the hips and knees in alignment.

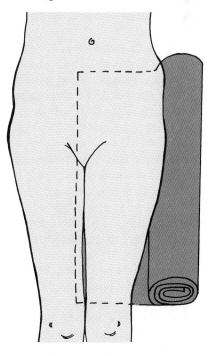

Fig. 18-5 Trochanter roll made from a bath blanket. It extends from the hip to the knee.

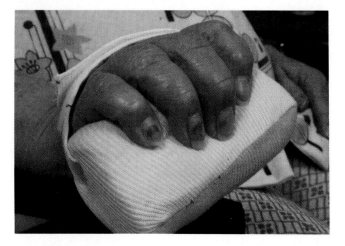

Fig. 18-6 Handroll.

Handrolls. The person can grasp a handroll to prevent contractures of the thumb, fingers, and wrist. Commercial handrolls are available (Fig. 18-6). One can be made by rolling up a washcloth (see Fig. 8-12). Foam rubber sponges and rubber balls can be used.

Bed cradles. The weight of linens on the foot can cause footdrop and decubiti. A bed cradle (see Fig. 13-41, p. 223) is often used to keep top linens off of the feet.

Exercise Exercise helps prevent contractures, muscle atrophy, and the other complications of bed rest. Some exercise occurs with activities of daily living and when turning and moving in bed without assistance. However, additional exercises are needed for muscles and joints.

Trapeze. A trapeze or trapeze bar is a swinging bar suspended from an overbed frame (see Fig. 25-10, page 397). The person grasps the bar with both hands to lift the trunk off the bed. The trapeze is also used to move up and turn in bed. If allowed, it can be used for pulling exercises to strengthen the arm muscles.

Range-of-motion exercises. The movement of a joint to the extent possible without causing pain is the *range of motion (ROM)* of that joint. Range-of-motion exercises involve exercising the joints through their complete range of motion. The exercises are done at least twice a day (b.i.d.). Range-of-motion exercises may be active, passive, or active-assistive. *Active* range-of-motion exercises are done by the person. *Passive* exercises involve having another person move the joints through their range of motion. *Active-assistive* range of motion is when the person does the exercises with some assistance from another person.

The following movements are involved in range-of-motion exercises:

Abduction—moving a body part away from the body
Adduction—moving a body part toward the body
Extension—straightening a body part
Flexion—bending a body part
Hyperextension—the excessive straightening of a body part
Dorsiflexion—bending backward
Rotation—turning the joint
Internal rotation—turning the joint inward
External rotation—turning the joint outward
Pronation—turning downward
Supination—turning upward

Range-of-motion exercises are done during activities of daily living. Patients on bed rest have few opportunities or cannot be active. Therefore range-of-motion exercises may be ordered. The nurse tells you which joints to exercise and if the exercises are to be active, passive, or active-assistive.

General rules. Range-of-motion exercises can cause injury if not performed properly. The following rules are practiced when performing or assisting with range-of-motion exercises.

1. Exercise only the joints that the nurse tells you to exercise.
2. Expose only the body part being exercised.
3. Use good body mechanics.
4. Support the extremity being exercised.
5. Move the joint slowly, smoothly, and gently.
6. Do not force a joint beyond its present range of motion or to the point of pain.

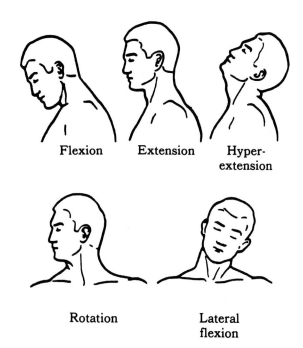

Fig. 18-7 Range-of-motion exercises for the neck.

PERFORMING RANGE-OF-MOTION EXERCISES

1 Identify the patient. Check the ID bracelet and call the patient by name.
2 Explain the procedure to the patient.
3 Wash your hands.
4 Obtain a bath blanket.
5 Provide for privacy.
6 Raise the bed to an appropriate level for good body mechanics.
7 Lower the side rails.
8 Position the patient supine and in good alignment.
9 Cover the patient with a bath blanket. Fanfold top linens to the foot of the bed.
10 Exercise the neck (Fig. 18-7):
   a Place your hands over the patient's ears to support the head.
   b Flexion—bring the head forward so that the chin touches the chest.
   c Extension—straighten the head.
   d Hyperextension—bring the head backward until the chin is pointing up.
   e Rotation—turn the head from side to side.
   f Lateral flexion—move the head to the right and to the left.
   g Repeat flexion, extension, hyperextension, rotation, and lateral flexion 5 to 6 times.
11 Exercise the shoulder (Fig. 18-8):
   a Grasp the wrist with one hand and the elbow with the other.
   b Flexion—raise the arm straight in front and over the head.
   c Extension—bring the arm down to the side.
   d Hyperextension—move the arm behind the body. (This can be done if the person is standing or sitting in a straight-backed chair.)
   e Abduction—move the straight arm away from the side of the body.
   f Adduction—move the straight arm to the side of the body.
   g Internal rotation—bend the elbow and place it at the same level as the shoulder. Move the forearm down toward the body.
   h External rotation—move the forearm toward the head.
   i Repeat flexion, extension, hyperextension, abduction, adduction, and internal and external rotation 5 to 6 times.

12 Exercise the elbow (Fig. 18-9):
   a Grasp the patient's wrist with one hand and the elbow with the other.
   b Flexion—bend the arm so that the same-side shoulder is touched.
   c Extension—straighten the arm.
   d Repeat flexion and extension 5 to 6 times.
13 Exercise the forearm (Fig. 18-10):
   a Pronation—turn the hand so that the palm is down.
   b Supination—turn the hand so that the palm is up.
   c Repeat pronation and supination 5 to 6 times.
14 Exercise the wrist (Fig. 18-11):
   a Hold the wrist with both of your hands.
   b Flexion—bend the hand down.
   c Extension—straighten the hand.
   d Hyperextension—bend the hand back.
   e Radial flexion—turn the hand toward the thumb.
   f Ulnar flexion—turn the hand toward the little finger.
   g Repeat flexion, extension, hyperextension, and radial and ulnar flexion 5 to 6 times.
15 Exercise the thumb (Fig. 18-12):
   a Hold the patient's hand with one hand and the thumb with your other hand.
   b Abduction—move the thumb out from the inner part of the index finger.
   c Adduction—move the thumb back next to the index finger.
   d Opposition—touch each fingertip with the thumb.
   e Flexion—bend thumb into hand.
   f Extension—move the thumb out to the side of the fingers.
   g Repeat flexion, extension, abduction, adduction, and opposition 5 to 6 times.
16 Exercise the fingers (Fig. 18-13):
   a Abduction—spread the fingers and the thumb apart.
   b Adduction—bringing the fingers and thumb together.
   c Extension—straighten the fingers so that the fingers, hand, and arm are straight.
   d Flexion—make a fist.
   e Repeat abduction, adduction, extension, and flexion 5 to 6 times.

NOTE: Figs. 18-7 to 18-18 are taken from Phipps WJ, Long BC, and Woods NF: *Medical-surgical nursing: concepts and clinical practice,* ed 2, St Louis, 1987, Mosby–Year Book.

Continued.

PERFORMING RANGE-OF-MOTION EXERCISES—cont'd

17   Exercise the hip (Fig. 18-14):
   a   Place one hand under the knee and the other under the ankle to support the leg.
   b   Flexion—raise the leg.
   c   Extension—straighten the leg.
   d   Abduction—move the leg away from the body.
   e   Adduction—move the leg toward the other leg.
   f   Internal rotation—turn the leg inward.
   g   External rotation—turn the leg outward.
   h   Repeat flexion, extension, abduction, adduction, and inward and outward rotation 5 to 6 times.

18   Exercise the knee (Fig. 18-15):
   a   Place one hand under the knee and the other under the ankle to support the leg.
   b   Flexion—bend the leg.
   c   Extension—straighten the leg.
   d   Repeat flexion and extension of the knee 5 to 6 times.

19   Exercise the ankle (Fig. 18-16):
   a   Place one hand under the foot and the other under the ankle to support the part.
   b   Dorsiflexion—pull the foot forward and push down on the heel at the same time.
   c   Plantar flexion—turn the foot down or point the toes.
   d   Repeat dorsal flexion and plantar flexion 5 to 6 times.

20   Exercise the foot (Fig. 18-17):
   a   Pronation—turn the outside of the foot up and the inside down.
   b   Supination—turn the inside of the foot up and the outside down.
   c   Repeat pronation and supination 5 to 6 times.

21   Exercise the toes (Fig. 18-18):
   a   Flexion—curl the toes.
   b   Extension—straighten the toes.
   c   Abduction—pull the toes together.
   d   Adduction—spread the toes apart.
   e   Repeat flexion, extension, abduction, and adduction 5 to 6 times.

22   Cover the leg and raise the side rail.
23   Go to the other side. Lower the side rail.
24   Repeat steps 11 through 21.
25   Make sure the patient is comfortable.
26   Cover the patient. Remove the bath blanket.
27   Raise the side rail.
28   Lower the bed to its lowest level.
29   Place the signal light within reach.
30   Unscreen the patient.
31   Return the bath blanket to its proper place.
32   Wash your hands.
33   Report the following to the nurse:
   a   The time the exercises were performed
   b   The joints that were exercised
   c   The number of times the exercises were performed on each joint
   d   Any complaints of pain or signs of stiffness or spasm
   e   The degree to which the patient participated in the exercises

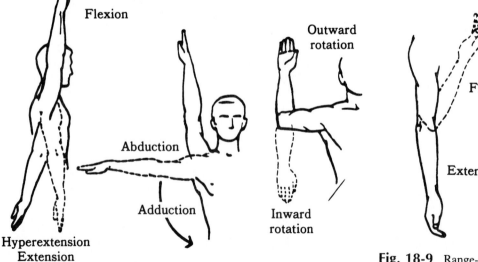

Fig. 18-8   Range-of-motion exercises for the shoulder.

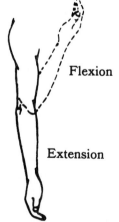

Fig. 18-9   Range-of-motion exercises for the elbow.

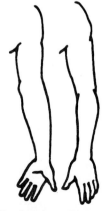

Fig. 18-10   Range-of-motion exercises for the forearm.

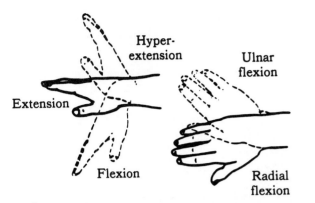

Fig. 18-11 Range-of-motion exercises for the wrist.

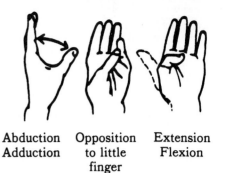

Fig. 18-12 Range-of-motion exercises for the thumb.

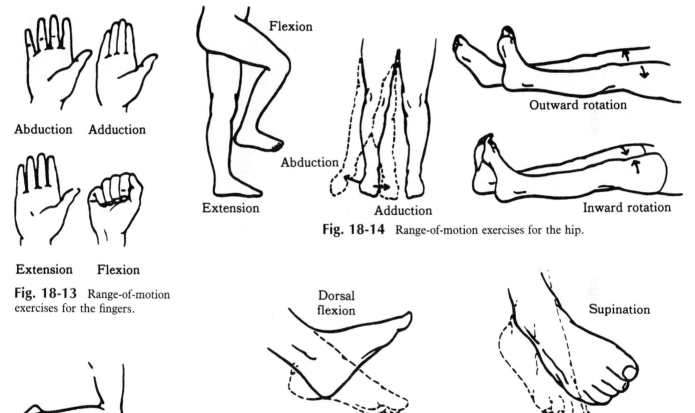

Fig. 18-13 Range-of-motion exercises for the fingers.

Fig. 18-14 Range-of-motion exercises for the hip.

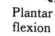

Fig. 18-15 Range-of-motion exercises for the knee.

Fig. 18-16 Range-of-motion exercises for the ankle.

Fig. 18-17 Range-of-motion exercises for the foot.

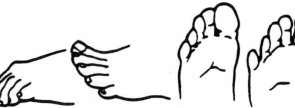

Flexion   Extension   Adduction   Abduction

Fig. 18-18 Range-of-motion exercises for the toes.

AMBULATION

Most patients on bed rest are able to increase activity. Activity is increased slowly and in steps. First the person dangles (sits on the side of the bed). The next step is to sit in a bedside chair. Next the person walks about in the room and then in the hallway. *Ambulation*, the act of walking, should not be a problem if complications have been prevented. Contractures and muscle atrophy are prevented by proper positioning and exercise.

Patients may be weak and unsteady from bed rest, surgery, or injury. You need to help them begin to walk after bed rest or illness. Use a gait (transfer or safety) belt if the person is weak or unsteady. For additional support, the person can use the hand rails along the wall.

The Falling Patient

Patients may begin to fall when standing or walking. They may be weak, lightheaded, or dizzy. Fainting may occur. Falling may be due to slipping or sliding on spills, waxed floors, throw rugs, or improper shoes (see Chapter 8). When a person is falling, there is a tendency to try to prevent the fall. However, trying to prevent a fall could cause greater harm. Twisting and straining to stop the fall could cause injuries to

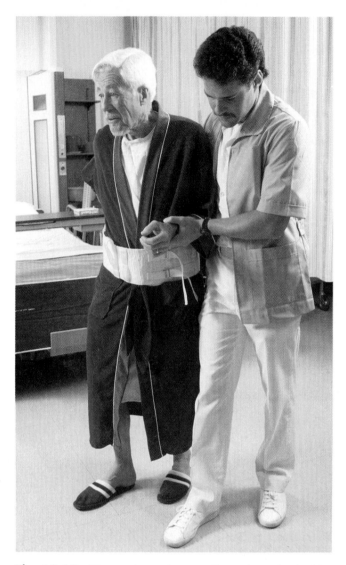

Fig. 18-19 The nursing assistant walks at the patient's side. A transfer (safety) belt is used for the patient's safety.

HELPING THE FALLING PATIENT

1 Stand with your feet apart. Keep your back straight.
2 Bring the patient close to your body as quickly as possible. Use the gait belt if one is worn. If not, wrap your arms around the patient's waist. You can also hold the patient under the arms (Fig. 18-20).
3 Move your leg so that the patient's buttocks rest on it (Fig. 18-21). Move the leg near the patient.
4 Lower the patient to the floor. Let him or her slide down your leg to the floor (Fig. 18-22). Bend at your hips and knees as you lower the patient.

5 Call a nurse to check the patient.
6 Help the nurse return the patient to bed. Get other workers to help if necessary.
7 Report the following to the nurse:
  a What time the patient got up
  b The patient's pulse before getting out of bed
  c How far the patient walked
  d How activity was tolerated before the fall
  e Any complaints before the fall
  f The amount of assistance needed by the patient while walking

HELPING THE PATIENT TO WALK

1 Explain the procedure to the patient.
2 Wash your hands.
3 Collect the following equipment:
   a Robe and shoes
   b Paper or sheet to protect bottom linens
   c Transfer (gait or safety) belt
4 Identify the patient. Check the ID bracelet and call the patient by name.
5 Provide for privacy.
6 Move furniture if necessary to allow moving space for you and the patient.
7 Lower the bed to its lowest position. Lock the bed wheels.
8 Fanfold top linens to the foot of the bed.
9 Place the paper or sheet under the patient's feet. This protects the bottom sheet from the shoes. Put the shoes on the patient.
10 Help the patient to dangle. (See *Helping the Patient to Sit on the Side of the Bed*, page 157.)
11 Help the patient put on the robe.
12 Apply the transfer belt. (See *Applying a Transfer [Gait] Belt*, page 159.)
13 Assist the patient to a standing position:
   a Stand so that you face the patient.
   b Have the patient place his or her hands on your shoulders.
   c Grasp the transfer belt at each side.
   d Brace your knees against the patient's knees. Block his or her feet with your feet (see Fig. 10-25).
   e Pull the patient up into a standing position as you straighten your knees (see Fig. 10-26).
14 Stand at the patient's side while he or she gains balance. Do not let go of the transfer belt. Grasp the belt at the side and back.
15 Encourage the patient to stand erect with the head up and back straight.
16 Assist the patient to walk. Walk at his or her side and provide support with the transfer belt (Fig. 18-19).

17 Encourage the patient to walk normally. The heel of the foot strikes the floor first. Discourage shuffling, sliding, or walking on tiptoes.
18 Walk the required distance if the patient can tolerate the activity. Do not rush the patient.
19 Help the patient return to bed:
   a Have the patient stand at the side of the bed.
   b Pivot him or her a quarter turn. The backs of the knees should touch the bed.
   c Have the patient place his or her hands on your shoulders. Grasp the sides of the transfer belt.
   d Lower the patient onto the bed as you bend your knees. Remove the transfer belt and robe.
   e Help the patient lie down. (See *Helping the Patient to Sit on the Side of the Bed*, page 157.)
20 Lower the head of the bed. Help the patient to the center of the bed.
21 Remove the shoes and the paper or sheet over the bottom sheet.
22 Make sure the patient is comfortable. Cover the patient.
23 Place the signal light within reach. Raise the side rails.
24 Return the robe and shoes to their proper place.
25 Return furniture to its proper location.
26 Unscreen the patient.
27 Wash your hands.
28 Report the following to the nurse:
   a How well the patient tolerated the activity
   b The distance walked

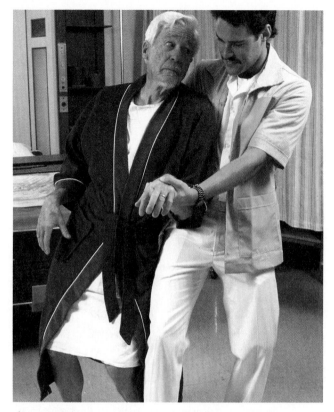

Fig. 18-20 Support the falling patient by holding the patient under the arms.

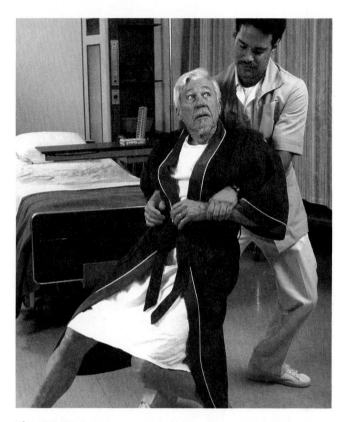

Fig. 18-21 The patient's buttocks are on the orderly's leg.

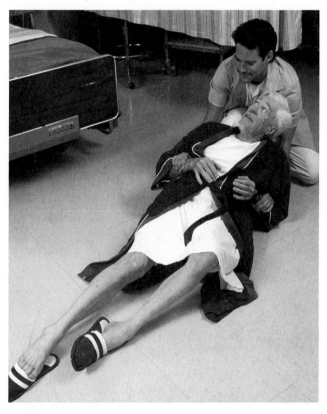

Fig. 18-22 The textbent is eased to the floor on the orderly's leg.

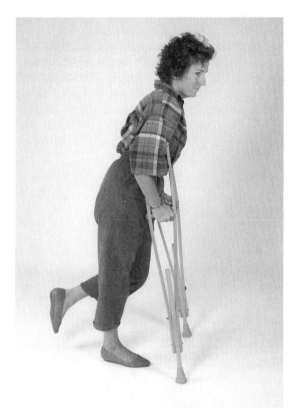

Fig. 18-23 A person using crutches.

yourself and the patient. Head injuries are common from falls. Balance is lost as a person is falling. If you try to prevent the fall, you could lose your balance. Thus both you and the patient could fall or cause the other person to fall.

If a patient begins to fall, ease him or her to the floor. This lets you control the direction of the fall. You can also protect the patient's head.

Walking Aids

Walkings aids support the body. They are ordered by the doctor. The type ordered depends on the person's physical condition, the amount of support needed, and the type of disability. The physical therapist or nurse teaches the patient to use the walking aid. It may be needed temporarily or permanently.

Crutches Crutches (Fig. 18-23) are used when the person cannot use one leg or when one or both legs need to gain strength. Some patients with permanent leg weakness are able to use crutches.

Safety must be considered when crutches are used. The person on crutches is at risk of falling. Though crutches provide support, certain safety measures must be followed.

1. The crutches must fit. The person is measured and fitted with crutches by a nurse or physical therapist. If they do not fit properly, the person may fall and suffer further injury. The person is also at risk for back pain, nerve damage, and injuries to the underarms and palms.
2. Crutch tips must be attached to the crutches. They must not be worn down or wet.
3. Crutches are checked for flaws. Wooden crutches are checked for cracks, and aluminum crutches are checked for bends. Bolts on both types must be tight.
4. Street shoes are worn. They should be flat and have non-skid soles.
5. Clothes must fit well. Loose clothing may get caught between the crutches and underarms. Clothing that is loose can also hang forward and block the person's view of the feet and crutch tips.
6. Safety rules to prevent falls must be followed (see Chapter 8).

Canes Canes are used when there is weakness on one side of the body. They help provide balance and support. There are single-tipped canes and canes with three and four points (Fig. 18-24). A cane is held on the strong side of the body. (If the left leg is weak, the cane is held in the right hand.) Three-point and four-point canes give more support than single-tipped canes. However, they are harder to move.

The tip of the cane should be about 6 to 10 inches (15 to 25 cm) to the side of the foot. The grip is level

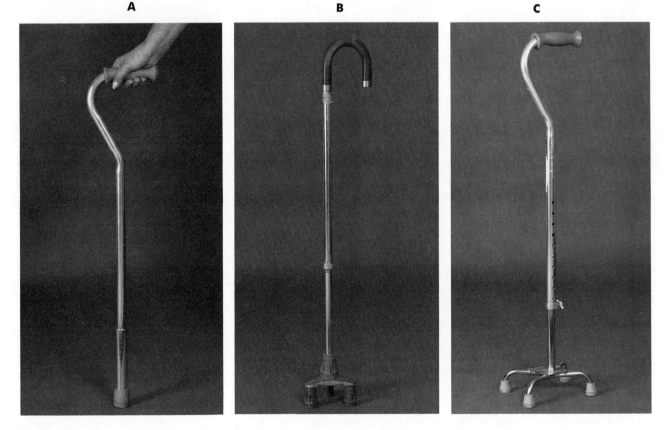

Fig. 18-24 **A,** Single-tipped cane. **B,** Tri-pod cane. **C,** Four-point (quad) cane.

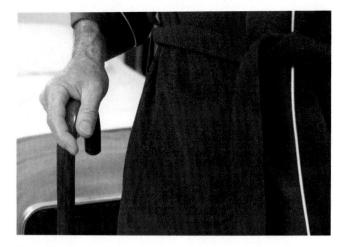

Fig. 18-25 The cane grip is held level with the hip.

with the hip (Fig. 18-25). When the patient walks, the cane is moved first. It is moved forward about 12 inches (Fig. 18-26, *A*). The weak leg (opposite the cane) is then moved forward even with the cane (Fig. 18-26, *B*). Then the strong leg is brought forward and ahead of the cane and the weak leg (Fig. 18-26, *C*).

Walkers A walker is a four-point walking aid (Fig. 18-27). It gives more support than a cane. Many people feel safer and more secure with a walker than with a cane. There are many kinds of walkers. The standard walker is picked up and moved about 6 inches in front of the person. The person then moves the right foot and then the left foot up to the walker (Fig. 18-28).

Baskets, pouches, and trays can be attached to walkers (Fig. 18-29). The attachments allow people to carry needed items rather than rely on others to do so. This allows greater independence. The attachment also keeps the hands free to grip the walker.

Braces Braces support weak body parts. They are also used to prevent or correct deformities or to prevent the movement of a joint. Metal, plastic, or leather may be used for braces. A brace is applied over the ankle, knee, or back (Fig. 18-30). An ankle-foot orthosis (AFO) is positioned in the shoe (Fig. 18-31). Then the foot is inserted. The device is secured in place with the Velcro calf strap. Bony points under braces must be protected, or skin breakdown can occur.

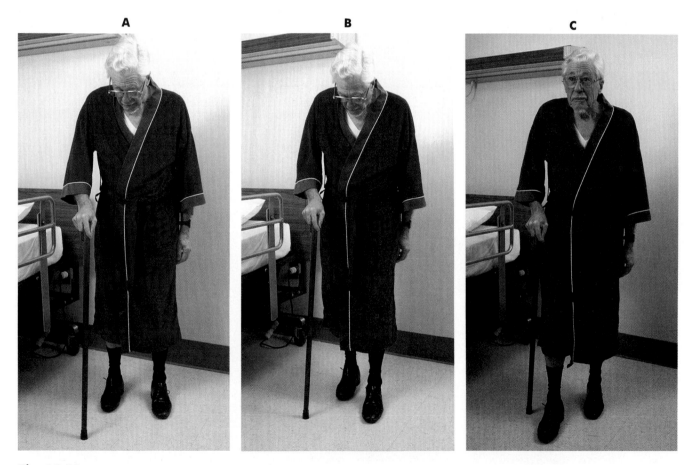

A **B** **C**

Fig. 18-26 Walking with a cane. **A,** The cane is moved forward about 1 foot. **B,** The leg opposite the cane (weak leg) is brought forward even with the cane. **C,** The leg on the cane side (strong leg) is moved ahead of the cane and the weak leg.

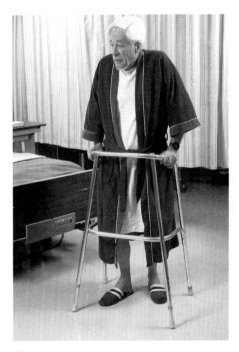

Fig. 18-27   A walker.

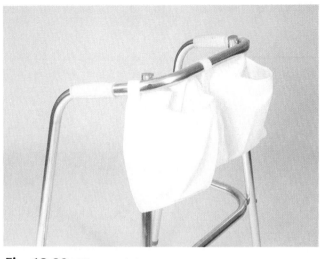

Fig. 18-29   The pouch is a walker attachment.

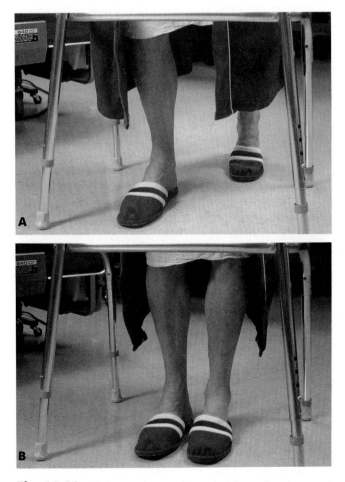

Fig. 18-28   Walking with a walker. **A,** The walker is moved about 6 inches in front of the patient. **B,** Both feet are moved up to the walker.

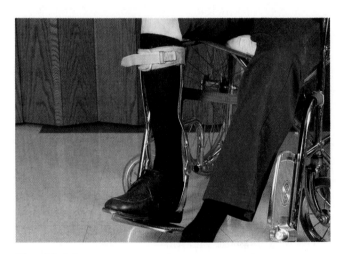

Fig. 18-30   Leg brace.

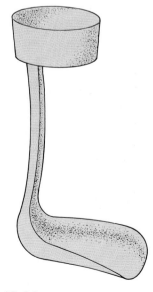

Fig. 18-31   Ankle-foot orthosis (AFO).

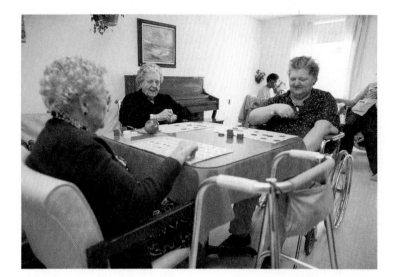

Fig. 18-32 Recreational activities are important for the elderly.

RECREATIONAL ACTIVITIES

Recreational activities are important for the elderly, both physically and psychologically. Joints and muscles are exercised, and circulation is stimulated. Recreational activities also provide social opportunities and are mentally stimulating (Fig. 18-32).

Bingo, movies, dances, exercise groups, shopping trips, museum trips, concerts, and guest speakers are often arranged by nursing facilities. Some facilities arrange fashion shows, have gourmet meal nights and family cook-outs, and provide gardening activities. Grade school and high school music groups often perform in nursing facilities.

Residents may require help getting to an activity. Some also need help in participating. You must provide assistance as necessary.

SUMMARY

Exercise and activity are necessary for physical and psychological well-being. Complications from a lack of activity or exercise can occur when a person is confined to bed. You will position and exercise patients. Exercises prevent the complications of bed rest, especially muscle atrophy and contractures. Muscle atrophy can make ambulation difficult. A contracture results in loss of function and movement of the body part. A leg contracture may make normal ambulation impossible. Supportive devices and range-of-motion exercises also help prevent muscle atrophy and contractures.

Most patients eventually ambulate after illness, surgery, or injury. A weak patient may need some assistance with walking at first. Some people need walking aids on a permanent or temporary basis. Doctors may prescribe crutches, canes, walkers, or braces.

REVIEW QUESTIONS

Circle the best answer.

1 Which statement about bed rest is *false?*
   a Persons on bed rest are never allowed to perform activities of daily living.
   b Bed rest helps reduce pain and promotes healing.
   c Complications of bed rest include decubiti, constipation, fecal impaction, blood clots, urinary infections, and pneumonia.
   d Contractures and muscle atrophy can occur.

2 Which helps to prevent plantar flexion?
   a Bed boards
   b A footboard
   c Trochanter rolls
   d Handrolls

3 Which prevents the hip from turning outward?
   a Bed boards
   b A footboard
   c Trochanter roll
   d Handroll

4 A trapeze can be used to
  a Lift the trunk off the bed
  b Move up or turn in bed
  c Strengthen arm muscles
  d All of the above

5 Passive range-of-motion exercises are performed by
  a The patient
  b A health team member
  c The patient with the assistance of another
  d The patient with the use of a trapeze

6 To safely perform ROM exercises, you should do the following *except*
  a Support the extremity being exercised
  b Move the joint slowly, smoothly, and gently
  c Force the joint through full range of motion
  d Exercise only the joints indicated by the nurse

7 Flexion involves
  a Bending the body part
  b Straightening the body part
  c Moving the body part toward the body
  d Moving the body part away from the body

8 Which statement about ambulation is *false*?
  a A transfer belt is used if the patient is weak or unsteady.
  b The patient is allowed to shuffle or slide when beginning to walk after bed rest.
  c Walking aids may be needed permanently or temporarily.
  d Crutches, canes, walkers, and braces are common walking aids.

9 A single-tipped cane is used
  a At waist level
  b On the strong side
  c On the weak side
  d On either side

10 You are getting a patient ready to crutch walk. You should do the following *except*
  a Check the crutch tips
  b Have the patient wear street shoes
  c Get any pair of crutches from physical therapy
  d Tighten the bolts on the crutches

Circle T *if the answer is true and* F *if the answer is false.*

T F **11** A single-tipped cane and a four-point cane give equal support.
T F **12** When using a cane, the feet are moved first.
T F **13** A walker is moved in front of the patient. Then the right and left feet are moved.
T F **14** You feel a patient falling. You should try to prevent the fall.
T F **15** A patient has a brace. Bony areas need to be protected from skin breakdown.
T F **16** Recreational activities exercise only muscles and joints.

Answers

1	a	7	a
2	b	8	b
3	c	9	b
4	d	10	c
5	b	11	False
6	c	12	False
		13	True
		14	False
		15	True
		16	False

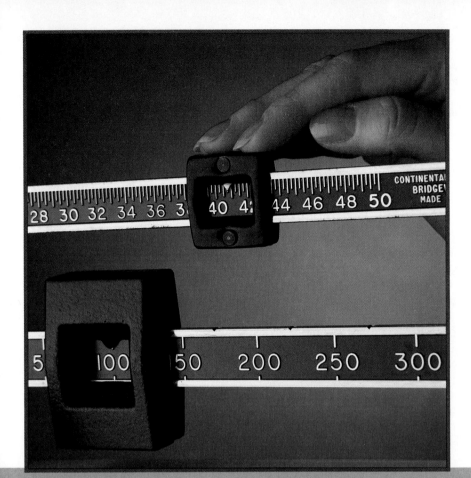

Admissions, Transfers, and Discharges

OBJECTIVES

19

- Describe what occurs in the admitting office
- Prepare the patient's room
- Explain how to admit a patient to the nursing unit
- Admit a patient to the nursing unit
- Measure height and weight
- Know how to handle the patient's clothing and valuables
- Dress and undress a patient
- Explain why a person may be transferred to another nursing unit
- Transfer a patient to another nursing unit
- Explain how a patient is prepared for discharge
- Discharge a patient

KEY TERMS

admission Official entry of a person into a facility or nursing unit
discharge Official departure of a patient from a facility or nursing unit
transfer Moving a patient from one room, nursing unit, or facility to another

Admission to a health care facility causes anxiety and fear. Patients and families may worry about the need for treatment or surgery and its outcome. They may be afraid that a serious health problem will be found. The fear of pain is very common. Never returning home is a common fear of many people admitted to nursing facilities. Many people are unfamiliar with health care facilities. They worry about where to go, what to expect, and the strange sights and sounds. Individuals may have similar concerns if transferred to another nursing unit. Discharge usually brings relief and happiness. However, the person may be going to another facility or may need home care.

Admission, transfer, and discharge are critical events for patients and families. They need to feel comfortable and secure. You must function competently and efficiently and show courtesy, kindness, and respect.

ADMISSIONS

Except in emergencies, the admission process begins in the admitting office. *Admission* is the official entry of a person into a facility or nursing unit. An admitting clerk or nurse obtains identifying information from the patient. This includes the person's full name, age, date of birth, doctor's name, social security number, and religion. The information is recorded on the admission record. The patient is given an identification number and an identification bracelet. A general consent for treatment is signed at this time.

Admitting office personnel notify the nursing unit that a new patient is being admitted. They tell the nursing staff what room and bed the patient will be in. The patient is taken to the nursing unit by admitting office personnel. Some facilities let patients walk to the nursing unit if they are able. Most require transport by wheelchair or stretcher.

Preparing the Room

The room must be ready for the new patient. This is usually the nursing assistant's responsibility. Figure 19-1 shows a room prepared for a patient's arrival.

Admitting the Patient

The patient is usually greeted and admitted by a nurse. However, this may be your responsibility if the patient is in no apparent discomfort or distress. The patient and the admission record are brought to the nursing unit by admitting office personnel. Use this record to find out the person's name. When you greet the person, call him or her by name. Be sure to introduce yourself by name and title. Also introduce yourself to family members who may be present (Fig. 19-2).

Admission procedures involve completing an admission checklist. The patient is weighed and measured, and a urine specimen is obtained. The patient is oriented to the room and told about the nursing unit and the facility.

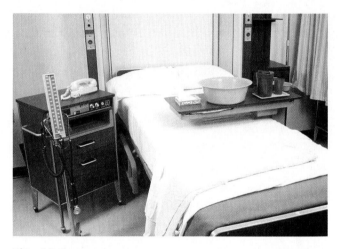

Fig. 19-1 The room is ready for a patient to be admitted.

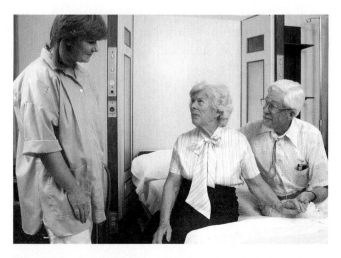

Fig. 19-2 The nursing assistant introduces herself to the patient and family member.

322

PREPARING THE PATIENT'S ROOM

1 Know which room and bed should be prepared. Find out if the person is arriving by wheelchair or stretcher.
2 Wash your hands.
3 Collect the following equipment:
   a Patient pack (contains bath basin, pitcher, cup, and personal care items)
   b Admission checklist
   c Urine specimen container
   d Sphygmomanometer
   e Stethoscope
   f Gown or pajamas
   g IV pole if indicated
4 Open the bed.
5 Lower the bed if the patient is ambulatory or arriving by wheelchair. Raise the bed to its highest level for a patient arriving by stretcher.
6 Attach the signal light to the bed linens.
7 Place the sphygmomanometer, stethoscope, and admission checklist on the overbed table.
8 Place the gown or pajamas on the bed.
9 Place the patient pack and specimen container on the bedside stand or overbed table.
10 Make sure a bedpan, emesis basin, and urinal (for a male) are in the bedside stand. Get missing equipment.
11 Wash your hands.

ADMITTING THE PATIENT—ADMISSION CHECKLIST

1 Wash your hands.
2 Prepare the room.
3 Greet the patient by name. Ask if he or she prefers a certain name.
4 Introduce yourself to the patient and relatives or friends who may be present. Explain that you are a nursing assistant and that you assist the staff nurses in giving care.
5 Introduce the patient to the roommate.
6 Call for a nurse immediately if the patient complains of any severe pain or appears to be in distress.
7 Proceed if the person's condition does not present an immediate or serious problem.
8 Provide for privacy. Ask family members or friends to leave the room. Tell them how long the procedure will take and where they can wait comfortably.
9 Have the person put on a gown or pajamas. Assist as indicated.
10 Make sure the patient is comfortable. He or she should be in bed or in a chair as directed by the nurse.
11 Hang clothes in the closet. Put personal items in the bedside stand and dresser drawers.
12 Complete the admission checklist (Fig. 19-3).
13 Complete a clothing and valuables list.
14 Explain activity limitations that have been ordered.
15 Explain that a urine specimen is needed and describe the procedure. Help the person to the bathroom or onto the bedpan.
16 Take the specimen to the nurses' desk. Clean the equipment.
17 Orient the patient to the new environment:
   a Give names of the head nurse and the primary nurse or team leader.
   b Identify equipment in the bedside stand. Explain the purpose of each item.
   c Demonstrate use of the call system.
   d Demonstrate how to operate the bed and television controls.
   e Explain how to make telephone calls and place the phone within reach.
   f Explain visiting hours and policies.
   g Describe the location of the nurses' station, lounge, chapel, dining room, gift shop, and other important areas.
   h Identify patient services: newspaper, library, diversional activities, educational programs, religious services, and others.
   i Identify other personnel who will be involved with the patient: workers from x-ray, laboratory, housekeeping, dietary, and physical therapy, as well as students and others.
   j Explain when meals and nourishments are served.
18 Fill the water pitcher if oral fluids are allowed.
19 Place the signal light within reach. Place other controls and equipment within reach.
20 Make sure the bed is in its lowest position and the side rails are up. Unscreen the patient.
21 Clean any used equipment. Discard used disposable items.
22 Take the urine specimen to the laboratory with the requisition slip. Wash your hands.
23 Provide a denture container if needed. Label it with the patient's name and room number.
24 Report your observations to the nurse.

Date:_____ Time:_____ Introduced: Self_____ Roommate_____

Admitted per: Wheelchair_____ Cart_____ Ambulatory_____ Carried by_____

Age:_____ Sex: M_____ F_____

Condition on admission:

Ambulatory ☐	Feeds self ☐	Admitted by ambulance ☐	Alert ☐
Semiambulatory ☐	Requires help with feeding ☐	From hospital ☐	Forgetful ☐
Chairridden ☐	Continent ☐	From home ☐	Confused ☐
Bedridden ☐	Incontinent ☐	From nursing home ☐	

State of consciousness: Alert_____ Confused_____ Semiconscious_____ Unconscious_____

Emotional state: Calm_____ Nervous_____ Fearful_____ Angry_____ Depressed_____

Pain: No_____ Yes_____ Where_____

Vital signs: BP_____ T_____ P_____ R_____ Ht_____ Wt_____

Glasses: Yes_____ No_____ Contact lenses: Yes_____ No_____ Hearing aid: Yes_____ No_____

Dentures: Yes_____ No_____ Artificial limb: Yes_____ No_____

Artificial eye: Yes_____ No_____ Right_____ Left_____ Pacemaker: Yes_____ No_____

Orientation to environment:

Call light_____ Emergency light_____ Bed controls_____ Bedside stand_____ Closet_____

Drawers_____ Bathroom_____ Mealtime_____ Visiting hours_____

Information obtained from: Patient_____ Spouse_____ Parent: M_____ F_____ Other_____

Other observations and comments:_____

_____

Show all body marks: scars, bruises, cuts, decubiti, ulcers, and discolorations (birth marks should not be shown).

Signed_____

Fig. 19-3 An admission checklist.

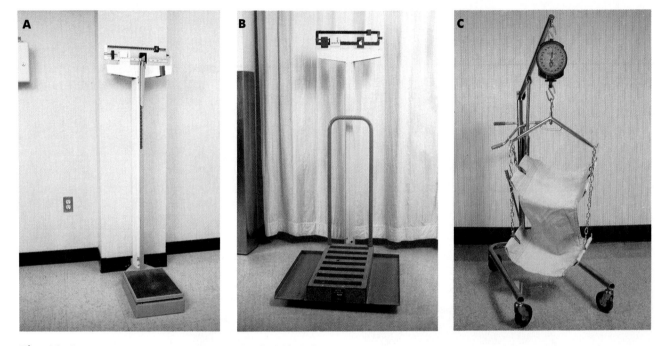

Fig. 19-4 **A,** Standing scale. **B,** Chair scale. **C,** Lift scale.

Measuring height and weight Height and weight are measured on admission. The person wears a gown or pajamas. Shoes or slippers add weight. They also cause inaccurate height measurements. The person should urinate before being weighed. A full bladder can affect the weight measurement. If a urine specimen is needed, collect it at this time.

Standing, chair, and lift scales are available (Fig. 19-4). Chair and lift scales are used for persons who cannot stand. You need to follow the manufacturer's instructions when using a chair or lift scale.

Clothing and valuables A list is made of the patient's clothing and valuables. Valuables, including money and jewelry, must be kept in a safe place. They may also be sent home with the family. A clothing list is completed by the staff member admitting the patient. Each item is identified and described on the list. The staff member and patient each sign the completed list. It may be signed by the person responsible for the patient.

A valuables envelope is used for money and jewelry. Each piece of jewelry is listed and described on

---

MEASURING HEIGHT AND WEIGHT

1 Explain the procedure to the patient.
2 Ask the patient to urinate.
3 Wash your hands.
4 Collect the following equipment:
  a Portable balance scale
  b Paper towels
5 Identify the patient. Check the ID bracelet and call the patient by name.
6 Provide for privacy.
7 Place the paper towels on the scale platform.
8 Raise the height measurement rod.
9 Have the patient remove the robe and slippers. Assist if necessary.
10 Assist the patient to stand on the scale platform. Arms should be to the sides.

11 Move the weights until the balance pointer is in the middle (Fig. 19-5).
12 Record the weight.
13 Ask the patient to stand very straight.
14 Lower the height measurement rod until it rests on the patient's head.
15 Record the height.
16 Help the patient put on the robe and slippers if he or she will be up. Help the patient back to bed if necessary. Make sure he or she is comfortable and the signal light is within reach. Unscreen the patient.
17 Discard the paper towels. Return the scale to its proper location.
18 Wash your hands.
19 Report and record the measurements.

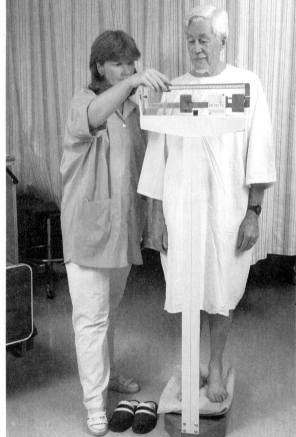

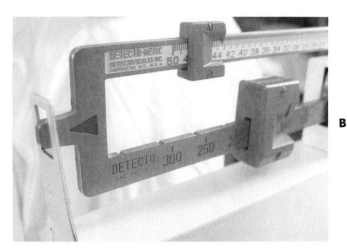

Fig. 19-5 **A,** The patient is weighed. **B,** The weight is read when the balance pointer is in the middle.

the envelope and placed in the envelope while the patient is watching. Money is counted with the patient before being put in the envelope. The envelope is sealed and signed like the clothing checklist. The envelope is given to the nurse. The nurse takes it to the safe or sends it home with the family.

Some valuables are kept at the bedside. These include dentures, eyeglasses, contact lenses, watches, and radios. Valuables kept at the bedside are listed in the patient's record. Some patients keep money for newspapers and gift cart items. The amount of money kept by the patient is noted in the patient's record.

Dressing and undressing patients Clothing changes are usually necessary on admission and discharge. Some people enter and leave the facility in a gown or pajamas. However, most wear street clothes.

Dressing and undressing occur at least daily and sometimes more often. Residents of nursing facilities and patients receiving home care probably wear street clothes during the day. Some patients and residents cannot dress and undress themselves. Others need some help. Certain rules are followed when dressing or undressing individuals.

1. Provide for privacy. Do not expose the patient.
2. Encourage the patient to do as much as possible.
3. Remove clothing from the strong or "good" side first.
4. Put clothing on the weak side first.

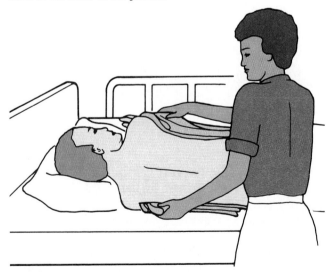

Fig. 19-6 The sides of the garment are brought from the back to the sides of the patient.

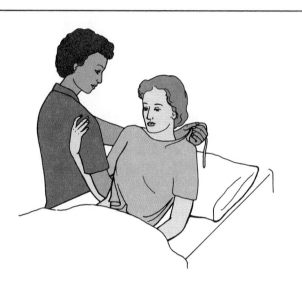

Fig. 19-7 A garment that opens in the back is removed from the patient in the side-lying position. The far side of the garment is tucked under the patient. The near side is folded onto the patient's chest.

UNDRESSING THE PATIENT

1 Explain the procedure to the patient.
2 Wash your hands.
3 Get a bath blanket.
4 Identify the patient. Check the ID bracelet and call the patient by name.
5 Provide for privacy.
6 Raise the bed to an appropriate level for good body mechanics.
7 Lower the side rail on the person's weak side.
8 Position him or her in the supine position.
9 Cover the patient with the bath blanket. Fanfold linens to the foot of the bed. Do not expose the patient during the procedure.
10 Remove garments that open in the back.
   a Raise the patient's head and shoulders. If this cannot be done, turn him or her onto the side away from you.
   b Undo buttons, zippers, ties, or snaps.
   c Bring the sides of the garment to the sides of the patient (Fig. 19-6). Do the following if he or she is in a side-lying position.
      1 Tuck the far side under the patient.
      2 Fold the near side onto the chest (Fig. 19-7).
   d Place the patient in the supine position.
   e Slide the garment off the shoulder on the strong side. Remove it from the arm (Fig. 19-8).
   f Repeat step 10e for the weak side.
11 Remove garments that open in the front.
   a Undo buttons, zippers, snaps, or ties.
   b Slide the garment off the shoulder and arm on the strong side.
   c Raise the head and shoulders. Bring the garment over to the weak side (Fig. 19-9). Lower the head and shoulders.
   d Remove the garment from the weak side.
   e Do the following if you cannot raise the patient's head and shoulders.
      1 Turn the patient toward you. Tuck the removed part under the patient.
      2 Turn him or her onto the side away from you.
      3 Pull the side of the garment out from under the patient. Make sure he or she will not lie on it when supine.

4 Return the patient to the supine position.
5 Remove the garment from the weak side.
12 Remove pullover garments.
   a Undo any buttons, zippers, ties, or snaps.
   b Remove the garment from the strong side.
   c Raise the head and shoulders. You may need to turn him or her onto the side away from you. Bring the garment up to the patient's neck (Fig. 19-10).
   d Remove the garment from the weak side.
   e Bring the garment over the patient's head.
   f Position him or her in the supine position.
13 Remove pants or slacks.
   a Remove shoes or slippers.
   b Position the patient in the supine position.
   c Undo buttons, zippers, ties, snaps, or buckles.
   d Remove the belt if one is worn.
   e Ask the patient to lift the buttocks off the bed. Slide the pants down over the hips and buttocks (Fig. 19-11). Have the patient lower the hips and buttocks.
   f Do the following if the patient cannot raise the hips off the bed.
      1 Turn the patient toward you.
      2 Slide the pants off the hip and buttock on the strong side (Fig. 19-12).
      3 Turn the patient away from you.
      4 Slide the pants off the hip and buttock on the weak side (Fig. 19-13).
   g Slide the pants down the legs and over the feet.
14 Dress or put a clean gown on the patient.
15 Help the person get out of bed if he or she is to be up. Cover the patient and remove the bath blanket if the patient will not be up.
16 Lower the bed and raise the side rail. Place the signal light within reach.
17 Unscreen the patient.
18 Place soiled clothing in the appropriate place.
19 Report your observations to the nurse.

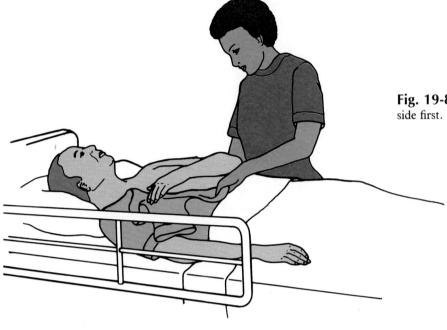

Fig. 19-8 The garment is removed from the strong side first.

Fig. 19-9 A front-opening garment is removed with the patient's head and shoulders raised. The garment is removed from the strong side first. Then it is brought around the back to the weak side.

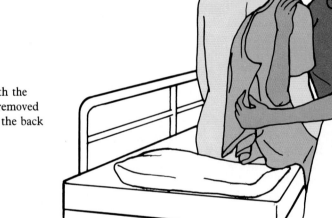

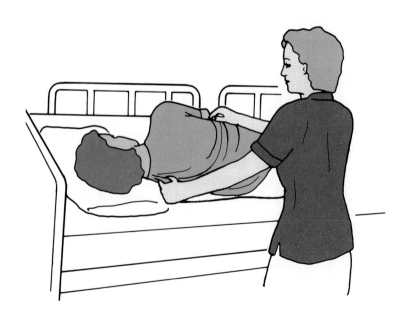

Fig. 19-10 A pullover garment is removed from the strong side first. Then the garment is brought up to the patient's neck so that it can be removed from the weak side.

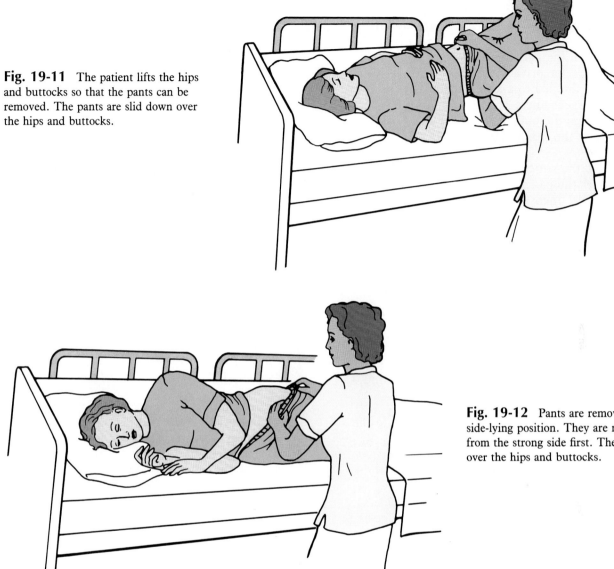

Fig. 19-11 The patient lifts the hips and buttocks so that the pants can be removed. The pants are slid down over the hips and buttocks.

Fig. 19-12 Pants are removed in the side-lying position. They are removed from the strong side first. They are slid over the hips and buttocks.

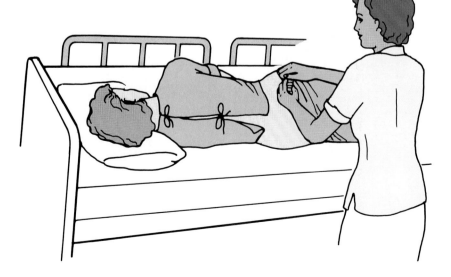

Fig. 19-13 The patient is turned onto the other side. The pants are removed from the weak side.

1 Explain the procedure to the patient.
2 Wash your hands.
3 Get a bath blanket and necessary clothing.
4 Identify the patient. Check the ID bracelet and call the patient by name.
5 Provide for privacy.
6 Raise the bed to a level appropriate for good body mechanics.
7 Undress the patient if indicated.
8 Lower the side rail on the patient's strong side.
9 Place the patient in the supine position.
10 Cover the patient with the bath blanket. Fanfold linens to the foot of the bed. Do not expose the patient during the procedure.
11 Put on garments that open in the back.
  a Slide the garment onto the arm and shoulder of the weak side.
  b Slide the garment onto the arm and shoulder of the strong side.
  c Raise the patient's head and shoulders.
  d Bring the sides to the back if he or she is in a semi-sitting position.
  e Do the following if the patient is in a side-lying position:
    1 Turn the patient toward you.
    2 Bring one side of the garment to the patient's back (Fig. 19-14, *A*).
    3 Turn the patient away from you.
    4 Bring the other side to the patient's back (Fig. 19-14, *B*).
  f Fasten buttons, snaps, ties, or zippers.
  g Position the patient in the supine position.
12 Put on garments that open in the front.
  a Slide the garment onto the arm and shoulder on the weak side.
  b Raise the patient's head and shoulders. Bring the other side of the garment around to the back. Lower the patient to the supine position. Slide the garment onto the arm and shoulder of the strong arm.
  c Do the following if the patient cannot raise the head and shoulders.
    1 Turn the patient toward you.
    2 Tuck the garment under him or her.
    3 Turn the patient away from you.
    4 Pull the garment out from under him or her.
    5 Turn the patient back to the supine position.
    6 Slide the garment over the arm and shoulder of the strong arm.
  d Fasten buttons, snaps, ties, or zippers.

13 Put on pullover garments.
  a Position the patient in the supine position.
  b Bring the neck of the garment over the head.
  c Slide the arm and shoulder of the garment onto the patient's weak side.
  d Raise the patient's head and shoulders.
  e Bring the garment down.
  f Slide the arm and shoulder of the garment onto the patient's strong side.
  g Do the following if the patient cannot assume a semi-sitting position:
    1 Turn the patient toward you.
    2 Tuck the garment under him or her.
    3 Turn the patient away from you.
    4 Pull the garment out from under him or her.
    5 Return the patient to the supine position.
    6 Slide the arm and shoulder of the garment onto the strong side.
  h Fasten buttons, snaps, ties, or zippers.
14 Put on pants or slacks.
  a Slide the pants over the feet and up the legs.
  b Ask him or her to raise the hips and buttocks off the bed.
  c Bring the pants up over the buttocks and hips.
  d Ask the patient to lower the hips and buttocks.
  e Do the following if the patient cannot raise the hips and buttocks.
    1 Turn patient onto strong side.
    2 Pull the pants over the buttock and hip on the weak side.
    3 Turn the patient onto the weak side.
    4 Pull the pants over the buttock and hip on the strong side.
    5 Return him or her to the supine position.
  f Fasten buttons, ties, snaps, the zipper, and the belt buckle.
15 Put socks and shoes or slippers on the patient.
16 Help the patient to the chair if he or she can be up. Otherwise, help the patient assume a comfortable position in bed.
17 Cover the patient and remove the bath blanket. Raise the side rails and lower the bed to its lowest position.
18 Make sure the signal light is within reach.
19 Unscreen the patient.
20 Place soiled clothing where appropriate.
21 Report your observations to the nurse.

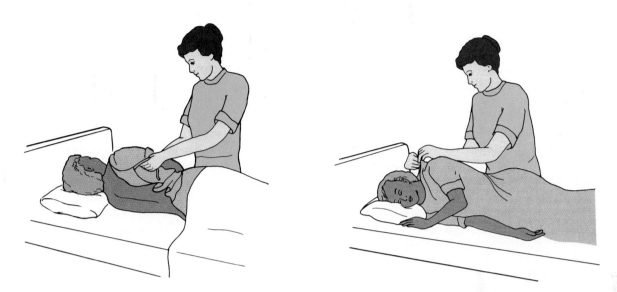

Fig. 19-14 A, The side-lying position can be used to put on garments that open in the back. The patient is turned toward the nursing assistant after the garment is put on the arms. The side of the garment is brought to the patient's back. **B,** The patient is then turned away from the nursing assistant. The other side of the garment is brought to the back and fastened.

TRANSFERS

A patient may be transferred to another room, nursing unit, or facility. A *transfer* is moving a patient from one room, nursing unit, or facility to another. Transfers are usually related to changes in condition. The patient may or may not welcome the transfer. The reasons for the transfer are explained by the doctor or nurse. The nurse also notifies the family and business office. You may assist in the transfer or carry out the entire procedure. The patient is usually transported by wheelchair or stretcher. Sometimes the bed is used. (See the box on page 332.)

DISCHARGES

Discharge is usually planned a few days in advance. *Discharge* is the official departure of a patient from a facility or nursing unit. This is usually a happy time if the person is going home. Some people are discharged to another hospital or to a nursing facility. Some require home care. They may have other fears and concerns. The doctor, nurse, dietician, social worker, and other health team members plan the person's discharge. They teach the patient and family about diet, exercise, and medications that must be taken. They provide teaching about dressing changes and treatments. A doctor's appointment may be given.

Nursing assistants usually help patients gather and pack belongings and change into street clothes. They also transport patients out of the facility. The nurse tells you when to begin the discharge procedure. The doctor must write a discharge order before the patient or resident is allowed to leave. The nurse tells you when the person can leave and how to transport him or her. Usually a wheelchair is used. Some facilities let the person walk. Occasionally a patient or resident leaves by ambulance. The ambulance attendants bring the stretcher to the room.

Financial arrangements are usually made on admission or before discharge. Before leaving the facility, the patient or family makes arrangements for payment at the business office.

A patient may wish to leave the facility without the doctor's permission. You must notify the nurse immediately if the patient expresses the wish or intent to leave. This situation is handled by the nurse. (See the box on page 332.)

TRANSFERRING THE PATIENT TO ANOTHER NURSING UNIT

1 Check with the nurse to find out where the patient is going. Find out if the bed, a wheelchair, or a stretcher will be used.
2 Obtain a stretcher or wheelchair, bath blanket, and a utility cart if needed.
3 Wash your hands.
4 Identify the patient. Check the ID bracelet with the transfer slip.
5 Explain the procedure to the patient.
6 Collect the patient's personal belongings and bedside equipment. Place them on the utility cart for transport.
7 Assist the patient to the wheelchair or stretcher. Cover the patient with a bath blanket.
8 Transport the patient to the assigned place.
9 Introduce the patient to the receiving nurse.
10 Help the nurse transfer the patient from the wheelchair or stretcher into bed. Help position the patient.
11 Bring the patient's personal belongings and equipment to the new room. Help put them away.
12 Report the following to the receiving nurse:
   a How the patient tolerated the transfer
   b That a nurse will bring the patient's chart, care plan, Kardex, and medications
13 Return the wheelchair or stretcher and the utility cart to the storage area.
14 Wash your hands.
15 Report the following to the nurse:
   a The time of transfer
   b Where the patient was taken
   c How the patient was transferred (bed, wheelchair, or stretcher)
   d How the patient tolerated the transfer
   e Who received the patient
   f Any other observations
16 Strip the bed, clean the unit, and make a closed bed. (This may be done by the housekeeping department.)

DISCHARGING THE PATIENT

1 Make sure the patient is to be discharged. Find out if transportation arrangements have been made.
2 Explain the procedure to the patient.
3 Wash your hands.
4 Identify the patient. Check the ID bracelet with the discharge slip.
5 Provide for privacy.
6 Help the patient dress if assistance is needed.
7 Help the patient pack. Check all drawers and closets to make sure all items are collected.
8 Check off the clothing list. Ask the patient to sign the form indicating that all clothing has been returned.
9 Tell the nurse that the patient is ready for the final visit. The nurse:
   a Gives prescriptions written by the physician
   b Provides discharge instructions
   c Secures valuables from the safe
10 Get a wheelchair and a utility cart for the patient's belongings. Ask a co-worker to help you.
11 Bring the wheelchair to the bedside and lock the wheels. Lock the bed wheels. Lower the bed to its lowest position.
12 Assist the patient into the wheelchair.
13 Unlock the wheels.
14 Take the patient to the exit area. Lock the wheels of the wheelchair (Fig. 19-15).
15 Help the person out of the wheelchair and into the car. Help put the belongings into the car.
16 Return the wheelchair and cart to the storage area.
17 Wash your hands.
18 Report the following to the nurse:
   a The time of discharge
   b How the patient was transported
   c Who accompanied the patient
   d The patient's destination
   e Any other observations
19 Strip the bed, clean the unit, and make a closed bed. (This may be done by the housekeeping department.)

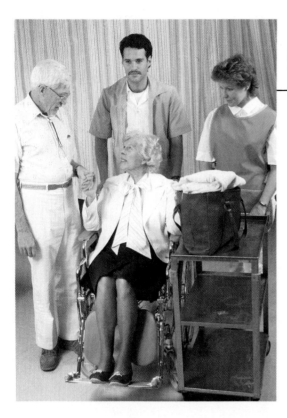

Fig. 19-15 The patient is taken to the exit by wheelchair. The patient's possessions are brought along at this time.

SUMMARY

Admission to a health care facility is usually a frightening time for the patient and family. Transfers can also cause fear and apprehension. This is particularly true when the transfer is due to a change in the patient's condition. Discharge is usually a happy and pleasant time. However, it may cause worries and concerns if more care and treatment are required. You can help the patient and family cope with these events. You need to be polite, courteous, caring, efficient, and competent. The person's property and valuables must be handled with care and respect. They should be kept in a safe place and protected from loss or damage. Always treat the patient and family the way you would like to be treated.

REVIEW QUESTIONS

Circle T *if the answer is true and* F *if the answer is false.*

T F **1** The patient's identifying information is obtained on arrival to the nursing unit.

T F **2** New patients are usually transported to the nursing unit in wheelchairs or on stretchers.

T F **3** The bed is opened when preparing the room for a new patient.

T F **4** The patient is greeted by name when being admitted to the nursing unit.

T F **5** A patient complains of pain. Report the complaint after the admission checklist has been completed.

T F **6** A urine specimen is needed on admission.

T F **7** You are never responsible for orienting the patient to the new environment.

T F **8** A robe and slippers are worn when the patient is being weighed and measured.

T F **9** A list is made of the patient's clothing and valuables during the admission process.

T F **10** Clothing is removed from the weak side first.

T F **11** Clothing is put on the weak side first.

T F **12** A patient's condition may require that he or she be transferred to another nursing unit.

T F **13** A doctor's order is required for discharge from the health care facility.

T F **14** You are responsible for providing the patient with instructions about diet and medications.

Answers

	10 False	**5** False
14 False	**9** True	**4** True
13 True	**8** False	**3** True
12 True	**7** False	**2** True
11 True	**6** True	**1** False

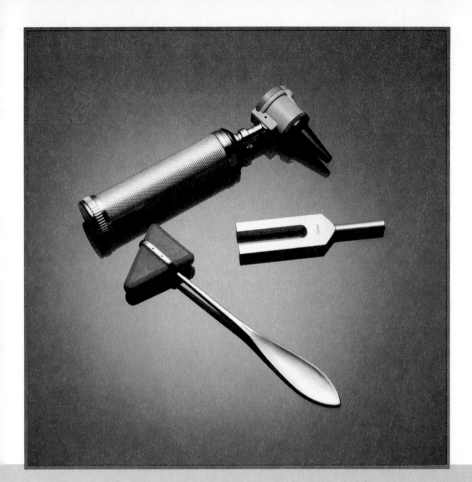

Assisting with the Physical Examination

OBJECTIVES

- Define the key terms listed in this chapter
- Identify the responsibilities of the nursing assistant as they relate to the physical examination
- Identify the equipment used during a physical examination
- Describe how to prepare a patient for an examination
- Describe four examination positions and how to drape the patient for each position
- Prepare the patient for an examination
- Describe the rules for assisting with a physical examination
- Identify the responsibilities of the nursing assistant after the physical examination
- Describe the differences between the examination of an infant or child and an adult

dorsal recumbent position The supine or back-lying examination position; the legs are together

horizontal recumbent position The dorsal recumbent position

knee-chest position The patient kneels and rests the body on the knees and chest; the head is turned to one side, the arms are above the head or flexed at the elbows, the back is straight, and the body is flexed about 90 degrees at the hips

laryngeal mirror An instrument used to examine the mouth, teeth, and throat

lithotomy position The patient is in a back-lying position, the hips are brought down to the edge of the examination table, the knees are flexed, the hips are externally rotated, and the feet are supported in stirrups

nasal speculum An instrument used to examine the inside of the nose

ophthalmoscope A lighted instrument used to examine the internal structures of the eye

otoscope A lighted instrument used to examine the external ear and the eardrum (tympanic membrane)

percussion hammer An instrument used to tap body parts for the purpose of testing reflexes

tuning fork An instrument used to test hearing

vaginal speculum An instrument used to open the vagina so that it and the cervix can be examined

Physical examinations are usually done by doctors. They are done for many reasons. Routine health examinations are done to promote health. Preemployment physicals are done to determine fitness for work. Physical examinations are also used to diagnose and treat disease. Today nurses are learning how to perform physical examinations. You may be asked to assist a doctor or nurse with a physical examination.

RESPONSIBILITIES OF THE NURSING ASSISTANT

Your responsibilities depend on the policies and procedures of the facility. The preferences of the examiner also affect what you are expected to do. You may perform some or all of the following functions.

1. Collect linens for draping the patient. Also collect other linens for the procedure.
2. Collect equipment to be used for the examination.
3. Prepare the examination room or patient unit for the examination.
4. Make sure there is adequate lighting.
5. Measure the patient's vital signs, height, and weight.
6. Position and drape the patient for the examination.
7. Hand the equipment and instruments to the examiner.
8. Label specimen containers.
9. Dispose of soiled linen and discard used disposable supplies. Clean reusable equipment after the examination.
10. Help the patient dress or assume a comfortable position after the examination.

EQUIPMENT

Some equipment and supplies used in the physical examination are used in patient care. You may recognize the other instruments. Some were probably used when you were examined. You need to know the instruments in Figure 20-1.

The *ophthalmoscope* is a lighted instrument used to examine the internal structures of the eye. The *otoscope* is used to examine the external ear and the eardrum (tympanic membrane). The otoscope is also a lighted instrument. Some scopes have interchangeable parts. Some can be changed into an ophthalmoscope or otoscope. The *percussion hammer* is used to tap body parts to test reflexes. The *vaginal speculum* is used to open the vagina so that it and the cervix can be examined. The *nasal speculum* is used to examine the inside of the nose. A *tuning fork* is vibrated to test hearing. The *laryngeal mirror* is needed to examine the mouth, teeth, and throat.

Many facilities have examination trays in the central supply department. If these are not available, the necessary items are collected. Items listed in *Preparing the Patient for an Examination* on page 338 are usually used for an examination. They are arranged on a tray or table for the examiner.

PREPARING THE PATIENT

The physical examination causes anxiety for many people. They are concerned about the possible findings. Other factors can add to their anxiety. These include discomfort, embarrassment, the fear of exposure, and unfamiliarity with the procedure. You need to be sensitive to the person's feelings and concerns. The person should be prepared physically and psychologically for the examination. The nurse explains the purpose of the examination and what to expect. This could be your responsibility, depending on the situation and the employer.

Usually all clothes are removed for a complete physical examination. The patient is covered with a drape. It may be a disposable paper drape, a bath blanket, a sheet, or a drawsheet. Sometimes a hospital gown is worn. It reduces the feeling of nakedness and the fear of exposure. Explain to the person that the amount of exposure during the examination is minimal. The patient needs to understand that some exposure is necessary to examine the body. However, only the body part being examined is exposed. You must screen the patient and close the door to the room. This further protects the person's right to privacy.

Patients are asked to urinate before the examination. The bladder must be empty so that the examiner can feel the abdominal organs. A full bladder can alter the normal position and shape of the organs. It can also cause discomfort, especially when the abdominal organs are felt. If a urine specimen is needed, it is obtained at this time. Explain how to collect the specimen and label the container properly (see Chapter 14).

Warmth is major concern during the examination. The patient must be protected from chilling, especially if the person is ill, elderly, or a child. An extra bath blanket should be nearby. Measures are also taken to prevent drafts.

The examiner may want you to measure the patient's height, weight, and vital signs. These are obtained before the examiner begins. They are recorded on the examination form. The patient is then positioned and draped for the examination.

Positioning and Draping

The patient may have to assume a special position for the physical examination. Some examination positions (Fig. 20-2) are uncomfortable and cause embarrassment. The examiner will tell you how to position the patient. You need to explain to the patient the need for the position and how it is assumed. Also explain how the body is draped and how long the patient can expect to stay in the position. Be sure to help the patient assume and maintain the position.

The *dorsal recumbent (horizontal recumbent)* or supine position is usually used to examine the abdomen, anterior chest, and breasts. The person is supine with the legs together. If the perineal area is to be examined, the knees are flexed and hips externally rotated (see Fig. 20-2, *A*). The patient is draped as for perineal care (see *Female Perineal Care*, page 211).

The *lithotomy* position (Fig. 20-2, *B*) is used to examine the vagina. The patient lies on her back, and her hips are brought to the edge of the examination table. The knees are flexed, and the hips are externally rotated. The feet are supported in stirrups. The patient is draped as for the dorsal recumbent position. Some facilities provide socks to cover the feet and calves.

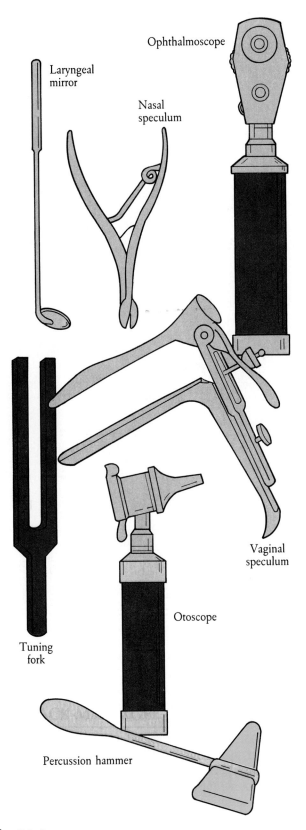

Fig. 20-1 Instruments used for the physical examination.

Ophthalmoscope

Laryngeal mirror

Nasal speculum

Vaginal speculum

Otoscope

Tuning fork

Percussion hammer

PREPARING THE PATIENT FOR AN EXAMINATION

1 Explain the procedure to the patient.
2 Wash your hands.
3 Assemble the following equipment on a tray at the bedside or in the examination room:
   a Flashlight
   b Sphygmomanometer
   c Stethoscope
   d Thermometer
   e Tongue depressors (blades)
   f Laryngeal mirror
   g Ophthalmoscope
   h Otoscope
   i Nasal speculum
   j Percussion (reflex) hammer
   k Tuning fork
   l Tape measure
   m Disposable gloves
   n Water-soluble lubricant
   o Vaginal speculum
   p Cotton-tipped applicators
   q Specimen containers and labels
   r Disposable bag
   s Emesis basin
   t Towel
   u Bath blanket
   v Tissues
   w Drape (sheet, bath blanket, drawsheet, or disposable drape)
   x Paper towels
   y Cotton balls
   z Disposable bed protector
   aa Eye chart (Snellen chart)
   bb Slides
   cc Gown
   dd Alcohol wipes
   ee Wastebasket
   ff Container for soiled instruments
   gg Marking pencils or pens
4 Identify the patient. Check the ID bracelet and call the person by name.
5 Provide for privacy.
6 Ask the patient to put on the gown. Instruct him or her to remove all clothes. Assist the patient as necessary.
7 Ask the patient to urinate. If the patient is not ambulatory, offer the bedpan or urinal. Provide for privacy.
8 Transport the patient to the examination room. Help the patient get on the examination table. Have him or her use a stool if necessary. Omit this step if the examination will be done in the patient's room.
9 Position the patient as directed. Raise the bed to its highest level.
10 Drape the patient. Untie the gown.
11 Place a bed protector under the buttocks.
12 Arrange for adequate lighting.
13 Put the signal light on for the nurse or examiner. Do not leave the patient unattended.

The *knee-chest* position (Fig. 20-2, *C*) is used to examine the rectum. Sometimes it is used to examine the vagina. The patient kneels on the bed or examination table. Then the patient rests his or her body on the knees and chest. The head is turned to one side, and the arms are above the head or flexed at the elbows. The back is straight and the body is flexed about 90 degrees at the hips. The patient wears a gown and sometimes socks. The drape is applied in a diamond shape to cover the back, buttocks, and thighs.

The *Sims' position* (Fig. 20-2, *D*) is sometimes used to examine the rectum or vagina (see page 169). The drape is applied in a diamond shape. The corner near the examiner is folded back to expose the rectum or vagina.

ASSISTING WITH THE EXAMINATION

You may be responsible for preparing, positioning, and draping the patient. You may also be asked to assist the doctor or nurse during the examination.

When assisting with the examination, you should follow these rules:
1. Wash your hands before and after the examination.
2. Provide for privacy throughout the examination. This is done by screening, closing doors, and draping. Expose only the body part being examined.
3. Assist the patient in assuming positions as directed by the examiner.
4. Place instruments and equipment in a convenient location for the examiner.
5. Stay in the room during the examination of a female patient (unless you are a male). When a woman is examined by a man, another female is in attendance. This is for the legal protection of the woman and the male examiner. A female attendant also adds to the psychological comfort of the patient.
6. Protect the patient from falling.
7. Anticipate the examiner's need for equipment.
8. Place paper or paper towels on the floor if the patient is asked to stand.

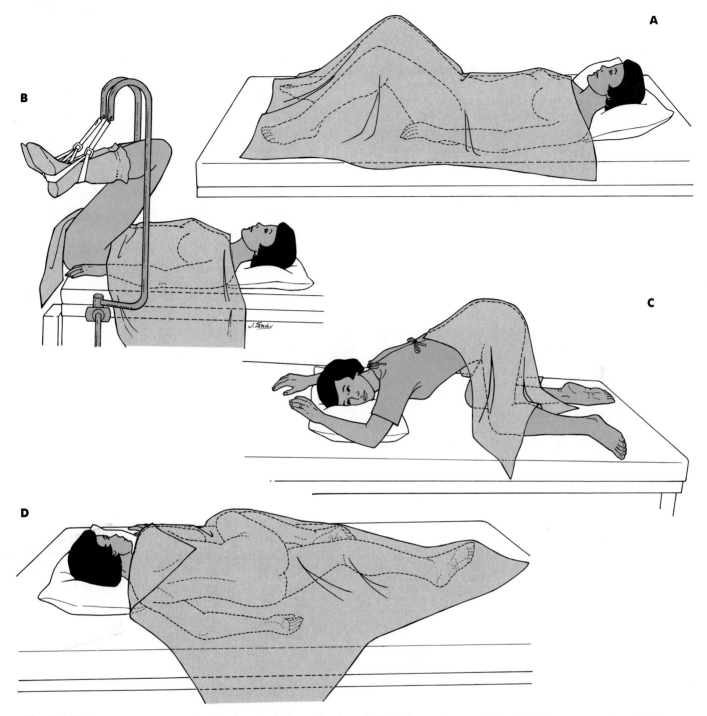

Fig. 20-2 Positioning and draping for the physical examination: **A,** Dorsal recumbent position. **B,** Lithotomy position. **C,** Knee-chest position. **D,** Sims' position.

After the Examination

After the examination the patient is taken back to the room. In a clinic, the person is allowed to dress. Assistance is given as necessary. Lubricant is used for the vaginal or rectal examination. The area should be wiped or cleaned before the patient dresses or returns to the room.

Used disposable supplies are put in a bag or waste container. Examples are bed protectors, paper drapes, tongue blades, applicators, and cotton balls.

These supplies are replaced so that the tray is ready for the next examination. Reusable equipment is cleaned and returned to the tray. This includes the otoscope and ophthalmoscope tips, speculum, and stethoscope. The examination table is covered with a clean drawsheet or paper. All specimens are labeled and sent to the laboratory with a completed requisition slip. The patient's unit or examination room should be neat and orderly after the examination. Soiled linens are taken to the "dirty" utility room.

EXAMINATION OF AN INFANT OR CHILD

The examination of an infant or child is similar to an adult examination. A parent is present during the examination. The parent may be asked to hold or restrain the infant or child during some parts of the procedure. Restraint may be necessary if the infant or child is uncooperative. However, restraining may frighten an infant. The child may also fear separation from the parent. Some children have a fear of physical harm during the examination. Maintaining a calm, comforting manner helps both the child or infant and the parent. Remember that the parent may also be anxious. The equipment needed is similar to that used for the adult examination. Toys may be used to assess development. Vaginal speculums are not used.

SUMMARY

Physical examinations are frightening to many people. Many fear body exposure or a serious diagnosis. Examinations may cause discomfort, especially for the ill, injured, or elderly. You may be asked to prepare patients for examinations. Collecting and arranging examination supplies and equipment are sometimes done by nursing assistants. You may also be asked to assist with the procedure. Feelings, fears, and sources of discomfort during the examination must be considered. This is essential for the patient's physical and psychological comfort. In addition, you must function efficiently and competently. This allows the examination to be performed smoothly and in a reasonable length of time.

REVIEW QUESTIONS

Circle the best *answer.*

1 The otoscope is used to
   a Examine the internal structures of the eye
   b Examine the external ear and the eardrum
   c Test reflexes
   d Open the vagina
2 You are preparing a patient for an examination. You should do the following *except*
   a Have the patient urinate
   b Ask the patient to undress
   c Drape the patient
   d Go tell the nurse the patient is ready
3 Which part of the physical examination can you do?
   a Examination of the eyes and ears
   b Inspection of the mouth, teeth, and throat
   c Measurement of height, weight, and vital signs
   d Observation of the perineum and rectum
4 A patient is supine. Hips are flexed and externally rotated. The feet are supported in stirrups. The patient is in the
   a Dorsal recumbent position
   b Lithotomy position
   c Knee-chest position
   d Sims' position
5 You are to assist with an examination. Which is *false?*
   a Handwashing is done before and after the examination.
   b Instruments are placed in a location convenient for the examiner.
   c The female nursing assistant leaves the room when a woman is being examined.
   d The patient's privacy is protected by screening, closing the door, and proper draping.
6 An infant is being examined. Which is *true?*
   a The examination is the same as for an adult.
   b Equipment is needed as for the adult examination.
   c The temperature is measured orally.
   d The parent is allowed to stay for the examination.

Answers
6 d   4 b   2 d
5 c   3 c   1 b

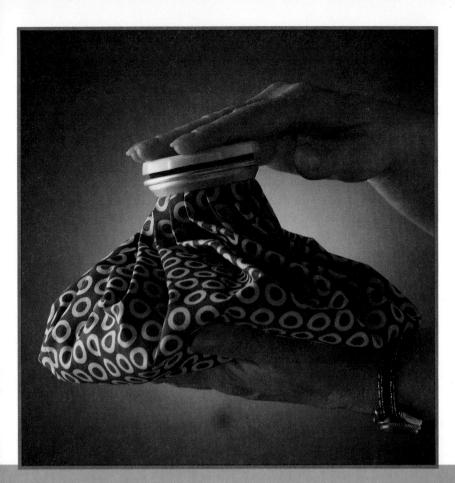

Heat and Cold Applications

21

OBJECTIVES

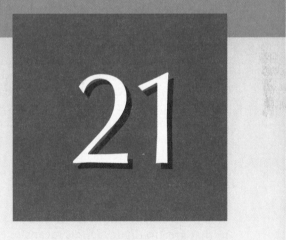

- Define the key terms listed in this chapter
- Identify the purposes, effects, and complications of heat applications
- Identify the persons at risk for complications from heat applications
- Explain the differences between moist and dry heat applications
- Describe the rules related to the application of heat
- Identify the purposes, effects, and complications of cold applications
- Identify the persons at risk for complications from cold applications
- Explain the differences between moist and dry cold applications
- Describe the rules related to the application of cold
- Perform the procedures described in this chapter

constrict To narrow
cyanosis Bluish discoloration of the skin
dilate To expand or open wider

Heat and cold applications are ordered by doctors. They promote healing and comfort and reduce tissue swelling. Heat and cold have opposite effects on body function. Serious injury can occur if safety precautions are not taken.

In many facilities the application of heat and cold is the responsibility of the nurse. Heat and cold applications are complex and more advanced nursing functions. This is because of the severe injuries and the changes in body function that can easily result. The risks are greater than those related to other procedures. Some facilities let nursing assistants apply heat and cold applications under the direction of a nurse. You are advised to perform these procedures only if you have a thorough understanding of their purposes, effects, and complications. Review the procedure with a nurse before you perform it. A nurse should closely supervise your work and the effects of the procedure on the patient.

HEAT APPLICATIONS

Heat applications are usually small and can be applied to almost any body part. "Local heat application" means that heat is applied to a body part. Heat applications have many therapeutic effects. Pain is relieved, muscles are relaxed, healing is promoted, and tissue swelling is reduced.

Effects

When applied to the skin, heat causes blood vessels in that area to dilate. *Dilate* means to expand or open wider (Fig. 21-1). More blood flows through the vessels. More oxygen and nutrients are available to the tissues for healing. There is faster removal of toxic (poisonous) substances and waste products. Excess fluid is removed from the area more rapidly. The skin feels warm and appears reddened in the area of the heat. These effects are from increased blood flow.

Complications

Complications can occur from heat applications. High temperatures can cause burns. Pain, excessive redness, and blisters are danger signs. These are reported to the nurse immediately. You must also observe for pale skin. When heat is applied for a long time, blood

vessels tend to *constrict*, or narrow (see Fig. 21-1). Blood flow decreases when vessels constrict. Decreased blood flow reduces the amount of blood available to tissues. Decreased blood supply causes tissue damage and gives the skin a pale color.

Certain persons are at greater risk for complications. They are infants, very young children, fair-skinned people, and the elderly. Their skin is very delicate and fragile, and is easily burned. Complications may also occur in those who have difficulty sensing (feeling) heat or pain. Many factors can interfere with sensation. They include circulatory disorders, central nervous system damage, aging, and loss of consciousness. Confused patients or those receiving strong pain medications may also have decreased sensation.

Moist and Dry Applications

Moist or dry applications may be ordered. A *moist heat application* means that water is in contact with the skin. Water is a good conductor of heat. Therefore the effects of the heat are greater and occur faster than with a dry application. Heat penetrates deeper with a moist application. There is less drying of the skin. Temperatures of moist heat applications are lower than those of dry heat applications to prevent patient injury.

Water is not in contact with the skin with *dry heat applications*. Dry heat has advantages. The application stays at the desired temperature longer. Heat is not lost through evaporation as with moist applications. The risk of burns is less because dry heat does not penetrate as deeply as moist heat. Also, water, which conducts heat, is not involved. Higher temperatures are used with dry heat to achieve the desired effect. Therefore burns are a risk.

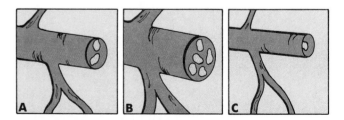

Fig. 21-1 A, Blood vessel under normal conditions.
B, Dilated blood vessel. **C,** Constricted blood vessel.

General Rules

Patients must be protected from injury during local heat applications. Those who cannot protect themselves need extra attention. The following rules are practiced to prevent burns and other complications.

1. Know how to operate equipment used in the procedure.
2. Use a bath thermometer to measure the temperature of moist heat applications.
3. Follow facility policies regarding the temperature ranges for heat applications.
4. Know the different temperature ranges for warm, hot, and very hot applications. The following ranges are guidelines:
   Warm—93° to 98° F (33.8° to 37° C)
   Hot—98° to 105° F (37° to 40.5° C)
   Very hot—105° to 115° F (40.5° to 46.1° C)
5. Ask the nurse what the temperature of the application should be for persons at risk for burns (see page 342). Lower temperatures are usually used for those at risk.
6. Cover dry heat applications with flannel covers before applying them.
7. Observe the skin for signs of complications. Immediately report any signs of complications or patient complaints of pain or burning.
8. Do not let the patient increase the temperature of the application.
9. Know how long to leave the application in place. Carefully watch the time.
10. Follow the rules of electrical safety when using electrical appliances to apply heat.
11. Expose only the body part where the heat is to be applied. Provide for privacy through proper draping and screening.
12. Make sure the signal light is within the patient's reach.

Hot Compresses and Packs

Hot compresses and packs are moist heat applications. They consist of a washcloth, small towel, or gauze dressing. A compress is usually applied to a small area. Packs are applied to large areas. Sterile or nonsterile compresses and packs may be ordered. Sterile applications are ordered for open wounds and for areas with a break in the skin. The nurse applies sterile hot compresses or packs.

Nonsterile applications are used for intact skin. The compress or pack is placed in a basin of hot water. After it is wrung out, it is applied to the body part. The application is left in place for 20 minutes and then removed.

Commercial Compresses

Commercial compresses are premoistened and packaged in foil. An ultraviolet light is used to heat the

APPLYING HOT COMPRESSES

1 Explain the procedure to the patient.
2 Wash your hands.
3 Collect the following equipment:
   a Basin
   b Bath thermometer
   c Small towel, washcloth, or gauze squares
   d Plastic wrap
   e Ties, tape, or rolled gauze
   f Bath towel
   g Waterproof bed protector
4 Identify the patient. Check the ID bracelet with the treatment card.
5 Provide for privacy.
6 Place the protector under the body part.
7 Fill the basin ½ to ⅔ full with hot water. Water temperature should be 105° to 115° F (40.5° to 46.1° C).
8 Place the compress in the hot water.
9 Wring out the compress (Fig. 21-2).
10 Apply the compress to the area. Note the time.
11 Cover the compress quickly with plastic wrap. Then cover it with the bath towel as in Figure 21-2.
12 Secure the towel in place with ties, tape, or rolled gauze.
13 Place the signal light within reach.
14 Check the area every 5 minutes. Check for redness and complaints of pain, discomfort, or numbness. Remove the compress if any occur. Notify the nurse immediately.
15 Change the compress if cooling occurs. Sometimes it is kept warm with a warm water bottle or heating pad.
16 Remove the compress after 20 minutes. Pat the area dry with a towel.
17 Make sure the patient is comfortable and unscreened, and the side rails are up. Place the signal light within reach.
18 Clean equipment. Discard disposable equipment and used linen.
19 Wash your hands.
20 Report the following to the nurse:
   a The time of the application
   b The site of the application
   c The length of the application
   d The patient's response
   e Your observations of the skin

APPLYING A COMMERCIAL COMPRESS

1 Explain the procedure to the patient.
2 Wash your hands.
3 Collect the following equipment:
  a Commercial compress
  b Ultraviolet light
  c Towel
  d Ties, tape, or rolled gauze
  e Waterproof bed protector
4 Place the compress under the ultraviolet light for 10 minutes.
5 Identify the patient. Check the ID bracelet with the treatment card.
6 Provide for privacy.
7 Place the bed protector under the body part.
8 Open the foil-wrapped compress.
9 Apply the compress quickly with the foil wrap.
10 Cover it with the towel.
11 Secure the towel in place with ties, tape, or rolled gauze.
12 Check the area every 5 minutes. Check for redness and complaints of pain, discomfort, or numbness. Remove the compress if any occur. Notify the nurse immediately.
13 Change the compress if cooling occurs. A warm water bottle or heating pad may be ordered to keep it warm.
14 Remove the compress after 20 minutes. Pat the area dry with the towel.
15 Make sure the patient is comfortable and unscreened, and the side rails are up. Place the signal light within reach.
16 Clean equipment. Discard disposable equipment and used linen in the "dirty" utility room.
17 Wash your hands.
18 Report the following to the nurse:
  a The time of the application
  b The site of the application
  c The length of the application
  d The patient's response
  e Your observations of the skin

THE HOT SOAK

1 Explain the procedure to the patient.
2 Wash your hands.
3 Collect the following equipment:
  a Small basin or an arm or foot bath
  b Bath thermometer
  c Bath blanket
  d Waterproof pads
4 Identify the patient. Check the ID bracelet with the treatment card.
5 Provide for privacy.
6 Assist the patient to a comfortable position for the treatment. Place the signal light within reach.
7 Place a waterproof pad under the area.
8 Fill the container ½ full with hot water. Measure the water temperature. It should be 105° to 110° F (40.5° to 43.3° C).
9 Expose the area without unnecessary patient exposure.
10 Place the part into the water. Pad the edge of the container with a towel if needed. Note the time.
11 Cover the patient with a bath blanket for extra warmth.
12 Check the area every 5 minutes. Check for redness and complaints of pain, numbness, or discomfort. Remove the part from the soak if any occur. Wrap the part in a towel and notify the nurse immediately.
13 Check water temperature every 5 minutes. Change water as necessary. Wrap the part in a towel while changing the water.
14 Remove the part from the water in 15 to 20 minutes. Pat dry with a towel.
15 Make sure the patient is comfortable and unscreened. Place the signal light within reach. Raise the side rails.
16 Clean and return equipment to its proper place. Discard disposable equipment and soiled linen.
17 Wash your hands.
18 Report the following to the nurse:
  a The time the procedure began
  b The site that was soaked
  c The length of the treatment
  d The patient's response
  e Your observations of the skin

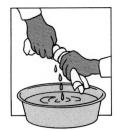
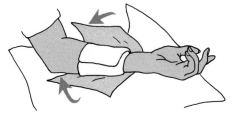

Fig. 21-2 A hot compress is covered with plastic and a bath towel. These keep the compress warm.

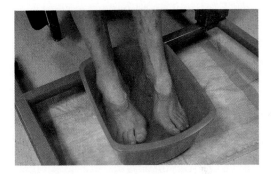

Fig. 21-3 The hot soak.

wrapped compress for 10 minutes. The ultraviolet light may be kept in the "clean" utility room, treatment room, medication room, or the patient's room.

Commercial compresses are sterile. Sometimes doctors order them for nonsterile compresses. Nurses may decide that they are necessary in certain situations. Commercial compresses are costly and should be used only when necessary.

Hot Soaks

A hot soak involves putting the body part into a container of water. This is usually used for smaller body parts, such as a hand, lower arm, foot, or lower leg (Fig. 21-3). Sometimes large areas are soaked, such as the torso or an entire arm or leg. A tub is used for a large area. The soak usually lasts 15 to 20 minutes. Patient comfort and good body alignment are maintained during the hot soak.

The Sitz Bath

The sitz bath (hip bath) involves immersing the pelvic area in warm or hot water for 20 minutes. Sitz baths are used to clean perineal wounds, relieve pain, increase circulation, or stimulate voiding.

The disposable plastic sitz bath fits onto the toilet seat (Fig. 21-4). It can be used in the home or health facility. A sitz tub is a built-in fixture with a deep seat. The patient sits in the seat that is filled with water (Fig. 21-5). A portable sitz chair is similar. The patient should flex the knees to keep the legs out of the water.

The sitz bath increases blood flow to the pelvic area. Therefore less blood flows to other body parts. As a result, the patient may become weak or feel faint. The relaxing effect of the treatment may cause drowsiness. Observe the patient frequently for signs of weakness, faintness, or fatigue. Also take precautions to keep the patient safe from injury.

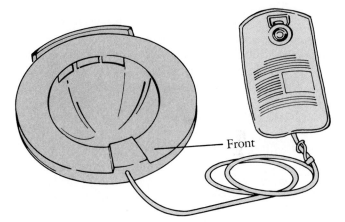

Fig. 21-4 The disposable sitz bath.

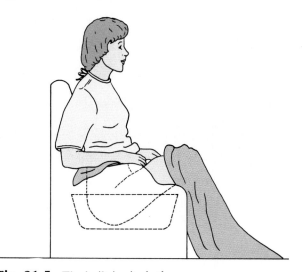

Fig. 21-5 The built-in sitz bath.

ASSISTING THE PATIENT TO TAKE A SITZ BATH

1 Explain the procedure to the patient.
2 Wash your hands.
3 Collect the following equipment:
 a Portable sitz bath or disposable sitz bath
 b Wheelchair if the patient will use a built-in sitz bath
 c Bath thermometer
 d Large water container
 e Two bath blankets
 f Footstool if the patient is short
 g Bath towels
 h Clean gown
 i Disinfectant solution
4 Identify the patient. Check the ID bracelet with the treatment card.
5 Provide for privacy.
6 Do one of the following:
 a Position the portable sitz bath at the bedside.
 b Place the disposable sitz bath on the toilet seat.
 c Transport the patient by wheelchair to the room where the sitz bath is.
7 Fill the sitz bath ⅔ full with water. Water temperature should be
 a 100° to 104° F (37.7° to 40° C) if used to clean the perineum
 b 105° to 110° F (40.5° to 43.3° C) if used to increase circulation
8 Lock the wheels of the portable sitz bath.
9 Use bath towels to pad the metal parts that will be in contact with the patient.
10 Raise the gown and secure it above the waist.

11 Help the patient sit in the sitz bath.
12 Place one bath blanket around the patient's shoulders. Place another over the legs to provide warmth.
13 Provide a footstool for the patient if the edge of the sitz bath causes pressure under the knees.
14 Make sure the signal light is within reach and the patient is comfortable.
15 Stay with a patient who is weak or unsteady.
16 Check the patient every 5 minutes for complaints of weakness, faintness, and drowsiness. If any occur, get assistance to help the patient back to bed.
17 Help the patient out of the sitz bath after 20 minutes.
18 Help the patient dry off and put on a clean gown.
19 Assist the patient back to bed. Make sure he or she is comfortable and unscreened. Place the signal light within reach and raise the side rails.
20 Clean the sitz bath with disinfectant solution.
21 Return reusable equipment to its proper place. Discard used linens.
22 Wash your hands.
23 Report the following to the nurse:
 a The time the sitz bath started and ended
 b The patient's response
 c The water temperature
 d Any other observations

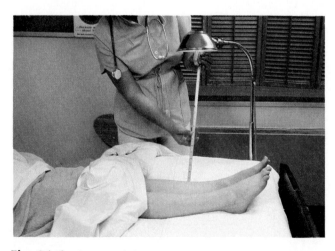

Fig. 21-6 Gooseneck lamp.

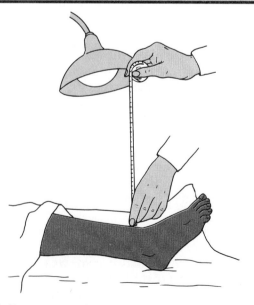

Fig. 21-7 The distance between the heat lamp and the patient is measured.

APPLYING A HEAT LAMP

1 Explain the procedure to the patient.
2 Wash your hands.
3 Collect the following equipment:
   a Gooseneck lamp
   b Bath blanket
   c Yardstick or tape measure
4 Identify the patient. Check the ID bracelet with the treatment card.
5 Provide for privacy.
6 Plug in the lamp and allow it to warm up.
7 Cover the patient with a bath blanket. Fanfold top linens to the foot of the bed.
8 Expose the body part.
9 Position the lamp a safe distance from the patient.
   a 25 watt bulb—14 inches
   b 40 watt bulb—18 inches
   c 60 watt bulb—24 inches
10 Note the time of application.
11 Measure the distance from the lamp to the patient. Use the tape measure or yardstick as in Figure 21-7.

12 Check the patient every 5 minutes. Check for redness or blistering of the skin. Ask about pain, burning, or decreased sensation. Stop the treatment if complications occur. Notify the nurse immediately.
13 Cover the body parts not being treated.
14 Remove the lamp after 20 to 30 minutes.
15 Return top linens to their proper position. Remove the bath blanket.
16 Make sure the patient is comfortable and unscreened. Place the signal light within reach.
17 Clean the lamp according to facility policy. Return it and other supplies to their proper place.
18 Wash your hands.
19 Report the following to the nurse:
   a The time the treatment started and ended
   b The site of application
   c Bulb wattage and the distance between the bulb and the patient
   d The patient's response
   e Any other observations

Heat Lamps

Dry heat can be applied with a heat lamp. A gooseneck lamp (Fig. 21-6) is used. The gooseneck is flexible. The lamp can be placed at various distances from the body part. First it is checked for breakage. The bulb wattage is also checked. The distance between the lamp and the body part is determined by the bulb wattage. The lamp is allowed to warm up before the treatment starts. It is not covered with bed linens. Heat from the lamp could burn the linens and cause a fire.

The Aquamatic Pad

The aquamatic pad is an electric heating pad. It is different from heating pads sold in stores. Those sold in stores have electric coils composed of wire. Tubes inside the aquamatic pad are filled with water. A heating unit placed at the bedside is also filled with distilled water. The water is heated and flows to the pad through a connecting hose (Fig. 21-8). Another hose returns water to the heating unit. The water is reheated and circulated back into the pad.

The heating unit is kept level with the pad and connecting hoses. Water must flow freely. Hoses should be free of kinks and air bubbles. The temperature is set at 105° F (40.5° C) with a key provided by the manufacturer. After the temperature is set, the key is removed. This prevents the temperature from being changed by the patient, a visitor, or other workers. The temperature may be preset in the central supply department. The key is kept in that department.

The aquamatic pad is an electrical device. Measures are taken to prevent equipment-related accidents.

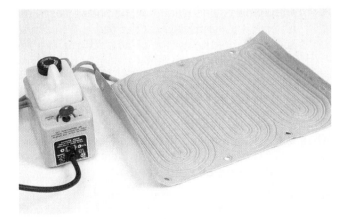

Fig. 21-8 The aquamatic pad and heating unit.

APPLYING AN AQUAMATIC PAD

1. Explain the procedure to the patient.
2. Wash your hands.
3. Collect the following equipment:
   a. Aquamatic pad and heating unit
   b. Distilled water
   c. Flannel cover
   d. Ties, tape, or rolled gauze
4. Identify the patient. Check the ID bracelet with the treatment card.
5. Provide for privacy.
6. Fill the heating unit ⅔ full with distilled water.
7. Remove any air bubbles. Place the pad and tubing below the heating unit. Then tilt the unit from side to side.
8. Set the temperature with the key. The nurse will tell you what the temperature should be (usually 105° F, or 40.5° C).
9. Place the pad in the flannel cover.
10. Plug in the unit. Let the water warm to the desired temperature.
11. Set the heating unit on the bedside stand. Keep the pad and connecting hoses level with the unit. Hoses must be free of kinks.
12. Apply the pad to the part. Note the time.
13. Secure the pad in place with ties, tape, or rolled gauze. Do not use pins.
14. Unscreen the patient. Make sure the signal light is within reach and the side rails are up.
15. Check the skin for redness, swelling, and blisters. Ask about pain, discomfort, or decreased sensation. Remove the pad if any occur. Notify the nurse immediately.
16. Remove the pad at the specified time.
17. Make sure the patient is comfortable and unscreened, and the side rails are up. Place the signal light within reach.
18. Clean and return equipment to its proper place.
19. Wash your hands.
20. Report the following to the nurse:
    a. The time of application and when it was removed
    b. The site of the application
    c. The temperature of the aquamatic pad
    d. The patient's response
    e. Any other observations

1. The cord is checked for fraying.
2. A three-pronged plug is used to ground the device.
3. The cord is kept out of the way of traffic.
4. The heating unit is placed on an uncluttered and even surface. This prevents it from being knocked over or knocked off of the surface.
5. Ties, tape, or rolled gauze are used to secure the pad in place. Pins are not used. They can puncture the pad and cause leaking.
6. A flannel cover is used to insulate the pad. It also absorbs perspiration at the application site.
7. The pad is not placed under the patient or under a body part. The weight of the body or extremity exerts pressure against the pad and mattress and prevents the escape of heat. Burns can result if heat cannot escape.

COLD APPLICATIONS

Cold applications reduce pain and prevent swelling. They also decrease circulation and cool the body when fever is present. Remember, heat and cold have opposite effects on body function.

Effects

When cold is applied to the skin, blood vessels constrict (see Fig. 21-1, *C*). Decreased blood flow results. Less oxygen and nutrients are carried to the tissues. Tissue metabolism also decreases. As a result, fewer toxic substances and waste products are produced. Cold applications are useful immediately after injuries. The decreased circulation reduces the amount of bleeding. The amount of fluid accumulation in tissues is also reduced. Cold has a numbing effect on the skin, which helps to reduce or relieve pain in the part. The skin appears pale and feels cool in the area of the cold because of decreased blood flow.

Complications

Complications can occur from local cold applications. They include pain, burns and blisters, and *cyanosis* (bluish discoloration of the skin). Burning and blistering tend to occur from intense cold. They also occur when dry cold applications are in direct contact with the skin. When cold is applied for a long time, blood vessels tend to dilate. Blood flow increases. Therefore the prolonged application of cold has the same effects as local heat applications.

Certain people have a greater risk for complications from local cold applications. They are infants, young children, the elderly, and fair-skinned persons.

Moist and Dry Applications

Cold applications can be moist or dry. The ice bag is a dry cold application. The cold compress and cold sponge bath are moist applications. Moist cold applications penetrate deeper than dry ones. Therefore temperatures of moist applications are not as cold as those of dry applications.

General Rules

Patients must be protected from injuries caused by cold applications. The general rules for the application of heat also apply for cold applications. The exceptions are:

1. Know the different temperature ranges for cool, cold, and very cold applications. The following ranges are guidelines:
   Cool—65° to 80° F (18.3° to 26.6° C)
   Cold—59° to 65° F (15° to 18.3° C)
   Very cold—59° F and below (15° C and below)
2. Do not let the patient lower the temperature of the application.
3. Report patient complaints of numbness, pain, or burning to the nurse immediately. Also immediately report blisters or burns; pale, white, or gray skin; cyanosis; and shivering.

Ice Bags

An ice bag is a dry cold application. The bag is filled with crushed ice or ice chips. Crushed ice is better because the bag can be molded to the body part more easily. Also, there is less air space between crushed ice for more even cooling. The ice bag is placed in a flannel cover before being applied. If the cover becomes moist, it is removed and a dry one is applied.

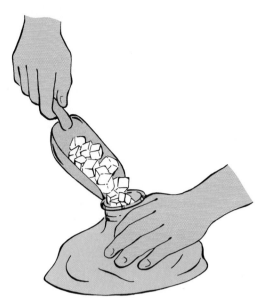

Fig. 21-9 The ice bag is filled with ice.

Ice bags are left in place for 30 minutes. If the bag is to be reapplied, wait 1 hour. This gives the tissues time to recover from the cold.

Ice collars are applied to the neck. Some facilities have commercial ice bags. They are filled with a special solution and are kept frozen until needed. Commercial ice bags can be refrozen for reuse. Flannel covers are also needed with ice collars or commercial ice bags.

APPLYING AN ICE BAG OR COLLAR

1 Explain the procedure to the patient.
2 Wash your hands.
3 Collect the following equipment:
  a Ice bag or collar
  b Crushed ice or ice chips
  c Flannel cover
  d Paper towels
4 Fill the ice bag with water. Put in the stopper. Turn the bag upside down to check for leaks.
5 Empty the bag.
6 Fill the bag ½ to ⅔ full with crushed ice or ice chips (Fig. 21-9).
7 Remove excess air. Bend, twist, or squeeze the bag, or press it against a firm surface.
8 Place the cap or stopper on securely.
9 Dry the bag with the paper towels.
10 Place the bag in the flannel cover.
11 Identify the patient. Check the ID bracelet with the treatment card.

12 Provide for privacy.
13 Apply the ice bag to the part.
14 Place the signal light within reach.
15 Check the skin every 10 minutes. Check for blisters; pale, white, or gray skin; cyanosis; and shivering. Ask about numbness, pain, or burning. Remove the bag if any occur. Notify the nurse immediately.
16 Remove the bag after 30 minutes.
17 Clean equipment. Discard the flannel cover.
18 Make sure the patient is comfortable and unscreened, and the side rails are up. Place the signal light within reach.
19 Wash your hands.
20 Report the following to the nurse:
  a The time of the application
  b The site of the application
  c The length of the application
  d The patient's response
  e Your observations of the skin

APPLYING DISPOSABLE COLD PACKS

1 Explain the procedure to the patient.
2 Wash your hands.
3 Collect the following equipment:
   a Disposable cold pack
   b Flannel cover
   c Ties, tape, or rolled gauze
4 Identify the patient. Check the ID bracelet with the treatment card.
5 Provide for privacy.
6 Squeeze, knead, or strike the cold pack as directed by the manufacturer. This causes a chemical reaction, which releases cold.
7 Cover the pack with the flannel cover.
8 Apply the cold pack to the part. Secure it in place with ties, tape, or rolled gauze. Note the time.
9 Place the signal light within reach.
10 Check the skin every 10 minutes. Check for blisters; pale, white, or gray skin; cyanosis; and shivering. Ask about pain, numbness, or burning. Remove the pack if any occur. Notify the nurse immediately.
11 Remove the pack after 30 minutes.
12 Discard the pack and other disposable equipment.
13 Make sure the patient is comfortable and unscreened, and the side rails are up. Place the signal light within reach.
14 Wash your hands.
15 Report the following to the nurse:
   a The time of the application
   b The site of the application
   c The length of the application
   d The patient's response
   e Your observations of the skin

Disposable Cold Packs

Disposable cold packs are dry cold applications. They are used once and then discarded. They come in various sizes to fit the different body parts. Some have an outer covering so that the pack can be applied directly to the skin. Use a flannel cover if there is no outer covering. A cold pack is left in place no longer than 30 minutes.

Cold Compresses

Applying a cold compress is similar to applying a hot compress. The cold compress is a moist application that may be sterile or nonsterile. As with hot compresses, the nurse applies sterile cold compresses. Sterile compresses are ordered for open wounds or breaks in the skin. Moist cold compresses are left in place no longer than 20 minutes.

APPLYING COLD COMPRESSES

1 Explain the procedure to the patient.
2 Wash your hands.
3 Collect the following equipment:
   a Large basin with ice
   b Small basin with cold water
   c Gauze squares, washcloths, or small towels
   d Waterproof pad
   e Bath towel
4 Identify the patient. Check the ID bracelet with the treatment card.
5 Provide for privacy.
6 Place the small basin with cold water into the large basin with ice.
7 Place the compresses into the cold water.
8 Place a bed protector under the area that is to receive the compress. Expose the area.
9 Wring out a compress so that water is not dripping.
10 Apply the compress to the part. Note the time.
11 Check the area every 5 minutes. Check for blisters; pale, white, or gray skin; cyanosis; or shivering. Ask about numbness, pain, or burning. Remove the compress if any occur. Notify the nurse immediately.
12 Change the compress when it becomes warm. Usually compresses are changed every 5 minutes.
13 Remove the compress after 20 minutes.
14 Pat dry the area with the bath towel.
15 Make sure the patient is comfortable and unscreened, and the side rails are up. Place the signal light within reach.
16 Clean equipment. Discard used linen.
17 Wash your hands,.
18 Report the following to the nurse:
   a The time of the application
   b The site of the application
   c The length of the application
   d The patient's response
   e Your observations of the skin

Cold Sponge Baths

The cold sponge bath is used to reduce body temperature when there is a high fever. A doctor's order is required. Sometimes the doctor orders that alcohol be added to the water. Alcohol evaporates quickly, causing rapid cooling. The cold sponge bath initially causes vasoconstriction, chilling, and shivering. These reactions to cold cause the body temperature to increase. As the body adjusts to the cold, body temperature decreases. The bath should last for 25 to 30 minutes to allow time for the body to adjust.

Body temperature and other vital signs are taken before, during, and after the procedure. Ice bags or moist cold compresses may be used to help lower the body temperature. They are applied to the forehead, axillae, and groin areas. The nurse may also request that they be placed on each side of the neck. A warm water bottle is sometimes applied to the feet to prevent chilling.

GIVING A COLD SPONGE BATH

1 Explain the procedure to the patient.
2 Wash your hands.
3 Collect the following equipment:
  a Bath basin
  b Bath thermometer
  c Equal amounts of 70% alcohol and water, if alcohol is ordered
  d Six ice bags or disposable ice packs
  e Bath blanket
  f Two or more bath towels
  g Two or more washcloths
  h Thermometer for body temperature
  i Hot water bottle
  j Sphygmomanometer and stethoscope
  k Ice chips
  l Seven flannel covers
4 Identify the patient. Check the ID bracelet with the treatment card.
5 Provide for privacy. Close the door to provide privacy and reduce drafts.
6 Measure and record vital signs. Note the time.
7 Raise the bed to a level appropriate for good body mechanics. Lower the side rail.
8 Cover the patient with a bath blanket. Remove top linens.
9 Remove the gown without exposing the patient. Raise the side rail.
10 Prepare the ice bags or packs for application. Place them in the flannel covers.
11 Prepare the hot water bottle for application. Place it in a flannel cover.
12 Lower the side rail. Move the patient to the side of the bed near you.
13 Apply the ice bags or packs to the forehead, axillae, and groin. Place one on each side of the neck if requested by the nurse. Apply the hot water bottle to the feet (Fig. 21-10).
14 Raise the side rail.
15 Fill the basin ⅔ full with cool water. Water (and alcohol if added) temperature should be 68° to 86° F (20° to 30° C). Add ice chips to cool the water if necessary.

16 Place the washcloths in the water. Alternate washcloths during the procedure. Make sure no ice chips stick to them.
17 Lower the side rail.
18 Place a bath towel under the patient's far arm.
19 Sponge the arm for 5 minutes using long, slow, gentle strokes. Pat the arm dry; do not rub dry.
20 Repeat steps 18 and 19 for the near arm.
21 Place the bath towel lengthwise over the patient's chest and abdomen. Fanfold the bath blanket to the pubic area.
22 Measure and record vital signs. Note the time.
23 Stop sponging and notify the nurse if one of the following occur:
  a Body temperature is reduced to normal or slightly above normal
  b Shivering
  c Cyanosis
  d Other signs and symptoms of cold. Check the skin under the ice bags and under the hot water bottle. Notify the nurse of signs of complications.
24 Place a towel under the far leg.
25 Sponge the leg with long, slow, gentle strokes for 5 minutes. Pat the leg dry, cover it, and remove the bath blanket.
26 Repeat steps 24 and 25 for the near leg.
27 Help the patient turn away from you.
28 Place a bath towel on the bed along the length of the patient's back and buttocks.
29 Sponge the back and buttocks with long, slow, gentle strokes for 5 minutes. Pat dry and remove the towel.
30 Position the patient supine in the center of the bed.
31 Remove the ice packs and hot water bottle.
32 Measure and record vital signs. Note the time.
33 Put a clean gown on the patient. Make the bed. Change damp or soiled linen.

Continued.

GIVING A COLD SPONGE BATH—cont'd

34 Make sure the patient is comfortable and the bed is in its lowest position. Place the signal light within reach. Unscreen the patient.

35 Clean and return equipment to its proper place.

36 Remove soiled linen and disposable equipment.

37 Measure vital signs 30 minutes after the procedure.

38 Wash your hands.

39 Report the following to the nurse:

   a The time the procedure was started and completed

   b Vital signs taken before, during, and after the procedure; and those taken 30 minutes after completion of the procedure

   c How the patient tolerated the procedure

   d Condition of the skin under the heat and cold applications

   e Other signs and symptoms

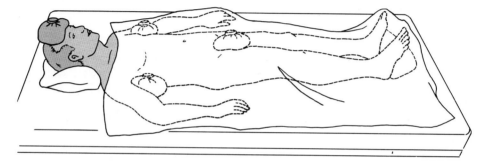

Fig. 21-10 Ice bags are applied to the forehead, axillae, and groin to help cool the body during the sponge bath. Ice bags may also be applied on each side of the neck. A hot water bottle is applied to the feet to prevent chilling.

SUMMARY

Heat and cold applications are often ordered by doctors. They have opposite effects on blood flow. However, both are used for healing, comfort, and tissue swelling. Extreme care must be taken to make sure the right temperature is used. The heat or cold must be applied properly. Close observation of the patient is also necessary. Complications can easily and quickly occur if necessary precautions are not taken. Of all the complications, burns are the most serious.

You may not be allowed to apply heat or cold. Only RNs or LPNs may be allowed to do so. If you are allowed to apply heat and cold, extreme caution must be taken. The dangers to the patient are severe. Therefore greater knowledge and judgment are required. The purpose and steps of the procedure need to be reviewed with the nurse. Also ask the nurse to closely supervise the procedure and its effects on the patient. The patient's safety is the most important consideration.

REVIEW QUESTIONS

Circle the best *answer.*

1 Local heat applications have the following effects *except*
   a Pain relief
   b Muscle relaxation
   c Healing
   d Decreased blood flow
2 The major complication of local heat applications is
   a Infection
   b Burns
   c Chilling
   d Decubiti
3 Which person has the greatest risk of complications from local heat applications?
   a A 10-year-old boy
   b A teenager
   c A 40-year-old woman
   d An elderly person
4 These statements are about moist heat applications. Which is *false?*
   a Water is in contact with the skin.
   b The effects of heat are less than with a dry heat application.
   c Heat penetrates deeper than with a dry heat application.
   d The temperature of the application is lower than a dry heat application.
5 The temperature of a hot application is usually between
   a 65° and 80° F
   b 93° and 98° F
   c 98° and 105° F
   d 105° and 115° F
6 An extremity is in a basin of hot water. This is a
   a Hot compress
   b Hot pack
   c Hot soak
   d Sitz bath
7 These statements are about sitz baths. Which is *false?*
   a The pelvic area is immersed in warm or hot water for 20 minutes.
   b The patient may become weak or faint.
   c The sitz bath lasts 25 to 30 minutes.
   d They can be used to clean the perineum, relieve pain, increase circulation, or stimulate voiding.
8 You are applying a heat lamp. You should do the following *except*
   a Cover the lamp with bed linens
   b Let the lamp warm up before starting the procedure
   c Check the bulb wattage
   d Measure the distance between the bulb and the patient's body
9 These statements are about aquamatic pads. Which is *false?*
   a The aquamatic pad is a dry heat application.
   b The temperature is usually set at 105° F.
   c Electrical safety precautions must be practiced.
   d Pins secure the aquamatic pad in place.
10 Local cold applications are used to
   a Reduce pain, prevent swelling, and decrease circulation
   b Dilate blood vessels
   c Prevent the spread of microorganisms
   d All of the above
11 Which is *not* a complication of local cold applications?
   a Pain
   b Burns and blisters
   c Cyanosis
   d Infection
12 Which is a dry cold application?
   a The ice bag
   b The cold compress
   c The cold sponge bath
   d All of the above
13 Before applying an ice bag
   a The bag is placed in a freezer
   b The temperature of the bag is measured
   c The bag is placed in a flannel cover
   d The patient is asked to void
14 Moist cold compresses are left in place no longer than
   a 20 minutes
   b 30 minutes
   c 45 minutes
   d 60 minutes
15 The cold sponge bath is ordered to
   a Reduce swelling
   b Relieve pain
   c Decrease circulation
   d Lower body temperature
16 The cold sponge bath should last
   a 15 to 20 minutes
   b 25 to 30 minutes
   c 45 to 50 minutes
   d 60 minutes or longer

Answers

16	b	12	a	8	a	4	b
15	d	11	d	7	c	3	d
14	a	10	a	6	c	2	b
13	c	9	d	5	c	1	d

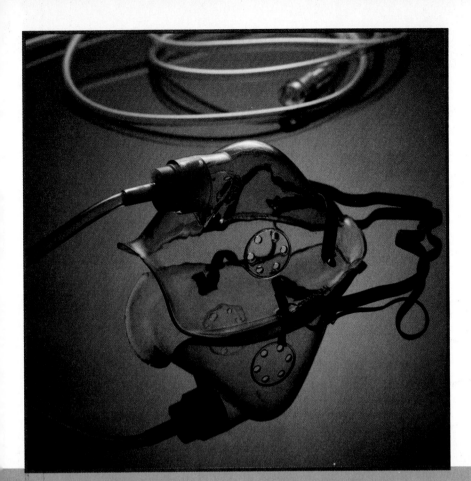

Special Procedures and Treatments

OBJECTIVES

- Define the key terms listed in this chapter
- Describe the safety measures that need to be practiced when caring for a patient with an IV infusion
- Identify common routes and reasons for suctioning
- Describe the rules related to suctioning
- Explain the purpose of oxygen therapy
- Describe the two sources of oxygen and four devices used to administer oxygen
- Describe the rules related to oxygen therapy
- Collect a sputum specimen
- Give a vaginal irrigation

22

face mask A device used in the administration of oxygen; it covers the nose and mouth

nasal cannula A two-pronged device used to administer oxygen; the prongs are inserted into the nostrils

nasal catheter A device used to administer oxygen; it is inserted through a nostril to the back of the throat

oxygen tent A device used to administer oxygen; it is made of clear plastic and covers all or the upper part of the bed

sputum Mucus secreted by the lungs, bronchi, and trachea during respiratory illnesses or disorders

suction The process of withdrawing or sucking up fluids

Most of the subjects and procedures presented in this chapter are the responsibility of RNs or LPNs. The principles involved are complex, and the risks to the patient are great. Nursing assistant education usually provides only very basic knowledge about biology, body structure and function, and disease processes. More knowledge and practice are needed to perform the procedures in this chapter. Educational programs for nursing assistants are usually not long enough to include content from this chapter.

IV therapy, suctioning, and oxygen therapy are never the responsibility of nursing assistants. However, you may be asked to collect a sputum specimen or give a vaginal irrigation. These procedures are performed only if you thoroughly understand them. You must understand the purpose, the procedure, and the possible complications. The procedure should be reviewed with the nurse. The nurse should closely supervise the procedure and its effect on the patient.

THE PATIENT WITH AN INTRAVENOUS INFUSION

An intravenous infusion is the administration of fluid through a needle within a vein. Nursing assistants are never responsible for IV therapy. However, you may care for patients receiving IV infusions. You must give safe care to these patients. Therefore you must understand the basic purposes of IV therapy. You also need to know the measures that are taken to assist the patient and the nurse.

Purposes

Intravenous infusions are ordered by doctors. They provide needed fluids to patients unable to take fluids by mouth. Minerals and vitamins lost because of illness or injury can be replaced through IVs. They are also used to provide sugar for energy and to administer medications and blood. The doctor orders the amount and type of IV solution to be administered.

Safety Measures

RNs are responsible for starting and maintaining IV infusions. An RN inserts a needle into a vein and connects IV tubing from the IV bottle (or bag) to the needle. RNs also regulate the flow rate (the number of drops per minute). They change the bottles or bags, tubing, and dressings at insertion sites. These are changed when necessary. Blood or medications ordered by the doctor are also administered by RNs.

You need to know two parts of the IV infusion (see Fig. 16-11, page 283). One is the drip chamber. Fluid drips from the bottle into the drip chamber. You can tell if the fluid is flowing by looking at the chamber. If no fluid is dripping, tell the nurse immediately. The second part is the clamp on the tubing. The RN uses the clamp to regulate the flow rate. *Never change the position of the clamp.*

You are never responsible for starting or maintaining the IV infusion. Nor are you responsible for regulating the flow rate or for changing bottles, tubing, or dressings. Nursing assistants never administer blood or medications. You may assist patients with

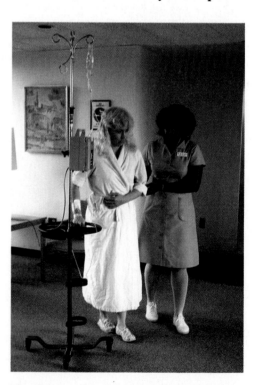

Fig. 22-1 A patient ambulating with an IV.

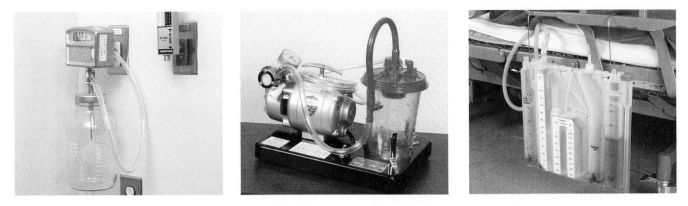

Fig. 22-2 **A,** Wall suction. **B,** Suction machine. **C,** Disposable suction apparatus.

IVs to meet personal hygiene and activity needs. Care must be taken to maintain the position of the IV needle when assisting a patient. If the needle is moved, it may come out of the vein. The fluid may flow into the tissues (infiltration), or the flow may stop. Sometimes a nurse has to splint or restrain the extremity to prevent movement of the part. This helps prevent the needle from moving. You must follow safety measures for the use of restraints (see Chapter 8). When changing a gown, be careful not to move the needle (see *Changing the Gown of a Patient with an IV*, page 220).

The IV bottle, tubing, and needle are protected when ambulating the patient. Portable IV standards are rolled along next to the patient (Fig. 22-1). The patient also needs help with turning and repositioning. The bottle is moved to the side of the bed on which the patient is lying. Always allow enough slack in the tubing. The needle will dislodge if pressure is exerted by the tubing.

SUCTIONING

Injury and illness often cause secretions to accumulate in body parts. Common areas are the upper airway, stomach, and surgical wounds. The secretions need to be removed for the patient's recovery and physical well-being. Suction is a method ordered by the doctor to remove excess secretions. *Suction* is the process of withdrawing or sucking up fluid (secretions). A tube is connected to a wall suction outlet, a suction machine, or a disposable suction apparatus (Fig. 22-2). The other end is inserted into the body part. The secretions are withdrawn through the tube (or catheter) into a collecting container.

Nursing assistants are never responsible for inserting tubes or suctioning patients. However, you may care for a patient who needs suctioning.

Upper Airway Suctioning

The airway must be clear of secretions for normal breathing. Secretions collect in the upper airway be-

cause of certain illnesses. Some patients cannot remove them by coughing. The upper airway needs to be suctioned to remove the secretions. A nurse inserts the suction catheter through the mouth or nose into the trachea when suctioning is needed (Fig. 22-3). When the procedure has been completed, the catheter is removed. You must be alert for signs and symptoms that indicate the need for suctioning. They are tachypnea, dyspnea, moist sounding respirations or gurgling, restlessness, or cyanosis. The signs and symptoms must be reported to the nurse immediately.

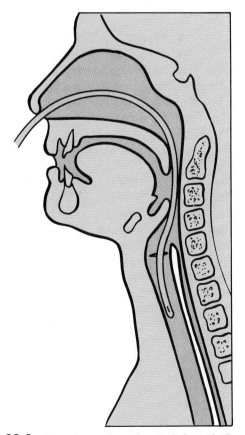

Fig. 22-3 A suction catheter inserted through the patient's nose into the trachea. Tubing connects the catheter to wall suction.

Nasogastric Suctioning

A nasogastric tube (Levine tube) is inserted to remove stomach contents and to keep the stomach empty. Gastrointestinal injuries, illnesses, and surgeries often require nasogastric suctioning. A nurse inserts the tube through the patient's nose, the esophagus, and into the stomach (see Fig. 16-8, page 283). The tube is connected to the suction source. The NG tube is left in place until the doctor orders its removal.

The NG tube can be very irritating to the patient's nose and mouth. Most patients breathe through their mouths when an NG tube is in place. Patients are also NPO when the tube is attached to suction. Frequent oral hygiene is necessary. The lips and oral mucous membranes can become dry and may crack. A bad taste in the mouth and mouth odor may develop. The nose also must be kept clean. Pressure and friction from the tube can irritate the nostril. Nasal secretions may harden and form crusts. The tube should not cause pressure on the nose.

Wound Suctioning

After surgery it may be necessary to suction blood and other drainage from a wound. A drain or catheter is inserted during surgery and attached to suction. Chest and abdominal surgeries usually require wound suction.

General Rules

The patient is protected from harm during suctioning. The suction tubing or catheter and the suction source are handled carefully. You need to practice the following safety rules.

1. Never suction a patient.
2. Make sure the patient is not lying on the catheter or tubing.
3. Make sure there are no kinks in the catheter or tubing.
4. Never turn off the suction source.
5. Do not raise the drainage container above the insertion site.
6. Do not empty the drainage container.
7. Do not disconnect any part of the suction system.
8. Report the appearance of bright red drainage or an increase in the amount of blood to the nurse immediately.
9. Observe the amount and appearance of drainage in the container. Report your observations to the nurse at regular intervals. Report unusual observations immediately.
10. Make sure there is enough slack in the tubing. There should not be any pull or pressure at the insertion site.

OXYGEN THERAPY

Oxygen is a tasteless, odorless, and colorless gas. Oxygen is necessary for survival. Death occurs within 4 minutes if a person stops breathing. Serious health problems develop if a person's oxygen supply is inadequate. During illness, the amount of oxygen carried in the blood may be less than normal. If so, the doctor will probably order supplemental oxygen. Surgical patients, the acutely ill, patients with respiratory disorders, and patients with heart disease often need supplemental oxygen.

Oxygen is a drug. The doctor orders the amount of oxygen to be administered and whether it is to be given continuously or intermittently (periodically). The orders also include the device used to give the oxygen. You are never responsible for administering oxygen. However, you may care for patients receiving oxygen therapy. Therefore you need to know how to give safe care to these patients.

Devices Used to Administer Oxygen

Oxygen is supplied through wall outlets and from oxygen tanks. With the wall outlet (Fig. 22-4), oxygen is piped into each patient unit. Each patient unit is connected to a centrally located oxygen supply.

The oxygen tank is portable (Fig. 22-5). It is brought to the patient unit when oxygen therapy is ordered by the doctor. Small oxygen tanks are used for emergency purposes. They are also used during transfers. Some ambulatory patients require continuous oxygen. They use small portable oxygen cylinders when walking (Fig. 22-6). The large oxygen tank or cylinder is more common in patient homes.

There are several devices used to administer oxygen. The *nasal catheter* (Fig. 22-7, *A*) is inserted by the doctor, nurse, or respiratory therapist. The cath-

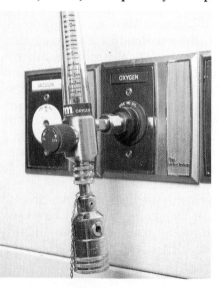

Fig. 22-4 Wall oxygen outlet.

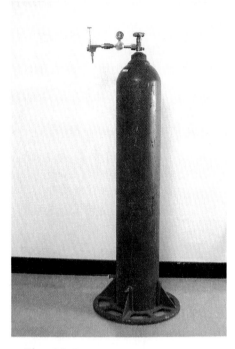

Fig. 22-5 Oxygen tank.

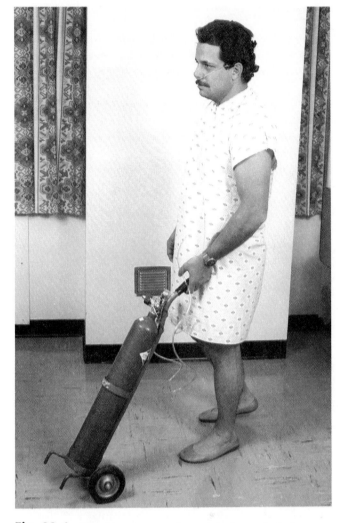

Fig. 22-6 Portable oxygen tank used during ambulation.

eter is inserted through the patient's nose until it can be seen in the back of the throat. It can be uncomfortable. Patients with NG tubes and those with nasal catheters have similar needs. Frequent oral hygiene and nasal care must be given.

The *nasal cannula* (Fig. 22-7, *B*) is the most common device used to administer oxygen. Two prongs project from the tubing and are inserted a short distance into the nostrils. The cannula is simple to use. The patient can eat and talk with it in place. Nasal irritation is possible if the prongs are too tight.

A *face mask* (Fig. 22-7, *C*) covers the nose and mouth. There are small holes in the sides of the mask. The holes allow the escape of carbon dioxide during exhalation and the entry of room air during inhalation. The mask must be removed for eating and drinking. A nasal cannula is usually used during meals. Many patients experience fright and feelings of suffocation with face masks. Talking can be difficult. The patient's face must be kept clean and dry to help prevent irritation from the mask.

Oxygen tents are not often used (Fig. 22-7, *D*). The other devices are more efficient. The tent is made of clear plastic and covers all or the upper part of the bed. Cool air that is rich in oxygen is circulated through the tent by a motor.

General Rules

The nurse and respiratory therapist are responsible for starting and maintaining oxygen therapy. You need to practice the safety precautions related to oxygen therapy.

1. Follow the safety precautions related to fire and the use of oxygen (see Chapter 8).
2. Never remove the device (cannula, catheter, mask, or tent) used to administer oxygen.
3. Never shut off the flow of oxygen from the wall outlet or tank.
4. Give oral hygiene as directed by the nurse.
5. Make sure the connecting tubing is taped or pinned to the patient's gown. The tubing must be secured in place.
6. Make sure there are no kinks in the tubing.
7. Make sure the patient is not lying on any part of the tubing.
8. Report signs and symptoms of respiratory distress or abnormal breathing patterns to the nurse immediately (see Chapter 17).
9. Observe the gauge to ensure that adequate oxygen is in the tank (Fig. 22-8).

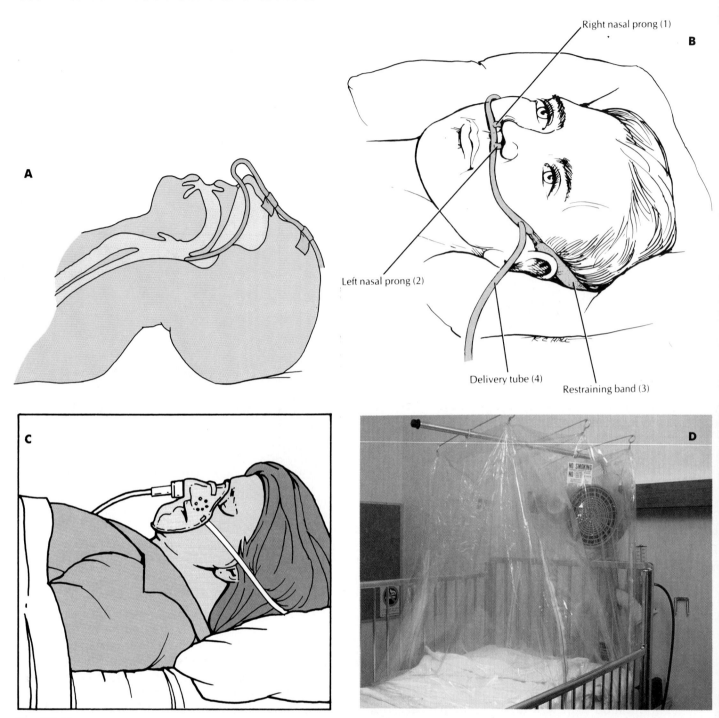

Fig. 22-7 **A,** Nasal catheter. **B,** Nasal cannula. **C,** Oxygen face mask. **D,** Oxygen tent. (**A** and **B** from Eubanks DH and Bone RC: *Comprehensive respiratory care: a learning system*, St Louis, 1985, Mosby–Year Book.)

Collecting Sputum Specimens

Respiratory disorders cause the lungs, bronchi, and trachea to secrete mucus. This mucous secretion is called *sputum* when it is expectorated (expelled) through the mouth. Sputum should not be mistaken for saliva. Saliva is a thin, clear liquid produced by the salivary glands in the mouth. Saliva is often called "spit."

Sputum specimens are studied for the presence of blood, microorganisms, and abnormal cells. The patient needs to cough up the sputum from the bronchi and trachea. Coughing and raising sputum can be very painful and difficult. It is usually easier to collect a specimen in the early morning. Secretions are usually coughed up after the patient wakes. The patient is allowed to rinse his or her mouth with water. Rinsing decreases the amount of saliva and removes food particles. Mouthwash is not used before collecting a

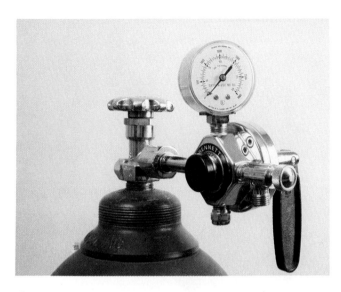

Fig. 22-8 The oxygen tank gauge shows the amount remaining.

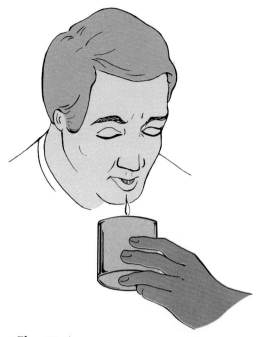

Fig. 22-9 The patient expectorates directly into the center of the specimen container.

sputum specimen. Mouthwash can destroy some of the microorganisms that may be present.

Collecting a sputum specimen can be embarrassing for the patient. Nearby patients may find that the sound of the coughing and expectorating is upsetting or nauseating. Also, the appearance of sputum can

be disagreeable to the patient and others. For these reasons the patient should be allowed privacy during the procedure. The specimen container should be immediately covered and placed in a paper bag. Some facilities have paper-covered sputum containers that conceal the contents.

COLLECTING A SPUTUM SPECIMEN

1 Explain the procedure to the patient.
2 Wash your hands.
3 Collect the following equipment:
   a Sputum specimen container with cover
   b Tissues
   c Label
   d Laboratory requisition slip
   e Paper bag
4 Write the requested information on the label. Put it on the container.
5 Identify the patient. Check the ID bracelet with the requisition slip.
6 Provide for privacy. Let the patient use the bathroom to obtain the specimen if able.
7 Ask the patient to rinse the mouth out with clear water.
8 Have the patient hold the container. Only the outside of the container is touched.
9 Ask the patient to cover the mouth and nose with tissues when coughing.
10 Ask him or her to take 2 or 3 deep breaths and cough up the sputum.

11 Have the patient expectorate directly into the container (Fig. 22-9). Sputum should not touch the outside of the container.
12 Collect 1 to 2 tablespoons of sputum unless directed to collect more.
13 Put the lid on the container immediately.
14 Place the container in the paper bag. Attach the requisition slip to the bag.
15 Make sure the patient is comfortable and unscreened.
16 Take the bag to the laboratory.
17 Wash your hands.
18 Report the following to the nurse:
   a The time the specimen was collected and taken to the laboratory
   b The amount of sputum collected
   c How easily the patient raised the sputum
   d The consistency and appearance of the sputum (thick, clear, white, green, yellow, or blood-tinged)
   e Any other observations

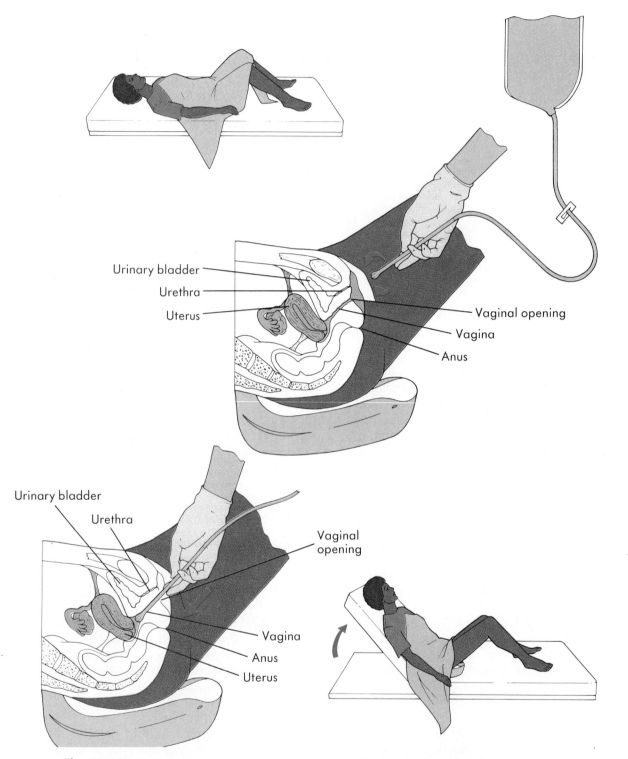

Fig. 22-10 Vaginal irrigation. **A,** Position of the patient. **B,** Solution is used to cleanse the vulva. **C,** Solution flows into the vagina through a nozzle that has been inserted 3 to 4 inches. **D,** Elevating the head of the bed allows the solution to drain from the vagina. (From Dison N: *Clinical nursing techniques*, ed 4, 1979, Mosby–Year Book.)

THE VAGINAL IRRIGATION

A vaginal irrigation (douche) is the introduction of a fluid into the vagina and the immediate return of the fluid. Vaginal douches are ordered by doctors to relieve pain and inflammation. They may be done to clean the vagina preoperatively or because of discharge. Medications and heat and cold can be applied with a vaginal irrigation. You should not perform the procedure if heat, cold, or a medication is being applied.

Vaginal irrigations are not done during menstruation. Nor are they done during the late part of pregnancy or during the first 6 to 8 weeks after childbirth. Douching after sexual intercourse is not a method of birth control. Normally, douching is not necessary. The vaginal secretions cleanse the vagina naturally and protect it from infection.

A disposable kit is used. It consists of a container, connecting tubing, and nozzle. The nozzle is made of plastic and is checked for chips and cracks, which could cause vaginal injury. The patient is positioned

GIVING A VAGINAL IRRIGATION

1 Explain the procedure to the patient.
2 Wash your hands.
3 Collect the following equipment:
 a Disposable vaginal irrigation kit
 b 1000 ml of the irrigation solution
 c Bath thermometer
 d Bath blanket
 e Bedpan
 f Toilet tissue
 g Waterproof pad
 h Disposable gloves
 i IV pole
 j Water pitcher
 k Equipment for perineal care
4 Identify the patient. Check the ID bracelet with the treatment card.
5 Provide for privacy.
6 Raise the bed to a level appropriate for good body mechanics.
7 Offer the bedpan and ask the patient to urinate. Her bladder should be empty for the procedure. Provide toilet tissue and ensure privacy.
8 Empty the bedpan. Measure I&O if ordered. Clean and return the bedpan. (Wear gloves for this step.)
9 Wash your hands.
10 Warm the irrigation solution. It should be body temperature or 105° F (40.5° C) as directed by the nurse. If the solution was prepared by central supply, set the container in a basin of hot water. Allow it to warm.
11 Do the following to warm a tap water solution. Fill the pitcher with 1000 ml of warm water. Measure the water temperature. Adjust the water temperature accordingly.
12 Cover the patient with a bath blanket. Fanfold the top linens to the foot of the bed.
13 Help the patient assume a back-lying position. Drape her with the bath blanket as for perineal care.
14 Place the waterproof pad under her buttocks.

15 Put on the gloves.
16 Provide perineal care (see *Giving Female Perineal Care*, page 211).
17 Position the patient on the bedpan.
18 Clamp the irrigation tubing. Pour the solution into the irrigation container.
19 Hang the container from the IV pole. It should be 12 inches above the level of the vagina.
20 Position the nozzle over the vulva. Unclamp the tubing. Let some solution run over the perineal area.
21 Insert the nozzle 3 to 4 inches into the vagina as in Figure 22-10. Rotate the nozzle gently during the procedure.
22 Clamp the tubing when the container is empty. Remove the nozzle.
23 Place the tubing in the irrigation container.
24 Assist the patient to sit up on the bedpan. This allows the rest of the solution to drain from the vagina into the bedpan.
25 Help her lie down again.
26 Remove the bedpan. Dry the perineal area with toilet tissue.
27 Take the bedpan into the bathroom. Clean and return it to its proper place.
28 Remove the waterproof pad.
29 Discard used disposable supplies.
30 Change damp linen. Remove the gloves.
31 Make sure the patient is comfortable.
32 Return top linens and remove the bath blanket.
33 Raise the side rail and lower the bed to its lowest position. Place the signal light within reach. Unscreen the patient.
34 Wash your hands.
35 Report the following to the nurse:
 a The time the irrigation was given
 b The amount, type, and temperature of the solution
 c The patient's response
 d The character of the returned solution
 e Any other observations

on her back for the procedure. The nozzle is gently inserted backward and upward (Fig. 22-10). This follows the angle of the vagina when the patient is in the back-lying position.

SUMMARY

Intravenous therapy, suction, and oxygen therapy are never the responsibility of nursing assistants. However, you may care for a patient receiving one of these therapies. You need to have a sound, basic understanding of their purposes and general safety rules.

Patient safety must never be overlooked. Careful observation of the patient is necessary. You must promptly report observations and patient complaints. The side effects and complications of some of the treatments and procedures can be severe. Every sign, symptom, or patient complaint is important.

Finally, you need to know your own limitations. Do not perform any procedure you do not understand or with which you are unfamiliar. Remember your legal and ethical responsibilities. You have the right to say no. Do not do anything that is beyond your legal scope, preparation, and skill level.

REVIEW QUESTIONS

Circle the best *answer.*

1 A patient has an IV infusion. You should
  a Add a new bottle if necessary
  b Check the drip chamber to see if fluid is dripping
  c Use the clamp to regulate the flow rate
  d Change the tubing daily
2 These statements are about suctioning the upper airway. You can
  a Suction the patient whenever necessary
  b Set up the suction system
  c Observe for signs and symptoms that indicate a need for suction
  d Turn on the suction source
3 A patient has nasogastric suction. You should
  a Give frequent oral hygiene
  b Turn off the suction when transferring the patient to the chair
  c Irrigate the tube
  d Empty the drainage container
4 These devices are used to administer oxygen. Which is the simplest and most often used?
  a Nasal catheter
  b Nasal cannula
  c Face mask
  d Oxygen tent
5 A patient is receiving supplemental oxygen. You should do the following *except*

  a Follow the safety measures related to fire and the use of oxygen
  b Remove the administration device for meals
  c Give oral hygiene as directed by the nurse
  d Make sure there are no kinks in the tubing
6 You are to collect a sputum specimen. Which is *false?*
  a An early morning specimen is best.
  b Provide for the patient's privacy.
  c The patient can use mouthwash before raising the sputum.
  d The sputum is expectorated directly into the specimen container.
7 You are to give a vaginal irrigation. You should do the following *except*
  a Have the patient void before beginning the procedure
  b Warm the solution to body temperature or to 105° F
  c Check the nozzle for chips or cracks
  d Hang the container 18 to 24 inches above the vagina

Answers

		3 a
7 d	5 b	2 c
6 c	4 b	1 b

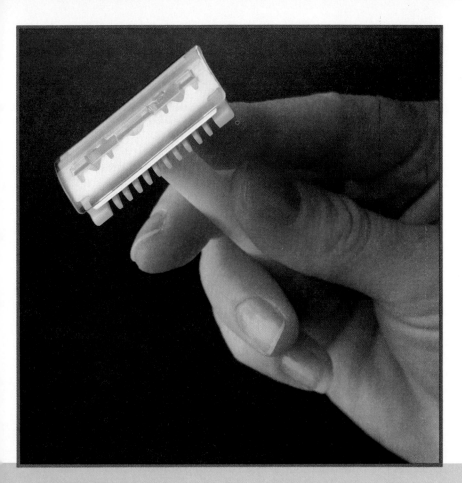

The Patient Having Surgery

23

OBJECTIVES

- Define the key terms listed in this chapter
- Describe the common fears and concerns of surgical patients
- Explain how patients are psychologically prepared for surgery
- Describe how to prepare a room for the postoperative patient
- Identify the signs and symptoms that must be immediately reported to the nurse during the postoperative period
- Explain the importance of turning and repositioning patients after surgery
- Explain the importance of coughing and deep breathing
- Explain the purpose of leg exercises
- Perform the procedures described in this chapter

anesthesia The loss of feeling or sensation produced by a drug given before surgery

atelectasis The collapse of a portion of the lung

elective surgery Scheduled surgery that the person chooses to have at a particular time

embolus A blood clot that travels through the vascular system until it lodges in a distant blood vessel

emergency surgery Surgery that is unscheduled and is done immediately to save the person's life or limb

general anesthesia Unconsciousness and the loss of feeling or sensation produced by a drug

postoperative After the operation or surgery

preoperative Before the operation or surgery

regional anesthesia The loss of sensation or feeling in a part of the body, produced by the injection of a drug; the patient does not lose consciousness

thrombus A blood clot

Surgeries are performed for many reasons. Surgery may be done to remove a diseased organ or body part, to remove a tumor, or to repair injured tissue. Surgery can also be done to diagnose a disease, to improve appearance, or to relieve symptoms. Surgery may be *elective*—the doctor and patient agree on a time for the surgery. Elective surgery can be scheduled 1 day or 6 months in advance. For example, a school-age child needs a tonsillectomy (tonsils are removed [ectomy]). The parents will probably schedule the surgery during a school vacation.

Emergency surgery is done immediately to save a person's life or limb. The need for surgery is sudden and unexpected. Vehicle accidents, stabbings, and bullet wounds often require emergency surgery.

Patients must be prepared physically and psychologically for surgery. Nurses and doctors are responsible for preparing the patient. They prepare the patient for what to expect before and after surgery.

If you work in a hospital, you may have contact with patients before and after surgery. In nursing facilities you may care for residents recovering from surgery. Many postoperative patients need home care. Your role in caring for surgical patients depends on certain factors. One relates to the employer's policies. Another is whether the surgery was simple or complex. The patient's condition before and after surgery is also a factor.

PSYCHOLOGICAL CARE OF THE PATIENT

Illness or injury causes many fears and concerns in the patient. The need for surgery may increase these fears. The person's deepest and worst fears are often felt. How would you feel if tomorrow your body was going to be cut open? Would you fear cancer or the loss of function? Would you have fears about pain, nausea and vomiting, or death? Who will care for your children and your home? Who will earn money while you are hospitalized? Imagine you have been in an accident. You are taken to the emergency room by ambulance. You wake up several hours later. The doctor tells you your right leg was amputated during surgery.

Psychological preparation is important. The person's fears and concerns must be appreciated. The health team needs to show the patient warmth, sensitivity, and caring.

Fears and Concerns of the Patient

A person's feelings are influenced by past experiences. Some patients have had surgery before. Others have not. Family and friends who have had surgery usually share their experiences with the patient. Their experiences also affect the patient. Most people have heard about tragic surgical events. Such tragedies include surgery on the wrong patient or instruments left inside the body. The patient may not talk about his or her fears and concerns. Instead the person may be quiet and withdrawn, may cry, or may talk constantly. Some pace, are unusually cheerful, or show unusual behavior. These behaviors may be due to one or more fears.

1. The fear that cancer will be found
2. The fear that the body will be disfigured
3. The fear of disability
4. The fear of pain during surgery
5. The fear of dying during surgery
6. The fear of the effects of anesthesia
7. The fear of going to sleep or not waking up after surgery
8. The fear of body exposure
9. The fear of severe pain or discomfort after surgery
10. The fear of tubes, needles, and other equipment used for care
11. The fear of complications
12. The fear of a prolonged recovery
13. The fear that further surgery or other treatments will be needed
14. The fear of being separated from family and friends

The following concerns are also common among surgical patients. They may affect the patient's behavior:

1. Who will care for children and other family members?

2. Are the children being cared for properly?
3. Who will take care of pets or plants?
4. Who will take care of the house, do the cleaning and laundry, mow the lawn, and tend the garden?
5. How will monthly bills, loan payments, mortgages, or rent be paid?
6. Will insurance cover hospital and doctor bills?

What the Patient Has Been Told

The physician explains the need for surgery to the patient. The person is told about the surgical procedure, risks, and possible complications. Probable consequences of not having surgery are also explained. The patient is told who will do the surgery, when it is scheduled, and how long it will take. The doctor and nurse provide other information. The patient and family may need to know more about the surgery and what to expect. Questions and misunderstandings may need to be cleared up. Instructions about care are also given.

The doctor tells the patient and the family about the surgery results. The doctor decides what and when to tell them. Often the health team knows before the patient does. Patients and families are usually anxious to know the results. They often ask nurses, nursing assistants, and other health workers. Often they ask if the reports are back from the laboratory or what the reports say. Knowing what the patient has been told is very important. You must not tell of any diagnosis, nor should you give incomplete or inaccurate information. The nurse will tell you what and when the patient and family have been told.

Responsibilities of the Nursing Assistant

You can assist in the psychological care of the surgical patient. You should do the following if you are involved in preoperative care:

1. Listen to the patient who voices fears or concerns about surgery
2. Refer any questions about the surgery or its results to the nurse
3. Explain procedures to the patient and why they are being done
4. Follow the rules of communication (see Chapter 3)
5. Use verbal and nonverbal methods of communication to relate to the surgical patient (see Chapter 4)
6. Provide care and perform procedures in an efficient and competent manner
7. Report any verbal and nonverbal indications of patient fear or anxiety to the nurse
8. Report a patient's request to see a member of the clergy to the nurse

THE PREOPERATIVE PERIOD

The preoperative (before surgery) period may be several days or just a few minutes. The length of time depends on the urgency of the surgery. If time permits, the patient is prepared psychologically and physically for the effects of anesthesia and surgery. Good preoperative preparation can prevent postoperative complications.

Preoperative Teaching

The nurse is responsible for preoperative teaching. Explanations are given about what to expect before and after surgery. Preoperative activities are explained. These include the type and purpose of tests, skin preparation, personal care measures, and the purpose and effects of preoperative medications. The patient is taught and encouraged to practice deep breathing, coughing, and leg exercises. After surgery, these activities are done every 1 or 2 hours while the patient is awake. The importance of turning, repositioning, and early ambulation after surgery is also explained.

The nurse tells the patient about the sights and sensations to expect when consciousness is regained. The patient is told about the recovery room where he or she will wake up (Fig. 23-1). It is explained that vital signs are taken frequently until they are stable. The patient is told about the type and amount of pain to expect. The patient is also told that pain medications are given for comfort. Certain treatments and equipment may be needed, depending on the type of surgery. The patient may be told about an IV infusion, urinary catheter, NG tube, oxygen, or wound suction. Special devices, such as a cast or traction, may also be needed. Activity or positioning restrictions are explained by the nurse as indicated.

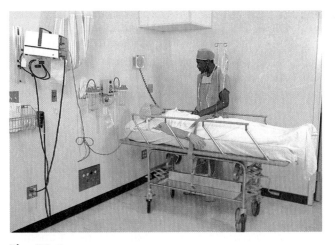

Fig. 23-1 Recovery room.

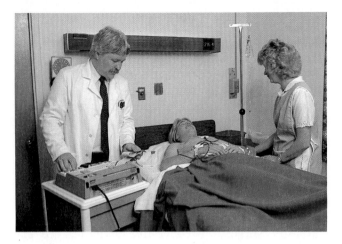

Fig. 23-2 An electrocardiogram is being taken.

Special Tests

Before surgery the doctor orders several tests. They are done to evaluate the patient's circulatory, respiratory, and urinary systems. These tests include a chest x-ray examination, a complete blood count (CBC), and urinalysis. An electrocardiogram (ECG or EKG) is done to detect any cardiac (heart) problems. The electrocardiogram is a recording of the electrical activity of the heart (Fig. 23-2). If blood loss is expected, the patient's blood is tested to determine the blood type. The blood is also tested for reactions with blood that may be given. This is called "type and crossmatch." Other tests may be done depending on the patient's condition and the surgery. A nurse prepares the patient for the tests. The nurse also makes sure the results are on the chart by the time of surgery.

Nutrition and Fluids

A light supper is usually allowed the evening before surgery. Then the patient is NPO from midnight until otherwise ordered. These measures reduce the risk of vomiting and aspiration during anesthesia and after surgery. Sometimes surgery is scheduled after noon. Then the patient is usually allowed a regular supper and a light breakfast. The NPO restriction begins after breakfast. You may be told to place the NPO sign in the patient's room. Remember to remove the water pitcher and glass when the patient is NPO.

Enemas

An enema may be given the evening before or the morning of surgery. A commercial enema or a cleansing enema may be ordered by the doctor. Abdominal surgeries almost always require a preoperative enema. If intestinal surgery is to be done, cleansing enemas are ordered. Cleansing enemas clear the colon of feces. Enemas are also given when straining or a

bowel movement could cause postoperative problems. Such problems include pain, severe bleeding (hemorrhage), or stress on the operative area. You may be assigned to give the preoperative enema.

Personal Care

You may be assigned to assist the patient with personal care. The patient should have a complete bed bath, shower, or tub bath the evening before or the morning of surgery. The bath reduces the number of microbes on the skin at the time of surgery. The doctor may order a shampoo for the evening before surgery. The patient's color and circulation must be observed during and after surgery. Therefore all makeup and nail polish are removed before surgery. Long hair is braided. All hair pins, clips, combs, and similar items are removed. Some facilities have both men and women wear surgical caps. A cap keeps hair out of the face and the operative area.

Oral hygiene is important before surgery. Because of being NPO, the patient will be very thirsty and will have a dry mouth. Good oral hygiene promotes comfort. However, the person must not swallow any water during the procedure. Dentures are not worn to the operating room. They are removed before preoperative medications are given. They are cleaned and kept moist in a denture cup. They are kept in a safe place. Some patients do not want to be seen without their dentures. If possible, let patients wear their dentures until they must be removed. This helps maintain the person's sense of dignity and esteem.

Other valuables are removed for safekeeping. These include glasses, contact lenses, hearing aids, and jewelry. These items can easily be lost or broken during surgery. They can also be lost or broken during transfers to the operating room, recovery room, and back to the patient's room. A note is made on the patient's chart about which valuables have been removed and where they are being kept. The patient may ask to wear a wedding band or religious medal. The item is secured in place with gauze or tape according to hospital policy.

Skin Preparation

The skin is prepared for surgery by thorough cleansing and shaving. The skin and hair shafts contain microorganisms that could enter the body through the surgical incision. A serious infection could result. The skin cannot be sterilized. However, the number of microbes can be reduced by the "skin prep."

The area to be prepared includes the site where the incision will be made. A large part of the surrounding area is also "prepped." This helps reduce the possibility of contamination during draping. Hospital policy and the surgeon's preferences determine the area to be prepared for a specific surgery (Fig. 23-3).

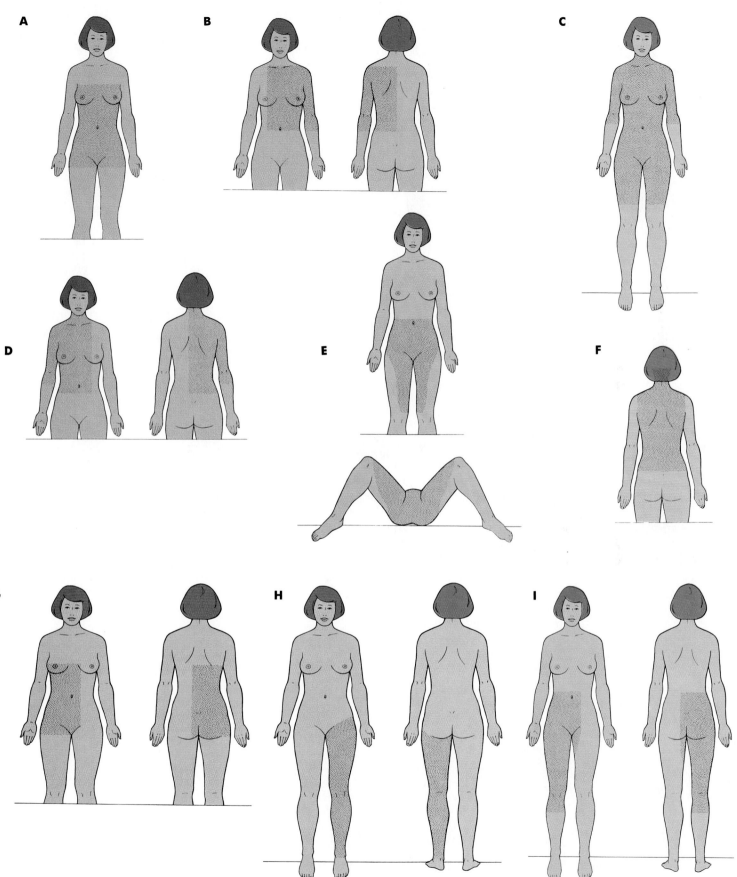

Fig. 23-3 Skin preparation sites for surgeries on various body areas. The shaded area indicates the area that should be shaved. **A,** Abdominal surgery. **B,** Chest or thoracic surgery. **C,** Open-heart surgery. **D,** Breast surgery. **E,** Perineal surgery. **F,** Cervical spine surgery. **G,** Kidney surgery. **H,** Knee surgery. **I,** Hip and thigh surgery.

Continued.

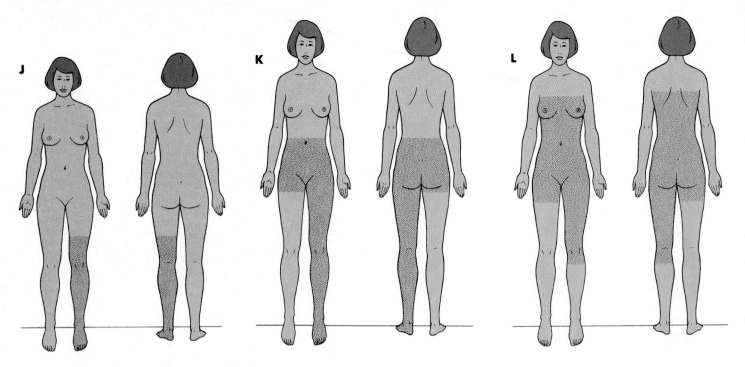

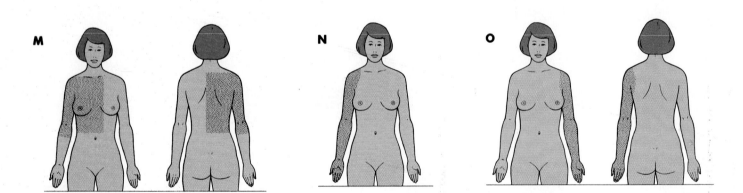

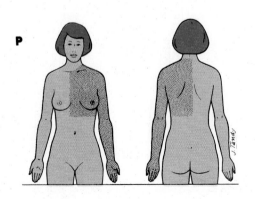

Fig. 23-3, cont'd **J,** Lower leg and foot surgery. **K,** Complete lower extremity surgery. **L,** Abdominal and leg surgery. **M,** Upper arm surgery. **N,** Lower arm surgery. **O,** Elbow surgery. **P,** Upper arm surgery.

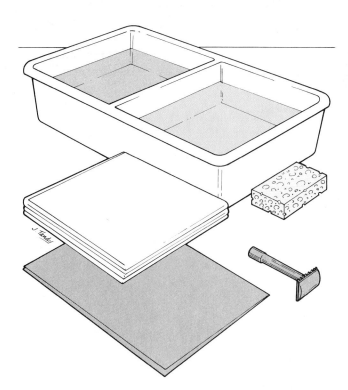

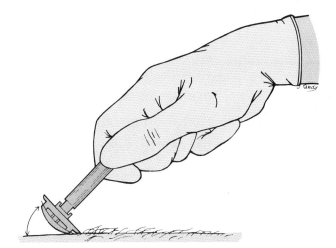

Fig. 23-5   The skin is held taut. Shaving is done in the direction of hair growth.

Fig. 23-4   Skin prep kit.

SHAVING THE PATIENT'S SKIN (SKIN PREP)

1 Explain the procedure to the patient.
2 Wash your hands.
3 Collect the following equipment:
   a Disposable skin prep kit
   b Bath blanket
   c Warm water
   d Disposable gloves
   e Waterproof pad
   f Bath towel
4 Identify the patient. Check the ID bracelet with the treatment card.
5 Provide for privacy.
6 Make sure you have good lighting. There should be no glares or shadows.
7 Raise the bed to a level appropriate for good body mechanics. Lower the side rail.
8 Cover the patient with a bath blanket. Fanfold top linens to the foot of the bed.
9 Place the waterproof pad under the area to be shaved.
10 Open the disposable skin prep kit.
11 Position the patient for the skin prep. Drape him or her with the disposable drape.
12 Add warm water to the basin. Put on the gloves.
13 Apply soap to the skin with the sponge. Work up a good lather.
14 Hold the skin taut. Shave in the direction of hair growth (see Fig. 23-5).
15 Shave outward from the center using short strokes.
16 Rinse the razor often.
17 Check to see that the entire area is free of hair. Make sure there are no cuts, scratches, or nicks.
18 Rinse the skin thoroughly. Pat dry.
19 Remove the drape and waterproof pad. Remove the gloves.
20 Return top linens. Remove the bath blanket.
21 Make sure the patient is comfortable.
22 Lower the bed to its lowest position. Place the signal light within reach. Unscreen the patient.
23 Return equipment to its proper place.
24 Discard used disposable equipment and soiled linen.
25 Wash your hands.
26 Report the following to the nurse:
   a The time the procedure was completed
   b The area prepared
   c Any cuts, nicks, or scratches
   d Any other observations

PREOPERATIVE CHECK LIST

ID BAND ON PATIENT_____

OPERATION CONSENT SIGNED____WITNESSED_____

HISTORY AND PHYSICAL_____

OPERATIVE AREA PREPARED_____

UA AND CBC DONE AND REPORT ON CHART_____

DENTURES IN OR OUT (CIRCLE)_____

BATH_____ORAL HYGIENE_____

VOIDED OR CATHETER_____

NPO MIDNIGHT_____

BREAKFAST (IF ORDERED)_____

ENEMA AS ORDERED_____

LEVINE INSERTED_____

CATHETER INSERTED_____

I & O SHEET ON CHART_____

PATIENT ABNORMALITIES_____

    DEAF, BLIND, DIABETES, AMPUTATION, COLOSTOMY, CARDIAC DISEASE, ETC._____

BED RAISED_____SIDE RAILS UP_____

HOSPITAL GOWN ON PATIENT_____

PREOPERATIVE MEDICATION GIVEN____TIME NOTED_____

TYPE AND CROSS MATCH COMPLETED_____

JEWELRY REMOVED OR SECURED_____

    WHERE PUT_____

MAKEUP REMOVED____MASCARA____LIPSTICK____NAIL POLISH____WIGS, WIGLETS,

    BOBBY PINS_____

CONTACT LENSES REMOVED_____

TEMPERATURE, PULSE, AND RESPIRATION_____

BLOOD PRESSURE_____

ALLERGIES_____

SIGNED _____

Fig. 23-6 Preoperative checklist.

The skin prep is done the evening before or the morning of surgery. The "skin prep" may be done in the patient's room by a nurse or nursing assistant. It may also be done in the operating room area by a member of the surgical team. Some hospitals have a "prep team" responsible for shaving all patients scheduled for surgery.

Disposable "prep kits" are used. A kit has a disposable razor, a sponge filled with soap, a basin, and a disposable drape and towel (Fig. 23-4). The skin is lathered with soap. Then the skin is shaved in the direction of hair growth (Fig. 23-5). Any break in the skin is a possible site of infection. You may be assigned to do a skin prep. Be very careful not to cut, scratch, or nick the skin during the procedure.

The Consent for Surgery

Before surgery can be done, the patient must give permission. The patient signs an "operative permit" or "surgical consent." The consent is signed when the person understands the information given by the doctor. Sometimes the patient's spouse or nearest relative is also required to sign the consent. A parent or legal guardian signs the surgical consent of a minor child. The legal guardian signs for a person who is mentally incompetent. The doctor is responsible for securing the patient's written consent. However, this responsibility is often delegated to the nurse. You are never responsible for obtaining the patient's written consent for surgery.

The Preoperative Checklist

A preoperative checklist (Fig. 23-6) is placed on the front of the patient's chart. The nurse makes sure the checklist is completed. Completion of the list means that the patient is ready for surgery. The nurse may ask you to do some of the things on the list. You need to promptly report when you have completed each activity. Observations are also reported. Except for the preoperative medication and side rails, the entire checklist is completed before preoperative medications are given.

Preoperative Medication

Medication is usually given the night before surgery to help the patient sleep. About 45 minutes to 1 hour before surgery, the preoperative medications are given. One medication helps the patient relax and feel drowsy. The other dries up respiratory secretions to prevent aspiration. Complaints of drowsiness, lightheadedness, thirst, and dry mouth are normal and expected.

Falls and accidents must be prevented after the preoperative medications are given. Side rails are raised and the patient is not allowed out of bed.

Therefore the patient is asked to urinate before the medications are given. Once the medications have been given, the bedpan or urinal is used for voiding. Smoking is not allowed. Dropping a cigarette or falling asleep can occur.

The bed is raised to the highest position at this time. The patient will be transferred from the bed to a stretcher. Furniture is moved out of the way to make room for the stretcher. The overbed table and bedside stand are cleaned off. This prevents damage to equipment and valuables.

Transporting the Patient to the Operating Room

A nurse or attendant from the operating room brings a stretcher to the patient's room. The patient is transferred onto the stretcher and covered with a bath blanket to provide warmth and prevent exposure. The patient is protected from falling. Safety straps are secured, and the side rails are raised. A small pillow may be placed under the patient's head for comfort.

Identification checks are made. Then the patient's chart is given to the staff member from the operating room.

The nurse responsible for preoperative care may go with the patient to the entrance of the operating room area. The family may be allowed to go also.

ANESTHESIA

There are two types of anesthetics: general and regional. *General anesthetics* produce unconsciousness and the loss of feeling or sensation. They are given in two ways. A drug is given intravenously, or a gas is inhaled (breathed in). *Regional anesthetics* (local anesthetics) produce loss of sensation or feeling in a body part. The patient does not lose consciousness. A drug is injected into a body part for regional anesthesia.

Anesthetics are given by specially educated doctors and nurses. An *anesthesiologist* is a doctor who specializes in the administration of anesthetics. An *anesthetist* is a nurse who has had advanced study in the administration of anesthetics.

THE POSTOPERATIVE PERIOD

After surgery (postoperative) the patient is taken to the recovery room or postanesthesia room (PAR). The recovery room is near the operating room. This is where the patient recovers from the anesthetic. The patient is watched very closely. Vital signs are taken, and other observations are made often. Certain conditions must be met before the patient leaves the recovery room. Vital signs must be stable. The patient must also be able to respond and call for help when it is needed. The doctor gives the transfer order when appropriate.

Preparing the Patient's Room

The room must be ready for the patient's return from the recovery room. A surgical bed is made. Equipment and supplies needed for the person's care are brought to the room. The nurse will tell you if special preparations and equipment are needed. The room is prepared after the patient is taken to the operating room. Preparations include:

1. Making a surgical bed
2. Placing equipment and supplies in the room:
   a. Thermometer
   b. Stethoscope
   c. Sphygmomanometer
   d. Emesis basin
   e. Tissues
   f. Waterproof bed protector
   g. Vital signs flow sheet
   h. Intake and output record
   i. IV pole
   j. Other equipment as directed by the nurse
3. Raising the bed to its highest position; the side rails must be down
4. Moving furniture out of the way so that the stretcher can be brought into the room

Receiving the Patient From the Recovery Room

The recovery room nurse calls the nursing unit when the patient is ready to be transferred. Sometimes special equipment is needed. If so, the recovery room nurse lists the needed equipment. The patient is transported to the room by the recovery room nurse. The nurse responsible for the patient's care receives the patient (Fig. 23-7). You may be asked to help transfer the patient from the stretcher to the bed. You may also need to help position the patient.

Vital signs are taken, and other important observations are made. They are compared with those reported by the recovery room nurse. Dressings are checked by the nurse for bleeding. The placement and functioning of tubes, catheters, and IV infusions are also checked. The side rails are raised, and the signal light is placed within the patient's reach. Necessary care and treatments are given. Then the family is allowed to see the patient.

Measurements and Observations

The patient's condition and hospital policies influence what care you give to a postoperative patient. You may be involved in some postoperative care. You may be assigned to measure vital signs and observe the patient's condition. These are usually done every 15 minutes during the first 1 or 2 hours after the patient's

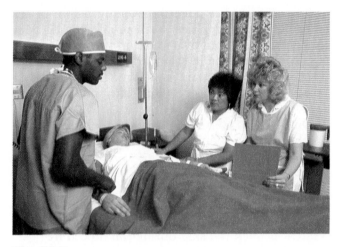

Fig. 23-7 A patient is brought to the nursing unit from the recovery room. A nurse meets the patient on return to the unit.

return from the recovery room. The nurse will tell you how often to check on the patient. This is an important responsibility. You must be alert for certain signs and symptoms. The following are reported to the nurse immediately:

1. A drop in blood pressure
2. A pulse rate of greater than 100 or less than 60 beats per minute
3. A weak or irregular pulse
4. A rise or drop in body temperature
5. Rapid, gasping, or difficult respirations
6. Patient complaints of thirst
7. Restlessness
8. Cold, moist, clammy, or pale skin
9. Cyanosis of the lips or nails
10. Increased drainage on or under dressings
11. The appearance of bright red blood from the incision, drainage tubes, or suction tubes
12. Patient complaints of pain or nausea
13. Vomiting
14. Choking
15. The amount, character, and time of the first voiding after surgery

Also measure intake and output. The IV is checked for dripping. The appearance of drainage from a urinary catheter, NG tube, or wound suction is also noted.

Positioning

Positioning is important for comfort and prevention of complications. The type of surgery affects positioning. Position restrictions may be ordered. The patient is usually positioned for easy and comfortable breathing. The patient is also positioned so that stress is not placed on the incision. When the patient is supine, the head of the bed is usually raised slightly.

COUGHING AND DEEP BREATHING EXERCISES

1 Explain the procedure to the patient.
2 Identify the patient. Check the ID bracelet with the treatment card.
3 Provide for privacy.
4 Help the patient to a comfortable position. Semi-Fowler's position is preferred.
5 Have the patient deep breathe:
   a Have the patient place the hands over the rib cage (Fig. 23-8).
   b Ask the patient to exhale. Explain that he or she should exhale until the ribs move as far down as possible.
   c Have the patient take a deep breath. It should be as deep as possible. Remind him or her to inhale through the nose.
   d Ask the patient to hold the breath for 3 to 5 seconds.
   e Ask the patient to exhale slowly through pursed lips (Fig. 23-9). He or she should exhale until the ribs move as far down as possible.
   f Repeat this step 4 more times.

6 Ask the patient to cough:
   a Ask the patient to interlace the fingers over the incision (Fig. 23-10, A). You may also have the patient hold a small pillow or folded towel over the incision (Fig. 23-10, B).
   b Have the patient take in a deep breath as in step 5.
   c Ask the patient to cough strongly twice with the mouth open.
7 Assist the patient to a comfortable position.
8 Raise the side rails and place the signal light within reach.
9 Unscreen the patient.
10 Report your observations to the nurse:
   a The number of times the patient coughed and deep breathed
   b How the patient tolerated the procedure

The patient's head may be turned to the side. These positions prevent aspiration if vomiting occurs.

Position changes are made at least every 2 hours. This helps prevent respiratory and circulatory complications. The patient may not want to turn because of pain. You need to provide support and turn the patient with smooth, gentle motions. Pillows and other devices are often used in positioning.

The nurse tells you when to reposition the patient and what positions are allowed. Usually you will assist the nurse. However, you may be responsible for turning and repositioning the patient. This may occur when the patient's condition is stable and care is simple.

Coughing and Deep Breathing

Postoperative patients can develop respiratory complications. There are two major complications. One is pneumonia, an infection in the lung. The other is *atelectasis*, the collapse of a portion of the lung. Atelectasis occurs when mucus collects in the airway. Air cannot get to a part of the lung, and the lung collapses. Coughing and deep breathing exercises help prevent these complications. Mucus is removed by coughing. Deep breathing promotes the movement of air into most parts of the lungs. These exercises may be ordered for patients on bed rest and for those with respiratory disorders.

The patient may be afraid to cough and deep breathe. The exercises may be painful. This is especially true after chest and abdominal surgeries. The patient may be afraid of breaking open the incision while coughing. However, coughing and deep breathing are necessary to prevent complications.

The frequency of coughing and deep breathing varies. Some doctors order the exercises every 1 or 2 hours while the patient is awake. Others want them done 4 times a day (q.i.d.). The nurse tells you when coughing and deep breathing need to be done. You will also be told how many deep breaths and coughs the patient should do. Remember that coughing and deep breathing are done only when directed by the nurse.

Leg Exercises

After surgery, it is important to stimulate circulation. This is especially true for blood flow in the extremities. If blood flow is sluggish, blood clots may form. Blood clots (*thrombi*) are more likely to form in the deep leg veins (Fig. 23-11, A). A blood clot (*thrombus*) can break loose and travel through the blood stream. It then becomes an embolus. An *embolus* is a blood clot that travels through the vascular system until it lodges in a distant vessel (Fig. 23-11, B). An embolus from a vein eventually lodges in the lungs (pulmonary embolus). A pulmonary embolus can cause severe respiratory problems and death.

Leg exercises increase venous blood flow. There-

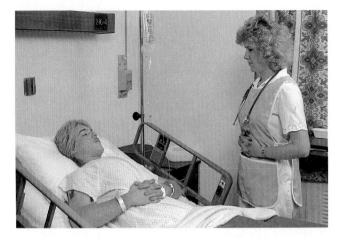

Fig. 23-8 The hands are placed over the rib cage for deep breathing.

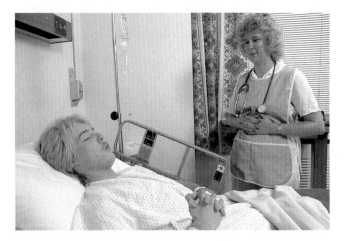

Fig. 23-9 The patient exhales through pursed lips during the deep breathing exercise.

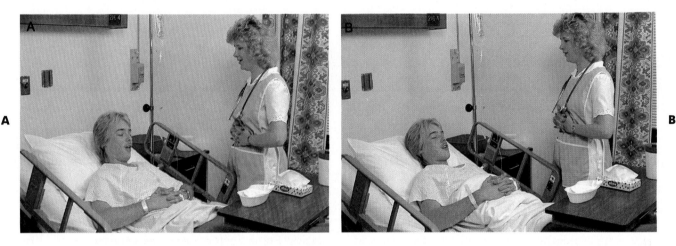

Fig. 23-10 The incision is supported for the coughing exercise. **A,** Fingers are interlaced over the incision area. **B,** A small pillow is held over the incision.

fore they help prevent thrombi. Leg exercises are easy to do. You may have to assist if the patient is weak. If the patient has had leg surgery, a doctor's order is needed for the exercises. Leg exercises are done while supine. They are done at least every 1 or 2 hours while the patient is awake. The following exercises are done 5 times:

1. Ask the patient to make circles with the toes. This rotates the ankles.
2. Have the patient dorsiflex and plantar flex the feet (see Chapter 18).
3. Have the patient flex and extend one knee and then the other (Fig. 23-12).
4. Ask the patient to raise and lower one leg off the bed (Fig. 23-13). Repeat this exercise with the other leg.

Bandages

Bandages are applied to an extremity. They promote comfort and circulation and provide support and pressure. They also promote healing and prevent injury. However, they must be applied properly. Incorrect application can cause severe discomfort, skin irritation, and circulatory and respiratory complications. Doctors often order elastic stockings and elastic bandages.

Elastic stockings Elastic stockings are frequently ordered for postoperative patients and for those with heart disease and circulatory disorders. Bed rest and pregnancy are also indications for elastic stockings. Affected persons can develop blood clots (thrombi).

Elastic stockings are often called TED hose or antiembolic stockings. They help prevent the devel-

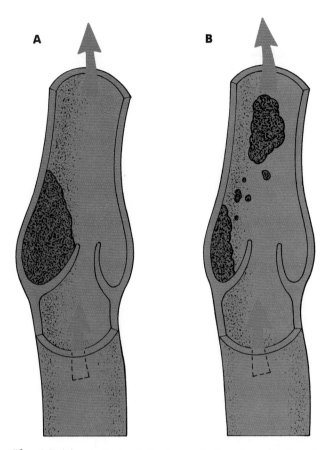

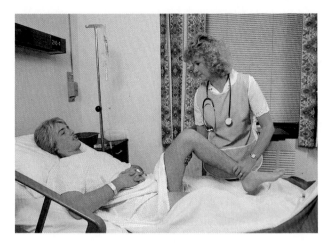

Fig. 23-12 The knee is flexed and then extended during postoperative leg exercises.

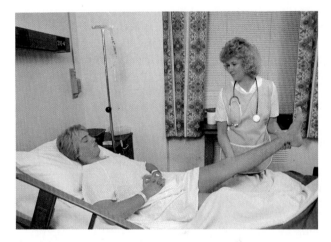

Fig. 23-11 **A,** A blood clot is attached to the wall of a vein. The arrows show the direction of blood flow. **B,** Part of the thrombus has broken off and has become an embolus. The embolus will travel in the bloodstream until it lodges in a distant vessel. (Modified from Phipps WJ, Long BC, and Woods NF: *Medical-surgical nursing: Concepts and clinical practice*, ed 3, St Louis, 1987, Mosby–Year Book.)

Fig. 23-13 The nursing assistant helps the patient raise and lower the leg in another postoperative leg exercise.

APPLYING ELASTIC STOCKINGS

1 Explain the procedure to the patient.
2 Wash your hands.
3 Obtain elastic stockings in the correct size.
4 Identify the patient. Check the ID bracelet with the treatment card.
5 Provide for privacy.
6 Raise the bed to a level appropriate for good body mechanics.
7 Lower the side rail.
8 Position the patient supine.
9 Expose the legs. Fanfold top linens back toward the patient.
10 Hold the foot and heel of the stocking. Gather the rest of the stocking in your hands.
11 Support the patient's foot at the heel.
12 Slip the foot of the stocking over the toes, foot, and heel (Fig. 23-14, *A*).
13 Pull the stocking up over the leg. It should be even and snug (Fig. 23-15, *B*).
14 Make sure the stocking is not twisted and has no creases or wrinkles.
15 Repeat steps 10 through 14 for the other leg.
16 Return top linens to their proper position.
17 Help the patient to a comfortable position and raise the side rail.
18 Lower the bed to its lowest position. Place the signal light within reach.
19 Unscreen the patient.
20 Wash your hands.
21 Tell the nurse that the stockings have been applied. Report the time of application.

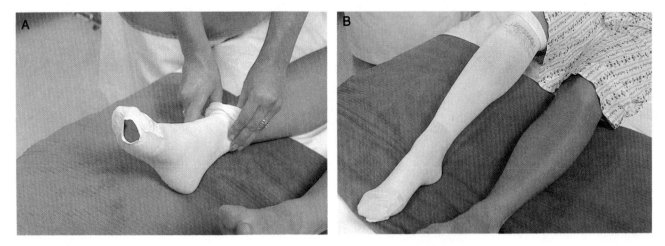

Fig. 23-14 **A,** The stocking is slipped over the toes, foot, and heel. **B,** The stocking is pulled up over the leg.

opment of thrombi. The elastic exerts pressure on the veins, promoting venous blood flow to the heart.

The stockings come in many sizes. Thigh-high or knee-high lengths are available. The nurse measures the patient to determine the proper size. The stockings are removed at least twice each day. They are applied before the patient gets out of bed.

Elastic Bandages Elastic bandages are used for the same purposes as elastic stockings. They also provide support and reduce swelling from musculoskeletal injuries. The bandage is applied from the lower (distal) part of the extremity to the top (proximal) part. The nurse will give you directions regarding the area to be bandaged.

General rules You need to follow these rules when applying elastic bandages:

1. Obtain the elastic bandage in the proper length and width to bandage the extremity.
2. Make sure the extremity is in good alignment.
3. Face the patient during the procedure.
4. Leave fingers or toes exposed if possible. This allows the circulation to be checked.
5. Apply the bandage with firm, even pressure.
6. Check the color and temperature of the extremity every hour.
7. Reapply a loose or wrinkled bandage.

APPLYING ELASTIC BANDAGES

1 Explain the procedure to the patient.
2 Wash your hands.
3 Collect the following equipment:
  a Elastic bandage as determined by the nurse
  b Tape, metal clips, or safety pins
4 Identify the patient. Check the ID bracelet with the treatment card.
5 Provide for privacy.
6 Raise the bed to a level appropriate for good body mechanics.
7 Help the patient to a comfortable position. Expose the part to be bandaged.
8 Make sure the area is clean and dry.
9 Hold the bandage with the roll up and the loose end on the bottom (Fig. 23-15, A).
10 Apply the bandage to the smallest part of the extremity (wrist, ankle, knee).
11 Make two circular turns around the part (Fig. 23-15, B).

12 Make overlapping spiral turns in an upward direction. Each turn should overlap about ⅔ of the previous turn (Fig. 23-15, C).
13 Apply the bandage smoothly with firm, even pressure. It should not be tight.
14 Pin, tape, or clip the end of the bandage to hold it in place.
15 Check the fingers or toes for coldness or cyanosis. Also check for complaints of pain, numbness, or tingling. Remove the bandage if any are noted. Report your observations to the nurse.
16 Make sure the patient is comfortable and the signal light is within reach. Lower the bed. Unscreen the patient.
17 Wash your hands.
18 Report the following to the nurse:
  a The time the bandage was applied
  b The site of the application
  c Any other observations

A   B   C

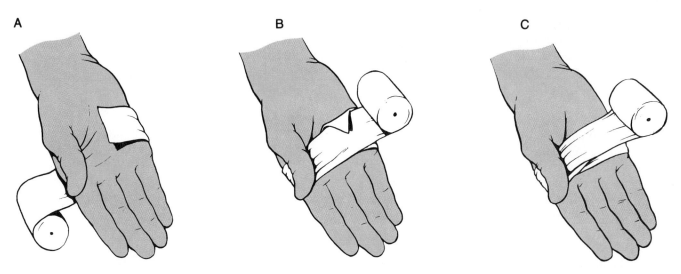

Fig. 23-15 **A,** The roll of the elastic bandage is up, and the loose end is on the bottom. **B,** The bandage is applied to the smallest part with two circular turns. **C,** The bandage is applied with spiral turns in an upward direction. (From Parcel GS, Rinear CE: *Basic emergency care of the sick and injured,* ed 4, St Louis, 1989, Mosby–Year Book.)

SUMMARY

Surgery is physically and psychologically unpleasant. The more urgent, serious, and complicated the surgery, the greater the effects on the patient. The doctor and nurse prepare the patient for the surgery. You may be asked to assist in certain preoperative activities. Always explain what you are going to do and why. This helps the patient psychologically.

After surgery, the patient recovers from the effects of anesthesia and the operation. Postoperative complications must be prevented. These include bleeding, respiratory distress or infection, thrombi and

emboli, and wound infection. Following the rules of patient safety and medical asepsis will help prevent complications. Turning, repositioning, coughing and deep breathing, and leg exercises will also help. You must be alert for signs and symptoms to report to the nurse. Your observations will help the nurse recognize and treat complications.

The nurse will tell you what care to give preoperatively and postoperatively. Remember that the patient has many fears and concerns about the surgery and its effects. A kind, caring, and sensitive nursing assistant is appreciated by the patient.

REVIEW QUESTIONS

Circle the best answer.

1 Which is *true* of elective surgery?
   a The surgery is done immediately.
   b The need for surgery is sudden and unexpected.
   c Surgery is scheduled for a later date.
   d General anesthesia is always used.
2 The fearful patient may
   a Be quiet and withdrawn
   b Cry
   c Pace or be unusually cheerful
   d All of the above
3 You can assist in the psychological preparation of the surgical patient by explaining
   a The reason for the surgery

   b Procedures and why they are being done
   c The risks and possible complications of surgery
   d What to expect during the preoperative and postoperative periods
4 Preoperatively, the surgical patient is usually
   a NPO
   b Allowed only water
   c Given a regular breakfast
   d Given a tube feeding
5 Enemas may be ordered preoperatively for the following reasons *except*
   a To clean the colon of all fecal material
   b To prevent postoperative bleeding

c To relieve flatus

d To prevent postoperative pain

6 The skin prep is done preoperatively to

a Completely bathe the body

b Sterilize the skin

c Reduce the number of microbes on the skin

d Destroy nonpathogens and pathogens

7 When shaving the skin before surgery,

a Shave in the direction opposite of hair growth

b Shave toward the center of the specific area

c Be careful not to cut, scratch, or nick the skin

d All of the above

8 Preoperative medication has been given. The patient

a Must remain in bed

b Is allowed to smoke with supervision

c Can use the commode for elimination

d Is allowed only sips of water

9 General anesthetics

a Is a specially educated nurse

b Produce unconsciousness and the loss of feeling or sensation

c Is a specially educated doctor

d Produce loss of sensation or feeling in a body part

10 Coughing and deep breathing exercises prevent

a Bleeding

b A pulmonary embolus

c Respiratory complications

d Pain and discomfort

11 Which is *true?*

a Leg exercises are done to stimulate circulation.

b Leg exercises are done to prevent thrombi.

c Leg exercises are done 5 times every 1 or 2 hours.

d All of the above.

12 Postoperatively, the patient's position is changed

a Every 2 hours

b Every 3 hours

c Every 4 hours

d Every shift

13 Elastic stockings are worn to

a Prevent blood clots

b Hold dressings in place

c Reduce swelling after musculoskeletal injury

d All of the above

14 When applying an elastic bandage,

a The extremity needs to be in good alignment

b The fingers or toes are covered if possible

c It is applied from the largest to smallest part of the extremity

d It is applied from the upper to the lower part of the extremity

Circle T *if the answer is true and* F *if the answer is false.*

T F 15 Hair is usually washed before surgery.

T F 16 Hair is kept out of the face for surgery by using pins, clips, or combs.

T F 17 Nail polish is removed before surgery.

T F 18 Women are allowed to wear makeup to surgery.

T F 19 Pajamas can be worn to the operating room.

T F 20 Valuables are removed preoperatively.

T F 21 A surgical bed is made for the patient's return from the recovery room.

T F 22 You are responsible for receiving the patient from the recovery room.

T F 23 A drop in a patient's blood pressure must be reported to the nurse immediately.

Answers

1	c	9	b	17	True
2	d	10	c	18	False
3	b	11	d	19	False
4	a	12	a	20	True
5	c	13	a	21	True
6	c	14	a	22	False
7	c	15	True	23	True
8	a	16	False		

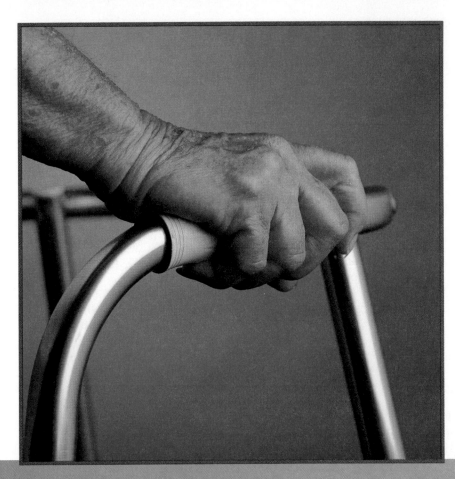

Rehabilitation and Restorative Care

24

OBJECTIVES

- Define the key terms listed in this chapter
- Describe rehabilitation in terms of the whole person
- Identify the complications that need to be prevented for successful rehabilitation
- Identify ways to help disabled individuals perform activities of daily living
- Identify the psychological reactions that are common during rehabilitation
- Describe the effects of a disability on a person's job status and how rehabilitation can help
- Identify the members of the rehabilitation team
- List the common rehabilitation services
- Describe the responsibilities of the nursing assistant in rehabilitation

activities of daily living Those self-care activities a person must perform daily to remain independent and to function in society

prosthesis An artificial replacement for a missing body part

rehabilitation The process of restoring the disabled person to the highest level of physical, psychological, social, and economic functioning possible

Disease, injury, and surgery can result in loss of body function or loss of a body part. Birth injuries and birth defects can also affect functioning. Often there is loss of more than one function. Everyday activities such as eating, bathing, dressing, and walking may be difficult or seem impossible. The individual may be unable to return to a job. The ability to care for children, family members, and the home may be seriously affected. The disabled or handicapped person may be totally or partially dependent on others to meet basic needs. The degree of disability present affects how much function is possible.

Health care is concerned with preventing disability and reducing the degree of disability. Helping the person adjust to the disability is also important. *Rehabilitation* is the process of restoring the disabled person to the highest level of physical, psychological, social, and economic functioning possible.

REHABILITATION AND THE WHOLE PERSON

The rehabilitation process involves the whole person. A physical illness or injury always has some psychological or social effect. A physical handicap has similar effects. How would you feel if a car accident left you paralyzed from the waist down? Would you be angry, afraid, or depressed? Would you deny that it happened to you? Would you be involved in your usual social activities? Could you dance, exercise, shop, or go to school? Could you attend church services or visit the homes of relatives and friends? Could you return to your present job? Could you find other employment with your remaining skills and abilities?

Rehabilitation helps a person adjust to the disability physically, psychologically, socially, and economically. Abilities are emphasized, not the disability. However, complications that can cause further disability must be prevented. Therefore rehabilitation begins when the individual first enters the health care facility.

Physical Considerations

Rehabilitation begins with preventing complications. Complications can occur from bed rest, prolonged illness, or recovery from injury. Contractures, decubitus ulcers, and bowel and bladder problems must be prevented. Contractures and decubitus ulcers can be prevented with good body alignment, frequent turning and repositioning, range-of-motion exercises, and the use of supportive devices (see Chapters 10 and 18). Good skin care is also very important in preventing decubiti (see Chapter 13).

Two methods of bladder training were described in Chapter 14. The method used depends on the physical problems, capabilities, and needs of the individual. The nurse will explain the method being used for an individual. The rules to be followed will also be explained.

Bowel training was described in Chapter 15. It involves gaining control of bowel movements and developing a regular pattern of elimination. Fecal impaction, constipation, and anal incontinence are prevented (see Chapter 15).

A major goal of rehabilitation is for the individual to be able to perform self-care activities. *Activities of daily living* (ADL) refer to self-care activities. Activities of daily living are performed daily by the individual in order to remain independent and to function in society. These activities include bathing, oral hygiene, eating, bowel and bladder elimination, and moving about. A person's ability to perform activities of daily living and the need for self-help devices are evaluated.

The hands, wrists, and arms may be affected by disease or injury. Self-help devices may be needed for various activities. Equipment can usually be changed or made to meet an individual's needs. Special eating utensils may be needed. Glass holders, plate guards, and silverware with curved handles or cuffs (Fig. 24-1) are available. Some devices are attached to a special splint (Fig. 24-2). Electric toothbrushes are helpful if the person cannot perform the back-and-forth motions necessary for brushing teeth. Longer handles can be attached to combs, brushes, and sponges (Fig. 24-3). Self-help devices are also available for preparing meals, using kitchen appliances, dressing, writing, dialing telephones, and for many other activities (Fig. 24-4).

Some individuals have lower-extremity involvement. They may have to learn how to walk with a supportive device or learn to use a wheelchair. If ambulation is possible, the person may be taught to use crutches or a walker, cane, or brace (Fig. 24-5). Both legs may be paralyzed or amputated. If so, a wheelchair is necessary. Persons paralyzed on one

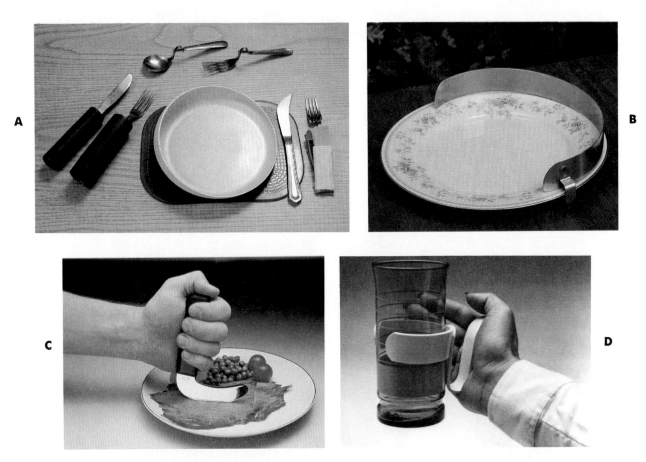

Fig. 24-1 Eating utensils for individuals with special needs. **A,** Note the cuffed fork, which fits over the hand. The rounded plate helps keep food on the plate. Special grips and swivel handles are helpful for some individuals. **B,** Plateguards help keep food on the plate. **C,** Knives with rounded blades are rocked back and forth to cut food. They eliminate the need to have a fork in one hand and a knife in the other. **D,** Glass or cup holder. (**B,C,** and **D** courtesy of BISSELL Healthcare Corporation/Fred Sammons, Inc. from Hoeman SP: *Rehabilitation/Restorative Care in the Community,* St Louis, 1990, Mosby–Year Book.)

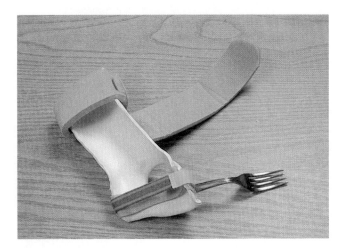

Fig. 24-2 Self-help devices can be attached to splints.

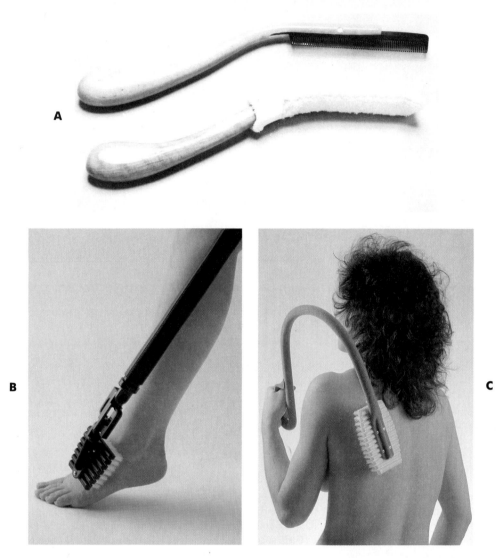

Fig. 24-3 **A,** A long-handled comb for hair care. **B,** The brush has a long handle for bathing. **C,** This brush has a curved handle. (Courtesy of Lumex, Division of Lumex, Inc. from Hoeman SP: *Rehabilitation/Restorative Care in the Community,* St Louis, 1990, Mosby–Year Book.)

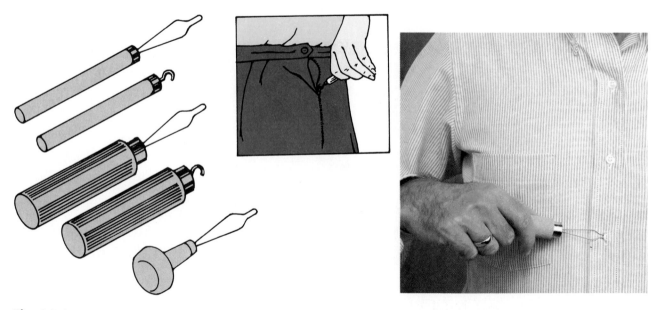

Fig. 24-4 For legend see opposite page.

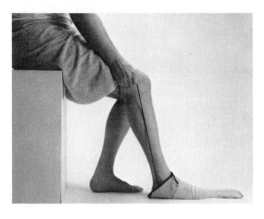

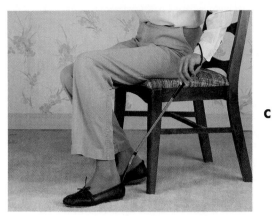

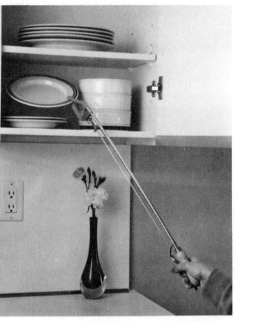

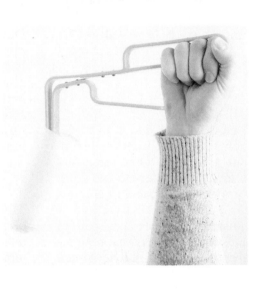

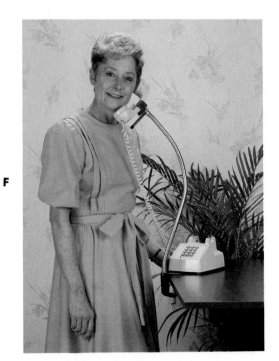

Fig. 24-4 **A,** A button hook is used to button and zip clothing. **B,** A sock puller is used to put on socks and stockings. **C,** A long-handled shoe horn for putting on shoes. **D,** Reachers are helpful for those in wheelchairs. **E,** A toilet paper holder is used for wiping. **F,** The telephone holder is for those who cannot hold a phone. (**A,** courtesy of Lumex, Division of Lumex, Inc. **B, C, E,** and **F** courtesy of BISSELL Healthcare Corporation/Fred Sammons, Inc. **D,** from Hoeman SP: *Rehabilitation/restorative care in the community,* St Louis, 1990, Mosby–Year Book.)

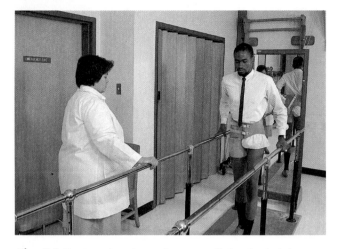

Fig. 24-5 A patient learns how to walk in physical therapy.

side of the body also need wheelchairs. If possible, the person is taught how to transfer from the bed to the wheelchair without assistance. Other transfers will be taught. These include transfers to and from the toilet, bathtub, sofas and chairs, and in and out of cars (Fig. 24-6).

The person with a missing body part may be fitted with a prosthesis. A *prosthesis* is an artificial replacement for the missing body part. An individual can usually be fitted with an artificial arm or leg and taught how to use the prosthesis (Fig. 24-7). Artificial eyes are available. Breast prostheses are available for women who have had a breast removed. Modern technology will result in more sophisticated prostheses.

The goal is to have a prosthesis that closely resembles the missing part in function and appearance.

Psychological and Social Considerations

Self-esteem and relationships with others are often affected by a disability. Changes in body appearance and function may cause the person to feel unwhole, unattractive, unclean, or undesirable to others. During the early stages of rehabilitation, the person may refuse to acknowledge the disability. The person may be depressed, angry, and hostile.

Successful rehabilitation depends on the person's attitude, acceptance of limitations, and motivation. The person must focus on the remaining abilities. Discouragement and frustration are common. Progress may be slow, or efforts may be unsuccessful. Each new task to be learned is a reminder of the disability. Old fears and emotions may again be experienced. The person needs help accepting the disability and the resulting limitations. Support, reassurance, encouragement, and sensitivity from the health team are necessary.

Economic Considerations

The person may be unable to return to a job held before the disease, injury, or surgery. Rehabilitation services can help the disabled person reenter the work force. The person is evaluated to determine work abilities, past work experiences, interests, and talents. Through the process of rehabilitation, a job skill may be restored or a new one may be learned. The goal is for the person to become gainfully employed. Assistance is often given in finding a job.

Fig. 24-6 **A,** A transfer board is used to transfer from one seat to another. **B,** The person transfers from the wheelchair to the bed. **C,** A transfer from the wheelchair to the bathtub. **D,** A transfer to the car. The person has left-side paralysis. (**A,** courtesy of BISSELL Healthcare Corporation/Fred Sammons, Inc. **A, B, C,** and **D** from Hoeman SP: *Rehabilitation/restorative care in the community,* St Louis, 1990, Mosby–Year Book.)

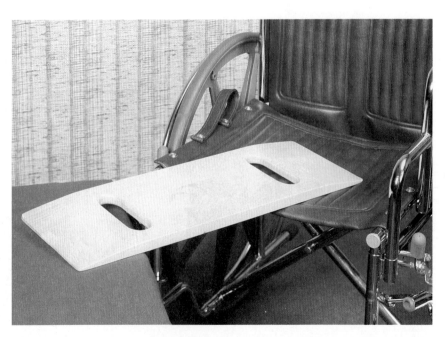

A

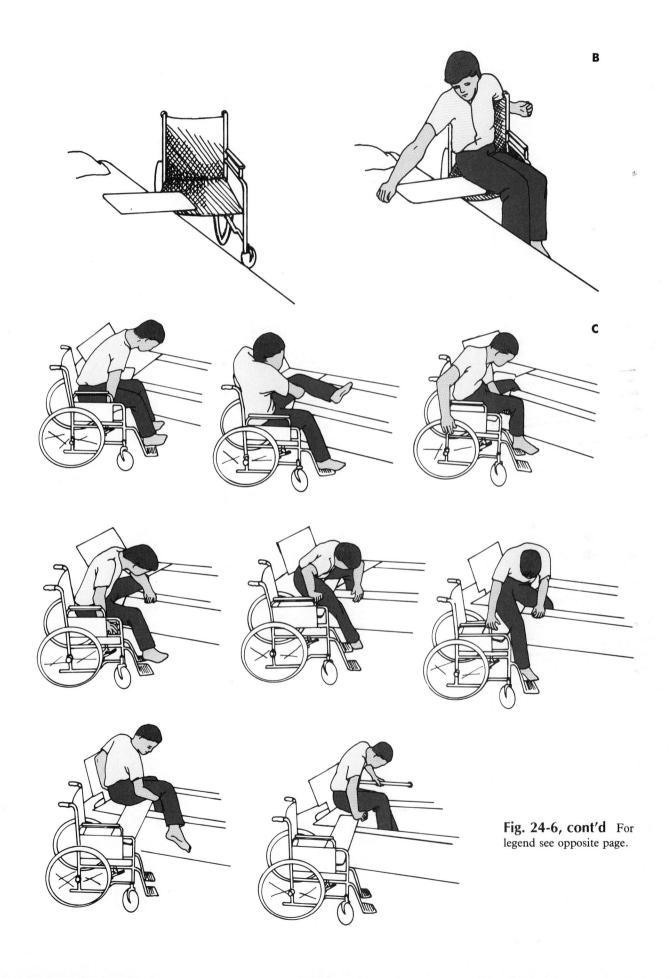

Fig. 24-6, cont'd For legend see opposite page.

D

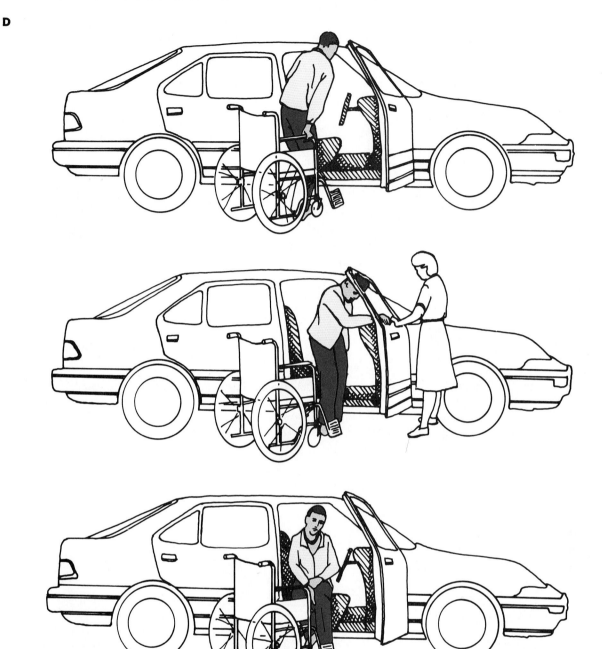

Fig. 24-6, cont'd For legend see page 386.

THE REHABILITATION TEAM

Rehabilitation is a team effort. The team consists of the patient, doctor, nursing team, other health professionals and workers, and the family. All assist the disabled person to achieve independence. A physical therapist, occupational therapist, psychiatrist, psychologist, speech therapist, social worker, member of the clergy, dietician, and others may be involved (Fig. 24-8). A vocational counselor evaluates the person's ability to perform a job skill and return to work.

The team meets regularly to discuss and evaluate the person's progress. Goals are set for the person.

Changes in the rehabilitation plan are made when indicated. Often the disabled individual and family members attend the meetings.

REHABILITATION SERVICES

Rehabilitation begins when the person enters the health care facility. Depending on the person's needs and problems, the process may be continued. The person may require extended hospitalization or care in a nursing facility. Some people are transferred to rehabilitation centers, where many specialized services are available. There are centers for the blind,

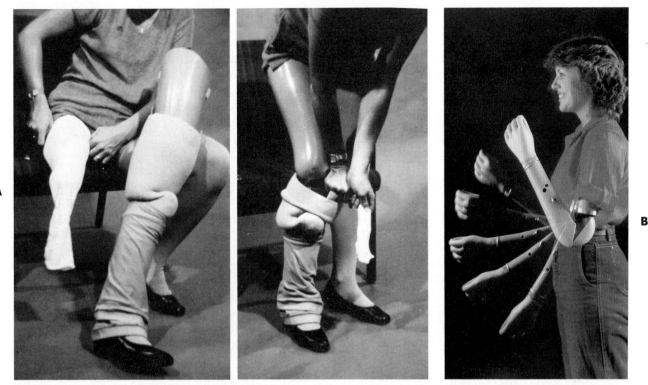

Fig. 24-7 **A,** Leg prosthesis. **B,** Arm prosthesis. (**A,** courtesy of Otto Bock Orthopedic Industry Inc., U.S.A. **B,** courtesy of Motion Control, division of IOMED. Inc., Salt Lake City, Utah. **A** and **B** from Hoeman SP: *Rehabilitative/restorative care in the community*, St Louis, 1990, Mosby–Year Book.)

deaf, mentally retarded, physically disabled, those with speech problems, and the mentally ill. Rehabilitation services are available to some people in their homes or in day-care centers.

RESPONSIBILITIES OF THE NURSING ASSISTANT

Nursing assistants are valuable members of the rehabilitation team. Some are employed in rehabilita-

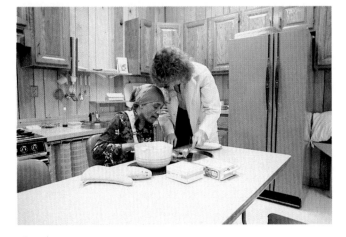

Fig. 24-8 The occupational therapist plans activities to meet the needs and interests of the disabled person.

tion centers. As in other situations, a nurse directs the nursing assistant in performing care activities. Many procedures and care measures already learned will be part of the care required by a disabled person. Safety, communication, legal, and ethical considerations apply in rehabilitation. The many rules described throughout this book also apply, regardless of the type of disability.

As a part of the rehabilitation team, you need to practice the following points:

1. Follow the instructions and directions given by the nurse very carefully.
2. Report early signs and symptoms of complications such as decubiti, contractures, and bowel and bladder problems.
3. Keep the person in good body alignment at all times (see Chapter 10).
4. Practice measures to prevent decubitus ulcers (see Chapter 13).
5. Turn and reposition the person as directed.
6. Perform range-of-motion exercises as instructed (see Chapter 18). They must be done as often as indicated by the nurse or the nursing care plan.
7. Encourage the person to perform as many activities of daily living as possible and to the extent possible.
8. Give praise when even a little progress is made.

9. Provide emotional support and reassurance.
10. Practice the techniques developed by other members of the rehabilitation team when assisting the person.
11. Know how to apply self-care devices used by the individual.
12. Try to understand and appreciate the person's situation, feelings, and concerns.
13. Do not pity the person or give sympathy.
14. Concentrate on the person's abilities, not the disabilities.
15. Remember that muscles will atrophy if they are not used.
16. Practice the task that the person must perform. This will help you guide and direct the individual.
17. Know how to use and operate special equipment used in the person's rehabilitation program.
18. Convey an attitude of hopefulness to the individual.

SUMMARY

Rehabilitation can be challenging and rewarding for the health team. Patience, understanding, and sensitivity are needed when working with the disabled person. Progress may be slow and difficult to see. The individual may become frustrated and discouraged. You must be able to give support, encouragement, and praise when needed. The disabled individual does not need pity or sympathy.

Emphasizing abilities is important. It is necessary to prevent disabling complications. Contractures, decubiti, and bowel and bladder problems must be prevented. Therefore good nursing care is necessary. Besides helping to prevent complications, you need to observe the techniques taught to the disabled person. This helps you to guide the person more effectively during care. If the person is expected to perform tasks in different ways, frustration takes the place of progress. Finally, remember that the more the person can do alone, the better off he or she will be.

REVIEW QUESTIONS

Circle the best *answer.*

1 Rehabilitation is concerned with
   a Physical disabilities
   b Physical capabilities
   c The whole person
   d Psychological, social, and economic functioning
2 Physical rehabilitation begins with the prevention of
   a Anger, frustration, and depression
   b Contractures and decubiti
   c Illness and injury
   d Loss of self-esteem
3 Mr. Williams has paralysis of both legs. ADL should be
   a Done by Mr. Williams to the extent possible
   b Done by the nursing assistant
   c Postponed until he regains use of his legs
   d Supervised by the physical therapist
4 The process of rehabilitation emphasizes
   a The disability
   b The individual's limitations
   c The person's abilities
   d All of the above
5 Which reaction may be experienced by a disabled person?
   a Feelings of being undesirable or unattractive
   b Anger and hostility
   c Depression
   d All of the above
6 Which statement is *false?*
   a Disabled people can never work again.
   b Disabled people may need to learn a new job skill.
   c The disabled person is evaluated to determine the ability to work.
   d Disabled people are often given help in finding a job.
7 The rehabilitation team consists of
   a The nursing team
   b The doctor
   c Various members of the health team
   d The disabled person and the nurse
8 The nursing assistant
   a Plans the rehabilitation program
   b Supplies prostheses
   c Gives praise when even slight progress is made
   d Does as much as possible for the disabled person
9 Which statement is *false?*
   a Sympathy and pity help the person adjust to the disability.
   b You should know how to apply self-care devices.
   c You should know how to use equipment used in the person's care.
   d An attitude of hopefulness must be conveyed to the individual.

Answers

9	a	6	a	3	a
8	c	5	d	2	b
7	c	4	c	1	c

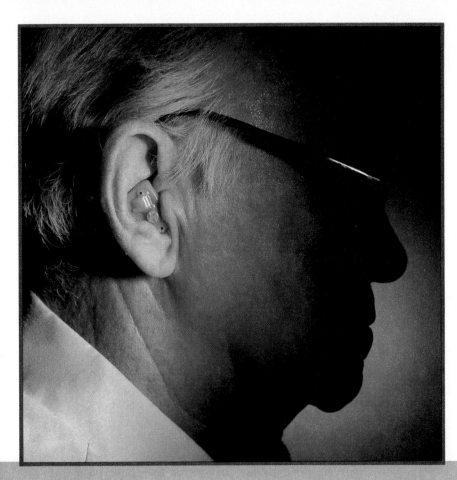

Common Health Problems

OBJECTIVES

- Define the key terms listed in this chapter
- Identify the warning signs of cancer
- List cancer treatments
- Explain how to maintain joint function in patients with arthritis
- Explain how to care for patients in casts, in traction, and with hip pinnings
- Describe osteoporosis and the care required
- Explain why loss of a limb requires psychological adjustment
- Describe cerebrovascular accident, its signs and symptoms, and the care required
- Describe Parkinson's disease and multiple sclerosis
- Identify the causes and effects of head and spinal cord injuries and the care required
- Describe how to communicate with the hearing impaired
- Describe glaucoma, cataract, and dealing with the blind
- Describe common respiratory disorders and the care required
- Identify the signs, symptoms, and treatment of hypertension
- List the risk factors for coronary artery disease
- Describe angina pectoris, myocardial infarction, congestive heart failure, and the care required
- Identify the signs, symptoms, and complications of diabetes
- Describe AIDS and hepatitis, their signs and symptoms, and necessary precautions.

alopecia Loss of hair

amputation The removal of all or part of an extremity

aphasia The inability (a) to speak (phasia)

arthritis Joint (arthr) inflammation (itis)

benign tumor A tumor that grows slowly and within a localized area

closed fracture The bone is broken but the skin is intact; simple fracture

compound fracture The bone is broken and has come through the skin; open fracture

fracture A broken bone

gangrene A condition in which there is death of tissue; tissues become black, cold, and shriveled

hemiplegia Paralysis on one side of the body

malignant tumor A tumor that grows rapidly and invades other tissues

metastasis The spread of cancer to other parts of the body

paraplegia Paralysis of the legs

quadriplegia Paralysis of the arms, legs, and trunk

stomatitis Inflammation (itis) of the mouth (stomat)

stroke A cerebrovascular accident (CVA); blood supply to a part of the brain is suddenly interrupted

tumor A new growth of cells; tumors can be benign or malignant

This chapter gives basic information about common health problems. People with these disorders are often cared for in health care facilities and in their own homes. Knowing something about a disorder makes the required care more meaningful. If more information is needed, ask a nurse for additional explanations.

Reviewing Chapter 5 (Body Structure and Function) will be helpful in studying this chapter.

CANCER

A tumor is a new growth of abnormal cells. Tumors can be benign or malignant (Fig. 25-1). *Benign* tumors grow slowly and within a localized area. They do not usually cause death. A malignant tumor is cancerous. *Malignant* tumors grow rapidly and invade other tissues. They cause death if not treated and controlled. The spread of cancer to other parts of the body is called *metastasis*. It occurs if the cancer is not treated and controlled. Cancer can occur in almost any body part. The most common sites are the lungs, colon and rectum, breast, prostate, and uterus.

The exact causes of cancer are unknown. However, certain factors are known to contribute to its development. These include a family history of cancer, exposure to radiation or certain chemicals, smoking, alcohol, food additives, and viruses.

Cancer can be treated and controlled with early detection. The American Cancer Society has identified seven early warning signs of cancer. They are:

1. A change in bowel or bladder habits
2. A sore that does not heal
3. Unusual bleeding or discharge from a body opening
4. A lump or thickening in the breast or elsewhere in the body
5. Difficulty swallowing or indigestion
6. An obvious change in a wart or mole
7. Nagging cough or hoarseness

The three cancer treatments are surgery, radiotherapy (radiation therapy), and chemotherapy. The treatment depends on the type of tumor, its location, and if it has spread. One treatment or a combination of treatments may be used.

Surgery involves removing malignant tissue. Surgery is done to cure cancer or to relieve pain from advanced cancer. Some surgeries are very disfiguring. Surgical patients require the care described in Chapter 23. A nurse plans measures for the patient's special needs.

Radiotherapy destroys living cells. X-rays are directed at the tumor. Cancer cells and normal cells are exposed to radiation. Both are destroyed. Radiotherapy is used to cure certain cancers or to control the growth of cancer cells. Pain can be relieved or prevented by controlling cell growth. Radiotherapy has side effects. "Radiation sickness" involves discomfort, nausea, and vomiting. Skin breakdown can occur in the exposed area. The doctor may order special skin care procedures.

Chemotherapy involves drugs that kill cells. Like radiotherapy, chemotherapy affects normal cells and cancer cells. It is used to cure cancer or control the rate of cell growth. Side effects can be severe. They are caused by the destruction of normal cells. The gastrointestinal tract is irritated. Nausea, vomiting, and diarrhea result. *Stomatitis*, an inflammation (itis) of the mouth (stomat), may also develop. Hair loss *(alopecia)* may occur. Decreased production of blood cells occurs. As a result, the patient is at risk for bleeding and infection. The heart, lungs, liver, kidneys, and skin may also be affected.

Cancer patients have many needs. Pain must be controlled. Adequate rest and exercise are needed. Fluid and nutritional status must be maintained. Skin breakdown and bowel elimination problems must be prevented. Constipation is a side effect of pain med-

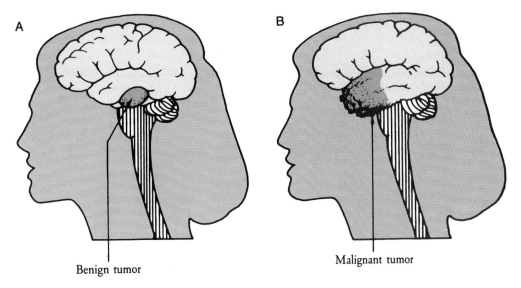

A

B

Benign tumor

Malignant tumor

Fig. 25-1 **A,** Benign tumors grow within a localized area. **B,** Malignant tumors invade other tissues.

ications. Diarrhea can occur because of chemotherapy. The side effects of radiotherapy and chemotherapy must be dealt with.

The patient's psychological and social needs are great. The patient may be angry, afraid, and depressed. There may be disfigurement from surgery. The patient may feel unwhole, unattractive, or unclean. The patient and family need much emotional support. The future may be uncertain. The possibility of death may be very real. Put yourself in the patient's position. How would you feel and what would you want if you had cancer? Do not be afraid to talk to the patient. Avoiding the patient because you are uncomfortable is one of the worst things you can do. Use touch to communicate the fact that you care. Listen to the patient. Often the patient needs to talk and needs someone to listen. Being there when your patient needs you is important. You may not have to say anything. Just be there to listen.

MUSCULOSKELETAL DISORDERS

Musculoskeletal disorders are common. They affect the ability to move about. Some are due to injury. Others result from aging.

Arthritis

Arthritis means joint (arth) inflammation (itis). It is the most common joint disease. Pain and decreased mobility occur in the affected joints. There are two basic types of arthritis.

Osteoarthritis   This type of arthritis occurs with aging. Joint injury is also a cause. The hips and knees are commonly affected. These joints bear the weight of the body. Joints in the fingers, thumbs, and spine can also be affected. Symptoms are joint stiffness and pain. Cold weather and dampness seem to increase the symptoms.

Osteoarthritis has no cure. Treatment involves relieving pain and stiffness. Doctors often order aspirin for the pain. Local heat applications may be ordered. When the condition is advanced, the patient may need help walking. A walking aid (cane, walker) may be needed. Assistance with ADL is given as necessary.

Rheumatoid arthritis   Rheumatoid arthritis is a chronic disease. It can occur at any age. Connective tissue throughout the body is affected. The disease affects the heart, lungs, eyes, kidneys, and skin. However, the joints are mainly affected. Smaller joints in the fingers, hands, and wrists are affected first. Eventually, larger joints are involved. Severe inflammation causes very painful and swollen joints. The patient will probably restrict movement because of severe pain.

Signs and symptoms are pain, redness, and swelling in the joint area; limitation of joint motion; fever; fatigue; and weight loss. As the disease progresses, more and more joints become involved. Changes in other organs eventually occur.

The goals in treating rheumatoid arthritis are:
1. Maintaining joint motion
2. Controlling pain
3. Preventing deformities

The patient needs a lot of rest. Bed rest may be ordered if several joints are involved and when fever is present. If the patient is on bed rest, turning and repositioning are done every 2 hours. The patient is positioned to prevent contractures. Adequate sleep—

8 to 10 hours—is needed each night. Morning and afternoon rest periods are also necessary. Rest is balanced with exercise. Range-of-motion exercises are done. Walking aids may be needed. Splints may be applied to the affected body parts. Safety measures to prevent falls are practiced.

Medications are ordered by the doctor for pain. Local heat applications may be ordered. A back massage is relaxing. Positioning to prevent deformities promotes comfort.

Patients need emotional support and reassurance. The disease is chronic. Death from other organ involvement is always possible. A good attitude is important. Patients should be as active as possible. The more patients can do for themselves, the better off they will be. A patient may need someone to talk to. You must be a good listener when the patient needs to talk.

Fractures

A *fracture* is a broken bone. Tissues around the fracture (muscles, blood vessels, nerves, and tendons) are usually injured also. Fractures may be open or closed (Fig. 25-2). A *closed fracture (simple fracture)* means the bone is broken but the skin is intact. An *open fracture (compound fracture)* means the broken bone has come through the skin.

Fractures are caused by falls and accidents. A bone disease called osteoporosis can also cause fractures (see page 398). Signs and symptoms of a fracture are pain, swelling, limitation of movement, bruising, and color changes at the fracture site. Bleeding may occur.

The bone has to heal. The two bone ends are brought into normal position. This is called reduc-

tion. *Closed reduction* involves manipulating the bone back into place. The skin is not opened. *Open reduction* involves surgery. The bone is exposed and brought back into alignment. Nails, pins, screws, metal plates, or wires may be used to keep the bone in place (Fig. 25-3). After reduction, the fracture is immobilized. In other words, movement of the two bone ends is prevented. A cast or traction may be used to immobilize the bone.

Cast care   Casts are made of plaster of paris, plastic, or fiberglass. The cast covers all or part of an extremity (Fig. 25-4). Before the doctor applies the cast, the extremity is covered with stockinette. Material for plaster of paris casts comes in rolls. A roll is moistened and wrapped around the extremity. Several rolls may be used. A plaster of paris cast needs 24 to 48 hours to dry. A dry cast is odorless, white, and shiny. A wet cast is gray, cool, and has a musty smell. The following rules apply to cast care:

1. Do not cover the cast with blankets, plastic, or other material. The cast gives off heat as it dries. Covers prevent the heat from escaping. Burns can occur if the heat cannot escape.
2. Turn the patient as directed by the nurse. All cast surfaces are exposed to the air at one time or another. Even drying is promoted by turning.
3. The cast must maintain its shape. It should not be placed on a hard surface while wet. A hard surface can flatten the cast. Pillows are used to support the entire length of the cast (Fig. 25-5). When turning and positioning the patient, support the cast with your palms (Fig. 25-6). Fingers can make dents in the cast. The dents can cause pressure areas that can lead to skin breakdown.
4. Protect the patient from rough edges of the cast. Cast edges may be covered with tape. This is called petaling (Fig. 25-7). If stockinette is used, the doctor pulls it up over the cast. The stockinette is then secured in place with a roll of cast material.
5. Keep the cast dry. A wet cast loses its shape. It must be protected from moisture from the perineal area. The nurse may apply a waterproof material around the perineal area once the cast is dry.
6. Do not let the patient insert anything into the cast. Itching often occurs under the cast and causes an intense desire to scratch. Skin can be broken by items used for scratching (pencils, coat hangers, knitting needles, back scratchers). The open area under the cast can become infected. Items used for scratching can also wrinkle the stockinette. The object can be lost into the cast. Both can cause pressure, which leads to skin breakdown.

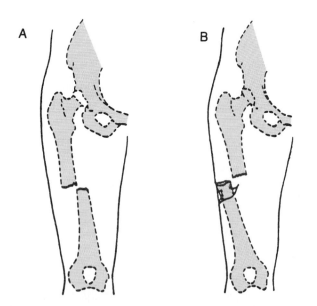

Fig. 25-2   **A,** Closed fracture. **B,** Open fracture. (From Hood GH, Dincher JR: *Total patient care: foundations and practice,* ed 6, St Louis, 1984, Mosby–Year Book.)

7. A casted extremity is elevated on pillows. Elevation of an arm or leg reduces swelling.
8. Have enough help when turning and repositioning the patient. A cast is heavy and awkward. Balance can be lost easily.
9. Lying on the injured side is usually not allowed. The nurse tells you what positions are allowed.
10. Report these signs and symptoms:
    a. Pain—a warning sign of a decubitus ulcer, poor circulation, or nerve damage.
    b. Swelling and a tight cast—blood flow to the part may be affected.
    c. Pale skin—reduced blood flow to the part.
    d. Cyanosis—reduced blood flow to the part.
    e. Odor—an infection may be present.
    f. Inability to move the fingers or toes—the cast may be causing presure on a nerve.
    g. Numbness—the cast may be causing pressure on a nerve. There may be reduced blood flow to the part.
    h. Temperature changes—cool skin means poor circulation. Hot skin means inflammation.
    i. Drainage on or under the cast—there may be an infection under the cast.
    j. Chills, fever, nausea, and vomiting—there may be an infection under the cast.

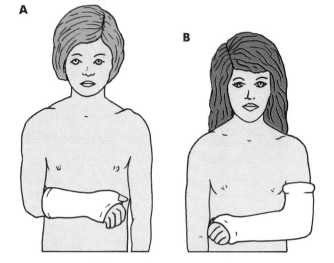

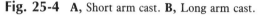

Fig. 25-4 A, Short arm cast. **B,** Long arm cast.

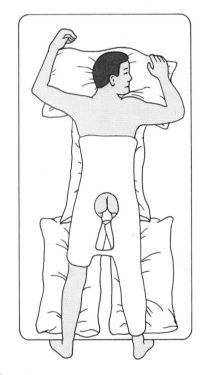

Fig. 25-5 Pillows support the entire length of the wet cast. (From Milliken ME, Campbell G: *Essential competencies for patient care,* St Louis, 1985, Mosby–Year Book.)

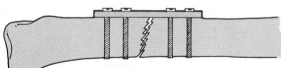

Screws and plate

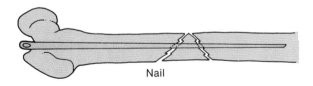

Nail

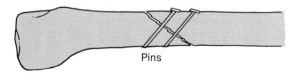

Pins

Fig. 25-3 Devices used to reduce a fracture. (From Milliken ME, Campbell G: *Essential competencies for patient care,* St Louis, 1985, Mosby–Year Book.)

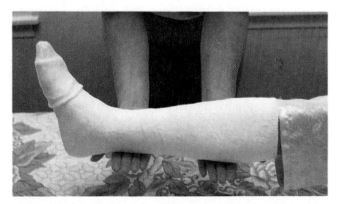

Fig. 25-6 The cast is supported with the palms during lifting.

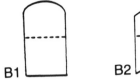
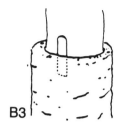
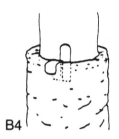
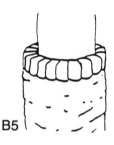
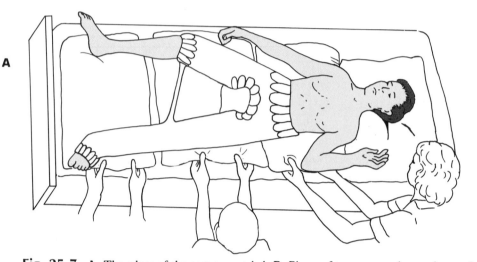

Fig. 25-7 A, The edges of the cast are petaled. **B,** Pieces of tape are used to make petals. The petal is placed inside the cast and then brought over the edge.
(From Billings DM, Stokes LG: *Medical-surgical nursing: common health problems of adults and children across the life span,* ed 2, St Louis, 1987, Mosby–Year Book.)

Traction Traction may be used to immobilize a fracture. Pull from two directions keeps the fractured bone in place. Weights, ropes, and pulleys are used (Fig. 25-8). Traction can be applied to the neck, arms, legs, or pelvis. Traction is also used for muscle spasms, to correct or prevent deformities, and for other musculoskeletal injuries.

Traction is applied by the doctor to the skin or to the bone. Skin traction involves applying bandages and strips of material to the skin. Weights are attached to the material or bandage (see Fig. 25-8). Traction applied directly to the bone is called skeletal traction. A pin is inserted through the bone. Special devices are attached to the pin. Weights are attached to the devices (Fig. 25-9).

Continuous or intermittent traction may be used. Continuous traction cannot be removed. Intermittent traction can be removed at times as ordered by the doctor.

The following rules apply when caring for a patient in traction:

1. Find out if the traction is continuous or intermittent.
2. Keep the patient pulled up in bed. This is necessary to maintain the proper pull of the traction.
3. Keep the weights off the floor. Weights should hang from the traction set-up (see Fig. 25-8).
4. Do not remove the weights.

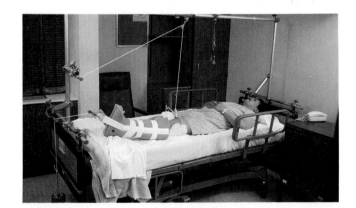

Fig. 25-8 Traction setup. Note the weights, pulleys, and ropes.
(From Thompson JM, et al: *Mosby's manual of clinical nursing,* ed 2, St Louis, 1989, Mosby–Year Book.)

5. Perform range-of-motion exercises for the uninvolved body parts as directed by the nurse.
6. Check with the nurse about positioning. Usually only the back-lying position is allowed.
7. The fracture pan is used for elimination.
8. Give skin care at frequent intervals.
9. Bottom linens are usually put on from the top down. The patient can use the trapeze to raise the body off the bed (Fig. 25-10).
10. Observe for the signs and symptoms listed under cast care. Report these observations to the nurse immediately.

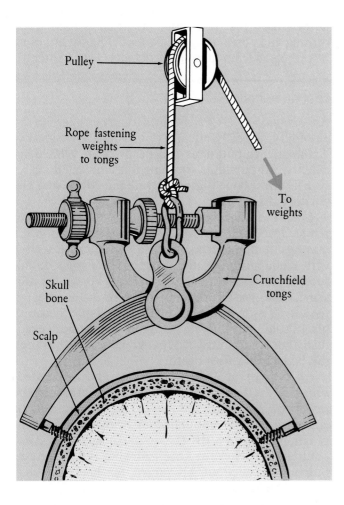

Fig. 25-9 Skeletal traction is attached to the bone.

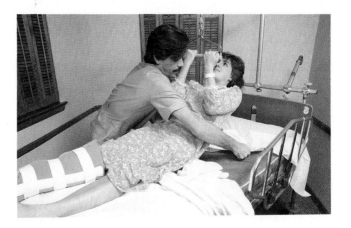

Fig. 25-10 A bed is made from the top down with traction. The patient uses the trapeze to lift the buttocks off the bed. Then the linens are pulled down over the bed.

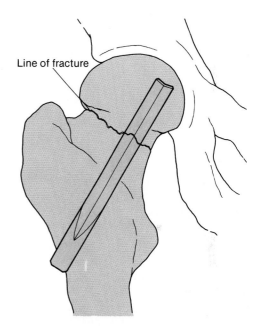

Fig. 25-11 A hip fracture is pinned in place. (From Milliken ME, Campbell G: *Essential competencies for patient care*, St Louis, 1985, Mosby–Year Book.)

Hip fractures Fractured hips are common in the elderly. They are especially serious because healing is slower in older people. The person may have other disorders. These disorders and slow healing may complicate the patient's condition and care. The patient is also at great risk for postoperative complications.

Open reduction is required. The fracture is fixed in position with a pin (Fig. 25-11). This is called a "hip pinning." The patient needs preoperative and postoperative care as described in Chapter 23. A cast or traction is also used in some situations. Therefore care of the patient who has a cast or is in traction may also be required. The patient with a hip pinning also requires the following care:

1. Give good skin care. Skin breakdown can occur rapidly.
2. Turn and reposition the patient as directed by the nurse. The doctor's orders for turning and positioning depend on the type of fracture and the surgical procedure performed.
3. Keep the operated leg abducted at all times. The leg is abducted when the patient is supine, being turned, or in a side-lying position. Pillows or abductor splints can be used as directed.
4. Prevent external rotation of the hip (Fig. 25-12). Use trochanter rolls or sandbags as directed.
5. Provide a straight-backed chair with armrests when the patient is to be up. A low, soft chair is not used.
6. Place the chair on the unoperated side.
7. Assist the nurse in transferring the patient from the bed to the chair as directed.
8. Do not let the patient stand on the operated leg unless permitted by the doctor.
9. Support and elevate the leg as directed when the patient is in the chair.

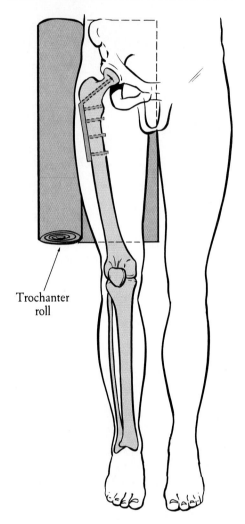

Fig. 25-12 A trochanter roll is used to prevent external rotation after a hip pinning.

Osteoporosis

Osteoporosis is a bone (osteo) disorder in which the bone becomes porous and brittle (porosis). It is common in the elderly and in women after menopause. A lack of dietary calcium is a major cause of osteoporosis. Bed rest and immobility are other causes because they do not allow for proper bone use. For bone to form properly, it must be used to bear weight. If it is not, calcium is absorbed and the bone becomes porous and brittle.

Signs and symptoms of osteoporosis include low back pain, gradual loss of height, and stooped posture. Fractures are a major threat. Bones are so brittle that the slightest stress can cause a fracture. Turning in bed or getting up from a chair can cause a fracture. Fractures are a great risk if the patient falls or has an accident.

Osteoporosis is treated with calcium and vitamin supplements. The hormone estrogen may be given to women. Exercise, good posture, and a back brace or corset are also important. Walking aids may be needed. Bed rest is avoided. Caution is used when turning and positioning the patient. The patient must be protected from falls and accidents (see Chapter 8).

Loss of a Limb

An *amputation* is the removal of all or part of an extremity. Usually the part is removed surgically. Traumatic amputations can occur from vehicle accidents. Amputations are sometimes indicated for severe injuries, bone tumors, severe infections, and circulatory disorders.

Gangrene is a condition in which there is death of tissue. Infection, injuries, and circulatory disorders may result in gangrene. These conditions interfere with blood supply to the tissues. The tissues do not receive enough oxygen and nutrients. Poisonous substances and waste products build up in the affected tissues. Tissue death results. The tissue becomes black, cold, and shriveled (Fig. 25-13), and can eventually fall off. If untreated, gangrene spreads through the body and causes death.

All or part of an extremity may be amputated. Fingers, the hand, forearm, or entire arm may be removed. Toes, the foot, lower leg, upper leg, or entire leg may be amputated. A below-the-knee amputation is called a BK (below the knee) or an ABK (amputation below the knee). An above-the-knee amputation is called an AK (above the knee) or AKA (above the knee amputation).

The patient needs preoperative and postoperative care (see Chapter 23). Much psychological support is needed. The patient faces the loss of a limb. A major psychological adjustment will be necessary. The patient's life will be affected by the amputation. Appearance, activities of daily living, moving about, and the job are just a few areas that will be affected. Put yourself in the patient's position. How would you feel if you had to lose an arm or a leg?

Nurses are responsible for the patient's postoperative care. At some point most patients are fitted with a prosthesis (see Figs. 24-7, *A* and *B*, page 389). The stump must be conditioned for the prosthesis to fit properly. Stump conditioning involves shrinking and shaping the stump into a cone shape. Bandaging is used to shrink and shape the stump. Exercises are ordered to strengthen the other limbs. Physical therapy helps the patient learn to use the prosthesis. Occupational therapy is necessary if the patient has to learn how to perform activities of daily living with the stump or prosthesis.

The patient may feel that the limb is still there or may complain of pain in the amputated part. This is called *phantom limb pain*. The exact cause is unknown. However, it is a normal reaction. The sensation may be present only for a short time after surgery. However, some patients experience phantom limb pain for many years.

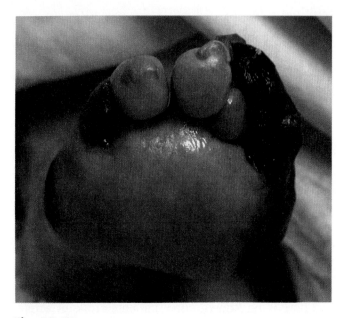

Fig. 25-13 Gangrene.

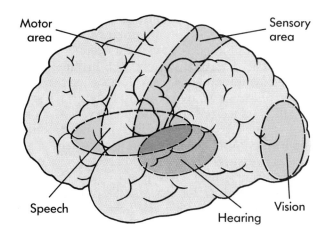

Fig. 25-14 Functions lost from a stroke depend on the area of brain damage.
(From Milliken ME, Campbell G: *Essential competencies for patient care*, St Louis, 1985, Mosby–Year Book.)

NERVOUS SYSTEM DISORDERS

Nervous system disorders can affect mental and physical functioning. The ability to speak, understand, feel, see, hear, touch, think, control bowels and bladder, or move may be affected. There are many causes and types of nervous system disorders. The common ones are described here.

Cerebrovascular Accident

A cerebrovascular accident (CVA) is commonly called a *stroke*. Blood supply to a part of the brain is suddenly interrupted. Brain damage occurs. The interruption can be due to the rupture of a blood vessel, which causes hemorrhage (excessive bleeding) into the brain. A blood clot can obstruct blood flow to the brain.

Stroke is more common among the elderly. However, persons in their 20s and 30s have had strokes. A common cause of stroke is hypertension (elevated blood pressure). Other risk factors include diabetes mellitus, obesity, birth control pills, a family history of stroke, hardening of the arteries, smoking, and stress.

Signs and symptoms vary. Sometimes there is a warning. The patient may be dizzy, have ringing in the ears, a headache, nausea and vomiting, and memory loss. The stroke may occur suddenly. Unconsciousness, noisy breathing, elevated blood pressure, slow pulse, redness of the face, seizures, and paralysis on one side of the body (*hemiplegia*) may occur. The stroke victim may lose bowel and bladder control and the ability to speak. *Aphasia* is the inability (a) to speak (phasia).

Emergency care of the stroke victim is described in Chapter 29. If the person survives, some brain damage is likely to occur. The functions lost depend on the area of brain damage (Fig. 25-14). Rehabilitation begins immediately. The patient may be partially or totally dependent on others for care. Care of the patient is as follows:

1. The patient is positioned in the lateral position to prevent aspiration.
2. Coughing and deep breathing are encouraged.
3. The bed is in semi-Fowler's position.
4. Side rails are kept up except when giving care.
5. Turning and repositioning are done every 2 hours.
6. Elastic stockings are usually ordered to prevent blood clots in the legs.
7. Range-of-motion exercises are performed to prevent contractures.
8. A catheter may be inserted, or a bladder training program may be started.
9. A bowel training program may be necessary.
10. Safety precautions are practiced.
11. Assistance is given for self-care activities. The patient is encouraged to do as much as possible.
12. Methods are established for communicating with the patient. Magic slates, pencil and paper, a picture board, or other methods may be used.
13. Good skin care is given to prevent decubitus ulcers.
14. Speech therapy, physical therapy, and occupational therapy may be ordered.
15. Emotional support and encouragement are given. Praise is given for even the slightest accomplishment.

Parkinson's Disease

Parkinson's disease is a slow, progressive disorder. Degeneration of a part of the brain occurs. There is no cure. The disease is usually seen in the elderly. Signs and symptoms are a masklike facial expression, tremors, pill-rolling movements of the fingers, a shuffling gait, stooped posture, stiff muscles, slow movements, slurred or monotone speech, and drooling. Mental function is usually not affected early in the disease process. As the disease progresses, confusion and forgetfulness may develop.

Drugs specifically for Parkinson's disease are ordered by the doctor. Physical therapy may also be ordered. The patient may need help with eating and other self-care activities. Measures to promote normal bowel elimination are practiced. There is a risk of constipation because of decreased activity and poor nutrition. Safety practices are carried out to protect the patient from injury. Remember that mental function may not be affected. Talk to and treat the person as an adult.

Multiple Sclerosis

Multiple sclerosis (MS) is a progressive disease. The myelin sheath (which covers the nerves), the spinal cord, and the white matter in the brain are destroyed. As a result, nerve impulses cannot be sent to and from the brain in a normal manner.

Symptoms begin in young adulthood. The onset is gradual. There is blurred or double vision. Difficulty with balance and walking occur. Tremors, numbness and tingling, weakness, dizziness, urinary incontinence, bowel incontinence or constipation, behavior changes, and incoordination eventually occur. Signs and symptoms progressively worsen over several years. Blindness, contractures, paralysis of all extremities (quadriplegia), loss of bowel and bladder control, and respiratory muscle weakness are among the patient's many problems. The patient is eventually totally dependent on others for care.

There is no known cure. Patients are kept active as long as possible. They are encouraged and allowed to do as much for themselves as possible. Nursing

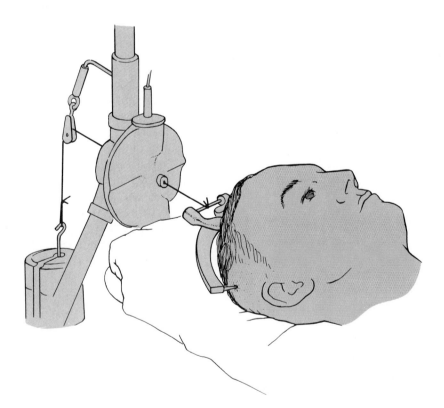

Fig. 25-15 Cervical traction. Screws are inserted into the skull. The weights are attached to the screws.
(From Long BC, Phipps WJ: *Essentials of medical-surgical nursing: a nursing process approach,* St Louis, 1985, Mosby–Year Book.)

care depends on the patient's needs and condition. Skin care, personal hygiene, and range-of-motion exercises are important. Patients are protected from injury. Measures are taken to promote bowel and bladder elimination. Turning, positioning, coughing, and deep breathing are also important. Measures are planned to prevent the complications of bed rest.

Head Injuries

The scalp, skull, and brain tissue can be injured. Sometimes injuries are minor. Minor injures may cause only a temporary loss of consciousness. Others are more serious. Permanent brain damage or death may result. Brain tissue can be bruised or torn. Skull fractures can cause brain damage. Hemorrhage from head injuries can occur in the brain or surrounding structures.

Head injuries are caused by falls, vehicle accidents, industrial accidents, and sport injuries. Other body parts may be injured also. Spinal cord injuries are likely. Birth injuries are another major cause of head trauma. If the person survives a severe head injury, some permanent damage is likely. Paralysis, mental retardation, personality changes, speech problems, breathing difficulties, and loss of bowel and bladder control may be permanent. Rehabilitation is required. Nursing care depends on the patient's needs and remaining abilities.

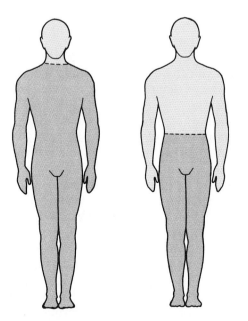

Fig. 25-16 The shaded areas indicate the areas of paralysis. (From Milliken ME, Campbell G: *Essential competencies for patient care,* St Louis, 1985, Mosby–Year Book.)

Spinal Cord Injuries

Spinal cord injuries can permanently damage the nervous system. These injuries usually occur from stab or bullet wounds, vehicle accidents, industrial accidents, falls, or sport injuries. Cervical traction (a form of skeletal traction) is often necessary (Fig. 25-15). The patient in cervical traction is placed on a Stryker frame.

The type of damage depends on the level of the injury. The higher the level of injury, the greater the loss of function (Fig. 25-16). If the injury is in the lumbar area, muscle function in the legs is lost. Injuries at the thoracic level cause loss of muscle function below the chest. Patients with injuries at the lumbar or thoracic levels are paraplegics. *Paraplegia* is paralysis of the legs. Cervical injuries may result in loss of function to the arms, chest, and all muscles below the chest. Patients with these injuries are quadriplegics. *Quadriplegia* is paralysis of the arms, legs, and trunk.

If the patient survives, rehabilitation is necessary. The patient's needs and the rehabilitation program depend on the functions lost and the abilities that remain. Emotional needs cannot be overlooked. These patients have severe emotional reactions to paralysis and the loss of function. Paralyzed patients generally need the following care:

1. Protect the patient from injury. Falls and burns are major risks. Keep side rails up, the bed in low position, and the call light within reach. Bath water, heat applications, and food must be at the proper temperature.
2. Turn and reposition the patient every 2 hours.
3. Give skin care and other measures to prevent decubitus ulcers.
4. Maintain good body alignment at all times. Pillows, trochanter rolls, foot boards, and other devices are used as needed.
5. Carry out bowel and bladder training programs.
6. Perform range-of-motion exercises to maintain muscle function and prevent contractures. Other exercises may be ordered.
7. Assist with food and fluids as needed. The patient may have to be fed. Self-help devices may be needed.
8. Give emotional and psychological support. Psychiatrists or psychologists may be involved in the patient's care.
9. Physical therapy, occupational therapy, and vocational rehabilitation may be ordered. They help the patient regain independent functioning to the extent possible.

Hearing Problems

Hearing losses range from slight hearing impairments to complete deafness. Hearing is required for many functions. Clear speech, responsiveness to others, safety, and awareness of surroundings all require hearing. Many people deny that they have difficulty hearing. This is because hearing loss is usually associated with aging.

Effects on the patient A person may be unaware of gradual development of difficulty in hearing. Others may notice changes in the person's behavior or attitude. However, they may not realize that the changes are due to hearing difficulties. The symptoms and effects of hearing loss vary. They are not always obvious to the person or to others.

There are some obvious signs of hearing impairment. These include speaking too loudly, leaning forward to hear, and turning and cupping the better ear toward the speaker. The person may answer questions or respond inappropriately or may ask for words to be repeated. Lack of attention and failing grades are early signs of poor hearing in children. Infants with hearing impairments often fail to start talking.

Psychological and social effects are less obvious. People with hearing problems may answer others inappropriately. Therefore they tend to avoid social situations. This is an attempt to avoid embarrassment. However, loneliness, boredom, and feelings of being left out often result. Only parts of conversations may be heard. People with hearing loss may become suspicious. They may think they are being talked about, or that others are intentionally talking softly. Some try to dominate conversations so that they do not have to respond or answer questions. Straining and working hard to hear can cause fatigue, frustration, and irritability.

People with hearing loss may develop speech problems. You hear yourself as you talk. How you pronounce words and the volume of your voice depend on how you hear yourself. Hearing loss may result in slurred speech and improper word pronunciation. Monotone speech and dropping word endings may also occur.

Communicating with the patient Hearing impaired persons may wear hearing aids or read lips. They also watch facial expressions, gestures, and body language to understand what is being said. Sign language may be necessary for the totally deaf. Some hearing impaired people have "hearing" dogs. The dogs alert the person to such things as ringing phones, door bells, sirens, or oncoming cars. Certain measures are necessary when communicating with the person with a hearing loss. The following measures can help the person hear or lip read:

1. Gain attention and alert the person to your presence in the room by lightly touching his or her arm. Do not startle or approach the person from behind.
2. Face the person directly when speaking. Do not turn or walk away while you are talking.
3. Stand or sit in good light. Shadows and glares affect the person's ability to see your face clearly.
4. Speak clearly, distinctly, and slowly.
5. Speak in a normal tone of voice. Do not shout.
6. Do not cover your mouth, smoke, eat, or chew gum while talking. These things affect mouth movements.
7. Stand or sit on the side of the better ear.
8. State the topic of conversation first.
9. Use short sentences and simple words.
10. Write out important names and words.
11. Keep conversations and discussions short to avoid tiring the person.
12. Repeat and rephrase statements as needed.
13. Be alert to the messages sent by your facial expressions, gestures, and body language.
14. Reduce or eliminate background noises.

The person with a hearing impairment may have speech problems. Understanding what the person is saying can be difficult. Do not assume that you understand what is being said. You should not pretend to understand to avoid embarrassing the person. Serious consequences can result if you assume or pretend to understand. The following guidelines will help you communicate with the speech impaired person:

1. Listen and give the person your full attention.
2. Ask the person questions to which you know the answer. This helps you to become familiar with the person's speech.
3. Determine the subject being discussed. This helps you to understand essential points.
4. Ask the person to repeat or rephrase statements if necessary.
5. Repeat what the person has said. Ask if you have understood correctly.
6. Ask the person to write down key words or the message.
7. Watch the person's lip movements.
8. Watch facial expressions, gestures, and body language for clues about what is being said.

Hearing aids A *hearing aid* amplifies sound. It does not correct or cure the hearing problem. The ability to hear is not improved. The person may hear better with a hearing aid. This is because the hearing aid makes sounds louder. Both background noise and speech are amplified. Noise must be minimized to help the person adjust to the hearing aid. Remember that the hearing aid does not make speech clearer, only louder. The measures for communicating with hearing impaired persons apply to those with hearing aids.

Hearing aids are operated by batteries. There is an on and off switch. Sometimes hearing aids do not seem to work properly. Several things need to be checked. Determine if the instrument is on. Proper battery position also should be checked. New batteries may be needed. The earpiece may need cleaning. The hearing aid may need repair.

Hearing aids are expensive. They must be handled carefully and cared for properly. The earpiece (Fig. 25-17) is the only part that can be washed. Soap and water are used daily to wash the earpiece. Thorough drying of the earpiece is necessary before it is snapped back into place.

Vision Problems

Vision problems occur at all ages. Problems range from very mild vision loss to complete blindness, and may be sudden or gradual in onset. One or both eyes may be affected. Surgery, eyeglasses, or contact lenses are often necessary.

Glaucoma   Glaucoma is an eye disease. Pressure within the eye is increased, which damages the retina and optic nerve. The result is visual loss with eventual blindness. The disease may be gradual or sudden in onset. Signs and symptoms include tunnel vision (Fig. 25-18), blurred vision, and blue-green halos around lights. With sudden onset, the patient also has severe eye pain, nausea, and vomiting. Glaucoma is a major cause of blindness. Persons over 40 years of age are at risk. The cause is unknown.

Treatment involves drug therapy and possibly surgery. The goal is to prevent further damage to the retina and optic nerve. Damage that has already occurred cannot be reversed.

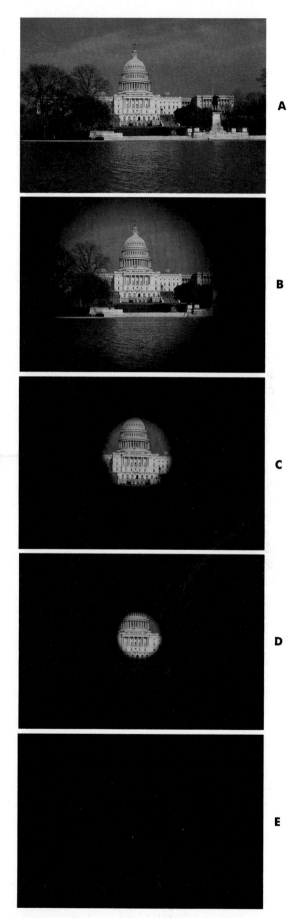

Fig. 25-18 **A,** Normal vision. **B,** Tunnel vision. **C, D, E,** Visual loss continues, with eventual blindness.

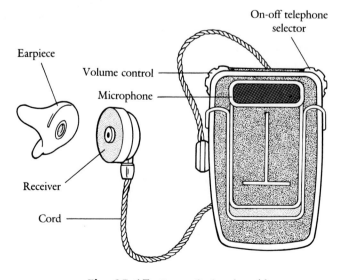

Fig. 25-17 Parts of a hearing aid.

Cataract Cataract is an eye disorder in which the lens becomes cloudy (opaque). The cloudiness prevents light from entering the eye. Gradual blurring and dimming of vision occurs. Sight is eventually lost. A cataract can occur in one or both eyes. Aging is the most common cause. Surgery is the only treatment.

The patient may have to wear an eye shield or patch for several days after surgery. The shield protects the eye from injury. One or both eyes may be covered. Measures for the blind person are practiced when an eye shield is worn. Even if only one shield is worn, there may be visual loss in the other eye from cataract or other causes.

A permanent implant is usually done during surgery. Some patients are fitted with corrective lenses after surgery. Even with corrective lenses or implants there will be some degree of impaired vision.

Corrective Lenses

Eyeglasses and contact lenses are prescribed to correct vision problems. Eyeglasses may be worn only for certain activities, such as reading or seeing at a distance. They may be worn continuously while awake. Contact lenses are usually worn continuously while awake.

Eyeglasses The person may be upset when glasses are first needed. However, adjustment is usually rapid. Most people accept the fact that they will need glasses sooner or later. Appearance is often a concern. Glasses come in many styles and shapes. Frames can be chosen that fit face shape, personality, and lifestyle.

Lenses are made of hardened glass or plastic. They are impact resistant to prevent shattering. Glass lenses are washed with warm water and dried with soft tissue. Plastic lenses are easily scratched. A special cleaning solution and special tissues and cloths are needed for cleaning and drying them.

Glasses are costly. They must be protected from breakage or other damage. When not being worn, they need to be put in their case. The case is put in the drawer of the bedside stand. Glasses are easily damaged or lost if not in the case and in the drawer.

Contact lenses Contact lenses fit directly on the eye. Hard and soft contacts are available. Many people prefer contacts because they cannot be seen. They do not break easily, so they can be worn for sports. However, contacts are more expensive than eyeglasses. They are also easily lost. Contacts are removed for activities like swimming, showering, and sleeping.

Persons with contact lenses are taught to insert, remove, and clean them. Patients should perform these activities personally. However, a patient may be unable to insert or remove the lenses. A nurse is responsible for meeting the person's needs in this area. The eye can easily be damaged when inserting or removing contact lenses. Therefore you should not perform these measures.

Special Needs of the Blind Patient

Blindness has many causes. Birth defects, accidents, and eye diseases are causes. It can also be a complication of diseases that affect other organs and body systems. Blindness is usually acquired later in life. A person's life is seriously affected by the loss of sight. Physical and psychological adjustments can be difficult and take a long time. Special education and training are required. Moving about, activities of daily living, reading braille, and using a Seeing Eye dog all require training.

Braille is a method of writing for the blind that uses raised dots. The dots are arranged to represent each letter of the alphabet. The first 10 letters also represent the numbers 0 through 9 (Fig. 25-19). The person feels the arrangement of dots with the fingers (Fig. 25-20). Many books, magazines, and newspapers are available in braille. There are also braille typewriters.

Braille is hard to learn, especially for many elderly people. Entire books and articles are available on records and tapes. These are often called "talking books." They can be bought or borrowed from libraries.

The blind person can be taught to move about using a white cane or a "Seeing Eye dog" or "guide dog." Both are recognized worldwide as signs that the person is blind. The dog serves as the eyes of the blind person. The dog recognizes danger and guides the person through traffic.

You must treat the blind person with respect and dignity—not with pity. Most blind people have adjusted to their blindness. They lead rather independent lives. Some have been blind for a long time and others for only a short time. Certain practices are necessary when dealing with a blind person. These

Fig. 25-19 Braille.

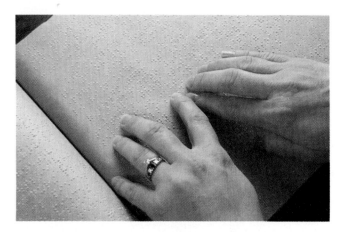

Fig. 25-20 Braille is "read" with the fingers.

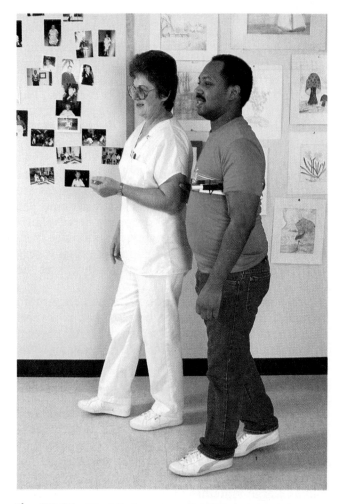

Fig. 25-21 The blind person walks slightly behind the nursing assistant and touches the assistant's arm lightly.

practices are necessary no matter how long the person has been blind.

1. Identify yourself promptly when you enter the room. Give your name, title, and reason for being there. Do not touch the person until you have indicated your presence in the room.
2. Orient the person to the room. Identify the location and purpose of furniture and equipment.
3. Allow the person to move about and touch and locate furniture and equipment if able.
4. Do not rearrange furniture and equipment.
5. Give step-by-step explanations of procedures as you perform them. Indicate when the procedure is over.
6. Tell the person when you are leaving the room.
7. Keep doors open or shut, never partially open.
8. Assist the person in ambulating by walking slightly ahead of him or her (Fig. 25-21). The person should touch your arm lightly. Never push or guide the blind person in front of you.
9. Inform the person of steps, doors, turns, furniture, curbs, and other obstructions when assisting with ambulation.
10. Assist in food selection by reading the menu to the person.
11. Explain the location of food and beverages on the tray. Use the face of a clock (see Fig. 16-5) or guide the person's hand to each item on the tray.
12. Cut the meat, open the containers, butter the bread, and perform other similar activities if needed.
13. Keep the signal light within the person's reach.
14. Provide a radio, "talking books," television, and braille books for entertainment.
15. Do not shout or speak in a loud voice. Just because a person is blind does not mean that hearing is impaired.
16. Let the person perform self-care if able.

RESPIRATORY DISORDERS

Patients with respiratory disorders are commonly seen in hospital and nursing facilities. Some need home care. The respiratory system brings oxygen into the lungs and removes carbon dioxide from the body. Respiratory disorders interfere with this function and threaten life.

Chronic Obstructive Pulmonary Disease (COPD)

Four disorders are grouped under chronic obstructive pulmonary disease (COPD). They are chronic bronchitis, asthma, bronchiectasis, and emphysema. These disorders interfere with the normal exchange of oxygen and carbon dioxide in the lungs.

Chronic bronchitis Chronic bronchitis occurs after repeated episodes of bronchitis (inflammation of the bronchi). Common causes are cigarette smoking and air pollution. "Smoker's cough" in the morning is usually the first symptom. At first the cough is dry. Eventually the patient coughs up mucus, which may contain pus and blood. The cough becomes more frequent as the disease progresses. The patient may have difficulty breathing and may tire easily. The mucus and inflamed breathing passages "obstruct" air flow into the lungs. Therefore the body cannot get normal amounts of oxygen.

Asthma   Air passages narrow with asthma. Difficult breathing results. Allergies and emotional stress are common causes. Episodes occur suddenly and are called asthma attacks. Besides dyspnea, there is shortness of breath, wheezing, coughing, rapid pulse, perspiration, and cyanosis. The patient is usually very frightened during the attack. Fear usually causes the attack to become worse.

Drugs are used to treat asthma. Emergency room treatment may be necessary if the attack is severe. The patient and family are taught ways to prevent asthma attacks. Repeated attacks can damage the respiratory system.

Bronchiectasis   Bronchiectasis is a disorder in which the bronchi dilate (enlarge). Pus collects in the dilated bronchi. There are many causes, including respiratory infections and aspiration. Bronchiectasis may be a complication of measles or whooping cough in young children. The patient has a chronic, productive cough. Large amounts of sputum are coughed up. The sputum contains pus and usually has a foul smell. The amount increases as the disease progresses. Eventually blood may be present in the sputum. Weight loss, fatigue, and loss of appetite can occur. The doctor may order drugs, respiratory therapy, rest, and measures to improve nutrition. The patient must be protected from others with respiratory infections. Cigarette smoking is not allowed. It may be necessary to remove the diseased part of the lung.

Emphysema   Emphysema is a disorder in which the alveoli become enlarged. Walls of the alveoli become less elastic. Therefore they do not expand and shrink normally with inspiration and expiration. As a result, some air is trapped in the alveoli during expiration. The trapped air is not exhaled. As the disease progresses, more alveoli are involved. The normal exchange of oxygen and carbon dioxide cannot occur in the affected alveoli.

Cigarette smoking is the most common cause. Signs and symptoms include shortness of breath and "smoker's cough." At first, shortness of breath occurs with exertion. As the disease progresses, it may occur at rest. Sputum may contain pus. As more air is trapped in the lungs, the patient develops a "barrel chest" (Fig. 25-22). Patients usually prefer to sit upright and slightly forward. Breathing is easier in this position.

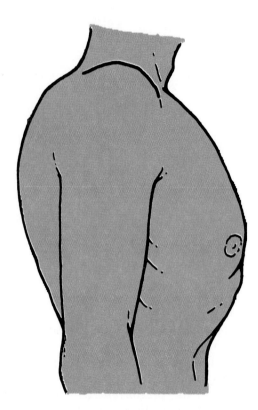

Fig. 25-22   Barrel chest from emphysema.

The patient must stop smoking. Respiratory therapy, breathing exercises, oxygen, and drug therapy are ordered.

Pneumonia

Pneumonia is an inflammation of lung tissue. The alveoli in the affected area fill with fluid. Because of fluid in the alveoli, oxygen and carbon dioxide cannot be exchanged normally.

Pneumonia is caused by bacteria, viruses, aspiration, or immobility. The patient is very ill. Signs and symptoms include fever, chills, painful cough, pain on breathing, and a rapid pulse. Cyanosis may be present. The color of sputum depends on the cause. Sputum may be clear, green, yellowish, or rust colored.

Drugs are ordered for the infection and for pain relief. The doctor may also order "force fluids" because of fever. Fluids also help to thin mucous secretions. Thin secretions are easier to cough up. Oxygen may be necessary. Most patients prefer semi-Fowler's position for breathing. Respiratory isolation may be necessary, depending on the cause. Mouth care is important. Frequent linen changes may be necessary because of fever.

CARDIOVASCULAR DISORDERS

Cardiovascular disorders are the leading causes of death in the United States. Problems may occur in the heart or in the blood vessels.

Hypertension

Hypertension is a condition in which the blood pressure is abnormally high. Narrowed blood vessels are a common cause of hypertension. When vessels are narrow, the heart has to pump with more force to move blood through the vessels. Kidney disorders, head injuries, certain complications of pregnancy, and tumors of the adrenal gland can also cause hypertension.

Hypertension can damage other body organs. The heart may enlarge so that it can pump with more force. Blood vessels in the brain may burst and cause a stroke. Blood vessels in the eyes and kidneys may be damaged.

At first, hypertension may not cause signs or symptoms. Usually it is discovered when the blood pressure is measured. Signs and symptoms develop as the disorder progresses. Headache, blurred vision, and dizziness may be reported. Complications of hypertension include stroke, heart attack, kidney failure, and blindness.

Medications to lower the blood pressure may be ordered by the doctor. The patient will be advised to quit smoking, exercise regularly, and get enough rest. A sodium-restricted diet may also be ordered. If the patient is overweight, a low-calorie diet is ordered.

Coronary Artery Disease (CAD)

Coronary artery disease is a disorder in which the coronary arteries become narrowed. One or all of the arteries may be affected. Because of narrowed vessels, blood supply to the heart muscle is reduced. Atherosclerosis is the most common cause. In atherosclerosis, fatty material collects on the arterial walls (Fig. 25-23). This causes the arteries to narrow and obstruct blood flow. Blood flow through an artery may be completely blocked. Permanent heart damage occurs in the part of the heart receiving its blood supply from that artery.

Risk factors for the development of CAD have been identified. They include obesity, cigarette smoking, lack of exercise, a diet high in fat and cholesterol,

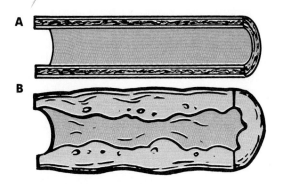

Fig. 25-23 A, Normal artery. **B,** Fatty deposits collect on the walls of arteries in atherosclerosis.

and hypertension. Age and sex (male or female) are other risk factors. CAD is more common in men and older people. The type A personality is also a risk factor. The person with a type A personality is aggressive, competitive, and works very hard. The person has difficulty relaxing, feels a sense of urgency, and does things at a rapid pace.

There are two major complications of coronary artery disease. They are angina pectoris and myocardial infarction (heart attack).

Angina pectoris Angina (pain) pectoris (chest) means "chest pain." The chest pain is due to reduced blood flow to a part of the heart muscle (myocardium). Angina pectoris is seen when the heart needs additional oxygen. Normally, blood flow to the heart increases when the heart's need for oxygen increases. Physical exertion, a heavy meal, emotional stress, and excitement increase the heart's need for oxygen. In CAD the narrowed vessels prevent increased blood flow.

Signs and symptoms of angina include chest pain. The pain may be described as a tightness or discomfort in the left side of the chest. The pain may radiate to the left jaw and down the inner aspect of the left arm (Fig. 25-24). The patient may be pale, feel faint, and may perspire. Dyspnea may be present. These signs and symptoms cause the patient to stop activity and rest. Rest often relieves the symptoms in 3 to 15 minutes. Rest reduces the heart's need for oxygen. Therefore normal blood flow is achieved and heart damage is prevented.

Besides rest, another treatment for angina pectoris is a medication called nitroglycerin. A nitroglycerin tablet is taken when an angina attack occurs. The nitroglycerin is put under the tongue. It dissolves under the tongue and is rapidly absorbed into the bloodstream. Most doctors allow the nitroglycerin to be kept at the bedside. The patient takes a tablet when one is needed and then tells the nurse. The patient does not have to wait for a nurse to answer the call light and then go get the tablet. The patient should have nitroglycerin tablets available at all times. This includes when the patient goes to physical therapy, occupational therapy, the x-ray department, the dining room, lounge, or other parts of the facility. Patients at home should keep the tablets close by.

Patients are taught to avoid situations that are likely to cause angina pectoris. These include overexertion, heavy meals and overeating, and emotional situations. They are advised to stay indoors during cold weather or during hot, humid weather. Exercise programs supervised by doctors may be developed. Some patients need coronary artery bypass surgery. The surgery bypasses the diseased part of the artery (Fig. 25-25) and increases blood flow to the heart.

Many patients with angina pectoris eventually have heart attacks. Chest pain that is not relieved by rest and nitroglycerin may have a more serious cause.

Fig. 25-24 Shaded areas show where the pain of angina pectoris is located.
(From Hood GH, Dincher JR: *Total patient care: foundations and practice,* ed 6, St Louis, 1984, Mosby–Year Book.)

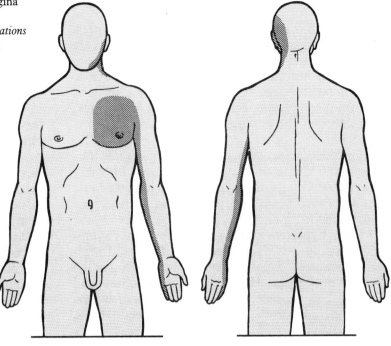

Myocardial infarction (MI)   A myocardial infarction is due to lack of blood supply to the heart muscle (myocardium). Tissue death occurs (infarction). Common terms for myocardial infarction are *heart attack, coronary, coronary thrombosis,* and *coronary occlusion.* Blood flow to the myocardium is suddenly interrupted. Usually a thrombus obstructs blood flow through an artery. The area of damage may be small or large. Cardiac arrest can occur (see Chapter 29).

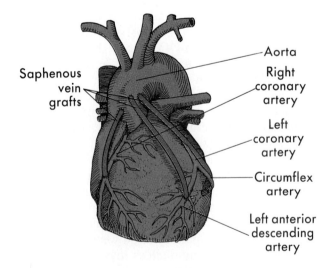

Fig. 25-25 Coronary artery bypass surgery. The diseased part of the area is bypassed with a vein graft.
(Modified from Long BC, Woods NF: *Medical-surgical nursing: concepts and clinical practice,* ed 3, St Louis, 1987, Mosby–Year Book.)

Signs and symptoms include sudden, severe chest pain. The pain is usually on the left side. It may be described as crushing, stabbing, or squeezing. Some have described the pain in terms of someone sitting on their chest. The pain may radiate to the neck and jaw, and down the arm. The pain is more severe and lasts longer than angina pectoris. It is not relieved by rest and nitroglycerin. Other symptoms include indigestion, dyspnea, nausea, dizziness, perspiration, pallor, cyanosis, cold and clammy skin, low blood pressure, and a weak and irregular pulse. The patient is very fearful and apprehensive. Some have described a feeling of doom. The patient may have all or some of these signs and symptoms.

Myocardial infarction is an emergency. Efforts are directed at relieving the pain, stabilizing vital signs, giving oxygen, and calming the patient. Many medications are given. The patient is treated in a coronary care unit (CCU), which has emergency equipment and drugs needed during a cardiac arrest. Measures are taken to prevent life-threatening complications.

The patient will be in the CCU for at least 3 days. When stable, the patient is transferred. Activity is increased gradually. Drug therapy and measures to prevent complications are continued. A cardiac rehabilitation program is developed for the patient. This includes an exercise program, teaching about medications, and dietary changes. Changes in lifestyle and sexual activity may be necessary. The goal of cardiac rehabilitation is to prevent another heart attack.

Congestive heart failure (CHF)

Congestive heart failure occurs when the heart cannot pump blood normally. Blood backs up and causes congestion of tissues. Left-sided heart failure, right-sided heart failure, or both, can occur.

When the left side of the heart fails to pump efficiently, blood backs up into the lungs. Signs and symptoms of respiratory congestion occur. These include dyspnea, increased sputum production, cough, and gurgling sounds in the lungs. In addition, blood is not pumped out of the heart to the rest of the body in adequate amounts. Organs receive an inadequate blood supply. Signs and symptoms occur because of the effects on the body's organs. For example, inadequate blood flow to the brain causes confusion, dizziness, and fainting. Inadequate blood flow to the kidneys causes reduced kidney function and decreased urinary output. The skin becomes pale or cyanotic. Blood pressure falls. A very severe form of left-sided failure is pulmonary edema (fluid in the lungs). Pulmonary edema is an emergency. Death can occur.

The right side of the heart may fail. Blood backs up into the venae cavae and into the venous system. The feet and ankles swell. Neck veins bulge. Congestion occurs in the liver, and liver function decreases. The abdomen may become congested with fluid. The right side of the heart cannot pump blood to the lungs efficiently. Therefore normal blood flow does not occur from the lungs to the left side of the heart. Less blood than normal is pumped from the left side of the heart to the rest of the body. As with left-sided failure, the body's organs will have a reduced blood supply. The signs and symptoms described in the previous paragraph eventually occur.

Congestive heart failure is usually caused by a weakened heart. Myocardial infarction and hypertension are common causes. Damaged heart valves can also cause CHF.

CHF can be treated and controlled. Drugs are given to strengthen the heart and to reduce the amount of fluid in the body. A sodium-restricted diet is ordered. Supplemental oxygen is given. Most patients prefer semi-Fowler's or Fowler's position for breathing. Many elderly people have CHF. They may need home care or care in a nursing facility. You may be involved in the following aspects of the person's care:

1. Maintaining bed rest or a limited activity program
2. Measuring intake and output
3. Measuring weight daily
4. Restricting fluids as ordered by the doctor
5. Giving good skin care to prevent skin breakdown
6. Performing range-of-motion exercises
7. Assisting with transfers or ambulation
8. Assisting with self-care activities
9. Maintaining good body alignment
10. Applying elastic stockings

TABLE 25-1 Insulin Shock and Diabetic Coma

	Insulin Shock	Diabetic Coma
Causes	Too much insulin	Undiagnosed diabetes
	Omitting a meal	Not enough insulin
	Eating an inadequate amount of food	Eating too much food
	Excessive physical activity	Insufficient amounts of exercise
	Vomiting	Stress from surgery, illness, emotional upset, etc.
Signs and symptoms	Hunger	Weakness
	Weakness	Drowsiness
	Trembling	Thirst
	Perspiration	Hunger
	Headache	Flushed cheeks
	Dizziness	Sweet breath odor
	Rapid pulse	Slow, deep, and labored respirations
	Low blood pressure	Rapid and weak pulse
	Confusion	Low blood pressure
	Convulsions	Dry skin
	Cold, clammy skin	Headache
	Unconsciousness	Nausea and vomiting
		Coma

THE ENDOCRINE SYSTEM

The most common endocrine disorder is diabetes mellitus. In this disorder, the body cannot use sugar properly. For proper use of sugar, there must be enough insulin. Insulin is secreted by the pancreas. In diabetes mellitus, the pancreas fails to secrete adequate amounts of insulin. Sugar builds up in the blood. Cells do not have enough sugar for energy. Therefore cells cannot perform their specific functions.

Diabetes mellitus occurs in children and adults. Persons at risk are those who have a family history of diabetes. Aging and obesity increase the risk.

Signs and symptoms include increased urine production, increased thirst, hunger, and weight loss. Urine testing shows sugar in the urine (see Chapter 14). If diabetes is not controlled, complications occur. These include changes in the retina that can lead to blindness, kidney damage, nerve damage, and circulatory disorders. Circulatory disorders can lead to a stroke, heart attack, and slow healing of wounds. Foot and leg wounds are especially serious. Infection and gangrene often occur and require amputation of the part.

Diabetes mellitus is treated with exercise, diet, and insulin therapy (see Chapter 16). Meals must be served on time. The patient needs to eat all foods served. Urine tests may be ordered (see Chapter 14). Good foot care is very important.

Insulin shock may develop if a patient gets too much insulin. Diabetic coma develops if a patient does not get enough insulin. Table 25-1 summarizes the causes, signs, and symptoms of insulin shock and diabetic coma. Both can lead to death if not corrected.

COMMUNICABLE DISEASES

Communicable diseases (contagious or infectious diseases) can be transmitted from one person to another. They can be transmitted in the following ways:

TABLE 25-2 Common Childhood Diseases (Communicable)

Disease	Signs and Symptoms	Mode of Transmission	Infective Material	Protective Measures
Bacterial Meningitis	Fever, severe headache, stiff neck, sore throat	Direct contact	Oral, nasal secretions	Mask
Chicken Pox (Varicella)	Fever, rash, cutaneous vesicles	Airborne, direct contact with drainage	Respiratory secretions, drainage from vesicles	Mask, handwashing
German Measles (Rubella)	Fever, rash	Airborne, direct contact with oral secretions	Oral secretions	Mask
Hepatitis A	Fever, loss of appetite, jaundice, fatigue	Direct contact Oral ingestion of virus	Urine, stool	Mask
Measles (Rubeola)	Fever, rash, bronchitis	Airborne, direct contact with secretions	Oral secretions	Gloves, handwashing
Mumps	Fever, swelling of salivary glands (parotid)	Airborne, direct contact	Saliva	Mask
Whooping Cough (Pertussis)	Violent cough at night, whooping sound when cough subsides	Airborne, direct contact	Oral secretions	Mask
Scarlet Fever	Fever, headache, nausea, vomiting	Airborne, direct contact	Oral secretions	Mask

*Reprinted and adapted with permission from Heckman James D: *Emergency Care and the Transportation of the Sick and Injured*, ed 4, Park Ridge, Il, 1987, American Academy of Orthopaedic Surgeons, pp 361-362.

Direct—from the infected person

Indirect—from dressings, linens, or surfaces

Airborne—from the patient through sneezing or coughing

Vehicle—through ingestion of contaminated food, water, drugs, blood, or fluids

Vector—from animals, fleas, and ticks

This section discusses AIDS and hepatitis. Tables 25-2 and 25-3 outline common childhood and adult communicable diseases. A review of Chapter 9 may be helpful in studying this section.

Acquired Immunodeficiency Syndrome (AIDS)

AIDS is caused by a virus. The virus attacks the body's immune system. It affects the person's ability to fight other diseases. There is presently no cure for AIDS and no vaccine to prevent the disease. AIDS eventually causes death.

Those at risk for AIDS are:

Homosexual or bisexual men with multiple sex partners

Intravenous drug users

Recent immigrants from Haiti or Central Africa

Sex partners of those who are homosexual, bisexual, intravenous drug users, or immigrants from Haiti or Central Africa

Children born to infected mothers

AIDS is transmitted mainly by blood or sexual contact. According to the Centers for Disease Control (CDC), the AIDS virus has been found in blood, semen, saliva, tears, urine, vaginal secretions, and breast milk. However, the AIDS virus is usually transmitted by contact with infected blood, semen, vaginal secretions, or breast milk.

The virus enters the bloodstream through the rectum, vagina, penis, or mouth. Small breaks in the mucous membrane of the vagina or rectum may occur when the penis, finger, or other objects are inserted. Gum disease can cause breaks in the mucous membrane of the gums. The breaks in the mucous membrane of the mouth, vagina, or rectum provide a route for the virus to enter the bloodstream.

TABLE 25-3 **Common Adult Diseases (Communicable)**

Disease	Signs and Symptoms	Mode of Transmission	Infective Material	Protective Measures
AIDS	Fever, night sweats, weight loss, cough	Sexual contact, blood, needles	Blood, semen, possibly saliva	Gloves, handwashing
Gonorrhea	Discharge from urethra or vagina, lower abdominal pain, fever	Sexual contact	Genital-urinary secretions	Gloves, if in contact with secretions
Hepatitis B	Fever, fatigue, loss of appetite, nausea, headache	Blood, oral secretions, sexual contact	Blood, saliva, semen	Gloves, handwashing
Hepatitis Non A Non B	Fever, headache, fatigue, jaundice	Blood	Blood	Gloves, handwashing
Malaria	Cyclic fever, chills, fever	Blood-mosquito vector	Blood	Handwashing
Mononucleosis	Fever, sore throat, fatigue	Mouth-to-mouth contact	Oral secretions	None
Pneumonia	Fever, cough	Airborne	Sputum	Mask
Syphilis	Genital and cutaneous lesions, nerve degeneration (late)	Sexual contact, blood	Drainage from genital lesions, blood	Gloves, handwashing
Tuberculosis	Fever, night sweats, weight loss, cough	Airborne	Sputum	Mask

*Reprinted and adapted with permission from Heckman James D: *Emergency Care and the Transportation of the Sick and Injured*, ed 4, Park Ridge, Il, 1987, American Academy of Orthopaedic Surgeons, pp 361-362.

Intravenous drug users transmit AIDS through the use of contaminated needles and syringes. The virus is carried in the contaminated blood that is left in the needles or syringes. When needles and syringes are used by others, the contaminated blood enters their bloodstreams.

Infection can also occur when infected body fluids come in contact with open areas on the skin. Babies can become infected during pregnancy or shortly after birth.

Some persons infected with the AIDS virus do not develop the disease for many years. They are carriers of the virus. Therefore they can spread the disease to others.

Some people carry the AIDS virus without showing signs or symptoms of the disease. They may not develop the illness for a long time. The signs and symptoms of AIDS include:

Loss of appetite
Weight loss greater than 10 pounds without reason
Fever
Night sweats
Diarrhea
Tiredness, extreme or constant
Skin rashes
Swollen glands in the neck, underarms, and groin
Dry cough
White spots in the mouth or on the tongue
Purple blotches or bumps on the skin that look like bruises; however, they do not disappear

Persons with AIDS develop other diseases. Their bodies do not have the ability to fight disease. The AIDS virus has damaged the immune system, which fights diseases. The person is at risk for pneumonia, Kaposi's sarcoma (a type of cancer), and central nervous system damage. The person with central nervous system damage may show memory loss, loss of coordination, paralysis, and mental disorders.

You may care for persons with AIDS or for AIDS carriers. You may have contact with the patient's body fluids. Mouth-to-mouth contact is possible during CPR. Certain precautions are necessary to protect yourself and others from the AIDS virus. Universal precautions have been recommended by the CDC (see Chapter 9, page 137). *These precautions apply to all patient contact.* Remember, you may care for a patient who has the AIDS virus but shows no symptoms. You may also care for a patient who has not yet been diagnosed as having AIDS.

Hepatitis

Hepatitis is an inflammatory disease of the liver. There are different types of hepatitis.

Type A (infectious hepatitis) is usually spread by the fecal-oral route. Food, water, or drinking or eating vessels can be contaminated with feces. The virus is ingested when the person eats or drinks contaminated food or water. It can also be ingested when a person eats or drinks from a vessel contaminated with the virus. Causes include poor sanitation, crowded living conditions, poor nutrition, and poor hygiene practices. The disease is more common in children. You must be careful when handling bedpans, feces, and rectal thermometers. Good handwashing is essential for you and the patient.

Type B (serum hepatitis) is usually transmitted by blood and sexual contact. The type B virus is present in blood, saliva, semen, and urine of infected persons. The virus is spread by contaminated blood or blood products and by sharing needles and syringes among IV drug users.

Hepatitis can be mild in severity or can cause death. The signs and symptoms of hepatitis include:

Loss of appetite
Weakness, fatigue, exhaustion
Nausea
Vomiting
Fever
Skin rash
Dark urine
Jaundice (yellowish skin color)
Light-colored stools
Headache
Chills
Abdominal pain

As with the AIDS virus, you must protect yourself and others from the hepatitis virus. Universal precautions are necessary to prevent the spread of hepatitis. Enteric precautions may be ordered (see Chapter 9, page 135).

SUMMARY

A patient may have one or more disorders. For example, a patient may have arthritis, diabetes, heart disease, chronic brain syndrome, and osteoporosis. Problems increase if a fracture occurs. The patient is then at risk for infection, pneumonia, and the complications of bed rest. The amount of care required relates to the nature of the problem and the number of problems a patient has.

Only very basic information was given about each disorder. Entire textbooks have been written on many of these disorders. You are not expected to have an in-depth understanding of your patients' diagnoses. However, the information in this chapter will help you better understand your patients' physical, psychological, and social needs.

REVIEW QUESTIONS

Circle the best *answer.*

1 The spread of cancer to other body parts is
   a A malignant tumor
   b Metastasis
   c Gangrene
   d A benign tumor

2 Which is *not* a warning sign of cancer?
   a Painful, swollen joints
   b A sore that does not heal
   c Unusual bleeding or discharge from a body opening
   d Nagging cough or hoarseness

3 A patient has arthritis. Care does *not* include
   a Measures to prevent contractures
   b Range-of-motion exercises
   c Local cold applications
   d Assistance with activities of daily living

4 Mr. Day's cast needs to dry. Which is *false?*
   a The cast should be covered with blankets or plastic.
   b He is turned as directed so that the cast dries evenly.
   c The entire length of the cast is supported with pillows.
   d The cast is supported by the palms when lifted.

5 A patient has a cast. Which are reported immediately?
   a Pain, numbness, or inability to move the fingers or toes
   b Chills, fever, or nausea and vomiting
   c Odor, cyanosis, or temperature changes of the skin
   d All of the above

6 Mrs. Matthews is in traction. You are assisting in her care. You should do the following *except*
   a Find out if traction is continuous or intermittent
   b Keep the weights off the floor
   c Remove the weights if she is uncomfortable
   d Give skin care at frequent intervals

7 A patient has had a hip pinning. The operated leg is
   a Abducted at all times
   b Adducted at all times
   c Externally rotated at all times
   d Flexed at all times

8 The patient with osteoporosis is at risk for
   a Fractures
   b An amputation
   c Phantom limb pain
   d All of the above

9 A patient has had an amputation. Why will the patient have a psychological adjustment?
   a Activities of daily living are affected.
   b Appearance is affected.
   c The patient's job may be affected
   d All of the above

10 Mr. Smith has had a CVA. Which is *false?*
   a Blood supply to part of his brain was interrupted.
   b Hemiplegia may occur.
   c Aphasia may occur.
   d Changes in brain tissue are progressive.

11 A patient has had a stroke. The nurse tells you to do the following. Which should you question?
   a Elevate the head of the bed to a semi-Fowler's position.
   b Do range-of-motion exercises every 2 hours.
   c Turn, reposition, and give skin care every 2 hours.
   d Keep the bed in the highest horizontal position.

12 A patient has Parkinson's disease. Which is *false?*
   a Parkinson's disease affects part of the brain.
   b The patient's mental function is affected first.
   c Signs and symptoms include stiff muscles, slow movements, and a shuffling gait.
   d The patient needs to be protected from injury.

13 A patient has multiple sclerosis. Which is *false?*
   a Nerve impulses are sent to and from the brain in a normal manner.
   b Symptoms begin in young adulthood.
   c There is no cure.
   d The patient is eventually paralyzed and totally dependent on others for care.

14 Patients with head or spinal cord injuries require
   a Rehabilitation
   b Speech therapy
   c Care in a long-term care facility
   d Psychiatric care

15 A quadriplegic has paralysis
   a Of the legs, arms, and trunk
   b On one side of the body
   c Of the legs
   d Of the legs and trunk

16 You are talking to a person with a hearing loss. You should do the following *except*
   a Speak clearly, distinctly, and slowly
   b Sit or stand where there is good light
   c Shout
   d Stand or sit on the side of the better ear

17 You are talking with a hearing impaired person. You can do the following *except*
   a State the topic of discussion
   b Chew gum while talking
   c Use short sentences and simple words
   d Write out important names and words

18 When eyeglasses are not being worn, they should be
   a Soaked in a cleansing solution
   b Kept within the person's reach
   c Put in the case and in the top drawer of the bedside stand
   d Placed on the overbed table

19 Mrs. Smith is blind. You should
   a Touch her to get her attention
   b Move equipment and furniture to provide for variety and relieve boredom
   c Explain procedures step by step
   d Have her walk in front of you as you guide from behind

20 Glaucoma and cataract result in
   a Decreased mental function
   b Paralysis
   c Loss of vision
   d Breathing difficulties

21 A patient has emphysema. Which is *false?*
   a The patient will have dyspnea only with activity.
   b Cigarette smoking is the most common cause.
   c The patient will probably breathe easier sitting upright and slightly forward.
   d Sputum may contain pus.

22 A patient has pneumonia. Respiratory isolation may be required.
   a True
   b False

23 A patient has hypertension. Which complication can occur?
   a Stroke
   b Heart attack
   c Kidney failure
   d All of the above

24 A patient has hypertension. Treatment will probably include the following *except*
   a No smoking and regular exercise
   b A high-sodium diet
   c A low-calorie diet if the patient is obese
   d Medications to lower the blood pressure

25 A patient has angina pectoris. Which is *true?*
   a Damage to the heart muscle occurs.

   b The pain is described as crushing, stabbing, or squeezing.
   c The pain is relieved with rest and nitroglycerin.
   d All of the above

26 A patient is having a myocardial infarction. You know that
   a The patient is having a heart attack
   b This is an emergency situation
   c The patient may have a cardiac arrest
   d All of the above

27 A patient has CHF. The following measures have been ordered. Which should you question?
   a Force fluids
   b Measure intake and output
   c Measure weight daily
   d Perform range-of-motion exercises

28 Which is not a sign of diabetes mellitus?
   a Increased urine production
   b Weight gain
   c Hunger
   d Increased thirst

29 AIDS and hepatitis require
   a Respiratory precautions
   b Enteric precautions
   c Universal precautions
   d Drainage/secretion precautions

30 AIDS is usually spread by contact with infected
   a Blood
   b Urine
   c Tears
   d Saliva

Answers

30	a	20	c	10	d
29	c	19	c	9	d
28	b	18	c	8	a
27	a	17	b	7	a
26	d	16	c	6	c
25	c	15	a	5	d
24	b	14	a	4	a
23	d	13	a	3	c
22	a	12	b	2	a
21	a	11	d	1	b

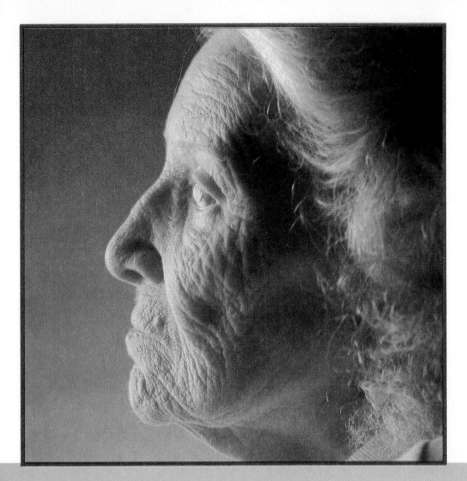

The Dementias

OBJECTIVES

- Define the key terms listed in this chapter
- Describe Alzheimer's disease
- Describe the signs, symptoms, and behaviors associated with Alzheimer's disease
- Explain the care required by persons with Alzheimer's disease
- Describe the effects of Alzheimer's disease on the family
- Explain chronic brain syndrome
- Describe the care required by persons with chronic brain syndrome

KEY TERMS

delusion A false belief
dementia The term used to describe mental disorders caused by changes in the brain
hallucination Seeing, hearing, or feeling something that is not real
sundowning Increased signs, symptoms, and behaviors of Alzheimer's disease during hours of darkness

Changes in the brain occur with aging. Certain diseases can also cause changes in the brain. These changes can affect the person's intellectual function. Intellectual functioning relates to memory, thinking, reasoning, ability to understand, judgment, and behavior. *Dementia* is the term used to describe such mental disorders that are caused by changes in the brain. Dementias are chronic. There is no cure, and they become progressively worse.

ALZHEIMER'S DISEASE

Alzheimer's disease is a brain disease (see the box on p. 417). Brain cells that control intellectual function are damaged. It occurs in both men and women. Though it is more common in the elderly, it also occurs in younger people. Some people in their 40s and 50s have Alzheimer's disease. The cause is unknown.

Stages of Alzheimer's Disease

Three stages of Alzheimer's disease have been described. Signs and symptoms become more severe with each stage. The disease ends in death.

Wandering, sundowning, hallucinations, and delusions also occur. Persons with Alzheimer's disease are disoriented to person, time, and place. They may wander from home and not be able to find their way back. They may be with caregivers one moment and gone the next. Remember, people with Alzheimer's disease have poor judgment and cannot tell what is safe or dangerous. They are in danger of accidents. A person may walk into traffic or into a nearby river or lake. If not properly dressed, they risk exposure in cold climates.

Sundowning occurs in the late afternoon and evening hours. As daylight ends and darkness occurs, confusion, restlessness, and other symptoms increase. The person's behavior is worse after the sun goes down. Sundowning may relate to being tired or hungry. Inadequate light may cause the person to see things that are not there. Like children, persons with Alzheimer's disease may be afraid of the dark.

Senses are dulled. The person may see, hear, or feel things that are not real. A *hallucination* is seeing, hearing, or feeling something that is not really there. People may see animals, insects, or people that are not present. Some hear voices. They may feel bugs crawling on their bodies or feel that they are being touched.

Delusions are false beliefs. People with Alzheimer's disease have thought that they were God, movie stars, or some other person. Some believe they are in jail, are going to be murdered, or are being attacked. A person may believe that the caregiver is actually someone else. Many other false beliefs can occur.

Care of the Person With Alzheimer's Disease

Alzheimer's disease is frustrating to the patient, family, and caregivers. Usually the person is cared for at home until symptoms become severe. Care in a nursing facility is often required. The person may develop other illnesses and need hospital care. Thus you may care for a person with Alzheimer's disease in a hospital, nursing facility, or private home. The person needs your support and understanding. The family does also.

You must remember that people with Alzheimer's disease do not choose to be forgetful, incontinent, agitated, or rude. Nor do they choose to have all of the other behaviors, signs, and symptoms of the disease. They have no control over what is happening to them. The disease causes the behaviors. Thus when a patient does something that a healthy person would not do, remember that the disease is responsible, not the person.

Care of persons with Alzheimer's disease is described in the following box. Such measures will probably be part of the person's care plan.

The Family

The family of the person with Alzheimer's disease has special needs. Caring for the loved one can be exhausting. They need much support and encouragement. Many join Alzheimer's disease support

416

STAGES OF ALZHEIMER'S DISEASE

Stage 1

Memory loss—forgetfulness; forgets recent events

Poor judgment; bad decisions

Disoriented to time

Lack of spontaneity—less outgoing or interested in things

Blames others for mistakes, forgetfulness, and other problems

Moodiness

Stage 2

Restlessness; increases during the evening hours

Sleep disturbances

Memory loss increases—may not recognize family and friends

Dulled senses—cannot tell the difference between hot and cold; cannot recognize dangers

Bowel and bladder incontinence

Needs assistance with activities of daily living—problems bathing, feeding, and dressing self; afraid of bathing; will not change clothes

Loses impulse control—may use foul language, have poor table manners, be sexually aggressive, or be rude

Movement and gait disturbances—walks slowly, has a shuffling gait

Communication problems—cannot follow directions; has problems with reading, writing, and math; speaks in short sentences or single words; statements may not make sense

Repeats motions and statements—may move things back and forth constantly; may say the same thing over and over again

Agitation—behavior may become violent

Stage 3

Seizures (see Chapter 29)

Cannot communicate—may groan, grunt, or scream

Does not recognize self or family members

Totally dependent on others for all activities of daily living

Disoriented to person, time, and place

Totally incontinent of urine and feces

Cannot swallow—choking and aspiration are risks

Sleep disturbances increase

Becomes bed bound—cannot sit or walk

Coma

Death

groups. These groups are sponsored by hospitals, nursing facilities, and the Alzheimer's Association. The Alzheimer's Association has chapters in cities and towns throughout the country. Support groups offer encouragement, advice, and ideas about care. People in similar situations share their feelings, anger, frustration, and other emotions.

The family often feels helpless. No matter what is done for the loved one, the person only gets worse. Much time, money, energy, and emotion are required to care for the person. Anger and resentment may result. The family may then feel guilty because of their anger and resentment. They know that the person did not choose to develop the disease. The family also knows that the person does not choose to have the signs, symptoms, and behaviors of the disease. They may be frustrated and angry that the loved one is no longer able to show love or affection. How would you feel if your mother, father, husband, or wife did not recognize you? Sometimes the person's behavior is embarrassing.

The family has to learn some of the same care measures and procedures that nursing assistants learn. They need to learn how to bathe, feed, dress, and give oral hygiene to the person. They also need to learn how to provide a safe environment. The nurse and support group will help them learn to give necessary care.

CHRONIC BRAIN SYNDROME

Chronic brain syndrome affects the ability to think and understand. Changes in brain cells occur. The changes may be due to decreased blood flow, atrophy, chemicals, infections, poor nutrition, or the aging process. This is common in the elderly.

Signs and symptoms of chronic brain syndrome develop slowly. They may go unnoticed for a long time. Usually the family realizes something is wrong when something drastic happens to the patient. There may be recent memory loss. The person may be unable to remember something that happened yesterday or a few minutes ago. However, events of the distant past are remembered. Disorientation occurs. The person may not know the date, time, or place. The patient may not recognize people or remember names. The ability to concentrate decreases. The person may be unable to follow simple instructions. Judgment is poor. The person may not recognize harmful situations. Attention to personal hygiene decreases.

Reality orientation is important for patients with chronic brain syndrome (see Chapter 7, page 100). The patient may be partially or totally dependent on others for basic needs. Supervision and assistance in activities of daily living are needed. The patient must also be protected from injury.

CARE OF THE PERSON WITH ALZHEIMER'S DISEASE

1 Safety
   a Remove sharp and breakable objects from the environment. This includes knives, scissors, glass, dishes, and razors.
   b Provide plastic eating and drinking utensils. This helps prevent breakage and cuts.
   c Place safety plugs in electrical outlets.
   d Keep cords and electrical equipment out of reach.
   e Childproof caps should be on medicine containers and household cleaners.
   f Store household cleaners and medicines in locked storage areas.
   g Practice safety measures to prevent falls (see Chapter 8, page 112).
   h Practice safety measures to prevent burns (see Chapter 8, page 112).
   i Practice safety measures to prevent poisoning (see Chapter 8, page 113).

2 Wandering
   a Make sure doors and windows are securely locked. Locks are often placed at the top and bottom of doors (Fig. 26-1). The person is not likely to look for a lock at the top or bottom of the door.
   b Make sure door alarms are turned on. The alarm goes off when the door is opened. These are common in nursing facilities.
   c Make sure the person wears an ID bracelet at all times.
   d Exercise the person as ordered. Adequate exercise often reduces wandering.
   e Do not restrain the person. Restraints require a doctor's order. They also tend to increase confusion and disorientation.
   f Do not argue with the person who wants to leave. Remember, the person does not understand what you are saying.
   g Go with the person who insists on going outside. Make sure he or she is properly dressed. Guide the person inside after a few minutes (Fig. 26-2).
   h Let the person wander in enclosed areas if provided. Many nursing facilities have enclosed areas where residents can walk about (Fig. 26-3). These areas provide a safe place for the person to wander.

3 Sundowning
   a Provide a calm, quiet environment late in the day. Treatments and activities should be done early in the day.
   b Do not restrain the person.
   c Encourage exercise and activity early in the day.
   d Make sure the person has eaten. Hunger can increase the person's restlessness.
   e Promote urinary and bowel elimination. A full bladder or constipation can increase restlessness.
   f Do not try to reason with the person. Remember, he or she cannot understand what you are saying.
   g Do not ask the person to tell you what is bothering him or her. The person's ability to communicate is impaired. He or she does not understand what you are asking. The person cannot think or speak clearly.

4 Hallucinations and delusions
   a Do not argue with the person. He or she does not understand what you are saying.
   b Reassure the person. Tell him or her that you will provide protection from harm.
   c Distract the person with some item or activity.
   d Use touch to calm and reassure the person (Fig. 26-4).

5 Comfort, rest, and sleep
   a Provide good skin care. Make sure the person's skin is free of urine and feces.
   b Promote urinary and bowel elimination (see Chapters 14 and 15).
   c Promote exercise and activity during the day. This helps reduce wandering and sundowning behaviors. The person may also sleep better.
   d Reduce the person's intake of coffee, tea, and cola drinks. These contain caffeine. Caffeine is a stimulant. The person's restlessness, confusion, and agitation can increase because of caffeine.
   e Provide a quiet, restful environment. Soft music is better in the evening than loud television programs.
   f Promote personal hygiene. Do not force the person into a shower or tub. People with Alzheimer's disease are often afraid of bathing. Try bathing the person when he or she is calm.
   g Provide oral hygiene.
   h Have equipment ready for any procedure ahead of time. This reduces the amount of time the person has to be involved in care measures.

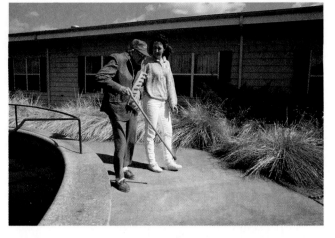

Fig. 26-2 The nursing assistant walks outside with the person who wanders. He is guided back into the facility.

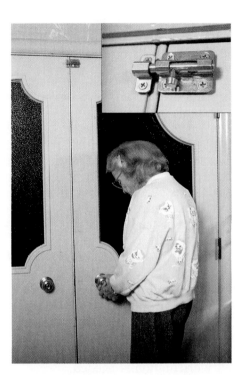

Fig. 26-1 A slide lock is at the top of the door. The person tries to open the lock on the knob.

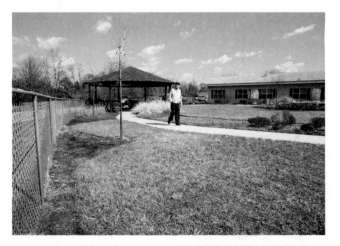

Fig. 26-3 An enclosed garden allows persons with Alzheimer's disease to wander in a safe environment.

SUMMARY

Dementia affects a person's ability to think, reason, and understand. Memory, judgment, and behavior are also affected. Therefore dementia affects the ability to meet basic needs. Physical, safety, love and belonging, esteem, and self-actualization needs are all affected.

Persons with dementia do not choose to be forgetful, to wander, or to have poor manners. The disease is responsible for their behaviors. As frustrating as their behaviors may be, you must remember that they have no control over their actions.

The patient and family need much encouragement and emotional support. Required care can be physically, emotionally, and financially draining. There are no cures. However, a kind, caring nursing assistant can be comforting.

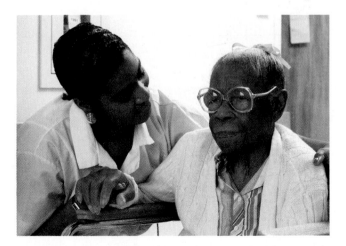

Fig. 26-4 The nursing assistant uses touch to calm a person with Alzheimer's disease.

REVIEW QUESTIONS

Circle the best *answer.*

1 Dementia describes
   a A false belief
   b Mental disorders caused by changes in the brain
   c Seeing, hearing, or feeling something that is not real
   d Alzheimer's disease

2 These statements are about Alzheimer's disease. Which is *true?*
   a It occurs only in the elderly.
   b Diet and medications can control the disease.
   c It is the same as chronic brain syndrome.
   d The disease ends in death.

3 Persons with Alzheimer's disease
   a Have memory loss, poor judgment, and sleep disturbances
   b Lose impulse control and the ability to communicate
   c May wander or have delusions and hallucinations
   d All of the above

4 Sundowning means that
   a The person becomes sleepy when the sun sets
   b Behaviors become worse in the late afternoon and evening hours
   c Behavior improves at night
   d The person is in the third stage of the disease

5 Alzheimer's disease support groups do the following *except*
   a Provide care
   b Offer encouragement and care ideas
   c Provide support for the family
   d Promote the sharing of feelings and frustrations

6 A person with Alzheimer's disease tends to wander. You should
   a Make sure doors and windows are locked
   b Make sure the person wears an ID bracelet
   c Exercise the person as ordered
   d All of the above

7 A person has Alzheimer's disease. Which is *false?*
   a Safety plugs should be placed in electrical outlets.
   b Cleaners and medications should be out of the person's reach.
   c The person can keep smoking materials.
   d Sharp and breakable objects are removed from the person's environment.

8 A person has Alzheimer's disease. Which is *false?*
   a It is possible to reason with the person.
   b Touch can calm and reassure the person.
   c A calm, quiet environment is important.
   d Assistance is needed with ADL.

9 Chronic brain syndrome
   a Is common in the elderly
   b Develops slowly
   c May be caused by decreased blood flow to the brain
   d All of the above

10 A person has chronic brain syndrome. Which is *false?*
   a Memory is not affected.
   b Concentration decreases.
   c Reality orientation is needed.
   d Supervision of ADL is needed.

Answers

10	a	5	a
9	d	4	b
8	a	3	d
7	c	2	d
6	d	1	b

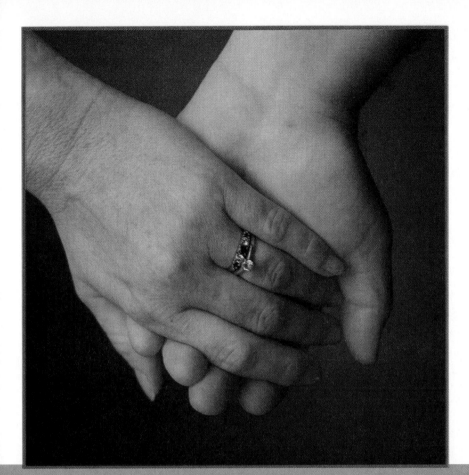

Sexuality

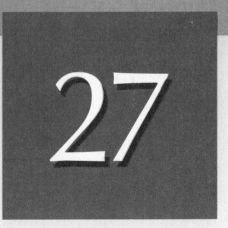

OBJECTIVES

- Define the key terms listed in this chapter
- Describe the differences between sex and sexuality
- Explain the importance of sexuality throughout life
- Describe five types of sexual relationships
- Explain how injury and illness can affect sexuality
- Identify the illnesses, injuries, and surgeries that often affect sexuality
- Explain how aging affects sexuality in the elderly
- Explain how the nursing team can promote a patient's sexuality
- List the reasons patients may become sexually aggressive
- Identify the ways you can deal with a sexually aggressive patient
- Explain how sexually transmitted diseases are spread
- Describe the common sexually transmitted diseases

bisexual   A person who is attracted to people of both sexes

heterosexual   A person who is attracted to individuals of the opposite sex

homosexual   A person who has a strong attraction to members of the same sex

impotence   The inability of the male to have an erection

menopause   The time when menstruation stops; it marks the end of the woman's reproductive years

sex   The physical activities involving the organs of reproduction; the activities are done for pleasure or to produce children

sexuality   That which relates to one's sex; those physical, psychological, social, cultural, and spiritual factors that affect a person's feelings and attitudes about his or her sex

transsexual   An individual who believes that he or she is really a member of the opposite sex

transvestite   An individual who becomes sexually excited by dressing in the clothes of the opposite sex

In the past, patients were viewed as having only physical problems. Therefore physical needs were the first and often the only concern. Little attention was given to the psychological or social effect of a disorder. The needs of love and belonging, esteem, and self-actualization were overlooked. Now attention is given to the total person. Physical, psychological, social, and spiritual aspects of the person are considered.

There is another part of the person that involves the physical, psychological, social, and the spiritual. That part is sexuality. The effect of illness and injury on a person's sexuality is now recognized. This chapter describes the effects of illness, injury, and aging on sexuality. A review of the reproductive system in Chapter 5 and growth and development in Chapter 6 will be helpful before studying this chapter.

SEX AND SEXUALITY

Sex and sexuality are different. *Sex* is the physical activities involving the reproductive organs. The activities are done for pleasure or to produce children. *Sexuality* involves the whole personality and the body. A person's attitudes and feelings are involved. Besides physical and psychological factors, sexuality is influenced by social, cultural, and spiritual factors. The way a person behaves, thinks, dresses, and responds to others is related to his or her sexuality.

Sexuality is present from birth. When the baby's sex is identified, a boy or girl name is given. Blue is used for boys, and pink is for girls. Toys reflect sexuality. Dolls are traditionally for girls. Trains and baseball bats are appropriate for boys. By 2 years of age, children know their own sex. A 3-year-old knows the sex of other children. Children learn male and female roles. They learn what boys or girls are to do from their parents (Fig. 27-1). Children learn early that there are certain behaviors for boys and certain ones for girls.

As children grow older, their interest about the human body and how it works increases. Body changes during adolescence bring a greater interest and curiosity about sex and the body. Adolescent boys usually feel a great need to have sex. Girls are usually less concerned about having sex and more concerned about their reputation.

Sexual activity is common in young adulthood. Sex takes on more meaning as young adults mature. Attitudes and feelings are important. Decisions about sexuality become increasingly important. Some decisions relate to selecting a sexual partner, having sex before marriage, and using birth control.

Sexuality continues to be important into adulthood and old age. Attitudes and the need for sex change as a person grows older. Life circumstances change. Changes may include divorce, death of a spouse, injury, and illness.

SEXUAL RELATIONSHIPS

Sex and sexuality usually imply that one partner is male and the other female. Most people are heterosexual. A *heterosexual* is a person who is attracted to people of the opposite sex. Sexual activities involve a member of the opposite sex. However, you may care for people who are not heterosexual.

A *homosexual* is attracted to members of the same sex. The person has sexual relationships and is aroused by a member of the same sex. Men are attracted to men, and women are attracted to women. The word "gay" is often used in reference to a homosexual. A female homosexual is called a "lesbian."

Homosexuality has existed for centuries. Since the 1960s and 1970s it has become more apparent in society. Before, it was hidden. Now many homosexuals are more open about their sexual preference and relationships.

Some people, *bisexuals*, are attracted to both sexes. They can be aroused and excited by men or women. Their pattern of sexual activity varies. Sometimes they are strictly heterosexual. At other times they are homosexual. Some alternate between homosexual and

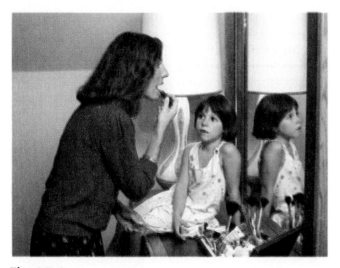

Fig. 27-1 This little girl is learning female roles from her mother.

heterosexual relationships. Bisexuals are often married and have children. They may seek a homosexual relationship or experience outside of marriage.

Some people believe that they are really members of the opposite sex. These people are *transsexuals*. A male believes he is really a woman in a man's body. A woman believes she is really a man in a woman's body. Transsexuals often describe feelings of being "trapped" in the wrong body. Most transsexuals have had these feelings for as long as they can remember. As children they usually show tendencies and interests of the opposite sex. Many transsexuals undergo psychiatric treatment. Some have sex-change operations. Neither psychiatric treatment nor sex-change operations have been very effective in helping these people.

Transvestites become sexually excited by dressing in clothes appropriate to the opposite sex. Most are male. They are usually married and heterosexual. They dress normally as men most of the time. Dressing as a woman is usually done in private. Some dress completely as women. Others focus on bras and panties. The wife may not know about the practice. Some wives know that their husbands are transvestites. If the wife agrees, she may be included in the transvestite's activities. Some transvestites have same-sex friends with similar interests.

INJURY AND ILLNESS

Sexuality and sex involve the mind and body. Injury and illness can affect the way the body works. The mind can also be affected. A person may feel unclean, unwhole, unattractive, or mutilated after disfiguring surgery. Attitudes about sex may change. The person may feel unattractive or incapable of being loved. These feelings affect the person's ability to be close and intimate. Therefore the person may develop sex-

ual problems that are psychological in nature. Time, understanding, and a caring partner are very helpful. Some people need counseling or psychiatric assistance.

Many illnesses, injuries, and surgeries cause changes in the nervous, circulatory, and reproductive systems. If one or more of these systems are affected, the patient may experience changes in sexual ability. Most chronic illnesses affect sexual functioning.

Impotence may occur. Impotence is the inability of the male to have an erection. Diabetes mellitus, spinal cord injuries, multiple sclerosis, and alcoholism are common causes. Circulatory disorders and medications can affect the male's ability to achieve an erection. Medications to control blood pressure often have impotence as a side effect.

Heart disease, stroke, chronic obstructive pulmonary disease, and nervous system disorders may also affect the ability to have sex. Surgeries done on the reproductive organs may have physical and psychological effects. Removal of the prostate or the testes affects a man's ability to achieve an erection. Removal of the uterus, ovaries, or a breast may affect a woman psychologically. A colostomy or ileostomy may psychologically affect both men and women.

You will care for patients with disorders that can affect sexual functioning. Changes in sexual functioning have a great impact on the patient. Fear, anger, worry, and depression often occur. These are evident in the patient's behavior and comments. You need to understand that the patient's feelings are very normal and are expected.

SEXUALITY AND THE ELDERLY

Many people think that sex, love, and intimacy are for the young. Young people fall in love, hold hands, embrace, and have sex. Older people are not supposed to need sex, love, and affection. There is also the idea that older people are not capable of sexual activities. Fortunately these ideas are untrue. Sexual relationships are psychologically and physically important to the elderly (Fig. 27-2).

Love, affection, and intimacy are needed throughout life. As the elderly person experiences other losses, feeling close to another human becomes more important. Children leave home. Friends and relatives die. Loss of the job occurs because of retirement. Health problems may develop. These losses may be compounded by a decrease in physical strength and changes in appearance.

Reproductive organs change during the aging process. However, the changes do not eliminate sexual needs or abilities. Changes in men are related to decreases of the male hormone testosterone. The hormone affects strength, sperm production, and the reproductive tissues. These changes affect sexual activity. It takes longer for an erection to occur. The

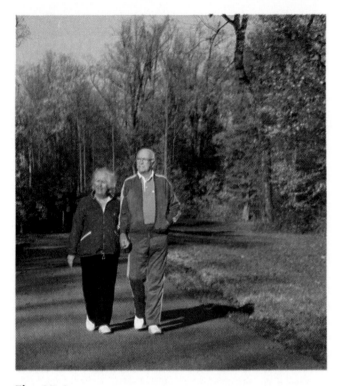

Fig. 27-2 Love and affection are important to the elderly.

phase between erection and orgasm is also longer. Orgasm is less forceful than in the younger years. After orgasm, the erection is lost quickly. The time between erections is also longer. Older men may need stimulation of the penis to become sexually excited. Younger men can become sexually excited by just thinking about sex or a sexual partner.

Elderly men usually experience decreased frequency in sexual activity. Decreased frequency can result from the physical changes just described. Other reasons include boredom with the sexual partner, mental and physical fatigue, overeating, and excessive drinking. A man may fear that he will be unable to perform. Therefore sexual activity is avoided. Pain and reduced mobility from illness and aging can affect frequency. One or both partners may have a chronic illness. The illness may result in decreased frequency or the complete absence of sexual activity.

Physical changes also occur in women. *Menopause* occurs around 50 years of age. Menopause is when a woman stops menstruating. It marks the end of her reproductive years. A related change is the decreased secretion of the female hormones (estrogen and progesterone). Reduced hormone levels affect reproductive tissues. The uterus, vagina, and external genitalia atrophy. The vagina can still receive the penis during intercourse. However, intercourse may be uncomfortable or painful. Pain and discomfort are due to thinning of the vaginal walls and vaginal dryness. Like elderly men, older women have changes in sexual excitement. It takes longer to become sexually

excited. The time between excitement and orgasm is longer. Orgasm is less intense, and the woman returns to a pre-excitement state more quickly.

Most elderly women experience decreased frequency of sexual activity. Reasons relate to weakness, mental and physical fatigue, pain, and reduced mobility. These may be due to the normal aging process or chronic illness.

Some elderly people do not have sexual intercourse. This does not mean that they do not have sexual needs or desires. Their needs may be expressed in other ways. Handholding, touching, caressing, and embracing are ways of expressing closeness and intimacy.

Having a sexual partner is also important. Death and divorce result in loss of a sexual partner. The partner may also be in a hospital or nursing facility. These situations are seen in adults of all ages.

MEETING THE PATIENT'S SEXUAL NEEDS

Sexuality is part of the total person. Illness or injury does not mean that sexuality is unimportant. Some patients are so ill that sexual activity is impossible. Others may want and be able to have sexual activity with their partners. Sexual activity does not always imply intercourse. It may be expressed in other ways. Nursing personnel used to discourage any form of sexual expression, especially among the elderly. Hand holding was okay. But two people were not to get any closer! The importance of sexuality in health and illness is now recognized. The nursing team has an important role in allowing patients and residents to meet their sexual needs. The following measures are appreciated by patients and residents. They are carried out in cooperation with the nurse supervising your work.

1. Allow the person to practice his or her grooming routines. This includes applying makeup, nail polish, and body lotion, and wearing cologne. Hair care and shaving are also important. Women may want to shave their legs and underarms and pluck their eyebrows. Men may wish to use after-shave lotion. The person may need help with these activities.
2. Let the person choose clothing. Hospital gowns are embarrassing to both men and women. Street clothes may be worn if the person's condition permits.
3. Avoid exposing the patient. Care and procedures are performed so that the patient is not exposed unnecessarily. The patient must be draped and screened appropriately.
4. Accept the person's sexual relationships. The person may not share your sexual attitudes, values, or practices. You cannot expect the person to behave according to your standards. The person may have a homosexual, pre-marital, or ex-

tra-marital relationship. There may be more than one sexual partner. Do not make judgments or gossip about relationships.

5. Allow privacy. You can usually tell when two people want to be alone. If the patient has a private room, close the door for privacy. Some facilities have "do not disturb" signs for doors. Let the patient and partner know how much time they can expect to have alone. For example, you can remind them when to expect a meal tray, medications, or a treatment. This gives them an idea of when to expect someone. Knocking before you enter any room is a common courtesy. It shows respect for privacy. Other staff members should be told that the patient wants some time alone. Other measures are necessary if there is a roommate. Consideration must be given to the roommate. The curtain between the two beds provides little privacy. Privacy can be arranged when the roommate is out of the room. Sometimes roommates volunteer to leave for a while when they sense that couples need time alone. If the roommate cannot leave, other areas on the nursing unit can be found for privacy.

6. Allow elderly individuals their right to be sexual. The measures described previously apply to the elderly and other age-groups.

7. Allow couples in nursing facilities to share the same room. This is now an OBRA requirement. The couple should not be separated. They may have lived together for years. Being in a nursing facility is no reason to separate them in male and female rooms. They should be allowed to share the same bed if their conditions permit. A double, queen-, or king-size bed may be provided by the facility or by the couple.

8. Allow single elderly people to develop new relationships. Death and divorce result in loss of a sexual partner. A widowed or divorced resident may develop a relationship with another resident. Instead of trying to keep them separated, measures should be taken to allow them time together (Fig. 27-3).

THE SEXUALLY AGGRESSIVE PATIENT

Some patients try to have their sexual needs met by health workers. They may flirt, make sexual advances or comments, expose themselves, or touch workers. Health workers usually become angry or embarrassed. These reactions are normal. Often there are reasons for the patient's behavior. Understanding this may help you to deal with the situation.

Illness, injury, surgery, or aging may threaten the male's sense of manhood. He may try to reassure or prove to himself that he is still attractive and capable of performing sexually. He may do so by behaving sexually toward health workers.

Some sexually aggressive behaviors are due to confusion or disorientation. Nervous system disorders, medications, fever, dementia, and poor vision are common causes of confusion and disorientation. The patient may confuse a worker with his or her sexual partner. The patient may be unable to control behavior because of changes in mental function. Normally the person would be able to control urges toward a worker. However, changes in the brain can make control difficult. Sexual behavior in these situations is usually innocent on the person's part.

Some patients do touch workers inappropriately. Their purpose is sexual. However, sometimes touch is the only way the patient can get the worker's attention. Consider the following situation. Mr. Green is a stroke patient. He is paralyzed on one side of his body and cannot speak. You have your back to him and are bending over. Your buttocks are the closest part of your body to him. To get your attention, he touches your buttocks. You should not consider his behavior to be sexual in this situation.

Sexual advances may be intentional. You need to deal with the situation in a professional manner. However, there is no ideal way to deal with the advances. The following suggestions may be helpful.

1. Discuss the situation with the nurse. The nurse can help you deal with or understand the person's behavior.
2. Ask the patient not to touch you in places where you were touched.
3. Explain to the patient that you have no intention of doing what he or she suggests.
4. Explain to the patient that his or her behavior makes you uncomfortable. Then politely ask the patient not to act in that way.
5. Allow privacy if the patient is becoming sexually aroused. Provide for safety (raise side rails, place the signal light within reach, etc.), and tell the person when you will return.

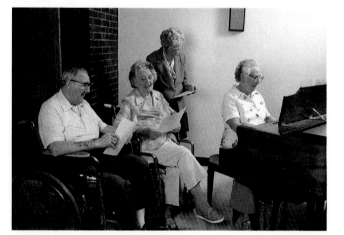

Fig. 27-3 Intimate relationships occur in nursing facilities.

TABLE 27-1   **Sexually Transmitted Diseases**

Disease	Signs and Symptoms	Treatment
Genital herpes	Painful, fluid-filled sores on or near the genitalia (Fig. 27-5) The sores may have a watery discharge Itching, burning, and tingling in the genital area Fever Swollen glands	No known cure Medications can be given to control discomfort
Venereal warts	Male—Warts appear on the penis, anus, or genitalia Female—Warts appear near the vagina, cervix, and labia	Application of special ointment that causes the warts to dry up and fall off Surgical removal may be necessary if the ointment is not effective
AIDS (Acquired Immunodeficiency Syndrome)	Seen most commonly in homosexual men, IV drug users, and those who have received contaminated blood prior to blood-screening procedures The patient is unable to fight off certain infections and cancers Death eventually occurs	No known treatment at this time
Gonorrhea	Burning on urination Urinary frequency and urgency Vaginal discharge in the female Urethral discharge in the male	Antibiotic medications
Syphilis	*Stage 1:* 10-90 days after exposure Painless chancre on the penis, in the vagina, or on genitalia (Fig. 27-4); the chancre may also be on the lips or inside of the mouth, or anywhere else on the body *Stage 2:* about two months after the chancre General fatigue, loss of appetite, nausea, fever, headache, rash, sore throat, bone and joint pain, hair loss, lesions on the lips and genitalia *Stage 3:* 3 to 15 years after infection Damage to the cardiovascular system and central nervous system, blindness	Antibiotic medications

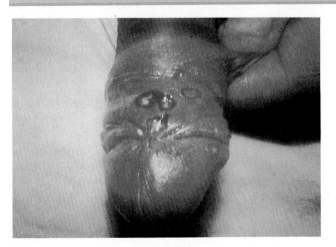

Fig. 27-4   Chancre caused by syphilis.

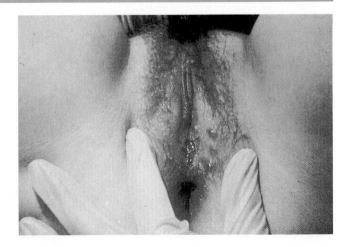

Fig. 27-5   Genital herpes sore.

SEXUALLY TRANSMITTED DISEASES

Some diseases are spread by sexual contact. They are grouped under the heading of sexually transmitted diseases (STDs) (see Table 27-1). Some people do not know that they have been infected. Others know but do not seek treatment. Embarrassment is a common reason for not seeking treatment.

The genital area is usually associated with STDs. However, other body areas may be involved. These areas include the rectum, ears, mouth, nipples, throat, tongue, eyes, and nose. Most STDs are spread by sexual contact. The use of condoms helps prevent the spread of STDs. Some are also spread through a break in the skin, by contact with infected body fluids (blood, sperm, saliva), or by contaminated blood or needles.

Infection precautions are necessary. Handwashing before and after patient care is essential.

SUMMARY

Sexuality is part of the total person. Ill or injured persons still need love, affection, and closeness with other people. Health workers should promote, not discourage, a patient's sexual expression. This is especially true for the elderly.

Illness, injury, and surgery may affect a person's sexuality. The problem may be temporary or permanent. Reproductive organs, the circulatory system, or the nervous system may be affected. Consequently, the patient may have problems in sexual performance. Some injuries and surgeries are disfiguring. Patients may feel unclean and unattractive to others. Their sexuality and sexual performance may be affected psychologically. Persons who have physical or psychological changes in sexuality need understanding and caring. You must try to understand the patient's situation. How would you feel if you had the patient's problem?

REVIEW QUESTIONS

Circle the best *answer.*

1 Sex involves
  a The organs of reproduction
  b Attitudes and feelings
  c Cultural and spiritual factors
  d All of the above

2 Sexuality is important to
  a Small children
  b Teenagers and young adults
  c Middle-aged adults
  d Persons of all ages

3 A person attracted to members of the opposite sex is a
  a Heterosexual
  b Homosexual
  c Bisexual
  d Transsexual

4 Either illness or injury can result in impotence. Impotence is
  a When menstruation stops
  b A psychological reaction to disfigurement
  c The inability of the male to achieve an erection
  d The complete absence of sexual activity

5 Reproductive organs change with aging. These changes make sexual activity difficult or impossible.
  a True
  b False

6 Which will *not* promote sexuality?
  a Allowing normal grooming routines
  b Having the person wear a hospital gown
  c Allowing the patient and his or her partner privacy
  d Accepting the patient's relationships

7 An elderly lady and an elderly gentleman seem to be developing a relationship. They live in a nursing facility. Nursing personnel should keep them separated.
  a True
  b False

8 Mr. Gibson requests time alone with his wife. The nurse tells you this is okay. You should
  a Close the door to the room
  b Put a "do not disturb" sign on the door
  c Tell them how long they can expect to be left undisturbed
  d All of the above

9 A married couple has been admitted to a nursing facility. They should be assigned to separate rooms.
  a True
  b False

10 Mr. Robinson is being sexually aggressive. The behavior may be
  a An attempt to prove he is still attractive and able to perform sexually
  b Due to confusion or disorientation

   c Done on purpose

   d All of the above

11 Mr. Robinson has made sexual advances to you. You should do the following *except*

   a Discuss the situation with the nurse

   b Do what the patient asks

   c Explain to the patient that his behavior makes you uncomfortable

   d Ask the patient not to touch you in places where you were touched

12 Which statement is *false?*

   a STDs are usually spread by sexual contact.

   b STDs can affect the genital area and other parts of the body.

   c Signs and symptoms of STDs are always obvious.

   d Some STDs result in death.

Answers

12	c	8	d	4	c
11	b	7	b	3	a
10	d	6	b	2	d
9	b	5	b	1	a

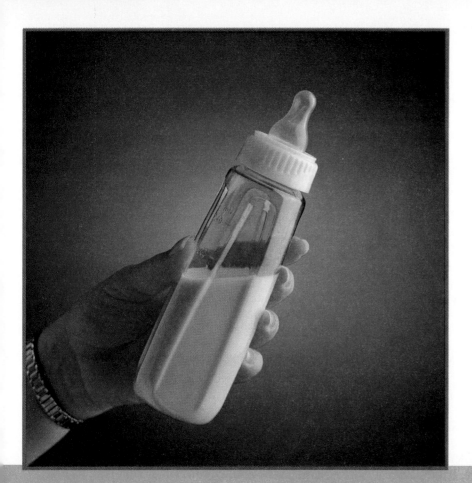

Caring for Mothers and Newborns

OBJECTIVES

- Describe how to meet an infant's safety and security needs
- Identify the signs and symptoms of illness in infants
- Explain how to help mothers with breast-feeding
- Describe three forms of baby formulas
- Explain how to bottle-feed babies
- Explain how to burp a baby
- Describe how to give cord care
- Describe the purposes of circumcision, the necessary observations, and the required care
- Identify planning, safety, temperature, and other factors related to bathing infants
- Perform the procedures described in this chapter

circumcision   The surgical removal of foreskin
rooting reflex   The baby turns his or her head in the direction of a stimulus
umbilical cord   The structure that carries blood, oxygen, and nutrients from the mother to the fetus

You may care for new mothers, infants, and children. New mothers and newborns are cared for in hospital maternity departments. Pediatric units are for infants and children. A mother or newborn may need home care.

Home care may be needed for many reasons. A mother may need help because of complications before or after childbirth. There may be other young children. A new baby and other children may be a lot of work. Sometimes mothers simply need help with home maintenance.

A review of growth and development will help you care for babies and children (see Chapter 6, page 79). Babies are helpless. They depend on others to meet their basic needs. Besides physical needs, babies also need to feel safe, secure, and loved, and that they belong. You can help meet the baby's basic needs.

INFANT SAFETY

Babies cannot protect themselves. Like adults, babies need safety and security. They feel secure when they are warm and when wrapped and held snugly. Responding to their cries and feeding them when they are hungry promote safety and security. Infant safety is discussed in Chapter 8. The following measures are also important in hospitals or home care.

1. Keep the baby warm. Room temperature should be 70° to 75° F during the day and 60° to 65° F at night. Check windows for drafts. Make sure windows are securely closed.
2. Keep your fingernails short. Do not wear rings or bracelets. Long nails and jewelry can scratch the baby.
3. Use both hands to lift a newborn.
4. Hold the baby securely. Use the cradle hold, football hold, or shoulder hold (Fig. 28-1).
5. Support the baby's head and neck when lifting or holding the baby (see Fig. 28-1). Neck support is necessary for the first 3 months after birth.
6. Handle the baby with gentle, smooth movements. Avoid sudden or jerking movements. Do not startle the baby.
7. Hold and cuddle infants. This is comforting and helps them learn to feel love and security.

8. Talk, sing, or play with the baby often. Be sure to talk to the baby during the bath, dressing, and diapering.
9. Respond to the baby's crying. Babies cry when they are hungry, uncomfortable, wet, frightened, or when they want attention. This is their way of communicating. Responding to their cry helps them feel safe and secure.
10. Do not leave a baby unattended on a table, bed, sofa, or other high surface. Keep one hand on the baby if you must look away (see Fig. 8-2, page 111).
11. Use safety straps for babies in infant seats or high chairs.
12. Make sure the crib is within hearing distance of the caregivers.
13. Keep crib rails up at all times.
14. Do not put a pillow in the crib. Pillows can cause suffocation.
15. Change the baby's position often. Do not always put the baby in the same position. Alternate between the prone and side-lying positions. Support the baby in the side-lying position with a rolled towel or small blanket (Fig. 28-2).
16. Do not lay babies on their backs after a feeding or for sleep. Aspiration can occur in the supine position.
17. Keep pins and small objects out of the baby's reach.

SIGNS AND SYMPTOMS OF ILLNESS

Your observations are important for the infant's safety. Signs and symptoms of illness can develop quickly in babies. Therefore you must tell the nurse if the baby cries continually or looks sick. You should tell the nurse immediately if the baby:

Is flushed, pale or perspiring
Has noisy, rapid, difficult, or slow respirations
Is coughing or sneezing
Has reddened or irritated eyes
Turns his or her head to one side or puts a hand to one ear (signs of an earache)
Is crying or screaming for a long time
Has skipped feedings
Has vomited most of the feeding or between feedings
Has hard, formed stools or watery stools
Has a rash

You may be asked for more information. You must be sure to tell your supervisor when a sign or symptom began. You may also be asked to take an infant's or child's temperature, pulse, and respirations (see Chapter 17). Rectal or axillary temperatures are taken

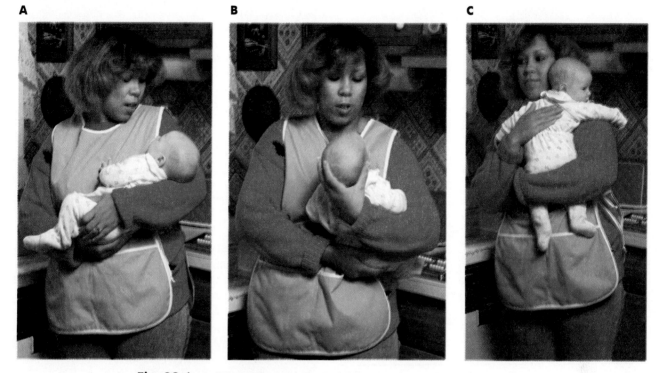

Fig. 28-1 **A,** The cradle hold. **B,** The football hold. **C,** The shoulder hold.

on children younger than 5 years of age. You should ask the nurse which method to use for the child. Apical pulses are taken on infants and young children.

HELPING MOTHERS BREAST-FEED

Many mothers breast-feed their babies. Breast-fed babies may need to nurse every 2 or 3 hours. They are fed on demand. In other words, they are fed when hungry rather than on a schedule. Babies nurse for a short time (5 minutes at each breast) at first. Even-

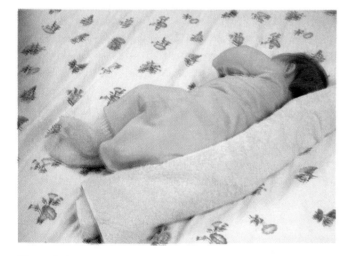

Fig. 28-2 The baby is supported in the side-lying position with a rolled towel.

tually, total nursing time may be 20 to 30 minutes.

Nurses will help mothers learn to breast-feed. They also teach breast care. Mothers and babies learn how to nurse in a very short time. If the mother or baby is having problems nursing, you should call the nurse.

The mother may need help getting ready to breast-feed. She may need help with hygiene. You may need to bring the baby to her. You must give help as necessary. Otherwise, you should make sure the signal light is within reach and leave the room. The mother and baby need privacy during breast-feeding. You must be sure to stay within hearing distance in case the mother needs help.

You can do the following to help with breast-feeding.

1. Help the mother wash her hands. Handwashing is necessary before she handles her breasts.
2. Help the mother wash her nipples. Nipples are washed with circular motions from the nipple outward to the breast (Fig. 28-3). Plain water is used. Soap has a drying effect. The nipples can dry and crack.
3. Help the mother to a comfortable position. She may want to sit up in bed or in a chair. Some mothers like to nurse in the side-lying position (Fig. 28-4).
4. Change the baby's diaper if necessary. Bring the baby to the mother.
5. Make sure the mother holds the baby close to her breast.

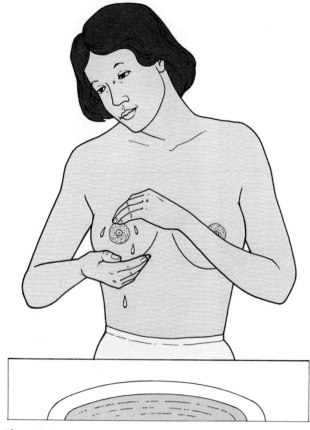

Fig. 28-3 The breast is washed from the nipple outward. Circular motions are used.

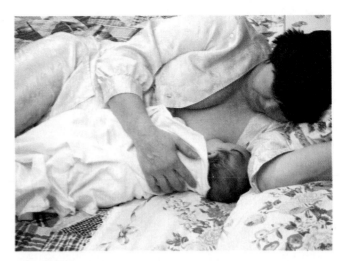

Fig. 28-4 A mother nursing in the side-lying position.

6. Have the mother stroke the baby's cheek closest to the breast (Fig. 28-5). This stimulates the *rooting reflex*. The baby turns his or her head toward the stimulus. If the right cheek is stroked, the baby turns his or her head to the right.

7. Have the mother keep breast tissue away from the baby's nose with her thumb (Fig. 28-6).

8. Give her a baby blanket to cover the baby and her breast. This promotes privacy during the feeding.

9. Encourage nursing from both breasts at each feeding. If the baby finished the last feeding at the right breast, the baby begins the next feeding at the right breast.

10. Remind her how to remove the baby from the breast. She needs to break the seal or suction between the baby and the breast. Ask her to insert a finger into a corner of the baby's mouth (Fig. 28-7). She can also press a finger down on her breast close to the baby's mouth.

11. Help the mother burp the baby if necessary (see page 436). The baby should be burped after nursing at each breast.

12. Have the mother put a diaper pin on the bra strap of the breast last used. This reminds her which breast to use first at the next feeding.

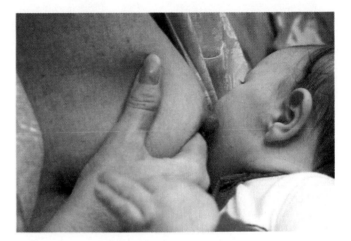

Fig. 28-5 The mother strokes the baby's cheek with her breast. This stimulates the rooting reflex.

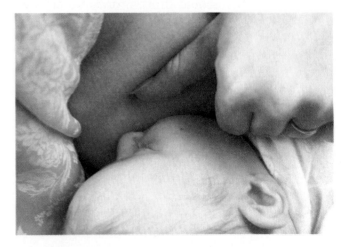

Fig. 28-6 The thumb is used to keep breast tissue away from the baby's nose.

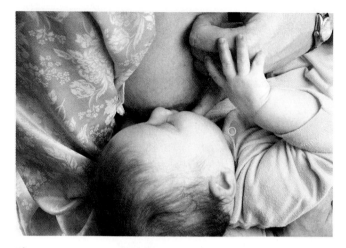

Fig. 28-7 The mother inserts a finger in the baby's mouth to remove the baby from the breast.

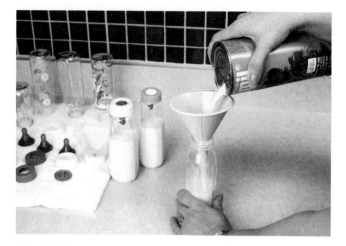

Fig. 28-8 Ready-to-feed formula is poured from the can into the bottle. A funnel is used to prevent spilling.

13. Change the baby's diaper after the feeding. Lay the baby in the crib if he or she has fallen asleep.
14. Encourage the mother to wear a nursing bra day and night. The bra supports the breasts and promotes comfort.
15. Encourage the mother to place cotton pads in the bra. The pads absorb leaking milk.
16. Have the mother apply cream (if prescribed) to her nipples after each feeding. The cream prevents nipples from drying and cracking.
17. Help the mother straighten clothing after the feeding if necessary.

The nursing mother needs good nutrition. If you are providing home care, you may need to plan meals and grocery shop (see Chapter 31). You must remember the following when planning meals or grocery shopping.

1. Calorie intake may be increased. Your supervisor will tell you how much to increase the mother's calorie intake.
2. The mother should drink 6 or more cups of milk a day. She can drink skim or whole milk.
3. Include foods high in calcium in the diet.
4. The mother should avoid spicy and gas-forming foods. They can cause cramping and diarrhea in the infant. She should avoid onions, garlic, spices, cabbage, brussel sprouts, asparagus, and beans. Chocolate, cola beverages, and coffee can also cause cramping and diarrhea.

BOTTLE-FEEDING BABIES

Formula is given to babies who are not breast-fed. The formula is prescribed by the doctor. Formula is commercially prepared. It provides the essential nutrients needed by the infant.

Formula comes in three forms. The *ready-to-feed* form is ready to use. It can be poured directly from the can into the baby bottle (Fig. 28-8). Water is added to *powdered* and *concentrated* formula. Container directions tell how much formula to use and how much water to add. Bottles can be prepared one at a time, or enough can be prepared for the whole day. Extra bottles are capped as in Figure 28-9 and stored in the refrigerator. These bottles should be used within 24 hours.

Babies must be protected from infection. Therefore baby bottles, caps, and nipples must be as clean as possible. Disposable equipment is used in hospitals. Reusable equipment may be used in homes. Reusable bottle-feeding equipment must be carefully washed in hot, soapy water. Complete rinsing is necessary to remove all soap. Some doctors tell mothers to sterilize bottle-feeding equipment. *Sterilization* is the process of killing all microorganisms (pathogens and nonpathogens). Some mothers like to use plastic nursers (Fig. 28-10). Plastic nursers do not have to be sterilized.

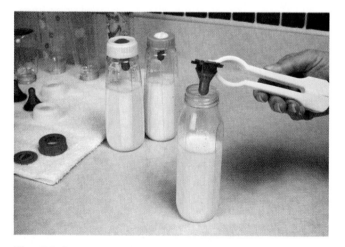

Fig. 28-9 Bottles are capped for storage in the refrigerator.

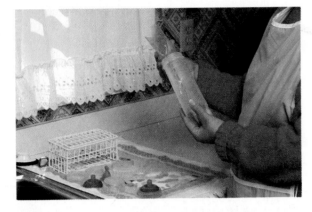

Fig. 28-10 Plastic nursers have disposable liners.

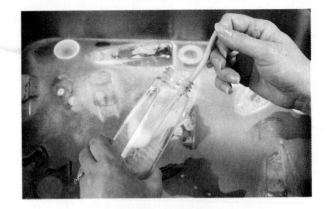

Fig. 28-11 A bottle brush is used to clean the inside of the bottle.

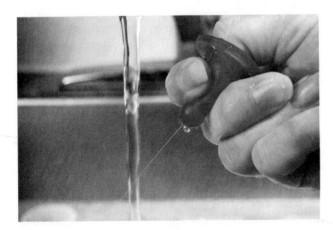

Fig. 28-12 Water is squeezed through the nipples during cleaning.

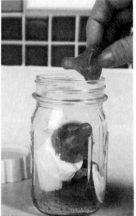

Fig. 28-13 Nipples and caps are placed in a jar for sterilization.

STERILIZING BOTTLES

1 Wash your hands.
2 Collect the following equipment:
  a Bottles, nipples, and caps
  b Funnel
  c Can opener
  d Tongs
  e Bottle brush
  f Sterilizer or large pot with cover
  g Dishwashing soap
  h Jar with openings in the lid
  i Other equipment used to prepare formula
  j Towel
3 Wash bottles, nipples, caps, funnel, can opener, and tongs in hot soapy water. Wash other equipment used to prepare formula.
4 Clean inside baby bottles with the bottle brush (Fig. 28-11).
5 Squeeze hot soapy water through the nipples (Fig. 28-12). This helps remove formula from them.
6 Rinse all equipment thoroughly in hot water. Be sure to squeeze hot water through the nipples to remove soap.
7 Place the nipples and caps in the jar. Put on the lid (Fig. 28-13).
8 Put all equipment into the sterilizer or pot. Stand the bottles and the jar upright.
9 Pour water into the pot. There should be about 2 inches of water in the bottom of the pot or sterilizer (Fig. 28-14).
10 Bring the water to a boil.
11 Cover the pot. Boil for 5 minutes.
12 Remove the pot from the heat. Let the pot cool. Do not remove the lid until the pot cools.
13 Lay a clean towel on the countertop.
14 Use the tongs to remove the remaining equipment. Stand the bottles upside down to drain. Open the jar. Remove the nipples with the tongs. Place the nipples and caps on the towel (Fig. 28-15).

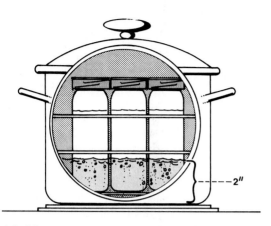

Fig. 28-14 Two inches of water is placed in the bottom of the pot for sterilizing bottles. (From Wernig J, Sorrentino SA: *The homemaker/home health aide*, St Louis, 1989, Mosby–Year Book.)

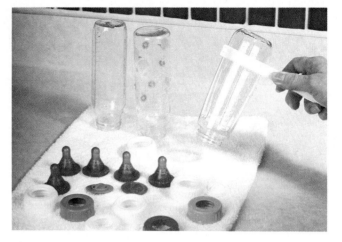

Fig. 28-15 Bottles, caps, and other equipment are allowed to dry after being sterilized.

Feeding the Baby

Babies generally want to be fed every 3 to 4 hours. The amount of formula they take increases as they grow older. The nurse or the mother will tell you how much formula a baby should have at each feeding. Babies usually take as much formula as they need. The baby will stop sucking and turn away from the bottle when satisfied.

Babies should not be given cold formula out of the refrigerator. A bottle is warmed before the baby is fed. You can warm the bottle in a pan of water. The formula should feel warm. You can test the temperature by sprinkling a few drops on your wrist (Fig. 28-16). You must not set the bottle out to warm at room temperature. This takes too long and allows the growth of microorganisms.

These guidelines will help you bottle-feed babies.
1. Warm the bottle so that the formula feels warm to your wrist.
2. Assume a comfortable position for the feeding.
3. Hold the baby close to you. Relax and snuggle the baby.
4. Tilt the bottle so that the neck and nipple are always filled (Fig. 28-17). Otherwise some air will be in the neck or nipple. The baby will suck air into the stomach. The air causes cramping and discomfort.
5. Do not prop the bottle and lay the baby down for the feeding (Fig. 28-18).
6. Burp the baby when he or she has taken half the formula (see page 436). Also burp the baby at the end of the feeding.
7. Do not leave the baby alone with a bottle.
8. Discard remaining formula.
9. Wash the bottle, cap, and nipple after the feeding (see *Sterilizing Bottles* on page 434).

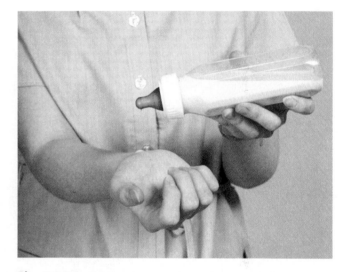

Fig. 28-16 A home health aide tests formula temperature. Formula should feel warm on her wrist.

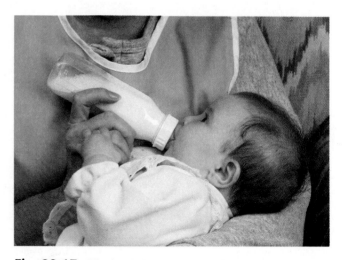

Fig. 28-17 The bottle is tilted so that formula fills the bottle neck and nipple.

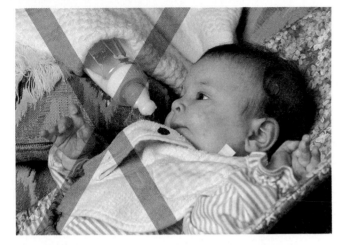

Fig. 28-18   Do not prop the bottle to feed the baby.

Burping the Baby

Babies take in air when they nurse. Bottle-fed babies take in more air than breast-fed babies do. Air in the stomach and intestines causes cramping and discomfort. This can lead to vomiting. Burping helps to get rid of the air. Burping a baby is sometimes called *bubbling.*

There are two ways to position the baby for burping (Fig. 28-19). One way is to hold the infant over your shoulder. You should place a clean diaper or towel over your shoulder. This protects your clothing if the baby "spits up." You can also support the baby in a sitting position on your lap. The towel or diaper should be held in front of the baby. To burp the baby, you will gently pat or rub the baby's back with circular motions.

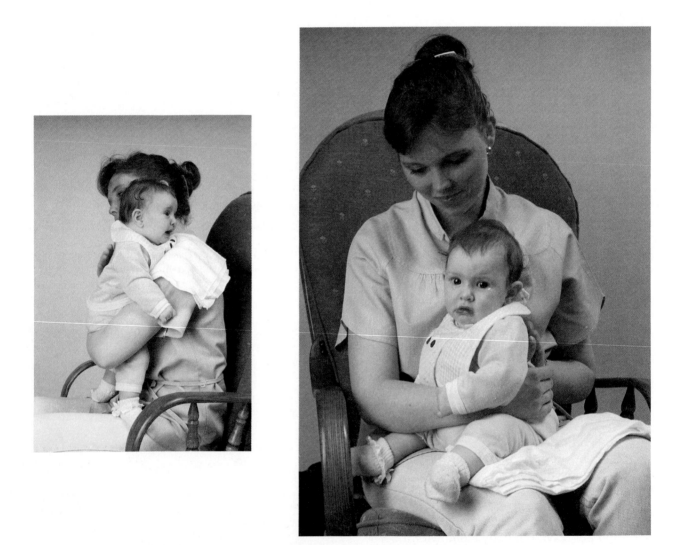

Fig. 28-19   A, The baby is held over the aide's shoulder for burping. **B,** The baby is supported in the sitting position for burping.

DIAPERING

Babies urinate 20 to 30 times a day. Breast-fed babies usually have bowel movements after feedings. Bottle-fed babies may have 3 bowel movements a day. A baby's stools are usually soft and unformed. Hard, formed stools mean the baby is constipated. This must be reported to the nurse immediately. Watery stools indicate diarrhea. Diarrhea is very serious in infants. Their water balance can be upset quickly (see Chapter 16, page 276). You must tell the nurse immediately if you suspect a baby has diarrhea.

Diaper changes are not necessary every time the baby wets. Changing the diaper after a feeding is usually sufficient. Cloth and disposable diapers are available. Cloth diapers are washed, dried, and folded for reuse. They are washed daily or every 2 days with a baby detergent. Putting them through the wash cycle a second time without detergent helps remove all soap. If possible, you should hang diapers outside to dry. This gives them a fresh, clean smell.

Disposable diapers are placed in the garbage. They are not flushed down the toilet. The use of disposable diapers is more expensive.

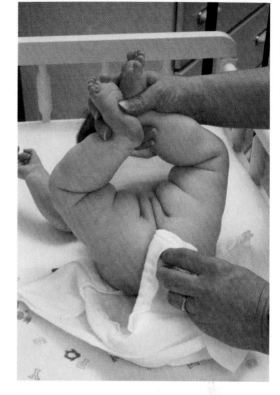

Fig. 28-20 The front of the diaper is used to clean the genital area.

DIAPERING A BABY

1 Wash your hands.
2 Unfasten the dirty diaper. If a cloth diaper is used, place diaper pins out of the baby's reach.
3 Wipe the genital area with the front of the diaper (Fig. 28-20). Wipe from the front to the back.
4 Fold the diaper so that urine and feces are well inside. Set the diaper aside.
5 Clean the genital area from front to back. Use a wet washcloth, disposable wipes, or cotton balls. Wash with mild soap and water if there is a lot of feces or if the baby has a rash. Rinse thoroughly and pat the area dry.
6 Give cord care and clean the circumcision at this time (see pages 438-439).
7 Apply cream or lotion to the genital area and buttocks. Do not use too much, because caking can occur.
8 Raise the baby's legs. Slide a clean diaper under the buttocks.
9 Fold a cloth diaper so that there is an extra thickness in front for a boy (Fig. 28-21, A). For girls, fold the diaper so that the extra

thickness is at the back (Fig. 28-21, B).
10 Bring the back of the diaper over the front.
11 Make sure the diaper is snug around the hips and abdomen. It should be loose near the penis if the circumcision has not healed. The diaper should be below the umbilicus if the cord stump has not healed.
12 Secure the diaper in place. Use the plastic tabs on disposable diapers (Fig. 28-22, A). Make sure the tabs stick in place. Use baby pins for cloth diapers. Pins should point away from the abdomen (Fig. 28-22, B).
13 Apply plastic pants if cloth diapers are worn. Do not use plastic pants with disposable diapers. They already have waterproof protection.
14 Put the baby in the crib, infant seat, or other safe location.
15 Rinse feces from the cloth diaper in the toilet.
16 Store used cloth diapers in a covered pail or plastic bag. Take the disposable diaper to the garbage.
17 Note and report your observations.

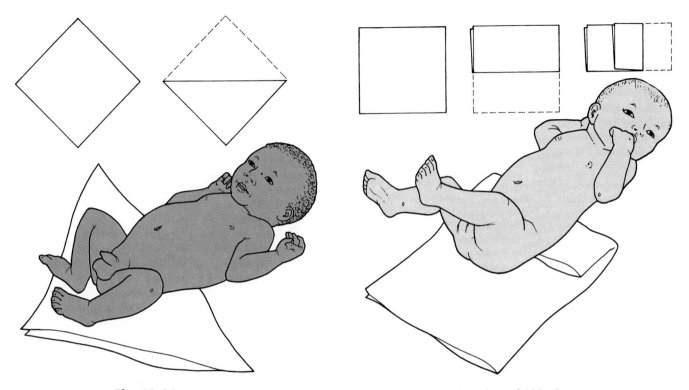

Fig. 28-21 **A,** A cloth diaper is folded in front for boys. **B,** The diaper has a fold in the back for girls.

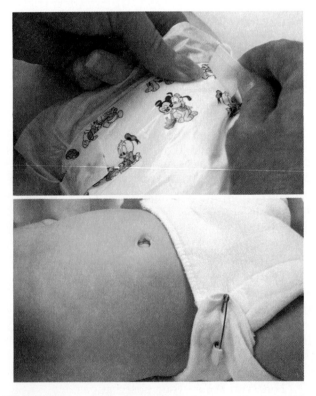

Fig. 28-22 **A,** A disposable diaper is secured in place with plastic tabs. **B,** Pins are used to secure cloth diapers. Pins point away from the abdomen.

CARE OF THE UMBILICAL CORD

The *umbilical cord* connects the mother and the fetus (unborn baby). It carries blood, oxygen, and nutrients from the mother to the fetus (Fig. 28-23). The umbilical cord is not needed after birth. Shortly after delivery, the doctor clamps and cuts the cord. A stump of cord is left on the baby. The stump dries up and falls off in 7 to 10 days. There may be a small amount of blood when the cord comes off.

The cord provides an area for the growth of microorganisms. Therefore it must be kept clean and dry. Cord care is done at each diaper change. Cord care is continued for 1 or 2 days after the cord comes off. It consists of the following:

1. Keep the stump dry. Do not get the stump wet.
2. Wipe the base of the stump with alcohol (Fig. 28-24). Use an alcohol wipe or a cotton ball moistened with alcohol. The alcohol promotes drying.
3. Keep the diaper below the cord as in Figure 28-22. This prevents the diaper from irritating the stump.
4. Report any signs of infection. These include redness or odor or drainage from the stump.
5. Give sponge baths until the cord falls off. Then the baby can have a tub bath.

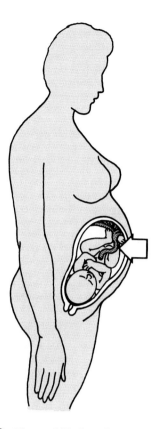

Fig. 28-23 The umbilical cord connects the mother and fetus. (From Wernig J, Sorrentino SA: *The homemaker/home health aide*, St Louis, 1989, Mosby–Year Book.)

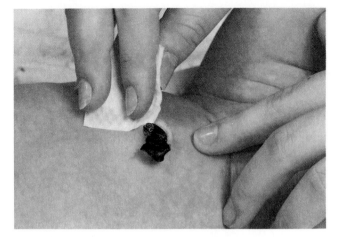

Fig. 28-24 The cord stump is wiped at the base with alcohol.

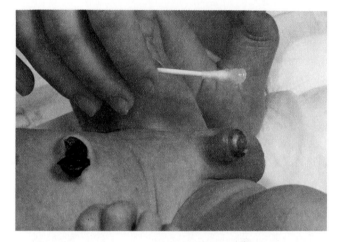

Fig. 28-25 Petrolatum is applied to the circumcised penis.

CIRCUMCISION

Boys are born with foreskin on the penis. The surgical removal of foreskin is called a *circumcision* (see Fig. 14-11 on page 237). The procedure allows good hygiene and is thought to prevent cancer of the penis. If a circumcision is done, it is usually performed in the hospital before the baby goes home. For those of the Jewish faith, circumcision is a religious ceremony.

The area will look red, swollen, and sore. However, the circumcision should not interfere with urination. You must carefully check for signs of bleeding and infection. There should be no odor or drainage. You should check the diaper for bleeding. The area should completely heal in 10 to 14 days.

The penis must be thoroughly cleaned at each diaper change. Cleaning is especially important if the baby has had a bowel movement. Mild soap and water or commercial wipes can be used. The diaper is loosely applied. This prevents the diaper from irritating the penis. Some doctors advise applying petrolatum to the penis. This protects the penis from urine and feces. It also prevents the penis from sticking to the diaper. A cotton swab is used to apply the petrolatum (Fig. 28-25). The nurse will tell you if other measures are needed.

BATHING AN INFANT

A bath is important for cleanliness. Though babies do not get very dirty, they need good skin care. Baths comfort and relax babies. They also provide a wonderful time to hold, touch, and talk to babies. Stimulation is important for development. Being touched and held helps babies learn safety, security, and love.

Planning is an important part of the bath. You cannot leave the baby unattended if you forget something. Therefore you need to gather equipment, supplies, and the baby's clothes before you begin the bath. Everything you will need should be within your reach.

Safety measures are also very important. You must never leave the baby alone on a table or in the bath tub. You must always keep one hand on the baby if you must look away for a moment. The baby must be held securely throughout the bath. Babies are very slippery when they are wet. A wet, squirming baby can be very hard to hold.

Room temperature should be 75° to 80° F for the bath. You may need to turn up the thermostat and close windows and doors about 20 minutes before the bath. The room temperature may be uncomfortable for you. You may want to remove a sweater or roll up your sleeves before starting the bath.

Water temperature needs special attention. Babies have delicate skin and are easily burned. Bath water temperature should be 90° to 100° F. Bath water temperature is measured with a bath thermometer. If one is not available, you may test the water temperature with the inside of your wrist (Fig. 28-26). The water should feel warm and comfortable to your wrist.

Bath time should be part of the baby's daily routine. Some mothers like to bathe their babies in the morning. Others prefer the evening. Evening baths have two important advantages. The bath is comforting and relaxing. This helps some babies sleep longer at night. Working fathers are usually available in the evening. The evening bath lets them be involved. Sometimes fathers will bathe the babies to give mothers time to rest or tend to other children. You must follow the family's routine when working in the home.

There are two bath procedures for babies. Sponge baths are given until the baby is about 2 weeks old.

GIVING A SPONGE BATH

1   Place the following equipment on your work area:
   a   Bath basin
   b   Bath thermometer
   c   Bath towel
   d   Two hand towels
   e   Receiving blanket
   f   Washcloth
   g   Clean diaper
   h   Clean clothing for the baby
   i   Cotton balls
   j   Baby soap
   k   Baby shampoo
   l   Baby lotion
   m   Cotton swabs
2   Fill the bath basin with warm water. Water temperature should be 90° to 100° F. Measure water temperature with the bath thermometer or use the inside of your wrist. The water should feel warm and comfortable on your wrist.
3   Provide for privacy.
4   Identify the baby. Check the ID bracelet.
5   Undress the baby. Leave the diaper on.
6   Wash the baby's eyes (Fig. 28-28):
   a   Dip a cotton ball into the water.
   b   Squeeze out excess water.
   c   Wash one eye from the inner part to the outer part.
   d   Repeat this step for the other eye with a new cotton ball.
7   Dip a cotton swab into the water. Tap the stick part gently against the basin to remove excess water.
8   Clean inside each nostril (Fig. 28-29). Be gentle and do not push the swab into the nose. Pat dry the baby's face.
9   Moisten the washcloth. Clean the outside of the ear and then behind the ear. Repeat this step for the other ear.

Be gentle. Do not use cotton swabs to clean inside the ears.
10   Rinse and squeeze out the washcloth. Make a mitt with the washcloth (see Fig. 13-10, page 203).
11   Wash the baby's face (Fig. 28-30). Pat dry.
12   Pick up the baby. Hold the baby over the bath basin using the football hold. Support the baby's head and neck with your wrist and hand.
13   Wash the baby's head (Fig. 28-31):
   a   Squeeze a washcloth onto the baby's head.
   b   Apply a small amount of baby shampoo to the head.
   c   Wash the head with circular motions.
   d   Rinse the head by squeezing a washcloth over the baby's head. Be sure to rinse thoroughly.
   e   Use a small hand towel to dry the head.
14   Lay the baby on the table. Remove the diaper.
15   Wash the front of the body. Use a soapy washcloth. You may also apply soap to your hands and wash the baby with your hands (Fig. 28-32) Do not get the cord wet. Rinse thoroughly. Pat dry. Be sure to dry all creases.
16   Turn the baby to the prone position. Repeat step 13 for the back and buttocks.
17   Give cord care and clean the circumcision.
18   Apply baby lotion to the baby's body.
19   Put a clean diaper and clean clothes on the baby.
20   Wrap the baby in the receiving blanket.
21   Clean and return equipment and supplies to the proper place. Do this step when the baby is settled.
22   Note and report your observations.

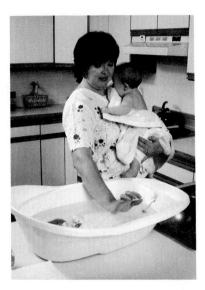

Fig. 28-26 The wrist is used to test the temperature of the bath water.

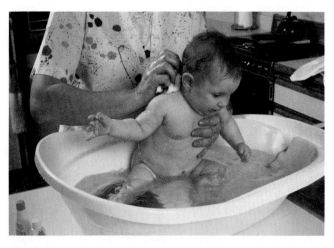

Fig. 28-27 The baby is given a tub bath.

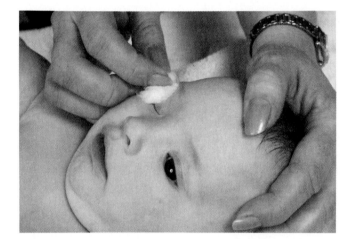

Fig. 28-28 The baby's eyes are washed with cotton balls. The eye is cleaned from the inner to the outer part.

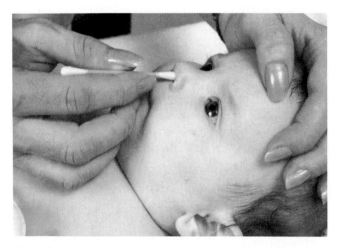

Fig. 28-29 The nostril is cleaned with a cotton swab.

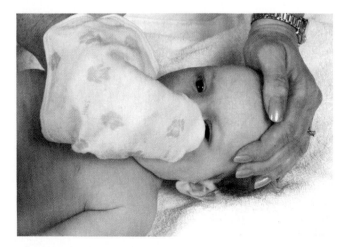

Fig. 28-30 The baby's face is washed with a mitted washcloth.

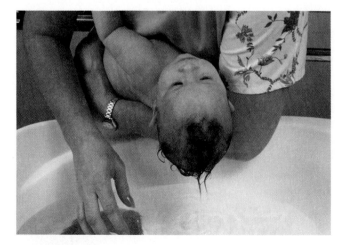

Fig. 28-31 The baby's head is washed over the basin.

GIVING A TUB BATH

1   Follow steps 1 through 14 in the sponge bath procedure (see page 440).
2   Hold the baby as in Figure 28-33:
    a   Place your right hand under the baby's shoulders. Your thumb should be over the baby's right shoulder. Your fingers should be under the right arm.
    b   Use your left hand to support the baby's buttocks. Slide your left hand under the thighs. Hold the right thigh with your left hand.
3   Lower the baby into the water feet first.
4   Wash the front of the baby's body. Be sure to wash all folds and creases. Rinse thoroughly.
5   Reverse your hold. Use your left hand to hold the baby.
6   Wash the baby's back as in Figure 28-27. Rinse thoroughly.
7   Reverse your hold again. Use your right hand to hold the baby.
8   Wash the genital area.
9   Lift the baby out of the water and onto a towel.
10 Wrap the baby in the towel. Also cover the baby's head.
11 Pat the baby dry. Be sure to dry all folds and creases.
12 Follow steps 18-22 of the sponge bath (page 440).

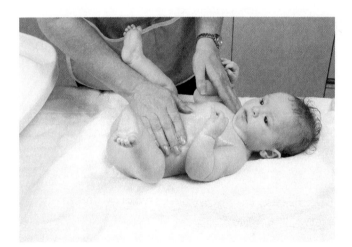

Fig. 28-32   The hands are used to wash the baby.

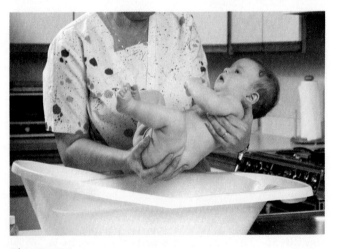

Fig. 28-33   The baby is held for the tub bath.

They are given until the cord stump falls off and the umbilicus and circumcision heal. The cord must not get wet. The tub bath is given after the cord and circumcision heal (Fig. 28-27).

SUMMARY

Caring for new mothers and infants can be a wonderful experience. Infant safety is very important. Babies cannot protect themselves. They depend on others for their physical needs. They must also feel safe, secure, and loved. Be sure to talk, sing, and play with babies while you meet their basic needs.

REVIEW QUESTIONS

Circle the best *answer.*

1 A baby's head must be supported for the first
   a 7 to 10 days
   b Month
   c 3 months
   d 6 months

2 When holding babies, you should
   a Hold them securely
   b Cuddle them
   c Sing and talk to them
   d All of the above

3 Which is *false?*
   a The crib should be within hearing distance of caregivers.
   b The baby should have a pillow for sleep.
   c The baby's position should be changed often.
   d Crib rails should be up at all times.

4 Report the following to your supervisor *except*
   a The baby looks flushed and is perspiring
   b The baby has watery stools
   c The baby's eyes are red and irritated
   d The baby spits up when burped

5 The breast-feeding mother should do the following *except*
   a Wash her breasts with soap and water
   b Hold the baby close to her breast
   c Stimulate the rooting reflex
   d Keep breast tissue away from the baby's nose

6 A breast-fed baby should be burped
   a Every 5 minutes
   b After nursing from one breast
   c After nursing from both breasts
   d After the feeding

7 A baby is bottle-fed. You do the grocery shopping. Which formula should you buy?
   a The one that is on sale
   b The ready-to-feed type
   c The one ordered by the doctor
   d The powdered form because it lasts longer

8 You are to sterilize baby bottles. How long should the water boil?
   a 5 minutes
   b 10 minutes
   c 15 minutes
   d 20 minutes

9 You are to warm a baby bottle. Which is *true?*
   a The bottle is warmed for 5 minutes in the microwave.
   b The formula should warm at room temperature.
   c The formula should feel warm on your wrist.
   d The formula is warmed in a pan for 5 minutes.

10 When bottle-feeding a baby, you should
    a Burp the baby every 5 minutes
    b Save remaining formula for the next feeding
    c Tilt the bottle so that formula fills the neck and nipple
    d All of the above

11 Diapers are changed whenever the baby urinates.
    a True
    b False

12 The cord has not yet healed. The baby's diaper should be
    a Loose over the cord
    b Snug over the cord
    c Below the cord
    d Disposable

13 The cord stump is cleaned with
    a Soap and water
    b Baby shampoo
    c Plain water
    d Alcohol

14 The cord and the circumcision are cleaned
    a Once a day
    b When the baby has a bowel movement
    c Three times a day
    d At every diaper change

15 The cord and circumcision have not healed. The baby should have a sponge bath.
    a True
    b False

16 Bath water for the baby should be
    a 60° to 65° F
    b 70° to 75° F
    c 75° to 80° F
    d 90° to 100° F

17 Which should you use to wash the baby's eyes?
    a A mitted washcloth
    b Alcohol wipes
    c A cotton swab
    d Cotton balls

18 Cotton swabs are used to clean inside the baby's ears.
    a True
    b False

Answers

18	b	12	c	6	b
17	d	11	b	5	a
16	d	10	c	4	d
15	a	9	c	3	b
14	d	8	a	2	d
13	d	7	c	1	c

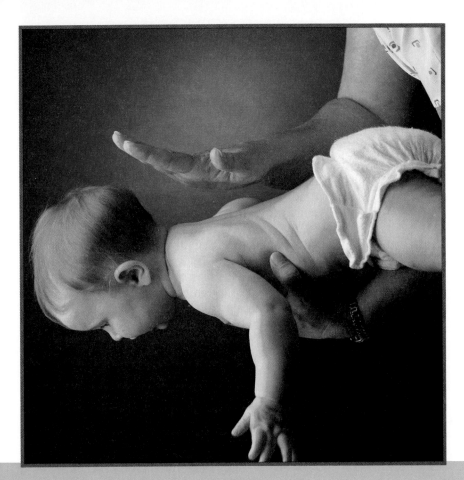

Basic Emergency Care

OBJECTIVES

- Define the key terms listed in this chapter
- Describe the general rules of emergency care
- Identify the signs of cardiac arrest and the signs of an obstructed airway
- Describe basic life support and basic life support procedures
- Explain the difference between internal and external hemorrhage and between arterial and venous bleeding
- Explain how to control hemorrhage
- Identify the signs of, and emergency care for, shock
- Describe two types of seizures and how to care for a person during a seizure
- Identify the common causes of, and emergency care for, fainting
- Describe the signs of, and emergency care for, stroke
- Describe the care given to help a person who is vomiting

cardiac arrest The sudden stoppage of breathing and heart action

convulsion Violent and sudden contractions or tremors of muscles; seizure

first aid Emergency care given to an ill or injured person before medical help arrives

hemorrhage The excessive loss of blood from a blood vessel

respiratory arrest Condition in which breathing stops but the heart continues to pump for several minutes

seizure A convulsion

shock A condition that results when there is an inadequate blood supply to the organs and tissues of the body

You may find emergency situations in health care facilities, in homes, in public places, or on the highway. Knowing what to do may mean the difference between life and death. This chapter describes some common emergencies and the basic care that should be given. You are encouraged to take a first aid course from the American Red Cross. A basic life support course given by the American Heart Association or the Red Cross is also recommended. These courses will prepare you to give care in emergency situations.

GENERAL RULES OF EMERGENCY CARE

First aid is the emergency care given to an ill or injured person before medical help arrives. The goals of first aid are to prevent death and to prevent injuries from becoming worse.

When an emergency occurs, the local Emergency Medical Services (EMS) system must be activated. The system involves emergency personnel (paramedics and emergency medical technicians) who have been trained and educated in emergency care. They have learned how to treat, stabilize, and transport persons in life-threatening situations. Their emergency vehicles have the equipment, supplies, and drugs used in emergencies. Emergency personnel communicate by two-way radio with doctors based in hospital emergency rooms. The doctors tell them what to do and when to transport the victim to the hospital. In many communities the EMS system can be activated by dialing 911. Calling the local fire or police department or the telephone operator can also activate the system.

Each emergency is different. However, the following rules apply to any emergency:

1. Know your limitations. Do not try to do more than you are able. Do not perform a procedure with which you are unfamiliar. Do what you can under the circumstances.
2. Stay calm. Calm and efficient functioning will help the victim feel more secure.
3. Make quick observations to detect life-threatening problems. Check for breathing, a pulse, and bleeding.
4. Keep the victim lying down or in the position in which he or she was found. You could make an injury worse if you move the victim.
5. Perform necessary emergency measures.
6. Call for help or tell someone to activate the EMS system. An operator will send emergency vehicles and personnel to the scene. Do not hang up until the operator has hung up. Give the operator the following information:
   a. Your location—include the street address and the city or town you are in. Give names of cross streets or roads and landmarks if possible. Also give the telephone number you are calling from
   b. What has happened (heart attack, accident, etc.)—police, fire equipment, and ambulances may be needed
   c. How many people need help
   d. The condition of the victims, any obvious injuries, and if there are life-threatening situations
   e. What aid is being given
7. Do not remove clothing from the victim unless you have to. If clothing must be removed, tear garments along the seams.
8. Keep the victim warm. Cover the victim with a blanket. Use coats and sweaters if there is no blanket.
9. Reassure the conscious victim. Explain what is happening and that help has been called.
10. Do not give the victim any food or fluids.
11. Do not move the victim. Emergency personnel have been trained to do so.
12. Keep bystanders away from the victim. Bystanders tend to stare, give advice, and comment about the victim's condition. The victim may think that the situation is worse than it really is. Also, the victim's privacy is invaded by onlookers.

BASIC LIFE SUPPORT

When the heart and breathing stop, the person is clinically dead. Blood and oxygen are not circulated through the body. Permanent brain damage and other organ damage occur within 4 to 6 minutes. Death may be expected. Death is expected in patients suffering from long illnesses for which there is no hope of recovery. However, the heart and breathing can stop suddenly and without warning. This is a state of *cardiac arrest.*

Cardiac arrest is a sudden, unexpected, and dramatic event. People have had cardiac arrests while driving, shoveling snow, playing golf or tennis, watching television, eating, and sleeping. Cardiac arrest can occur anywhere and at any time. Common causes include heart disease, drowning, electrical shock, severe injury, obstruction of the air passages, and drug overdose. The victim suffers permanent brain damage unless breathing and circulation are restored.

Respiratory arrest is when breathing stops but the heart continues to pump blood for several minutes. If breathing is not restored, cardiac arrest occurs. Causes of respiratory arrest include drowning, stroke, obstructed airway, drug overdose, electrocution, smoke inhalation, suffocation, injury from lightning, myocardial infarction, coma, and other injuries.

Basic life support involves preventing or promptly recognizing cardiac arrest or respiratory arrest. Basic life support procedures support breathing and circulation. These life-saving measures require speed, skill, and efficiency.

Cardiopulmonary Resuscitation

There are three major signs of cardiac arrest—no pulse, no breathing, and unconsciousness. The person's skin is cool, pale, and gray. The person has no blood pressure.

Cardiopulmonary resuscitation (CPR) must be started as soon as cardiac arrest occurs. CPR provides oxygen to the brain, heart, kidneys, and other organs until more advanced emergency care can be given. CPR has three basic parts (the ABCs of CPR): airway, breathing, and circulation.

Airway The respiratory passages (airway) must be open if breathing is to be restored. The airway is often blocked or obstructed during cardiac arrest. The victim's tongue falls toward the back of the throat and blocks the airway. The head-tilt/chin-lift maneuver is used to open the airway (Fig. 29-1). One hand is placed on the victim's forehead. Pressure is applied on the forehead with the palm to tilt the head back. The fingers of the other hand are placed under the bony part of the chin. The chin is lifted forward as the head is tilted backward with the other hand.

The head-tilt/chin-lift maneuver is used for infants and children. The head is not hyperextended as in the adult. Rather the head is tilted to a normal (neutral) or "sniffing" position (Fig. 29-2).

Breathing Oxygen is not inhaled when breathing stops. The victim must get oxygen. Otherwise, permanent brain and organ damage will occur. Because the victim cannot breathe, breathing is done for the victim. This is accomplished during CPR by *mouth-to-mouth* resuscitation (Fig. 29-3).

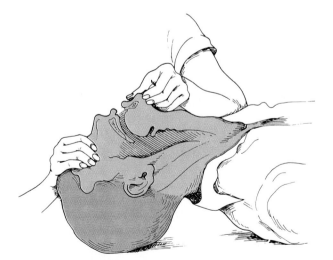

Fig. 29-1 The head-tilt/chin-lift maneuver is used to open the airway. One hand is on the victim's forehead, and pressure is applied to tilt the head back. The fingers of the other hand are placed under the chin. The chin is lifted forward with the fingers. (From Ellis PD, Billings DM: *Cardiopulmonary resuscitation: procedures for basic and advanced life support,* St Louis, 1979, Mosby–Year Book.)

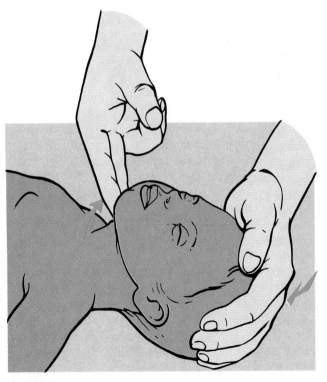

Fig. 29-2 The head-tilt/chin-lift maneuver is used for infants. The infant's head is not tilted as far back as that of the adult. The infant's head is in a neutral or "sniffing" position.

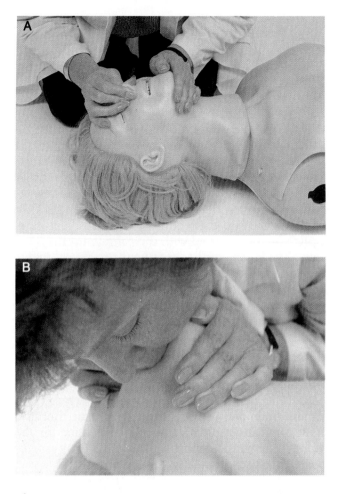

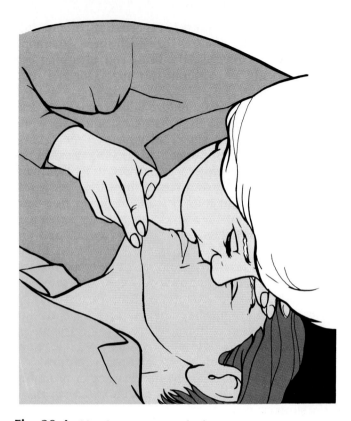

Fig. 29-3 Mouth-to-mouth resuscitation. **A,** The victim's airway is opened, and the nostrils are pinched shut. **B,** The victim's mouth is sealed by the rescuer's mouth.

Fig. 29-4 Mouth-to-nose resuscitation.

The airway is kept open to give mouth-to-mouth resuscitation. The victim's nostrils are pinched shut with the thumb and index finger of the hand on the forehead. Shutting the nostrils prevents air from escaping through the nose. After taking a deep breath, place your mouth tightly over the victim's mouth. Blow air into the victim's mouth as you exhale. You should see the victim's chest rise as the lungs fill with air. After you give a ventilation, remove your mouth from the victim's mouth. Then take in a quick, deep breath.

Mouth-to-mouth resuscitation is not always indicated or possible. The *mouth-to-nose* technique may be necessary. The mouth-to-nose technique is recommended when:
1. You cannot ventilate the victim's mouth
2. You cannot open the mouth
3. You cannot make a tight seal for mouth-to-mouth resuscitation
4. The mouth is severely injured

The mouth must be closed for mouth-to-nose resuscitation. The head-tilt/chin-lift method is used to open the airway. Pressure is placed on the chin to close the mouth. To give the ventilation, place your mouth over the victim's nose and blow air into the nose (Fig. 29-4).

Some people breathe through openings *(stomas)* in their necks (Fig. 29-5). They need *mouth-to-stoma* ventilation during cardiac or respiratory arrest. You will seal your mouth around the stoma and blow air into the stoma (Fig. 29-6). To see if a person is a "neck-breather," check for an opening at the front of the neck.

You will have contact with the victim's body fluids or body substances when giving artificial ventilation. If available, a pocket mask with a one-way valve is used for mouth-to-mouth resuscitation (Fig. 29-7). This provides a barrier between you and the victim's body fluids or body substances.

Circulation Blood flow to the brain and other organs must be maintained. Otherwise, permanent damage results. The heart has stopped beating in cardiac arrest. Therefore blood must be pumped through the body in some other way. Artificial circulation is accomplished by external chest compression. This is also called external cardiac massage. Each chest compression forces blood through the circulatory system.

The heart lies between the sternum (breastbone) and the spinal column. When pressure is applied to

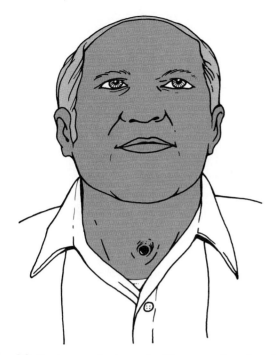

Fig. 29-5 A stoma in the neck. The person breathes air in and out of the stoma.

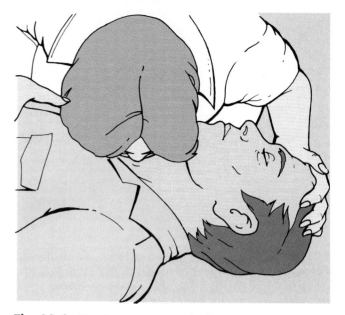

Fig. 29-6 Mouth-to-stoma resuscitation.

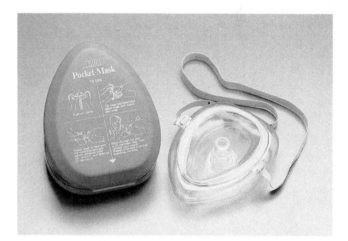

Fig. 27-7 A pocket mask with a one-way valve.

the sternum, the sternum is depressed. This compresses the heart between the sterum and spinal column (Fig. 29-8). For effective chest compressions, the victim must be supine and on a hard, flat surface.

Proper hand position is important for external chest compressions. The process for locating hand position for adults is shown in Figure 29-9.

1. Use your index and middle fingers to locate the lower part of the victim's rib cage on the side nearest you.
2. Then run your fingers up along the rib cage to the notch at the center of the chest. The notch is where the ribs and sternum meet.
3. Use your middle finger to mark the notch.
4. Place your index finger next to your middle finger on the lower end of the sternum.
5. Place the heel of your other hand on the lower half of the sternum next to your index finger.
6. Remove your index finger and middle finger from the notch.
7. Place that hand on the hand already on the sternum.
8. Extend or interlace your fingers to keep them off the chest.

You must be positioned properly for chest compressions. Your elbows must be straight. Your shoulders must be directly over the victim's chest (Fig. 29-10). Firm downward pressure is exerted to depress the sternum about 1½ to 2 inches. Then the pressure is released without removing your hands from the chest. Compressions are given in a regular, rhythmic fashion.

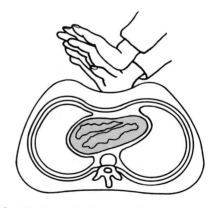

Fig. 29-8 The heart lies between the sternum and spinal cord. The heart is compressed when pressure is applied to the sternum. (From Rosen P, et al.: *Emergency medicine: concepts and clinical practice*, ed 2, St Louis, 1988, Mosby–Year Book.)

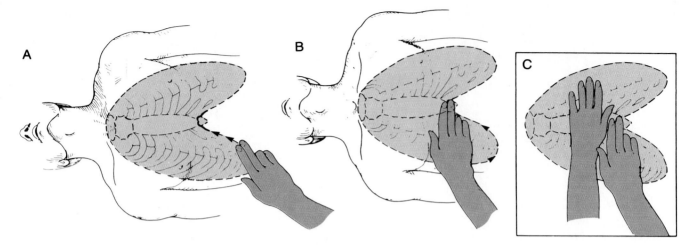

Fig. 29-9 Proper hand position for CPR. **A,** Locate the rib cage. **B,** Run the fingers along the rib cage to the notch. **C,** The heel of the hand is placed next to the index finger. (From Ellis PD, Billings DM: *Cardiopulmonary resuscitation: procedures for basic and advanced life support*, St Louis, 1979, Mosby–Year Book.)

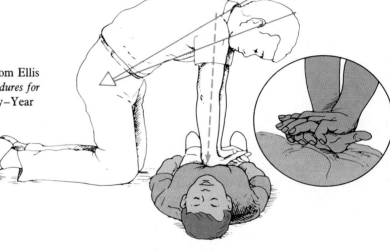

Fig. 29-10 Position of the shoulders for CPR. (From Ellis PD, Billings DM: *Cardiopulmonary resuscitation: procedures for basic and advanced life support*, St Louis, 1979, Mosby–Year Book.)

Performing CPR CPR is done only for cardiac arrest. You must determine if cardiac arrest or fainting has occurred. CPR is done when there is unresponsiveness, breathlessness, and pulselessness. Determine unresponsiveness by tapping or gently shaking the victim and shouting "Are you OK?" If there is no response, the victim is unconscious.

Establishing breathlessness involves three steps. *Look* at the victim's chest to see if it rises and falls. *Listen* for the escape of air during expiration. Place your ear near the victim's nose and mouth to listen for the escape of air. *Feel* for the flow of air. To feel for air, place your cheek near the victim's nose.

The carotid artery is used to check for pulselessness. To find the carotid pulse, place the tips of your index and middle fingers on the victim's trachea (windpipe). Then slide your fingertips down off the trachea to the groove of the neck on the side near you (Fig. 29-11).

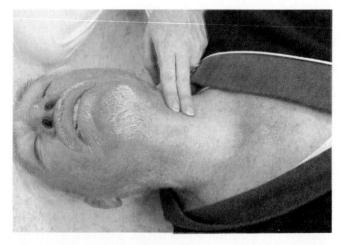

Fig. 29-11 Locating the carotid pulse. Index and middle fingers are placed on the trachea. The fingers are moved down into the groove of the neck where the carotid pulse is located.

ADULT CPR—ONE RESCUER

1 Check for unresponsiveness.
2 Call for help.
3 Position the victim supine. Logroll the victim so that there is no twisting of the spine. The victim must be on a hard, flat surface. Place the victim's arms alongside the body.
4 Open the airway. Use the head-tilt/chin-lift maneuver.
5 Check for breathlessness.
6 Give 2 ventilations. Each should be 1½ seconds long. Let the victim's chest deflate between ventilations.
7 Check for pulselessness. Check the pulse for 5 to 10 seconds. Use your other hand to keep the airway open with the head-tilt maneuver.
8 Have your helper activate the EMS system.

9 Give chest compressions at a rate of 80 to 100 per minute. Give 15 compressions and then 2 ventilations.
   a Establish a rhythm and count out loud (try: "1 and, 2 and, 3 and, 4 and, 5 and, 6 and, 7 and, 8 and, 9 and, 10 and, 11 and, 12 and, 13 and, 14 and, 15").
   b Open the airway and give 2 ventilations.
   c Repeat this step until 4 cycles of 15 compressions and 2 ventilations have been given.
10 Check for a carotid pulse (5 seconds).
11 Give 2 ventilations if pulselessness continues.
12 Repeat step 9. Check for a pulse every 4 to 5 minutes. Do not interrupt CPR for more than 7 seconds.

ADULT CPR—TWO RESCUERS

1 Perform one-person CPR until a helper arrives.
2 Continue chest compressions. The helper says, "I know CPR. Can I help?"
3 Indicate that you want help. Do not stop the chest compressions. The helper kneels on the other side of the victim. The two-rescuer procedure begins after you complete a cycle of 15 compressions and 2 ventilations.
4 Stop compressions for 5 seconds. The helper checks for a carotid pulse. The helper states "No pulse."
5 Perform two-person CPR (Fig. 29-12) as follows:
   a The helper gives 2 ventilations.
   b Give chest compressions at a rate of 80 to 100 per minute. Count out loud in a rhythm (try: "1 and, 2 and, 3 and, 4 and, 5").
   c The helper gives a ventilation immediately after the fifth compression. Pause for 1 to 1½ seconds for the ventilation. Continue chest compressions after the ventilation.
   d A ventilation is given after every fifth compression. Your helper checks for a pulse during the compressions.

6 Stop compressions after 1 minute. Your helper checks for breathing and a pulse. After the first minute, compressions are stopped every few minutes to check for breathing and circulation. Compressions are stopped for only 5 seconds.
7 Call for a switch in positions when you are tired.
8 Change positions quickly as follows:
   a Helper gives a ventilation after you give the fifth compression.
   b Helper moves down to kneel at the victim's shoulder and finds the proper hand position.
   c You move to the victim's head after giving the fifth compression.
   d Check for a pulse (5 seconds).
   e Say "No pulse."
   f Give 1 ventilation before your helper begins chest compressions.
9 Give 1 ventilation after every fifth compression.
10 Switch positions when the person giving the compressions is tired. Check for a pulse and breathing at every position change.

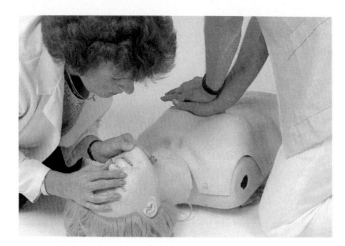

Fig. 29-12 Two people performing CPR.

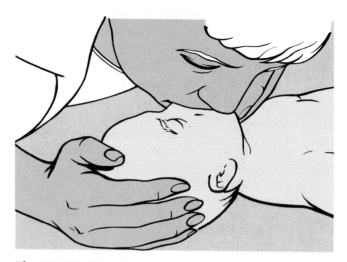

Fig. 29-13 The infant's mouth and nose are covered during mouth-to-mouth resuscitation.

CPR FOR INFANTS AND CHILDREN

1 Check for unresponsiveness.
2 Call for help.
3 Logroll the victim onto his or her back. Support the head and neck when turning the victim. Position the infant or child supine on a hard, flat surface.
4 Open the airway. Use the head-tilt/chin-lift maneuver. Do not hyperextend the head. Extension of the head usually opens an infant's or child's airway (see Fig. 29-2).
5 Check for breathlessness.
6 Give 2 gentle, slow ventilations. Each should take 1 to 1½ seconds. Cover an infant's nose and mouth with your mouth when giving a ventilation (Fig. 29-13). Let the chest deflate between ventilations.
7 Check for pulselessness. Use the brachial artery for infants and the carotid artery for children. Keep the airway open.
8 Have your helper activate the EMS system.
9 Give chest compressions to an *infant*:
  a Locate hand position (Fig. 29-14).
    1 Draw an imaginary line between the nipples.
    2 Place your index finger farthest from the infant's head just under the imaginary line.
    3 Place your middle and ring fingers next to your index finger. The area for chest compression is below your middle and ring fingers.

  b Give compressions using 2 or 3 fingers. The sternum is compressed ½ to 1 inch at least 100 times per minute. Release pressure after each compression. Do not remove your fingers from the chest.
  c Count out loud in a rhythm (try: "1, 2, 3, 4, 5").
  d Give 1 ventilation after every fifth compression.
  e Check for a pulse after 10 cycles of 5 compressions and 1 ventilation.
  f Continue chest compressions and ventilation if there is no pulse.
  g Check for a pulse every few minutes.
10 Give chest compressions to a *child*. (Use the adult method if the child is large or older than age 8.)
  a Locate proper hand position as for the adult.
  b Use the heel of one hand to depress the sternum 1 to 1½ inches (Fig. 29-15).
  c Give 80 to 100 compressions per minute. Count out loud in a rhythm (try: "1 and 2 and 3 and 4 and 5").
  d Give a ventilation after every fifth compression.
  e Check for a pulse after 10 cycles of 5 compressions and 1 ventilation.
  f Continue chest compressions and ventilations if there is no pulse.
  g Check for a pulse every few minutes.

Cardiopulmonary resuscitation can be done alone or with another person. CPR is given with the victim on a hard, flat surface. You need to kneel next to the victim's shoulders. CPR is *never* practiced on another person. Serious damage can be done. Mannequins are used for learning CPR.

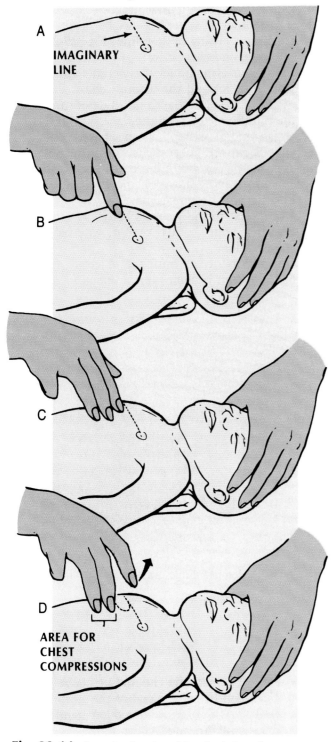

Fig. 29-14 Locating hand position for infant chest compressions. **A,** Draw an imaginary line between the nipples. **B,** The index finger is placed just under the line. **C,** The middle and ring fingers are placed next to the index finger. **D,** The area for chest compressions is under the middle and ring fingers.

Obstructed Airway

Airway obstruction (choking) can lead to cardiac arrest. Air cannot pass through the air passages to the lungs. This deprives the entire body of oxygen. Airway obstruction often occurs during eating. Meat is the most common food that causes airway obstruction. Choking often occurs on large, poorly chewed pieces of meat. Laughing and talking while eating can also cause choking. Adults can choke on dentures. Children have choked on small objects such as pieces of hot dogs, marbles, hard candy, coins, and

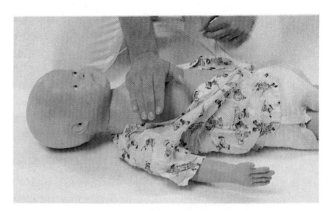

Fig. 29-15 The heel of one hand is used for CPR on a child. The heel is placed over the lower end of the sternum as for an adult.

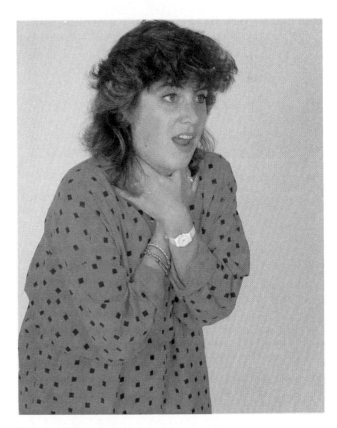

Fig. 29-16 A choking person will usually clutch the throat.

beads. Airway obstruction can occur in unconscious persons. Common causes are aspiration of vomitus and the tongue falling back into the airway.

When airway obstruction occurs, the victim clutches at the throat (Fig. 29-16). The person cannot breathe, speak, or cough. The victim is pale and cyanotic. If conscious, the victim is very apprehensive. The obstruction must be removed immediately before cardiac arrest occurs. The Heimlich maneuver is used to relieve an obstructed airway. It involves abdominal thrusts. The maneuver can be performed with the victim standing, sitting, or lying. The finger sweep

is another maneuver that is used when an adult victim is unconscious. You need to call for help when a victim has an obstructed airway. Have someone activate the EMS system.

The Heimlich maneuver is not effective in extremely obese persons and in pregnant women. Chest thrusts are used for them. Chest thrusts are performed as follows:
1. The victim is sitting or standing (Fig. 29-20):
   a. Stand behind the victim.
   b. Place your arms under the victim's arm. Wrap your arms around the victim's chest.
   c. Make a fist. Place the thumb side of the fist on the middle of the sternum.
   d. Grasp the fist with your other hand.
   e. Give backward chest thrusts until the object is expelled or the victim becomes unconscious.
2. The victim is lying down or unconscious:
   a. Position the victim supine.
   b. Kneel next to the victim's body.
   c. Position your hands as for external chest compression.
   d. Give chest thrusts until the object is expelled or the victim becomes unconscious.

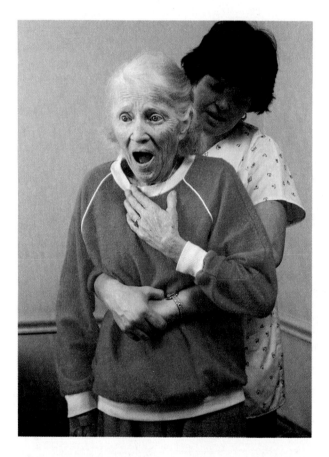

Fig. 29-17 Abdominal thrusts with the victim standing.

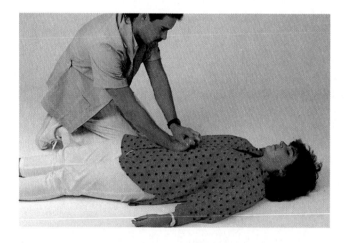

Fig. 29-18 Abdominal thrusts with the victim lying down.

CLEARING THE OBSTRUCTED AIRWAY—THE CONSCIOUS ADULT

1 Ask the victim if he or she is choking.
2 Determine if the victim can cough or speak.
3 Perform the Heimlich maneuver (abdominal thrusts) if the victim is standing or sitting (Fig. 29-17).
   a Stand behind the victim.
   b Wrap your arms around the victim's waist.
   c Make a fist with one hand. Place the thumb side of the fist against the abdo-

men. The fist is in the middle above the navel and below the end of the sternum.
   d Grasp your fist with your other hand.
   e Press your fist and hand into the victim's abdomen with a quick, upward thrust.
   f Repeat the abdominal thrust until the object has been expelled or the victim loses consciousness.

1 Check for unresponsiveness.
2 Call for help.
3 Logroll the victim to the supine position with his or her face up. The victim's arms should be at the sides.
4 Open the airway. Use the head-tilt/chin-lift maneuver.
5 Check for breathlessness.
6 Give 1 ventilation. Reposition the victim's head and open the airway if you could not ventilate. Give 1 ventilation.
7 Have your helper activate the EMS system.
8 Do the Heimlich maneuver if you could not ventilate the victim.
   a Kneel by the victim's thighs.
   b Place the heel of one hand against the victim's abdomen. It should be in the middle of the abdomen between the lower end of the sternum and the navel.
   c Place your other hand on top of the hand on the victim's abdomen (Fig. 29-18).
   d Give an abdominal thrust. Press inward and upward.
   e Give 6 to 10 abdominal thrusts.
9 Do the finger sweep maneuver to check for a foreign object.
   a Open the victim's mouth. Use the tongue-jaw lift maneuver (Fig. 29-19).
      1 Grasp the tongue and lower jaw with your thumb and fingers.
      2 Lift the lower jaw upward.
   b Insert your other index finger into the mouth along the side of the cheek and deep into the throat. Your finger should be at the base of the tongue.
   c Form a hook with your index finger.
   d Try to dislodge and remove the object. Do not push it deeper into the throat.
   e Grasp and remove the object if it is within reach.
10 Open the airway with the head-tilt/chin-lift method.
11 Give 1 ventilation.
12 Repeat steps 8 through 11 for as long as necessary.

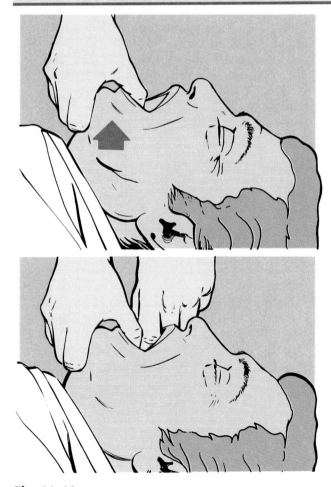

Fig. 29-19 Tongue-jaw lift maneuver. **A,** The victim's tongue is grasped, and the jaw is lifted forward with one hand. **B,** The index finger of the other hand is used to check for a foreign object.

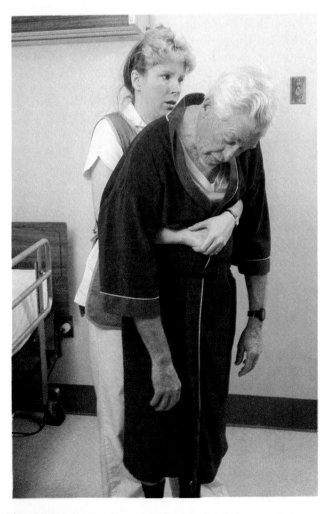

Fig. 29-20 Chest thrusts done with the victim standing.

RELIEVING AN OBSTRUCTED AIRWAY—THE CONSCIOUS CHILD

1 Ask "Are you choking?"
2 See if the child can cough or speak.
3 Do the Heimlich maneuver if the child is choking:
   a Stand behind the child.
   b Wrap your arms around the child's waist.
   c Make a fist with one hand. Place the thumb side of the fist against the child's abdomen. The fist should be in the middle, above the navel and below the end of the sternum.
   d Give a quick inward and upward thrust.
   e Repeat the abdominal thrusts until the object is expelled or the child loses consciousness.
4 Lay the child down if he or she loses consciousness. (See *Relieving an Obstructed Airway—the Unconscious Child*, below).

RELIEVING AN OBSTRUCTED AIRWAY—THE UNCONSCIOUS CHILD

1 Check for unresponsiveness.
2 Call for help.
3 Logroll the child if he or she is face down. Support the head and neck. Position the child supine on a hard, flat surface.
4 Open the airway. Use the head-tilt/chin-lift maneuver.
5 Check for breathlessness.
6 Give 1 ventilation. Reposition the child's head if you could not ventilate the child. Give 1 more ventilation.
7 Have your helper activate the EMS system.
8 Do the Heimlich maneuver if you could not ventilate the child (Fig. 29-21).
   a Kneel at the child's feet if he or she is on the floor. Stand at the child's feet if he or she is on a table.
   b Place the heel of one hand against the child's abdomen. The hand is in the middle and slightly above the navel and below the end of the sternum.
   c Place your other hand directly on top of the fist on the child's abdomen.
   d Give a quick, upward thrust.
   e Give 6 to 10 abdominal thrusts.
9 Check for a foreign object.
   a Open the child's mouth. Use the tongue-jaw lift maneuver.
   b Look into the child's mouth. Do the finger-sweep maneuver *only* if you see a foreign object.
   c Remove the foreign object if it is seen.
10 Open the airway. Use the head-tilt/chin-lift maneuver.
11 Give 1 ventilation.
12 Repeat steps 8 through 11 as often as necessary.

RELIEVING AN OBSTRUCTED AIRWAY—THE UNCONSCIOUS INFANT

1 Check for unresponsiveness.
2 Call for help.
3 Turn the infant as a unit. Place the infant on a hard, flat surface.
4 Open the airway. Use the head-tilt/chin-lift maneuver. The infant's head is in a "sniffing" position. The head is not hyperextended.
5 Check for breathlessness.
6 Give 1 ventilation. Reposition the infant's head if you could not ventilate. Give another ventilation.
7 Have your helper activate the EMS system.
8 Give 4 back blows (see *Relieving an Obstructed Airway—the Conscious Infant*, page 457).
9 Give 4 chest thrusts (see *Relieving an Obstructed Airway—the Conscious Infant*, page 457).
10 Check for a foreign body (see *Relieving an Obstructed Airway—the Unconscious Child*, above).
11 Open the airway. Use the head-tilt/chin-lift maneuver.
12 Give 1 ventilation.
13 Repeat steps 8 through 12 for as long as necessary.

RELIEVING AN OBSTRUCTED AIRWAY—THE CONSCIOUS INFANT

1 Determine if the infant has an airway obstruction.
2 Hold the infant face down over your forearm or thigh (Fig. 29-22) with one hand. The infant's head should be lower than the trunk.
3 Give 4 back blows with the heel of one hand. The blows are given between the infant's shoulder blades (Fig. 29-23).
4 Support the infant's back with your free hand. Your other hand supports the neck, jaw, and chest. Turn the infant.
5 Place the infant over your thigh with his or her head lower than the trunk (Fig. 29-24).
6 Give chest thrusts:
  a Locate hand position as for chest compressions.
  b Compress the chest 4 times as for chest compressions but at a slower rate (1 every 3 to 5 seconds).
7 Repeat back blows and chest thrusts until the object is expelled or the infant loses consciousness.

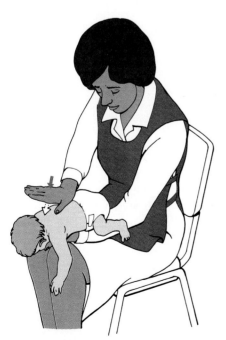

Fig. 29-21 The Heimlich maneuver performed on an unconscious child.

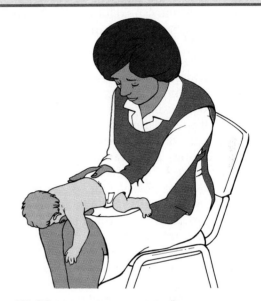

Fig. 29-22 The infant is held face down and supported with one hand. The rescuer supports her arm on her thigh.

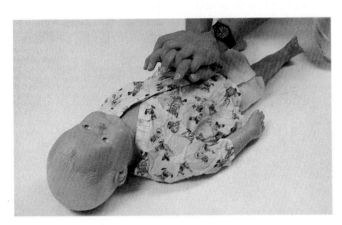

Fig. 29-23 Back blows are given with the heel of one hand. The blows are given between the infant's shoulder blades.

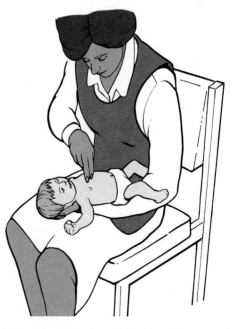

Fig. 29-24 The infant is positioned on the rescuer's thigh for chest thrusts. Hand position for chest thrusts in the infant is the same as for chest compressions.

HEMORRHAGE

Life and body functions require an adequate blood supply. Circulation of blood through the body is also needed. If a blood vessel is torn or cut, bleeding and blood loss occur. The larger the blood vessel, the greater the bleeding and blood loss. *Hemorrhage* is the excessive loss of blood from a blood vessel. If the bleeding is not stopped, death will result.

Hemorrhage may be internal or external. Internal hemorrhage cannot be seen. Bleeding occurs inside the body into tissues and body cavities. Pain, shock (see p. 458), vomiting blood, coughing up blood, and loss of consciousness are signs of internal hemorrhage. There is little you can do for internal bleeding. Keep the person warm, flat, and quiet until medical help arrives. Fluids are not given.

External bleeding is usually seen. However, it may be hidden by clothing. Hemorrhage may be from an injured artery or vein. Bleeding from an artery is bright red and occurs in spurts. There is a steady flow of blood when bleeding is from a vein. Basic emergency care for external hemorrhage involves stopping the bleeding. The treatment of choice is to apply direct pressure to the bleeding site. If direct pressure does not control bleeding, pressure is applied to the artery above the bleeding site. You can do the following to control external hemorrhage.

1. Practice universal precautions. Wear gloves if possible.
2. Place a sterile dressing directly over the wound. Any clean material (handkerchief, towel, cloth, or sanitary napkin) can be used if a sterile dressing is not available.
3. Apply pressure with your hand directly over the bleeding site (Fig. 29-25). Do not release the pressure until the bleeding is controlled.
4. If direct pressure does not control bleeding, apply pressure over the artery above the bleeding site (Fig. 29-26). Use your first three fingers. For example, if bleeding is from the lower arm, apply pressure over the brachial artery. The brachial artery supplies blood to the lower arm.

SHOCK

Shock results when there is an inadequate blood supply to organs and tissues. Blood loss, heart disease, and severe infection can cause shock. Signs and symptoms include a low or falling blood pressure; a rapid and weak pulse; cold, moist and pale skin; rapid respirations; thirst; and restlessness. Confusion and loss of consciousness occur as shock becomes worse.

Shock is possible in any person who is acutely ill or injured. Do the following to prevent and treat shock:

1. Keep the victim lying down.
2. Control hemorrhage.
3. Keep the victim warm. Place a blanket over and under the victim if possible.
4. Reassure the victim.
5. Summon medical assistance.

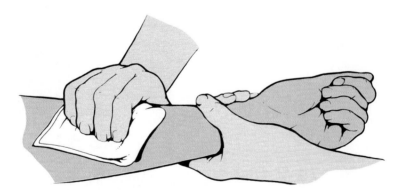

Fig. 29-25 Direct pressure is applied to the wound to stop bleeding. The hand is placed over the wound. (From Parcel GS, Rinear CE: *Basic emergency care of the sick and injured*, ed 4, St Louis, 1990, Mosby–Year Book.)

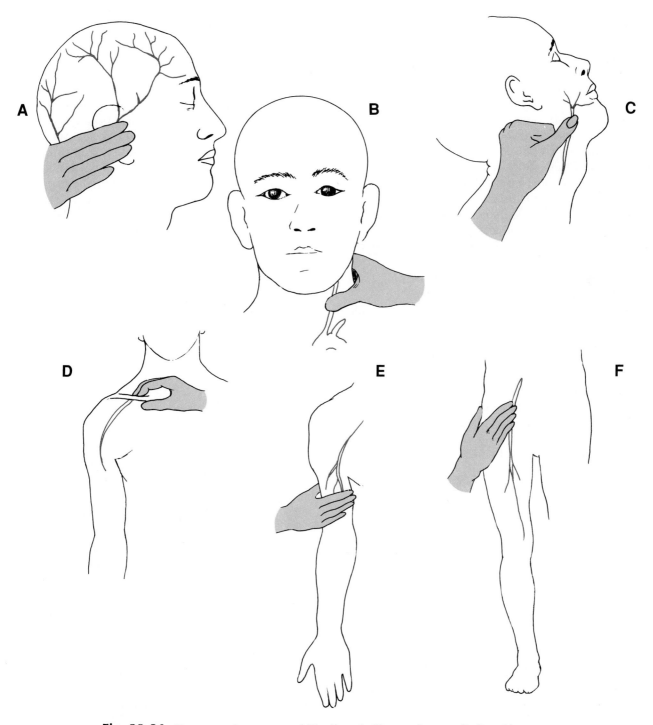

Fig. 29-26 Pressure points to control bleeding. **A,** Temporal artery. **B,** Carotid artery. **C,** External maxillary artery. **D,** Subclavian artery. **E,** Brachial artery. **F,** Femoral artery. (From Billings DM, Stokes LG: *Medical-surgical nursing: common health problems of adults and children across the lifespan*, St Louis, 1982, Mosby–Year Book.)

SEIZURES

Seizures (convulsions) are violent and sudden contractions or tremors of muscles. They are due to an abnormality within the brain. The abnormality may be caused by head injury during birth, high fever, brain tumors, poisoning, and central nervous system infections. Head trauma and lack of blood flow to the brain can also cause seizures. The terms "attack" and "fits" have been used by people outside the health care industry in referring to seizures. Do not use these terms. They have unpleasant and disturbing meanings.

There are many types of seizures. You need to be aware of two types. The *tonic-clonic (grand mal seizure)* has two phases. The tonic phase is first. The person loses consciousness. If standing or sitting, the person falls to the floor. The body is rigid. This is because all the muscles contract at once. The clonic phase is next. Muscle groups contract and relax. This causes jerking and twitching movements of the body. Urinary and fecal incontinence may occur during this phase of the seizure. After the seizure, the patient usually falls into a deep sleep. On awakening, confusion and headache may be experienced.

The *generalized absence (petit mal)* seizure usually lasts about 5 to 15 seconds. There is loss of consciousness, twitching of arm and face muscles, and rolling of the eyes. The person appears to be staring. These seizures occur in children and adolescents.

The person must be protected from injury during a seizure. The following measures are performed:

1. Call for help.
2. Lower the patient to the floor.
3. Place a folded bath blanket or towel under the person's head. You may cradle the person's head in your lap or on a pillow (Fig. 29-27). This prevents the person's head from striking the hard surface of the floor.
4. Turn the head to one side.
5. Loosen tight clothing.
6. Move furniture and equipment away from the person. The person may strike these objects during the uncontrolled body movements.
7. Do not try to restrain body movements during the seizure.
8. Position the person on one side if possible.
9. Summon medical help. Do not leave the person during the seizure.

FAINTING

Fainting is the sudden loss of consciousness from an inadequate blood supply to the brain. Hunger, fatigue, fear, and pain are common causes. Some people faint at the sight of blood or injury. Fainting can also be caused by standing in one position for a long time or being in a warm, crowded room. Dizziness, perspiration, and blackness before the eyes may occur before fainting. The person looks pale. The pulse is weak. Respirations are shallow if consciousness is lost. Emergency care for fainting includes the following:

1. Have the person sit or lie down before fainting occurs.
   a. If sitting, the person should bend forward and place his or her head between the knees (Fig. 29-28).

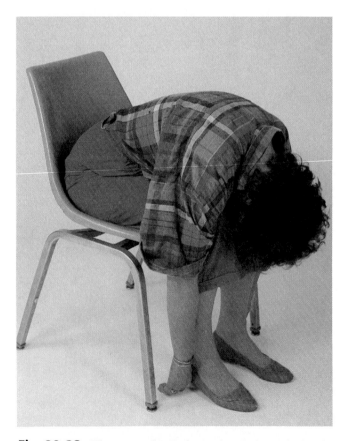

Fig. 29-28 The person bends forward and places the head between the knees to prevent fainting.

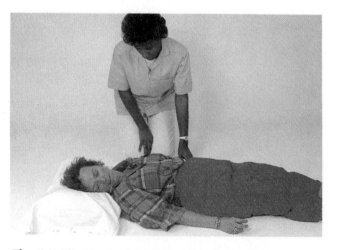

Fig. 29-27 The head is protected during a seizure.

b. If the victim is lying down, the legs should be elevated.
2. Loosen tight clothing.
3. Keep the person lying down if fainting has occurred.
4. Do not let the person get up until symptoms have subsided for about 5 minutes.
5. Help the person to a sitting position after recovery from fainting. Observe for symptoms of fainting.

STROKE

Stroke (cerebrovascular accident) was described in Chapter 25. A stroke occurs when the brain is suddenly deprived of its blood supply. Usually only a part of the brain is affected. A stroke may be caused by a thrombus, an embolus, or cerebral hemorrhage. Cerebral hemorrhage is due to the rupture of a blood vessel in the brain.

The signs of stroke vary. They depend on the size and location of brain injury. Loss of consciousness or semiconsciousness, rapid pulse, labored respirations, elevated blood pressure, vomiting, and hemiplegia are signs of stroke. The person may have aphasia (the inability to speak). Convulsions may occur.

Emergency care includes the following:
1. Turn the person onto the affected side. The affected side is limp and the cheek appears puffy.
2. Elevate the head without flexing the neck.
3. Loosen tight clothing.
4. Keep the person quiet and warm.
5. Reassure the person.
6. Summon medical help.

VOMITING

Vomiting is the act of expelling stomach contents through the mouth. Although it is not a true emergency, vomiting is a sign of illness or injury. It can be life threatening. The vomitus (material vomited) can be aspirated into the respiratory tract and may obstruct the airway. Shock can also occur if large amounts of bright red blood are vomited.

The following measures will help the vomiting patient:
1. Use universal precautions to protect yourself from the person's body fluids and body substances. Wear gloves if possible.
2. Turn the person's head well to one side. This prevents aspiration.
3. Place an emesis basin under the person's chin.
4. Remove the vomitus from the person's immediate environment.
5. Let the person use mouthwash and perform oral hygiene. This helps to eliminate the taste of vomitus.
6. Eliminate odors.
7. Change linens as necessary.

Observe vomitus for color, odor, and the presence of undigested food. Vomitus that looks like coffee grounds contains digested blood. This indicates bleeding. The amount of vomitus is measured. The amount is reported to the nurse and recorded on the I&O sheet. A specimen may be saved for laboratory study. Do not discard vomitus until it has been observed by the nurse.

SUMMARY

Emergencies are sudden and unexpected. They are frightening for the victim and others nearby. Quick action may be needed to save the victim's life and to prevent injuries from becoming worse. Emergencies can occur anywhere. You may be with the victim when an emergency occurs. Staying calm, knowing what to do, and calling for help are important for the victim's physical and psychological well-being.

Cardiac arrest and airway obstruction are deadly and frightening emergencies. They may occur anywhere and at any time. A basic life support course will prepare you for these emergencies. You may be able to save a person's life with the basic life support procedures.

A first aid course is also beneficial. A first aid course will prepare you to function if injuries occur. Examples include insect stings, fractures, frostbite, poisoning, and eye injuries. The general rules of emergency care apply to any emergency situation. You may not know how to care for the specific injury. However, you can help the victim by following the general rules of emergency care.

REVIEW QUESTIONS

Circle the best *answer.*

1 The goals of first aid are to
   a Call for help and keep the victim warm
   b Prevent death and prevent injuries from becoming worse
   c Stay calm and perform emergency measures
   d Reassure the victim and keep bystanders away

2 When giving first aid, you should
   a Be aware of your own limitations
   b Move the victim
   c Give the victim fluids
   d Perform any necessary emergency measures

3 Cardiac arrest is
   a The same as stroke
   b The sudden stopping of heart action and breathing
   c The sudden loss of consciousness
   d The condition that results when there is inadequate blood supply to the organs and tissues of the body

4 Which is *not* a sign of cardiac arrest?
   a No pulse
   b No breathing
   c A sudden drop in blood pressure
   d Unconsciousness

5 You are to give mouth-to-mouth resuscitation to an adult. You should do the following *except*
   a Pinch the victim's nostrils shut
   b Place your mouth tightly over the victim's mouth
   c Blow air into the victim's mouth as you exhale
   d Cover the victim's nose with your mouth

6 External chest compressions are performed on an adult. The chest is compressed
   a ½ to 1 inch with the index and middle fingers
   b 1 to 1½ inches with the heel of one hand
   c 1½ to 2 inches with two hands
   d With one hand in the middle of the sternum

7 Which does *not* determine breathlessness?
   a Looking to see if the chest rises and falls
   b Counting respirations for 30 seconds
   c Listening for the escape of air
   d Feeling for the flow of air

8 Which is used to feel for a pulse during adult CPR?
   a The apical pulse
   b The brachial pulse
   c The carotid pulse
   d The dorsalis pedis pulse

9 How many ventilations are given at the beginning of CPR?
   a 1
   b 2
   c 3
   d 4

10 You are performing CPR alone. Which is *false?*
    a Give 2 ventilations after every 15 compressions
    b Check for a pulse after 1 minute
    c Give 1 ventilation after every fifth compression
    d Count out loud

11 CPR is being given by two people. Ventilations are given
    a After every fifth compression
    b After every fifteenth compression
    c After every compression
    d Only when the positions are changed

12 External cardiac compressions are given to an infant at a rate of
    a 60 per minute
    b 75 per minute
    c 80 per minute
    d 100 per minute

13 The most common cause of obstructed airway in adults is
    a A loose denture
    b Meat
    c Marbles
    d Candy

14 If airway obstruction occurs, the victim usually
    a Clutches at the throat
    b Can speak, cough, and breathe
    c Is calm
    d Has a seizure

15 The Heimlich maneuver is used to relieve an obstructed airway. Which is *false?*
    a The victim can be standing, sitting, or lying down.
    b A fist is made with one hand.
    c The thrusts are given inward and upward at the lower end of the sternum.
    d The hands are positioned in the middle between the waist and lower end of the sternum.

16 A victim has an obstructed airway. You can use poking motions when using the finger-sweep maneuver.
    a True
    b False

17 Arterial bleeding
    a Cannot be seen
    b Occurs in spurts
    c Is dark red
    d Oozes from the wound

18 A victim is hemorrhaging from the left forearm. Your first action is to
    a Lower the body part
    b Apply pressure to the brachial artery
    c Apply direct pressure to the wound
    d Cover the victim

19 The signs of shock are
- a Rising blood pressure, rapid pulse, and slow respirations
- b Rapid pulse, rapid respirations, and warm skin
- c Falling blood pressure; rapid pulse and respirations; and skin that is cold, moist, and pale
- d Falling blood pressure; slow pulse and respirations; thirst; restlessness; and warm, flushed skin

20 A victim is in shock. You should
- a Give mouth-to-mouth resuscitation
- b Keep the victim lying down
- c Remove the victim's clothing
- d Place the victim in Trendelenburg position

21 These statements relate to tonic-clonic seizures. Which is *false?*
- a There is contraction of all muscles at once
- b The person may stop breathing
- c The seizure usually lasts about 10 to 20 seconds
- d There is loss of consciousness during the seizure

22 A person is about to faint. Which is *false?*
- a Take the person outside for some fresh air.
- b Have the person sit or lie down.
- c Loosen tight clothing.
- d Elevate the legs if the person is lying down.

23 Emergency care of the stroke victim includes the following *except*
- a Positioning the patient on the affected side
- b Giving the person sips of water
- c Loosening tight clothing
- d Keeping the person quiet and warm

24 Vomiting is dangerous because of
- a Aspiration
- b Cardiac arrest
- c Fluid loss
- d Stroke

Answers

24 a	**16** b	**8** c
23 b	**15** c	**7** b
22 a	**14** a	**6** c
21 c	**13** b	**5** d
20 b	**12** d	**4** c
19 c	**11** a	**3** b
18 c	**10** c	**2** a
17 b	**9** b	**1** b

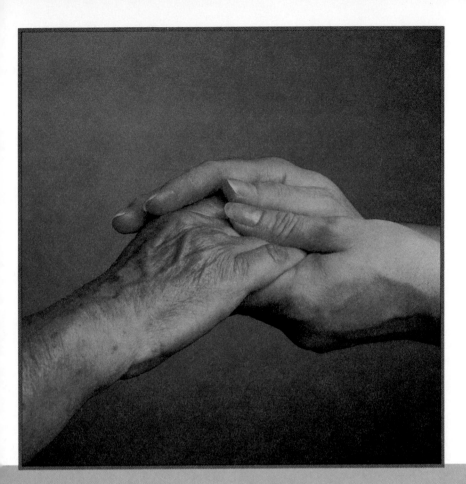

The Dying Patient

30

OBJECTIVES

- Define the key terms listed in this chapter
- Describe terminal illness
- Identify two psychological forces that influence living and dying
- Explain how religion influences attitudes about death
- Describe the beliefs about death held by different age-groups
- Describe the five stages of dying
- Explain how the dying person's psychological, social, and spiritual needs can be met
- Explain how you can help meet the physical needs of the dying patient
- Describe the needs of the family during the dying process
- Describe hospice care
- Explain what is meant by a "do not resuscitate" order
- Identify the signs of approaching death and the signs of death
- Assist in giving postmortem care

postmortem After (post) death (mortem)

reincarnation The belief that the spirit or soul is reborn in another human body or in another form of life

rigor mortis The stiffness or rigidity (rigor) of skeletal muscles that occurs after death (mortis)

terminal illness An illness or injury for which there is no reasonable expectation of recovery

Dying people are cared for in hospitals, nursing facilities, or in their homes. Many are part of hospice programs (see Chapter 1). Death may be sudden and without warning. Often it is expected.

Health workers see death often. However, many are unsure of their feelings about death. They are uncomfortable with dying patients and the subject of death. Dying patients represent helplessness and failure to cure. They are also reminders of our own eventual death.

You must examine your own feelings about death. Your attitude about death and dying affects the care you give. You will help meet the patient's physical, psychological, social, and spiritual needs. Therefore you need to understand the dying process. Then you can approach the dying person with care, kindness, and respect.

TERMINAL ILLNESS

Many illnesses and diseases can be cured or controlled. Others have no cure. Many injuries can be repaired. Others are so serious that the body cannot function. Recovery is not expected. The disease or injury will result in death. An illness or injury for which there is no reasonable expectation of recovery is a *terminal illness*.

Doctors cannot tell exactly when death will occur from a terminal illness. A person may have days, months, weeks, or years to live. Predictions have been wrong. People expected to live for only a short time have lived for years. Others have been expected to live for a longer time. They have died sooner than expected.

Modern medicine has resulted in cures or has prolonged life in many cases. Future research is likely to bring new cures. However, two very powerful psychological forces influence living and dying. They are hope and the will to live. People have died sooner than expected or for no apparent reason when they have lost hope or the will to live.

ATTITUDES ABOUT DEATH

Experiences, culture, religion, and age influence a person's attitude about death. Many people fear death. Others do not believe they will die. Some look forward to and accept death. Attitudes and beliefs about death often change as a person grows older. They are also affected by changing circumstances.

In the United States, dying people are usually cared for in health facilities. When death occurs, the funeral director is notified. The funeral director takes the body from the facility and prepares it for funeral practices and burial. Consequently, many adults and children have never had contact with a dying person. Nor have they been present when death occurred. The process of dying and death is not seen. Therefore it is viewed as frightening, morbid, and a mystery.

These practices and attitudes are different from those of other cultures. Dying people are cared for at home by family. The family is at the bedside to comfort the dying person and each other. Some families care for the body after death and prepare it for burial.

Attitudes about death are closely related to religion. Some believe that life after death will be free of suffering and hardship. They also believe there will be a reunion with family and loved ones. Many believe there is punishment and suffering in the afterlife for sins and misdeeds. Others do not believe in the afterlife. They believe that death is the end of life. There are also religious beliefs about the form of the human body after death. Some believe that the body keeps its physical form. Others believe that only the spirit or soul is present in the afterlife. Reincarnation is another belief. *Reincarnation* is the belief that the spirit or soul is reborn into another human body or into another form of life. Many people strengthen their religious beliefs during the process of dying. Religion is also a source of comfort for the dying person and the family.

Ideas about death change as people grow older. Infants and toddlers have no concept of death. Children between the ages of 3 and 5 start to be curious and have ideas about death. They recognize the death of family members or pets and notice dead birds or bugs. They think death is temporary. Children often blame themselves when someone or something dies. They see the event as punishment for being bad. When children ask questions about death, adults often give answers that cause fear and confusion. Children who are told, "He is sleeping," may be afraid to go to sleep.

Between the ages of 5 and 7 years, children view death as final. Children this age do not see death in relation to themselves. Death is something that happens to other people. They also think death can be avoided. Children associate death with punishment and mutilation of the body. It is also associated with witches, ghosts, goblins, and monsters. These ideas come from fairy tales, cartoons, movies, and television.

Adults have more fears about death than children do. They fear pain and suffering, dying alone, and the invasion of privacy. They also fear loneliness and separation from family and loved ones. They worry about who will care for and support those left behind. Adults often resent death. This is particularly true when it interferes with plans, hopes, dreams, and ambitions.

Elderly people usually have fewer fears than younger adults do. They are more accepting that death will occur. They have had more experiences with dying and death. Many have lost family members and friends. Some welcome death as freedom from pain, suffering, and disability. Like younger adults, elderly persons often fear dying alone.

THE STAGES OF DYING

Dr. Elisabeth Kübler-Ross has identified five stages of dying. They are denial, anger, bargaining, depression, and acceptance. During *denial*, persons refuse to believe they are dying. "No, not me," is a common response. The person believes a mistake has been made. Information about the illness or injury is not heard. The person cannot deal with any problem or decision about the illness or injury. This stage can last for a few hours, days, or much longer. Some people are still in denial when they die.

Anger is the second stage of dying. The person thinks, "Why me?" People in this stage feel anger and rage. They envy and resent those who have life and health. Family, friends, and the health team are usually targets of their anger. They blame others. Fault is found with those who are loved and needed the most. The health team and family may have a hard time dealing with patients during this stage. Remember that anger is a normal, healthy reaction. Do not take the person's anger personally. You must control any urge to attack back or avoid the patient.

The third stage is *bargaining*. The anger has passed. The person now says, "Yes, me, but. . ." Often there is bargaining with God for more time. Promises are made in exchange for more time. The person may want to see a child marry, see a grandchild, have one more Christmas, or live to see some important event. Usually more promises are made as the person makes "just one more" request. This stage may not be obvious to you. Bargaining is usually done privately and on a spiritual level.

Depression is the fourth stage. The person thinks, "Yes, me." The person is very sad. There is mourning over things that have been lost and the future loss of life. The person may cry or say little. Sometimes the person will talk about people and things that will be left behind.

The fifth and final stage of dying is *acceptance* of death. The person is calm and at peace. The person has said what needs to be said. Unfinished business is completed. The person is ready to accept death. A person may be in this stage for many months or years. Reaching the acceptance stage does not mean that death is near.

Dying persons do not always pass through all five stages. A person may never get beyond a certain stage. Some people move back and forth between stages. For example, a person who has reached acceptance may move back to bargaining. Then he or she may move forward to acceptance. Some people are in one stage until death.

PSYCHOLOGICAL, SOCIAL, AND SPIRITUAL NEEDS

Dying people continue to have psychological, social, and spiritual needs. They may want family and friends present. They may want to talk about the fears, worries, and anxieties of dying. Some want to be alone. Often they want to talk to a member of the nursing team. Patients often need to talk during the night. Things are quiet and there are few distractions at this time.

There are two very important aspects of communication when dealing with the dying patient. These are listening and touch. The patient is the one who needs to talk, express feelings, and share worries and concerns. Just being there and listening helps to meet the person's psychological and social needs. Do not worry about saying the wrong thing. Nor should you worry about finding the right words to comfort and cheer the person. Nothing really must be said. Being there for the patient is what counts. Touch can convey caring and concern when words cannot. Sometimes patients do not want to talk but need you nearby. Do not feel that you need to talk. Silence, along with touch, is a powerful and meaningful way to communicate.

Spiritual needs are important. The person may wish to see a priest, rabbi, or minister. The person may also want to participate in religious practices. Privacy is provided during spiritual moments. Courtesy is given to the clergy. The patient is allowed to have religious objects nearby, such as medals, pictures, statues, or Bibles. You must handle these items like other valuables.

PHYSICAL NEEDS

Dying may take a few minutes, hours, days, or weeks. There is general slowing of body processes, weakness, and changes in the level of consciousness. The patient is allowed to be as independent as possible. As the patient's condition weakens, the nursing team helps meet the patient's basic needs. The patient may totally depend on others for basic needs and activities of daily living. Every effort is made to promote the person's physical and psychological comfort. The person is allowed to die in peace and with dignity.

Vision, Hearing, and Speech

Vision becomes blurred and gradually fails during the dying process. The patient naturally turns toward light. A darkened room may frighten the patient. The eyes may be half open. Secretions may collect in the corners of the eyes. Because of failing vision, you need to explain what is being done to the patient or in the room. The room should be well lit. However, bright lights and glares are avoided. Good eye care is essential (see Chapter 13). If the eyes stay open, a nurse may apply a protective ointment. Then the eyes are covered with moistened pads to protect them from injury.

Speech becomes difficult. It may be hard to understand the patient. Sometimes the patient cannot speak. The nursing team needs to anticipate the patient's needs. The patient is not asked questions that have long answers. "Yes" or "no" questions can be asked. These are kept to a minimum. Though speech may be hard or impossible for the patient, you must still talk to him or her.

Hearing is one of the last functions to be lost during the dying process. Many people hear until the moment of death. Even if unconscious, the person may hear. Always assume that the dying patient, or any unconscious patient, can hear. Speak in a normal voice, provide reassurance and explanations about care, and offer words of comfort. Topics that could upset the patient are avoided.

Mouth, Nose, and Skin

Oral hygiene is very important for comfort. Routine mouth care is usually adequate if the patient can eat and drink. Frequent oral hygiene is given as death approaches and when there is difficulty taking oral fluids. Oral hygiene is also important if mucus collects in the mouth and the patient cannot swallow.

Crusting and irritation of the nostrils can occur. Common causes are increased nasal secretions, an oxygen cannula, or an NG tube. Careful cleansing of the nose is important. The nurse may have you apply a lubricant to the nostrils.

Circulation fails, and body temperature rises as death approaches. The skin is cool and pale. Perspiration increases. Good skin care, bathing, and the prevention of decubiti are necessary. Linens and gowns are changed as often as needed because of perspiration. Although the skin feels cool, only light bed coverings may be needed. Blankets may make the person feel warm and cause restlessness.

Elimination

Dying patients may have urinary and anal incontinence. Waterproof bed protectors are used. Perineal care is given as necessary. Some patients are constipated and have urinary retention. Doctors may order enemas. Foley catheters may be ordered for urinary retention or incontinence. You may be responsible for giving enemas and catheter care.

Comfort and Positioning

Measures are taken to promote comfort. Good skin care, personal hygiene, back massages, and oral hygiene help to increase comfort. Some patients have severe pain. They need strong pain medications, which are given by nurses. You can also promote comfort by frequent position changes. Good body alignment using supportive devices also promotes comfort. Care is taken when turning the patient. You may need help to turn the patient slowly and gently. Patients with breathing difficulties usually prefer semi-Fowler's position.

The Patient's Room

The patient's room should be as pleasant as possible. Besides being well lit, the room should be well ventilated. Unnecessary equipment is removed. Some equipment is upsetting to look at (suction machines, drainage containers). If possible, this equipment is kept out of the patient's sight. The room should be near the nurse's station. The patient can be watched more carefully.

Mementos, pictures, cards, flowers, religious objects, and other significant items comfort and reassure the patient. Arranging them within the patient's view is appreciated. The patient and family are allowed to arrange the room according to the patient's wishes. This helps meet the needs of love, belonging, and esteem. The room should be comfortable, pleasant, and reflect the person's choices. This promotes physical and psychological comfort.

THE PATIENT'S FAMILY

The family is going through a hard time. It may be very difficult to find the right words to comfort them. You can show your feelings to the family by being available, courteous, and considerate. Also use touch to show your concern.

The family is usually allowed to spend a lot of time with their loved one. Normal visiting hours usually do not apply if the patient is dying. You must respect the patient's and family's right to privacy. They need as much time together as possible. However, patient care cannot be neglected just because the family is present. Most facilities let family members help give care if they wish. If they do not want to help, you can suggest that they take a break. They can use the time to have a beverage or meal.

The family may be very tired, sad, and tearful. They need support and understanding. Watching a loved one die is very painful. Dealing with the eventual loss of that person is painful also. The family must be given every possible courtesy and respect. They may find comfort in a visit from a member of the clergy. You need to communicate this request to the nurse immediately.

HOSPICE CARE

Many patients seek hospice care (see Chapter 1) when they are dying. Hospices are concerned with the physical, emotional, social, and spiritual needs of dying patients and their families. Hospices are not concerned with cures or with life-saving procedures. Rather, they emphasize pain relief and comfort measures. The goal of hospice care is to improve the dying person's quality of life.

A hospice may be part of a health facility or a separate facility. Many hospices offer home care. Follow-up care and support groups for survivors are also part of hospice services.

"DO NOT RESUSCITATE" ORDERS

When death is sudden and unexpected, every effort is made to save the person's life. CPR is started, and an emergency "code" is called (see Chapter 29). Nurses, doctors, and other emergency personnel rush to the person's bedside. Emergency and life-saving equipment is also brought to the bedside. CPR and other life-support measures are continued until the person is resuscitated or until the doctor declares the person dead.

Doctors often write "do not resuscitate" (DNR) or "no code" orders for terminally ill patients. This means that no attempts will be made to resuscitate the person. The person will be allowed to die in peace and with dignity. The orders are often written after the patient or family has been consulted. Some patients have written instructions about life-prolonging measures. These are called "living wills." A living will usually states that the person does not want his or her life prolonged by extraordinary means if there is no reasonable expectation of recovery.

SIGNS OF DEATH

You need to know the signs of approaching death. These signs may occur rapidly or gradually.
1. Movement, muscle tone, and sensation are lost. This usually begins in the feet and legs. It eventually spreads to the rest of the body. When the

mouth muscles relax, the jaw drops. The mouth may stay open. There is often a peaceful facial expression.
2. Peristalsis and other gastrointestinal functions slow down. There may be abdominal distention, anal incontinence, impaction, nausea, and vomiting.
3. Circulation fails, and body temperature rises. The person feels cool or cold, looks pale, and perspires heavily. The pulse is fast, weak, and irregular. The blood pressure begins to fall.
4. The respiratory system fails. Cheyne-Stokes, slow, or rapid and shallow respirations may be observed. Mucus accumulates in the respiratory tract. This causes the "death rattle" that is heard.
5. Pain decreases as the patient loses consciousness. However, some people are conscious until the moment of death.

The signs of death include no pulse, respirations, or blood pressure. The pupils are fixed and dilated. A doctor determines that death has occurred and pronounces the person dead.

CARE OF THE BODY AFTER DEATH

Care of the body after (post) death (mortem) is called *postmortem* care. A nurse is responsible for postmortem care. You may be asked to assist. The care begins as soon as the doctor pronounces the patient dead. Universal precautions are followed when giving postmortem care. You may have contact with infected body fluids or body substances.

Postmortem care is done to maintain good appearance of the body. Discoloration and skin damage are prevented. Postmortem care also includes gathering valuables and personal possessions for the family. The right to privacy and the right to be treated with dignity and respect also apply after death.

Within 2 to 4 hours after death, rigor mortis develops. *Rigor mortis* is the stiffness or rigidity (rigor) of skeletal muscles. It occurs after death (mortis). Postmortem care involves positioning the body in normal alignment before rigor mortis sets in. There is another reason for placing the body in a normal position. The family may wish to see the body before it is taken to the morgue or funeral home. The body should appear in a comfortable and natural position for viewing by the family.

In some facilities the body is prepared only for viewing. Postmortem care is completed later by the funeral director.

SUMMARY

American society values youth, beauty, and life. The topic of death is usually avoided. Many people die in health facilities. Therefore health workers see death often.

ASSISTING WITH POSTMORTEM CARE

1 Wash your hands.
2 Collect the following equipment:
  a Postmortem kit if used in your facility (shroud, gown, two tags, gauze squares, and safety pins)
  b Valuables list
  c Waterproof bed protectors
  d Wash basin
  e Bath towels
  f Washcloth
  g Tape
  h Dressing
  i Disposable gloves
3 Provide for privacy.
4 Raise the bed to its highest level.
5 Make sure the bed is flat.
6 Put on the gloves.
7 Position the body supine. The arms and legs are straight. Place a pillow under the head and shoulders (Fig. 30-1).
8 Close the eyes. Gently pull the eyelids over the eyes. Apply a moistened cotton ball gently over the eyelid if the eye will not stay closed.
9 Insert dentures if it is facility policy. If not, put them in a labeled denture container.
10 Close the mouth. Place a rolled towel under the chin to support the mouth in the closed position if necessary.
11 Remove all jewelry except for wedding rings. List the jewelry that was removed. Place the jewelry and the list in an envelope to be given to the family.
12 Place a cotton ball over the ring. Secure it in place with tape.
13 Remove drainage bottles, bags, and containers. Leave tubes and catheters in place if an autopsy is to be performed. Ask the nurse about removal of tubes.
14 Bathe soiled areas with plain water. Dry thoroughly.
15 Place a bed protector under the buttocks.
16 Remove soiled dressings and replace them with clean ones.

17 Put a clean gown on the body. Make sure the body is positioned as in step 7.
18 Brush and comb the hair if necessary.
19 Fill out the identification tags. Tie one to an ankle or to the right big toe.
20 Cover the body to the shoulders with a sheet if the family is to view the body.
21 Gather all of the patient's belongings. Put them in a bag labeled with the person's name.
22 Remove all used supplies, equipment, and linens except the shroud and the other identification tag. Make sure the room is neat. Adjust the lighting so that it is soft.
23 Let the family view the body. Provide for privacy. Give the patient's belongings to the family.
24 Get a stretcher.
25 Place the body on the shroud or cover the body with a sheet after the family has left the room. Apply the shroud as in Figure 30-2.
  a Bring the top down over the head
  b Fold the bottom up over the feet
  c Fold the sides over the body
26 Secure the shroud in place with safety pins or tape.
27 Attach the second ID tag to the shroud.
28 Move the body onto the stretcher with the help of co-workers.
29 Have the doors to other patient rooms along the hallway closed.
30 Transport the body to the morgue. Leave the denture cup with the body.
31 Return the stretcher to its proper place.
32 Strip the patient's unit.
33 Remove the gloves.
34 Wash your hands.
35 Report the following to the nurse:
  a The time the body was taken to the morgue
  b What was done with jewelry and personal items
  c What was done with dentures

You may be uncomfortable with the subject of death. If so, you will be uncomfortable with the dying patient. Some people believe that medicine should be able to keep people alive. These people may be angry and frustrated with the dying patient. Certain behaviors are seen when health workers do not feel comfortable with death and dying. The behaviors include avoiding the patient, nervous talking, hurried care, rough handling, and minimizing the patient's needs. You may need to discuss your feelings about death with a nurse, other health workers, or a member of the clergy. This will help you develop a more positive attitude about death.

The terminally ill patient should be allowed to die with peace and dignity. The person is encouraged to be independent for as long as possible. As the person's

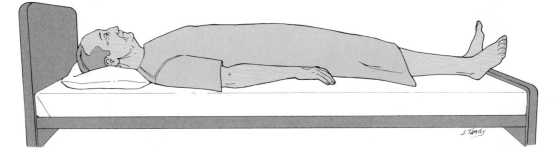

Fig. 30-1   The body is in the dorsal recumbent position. Arms are straight at the sides. There is a pillow under the head and shoulders.

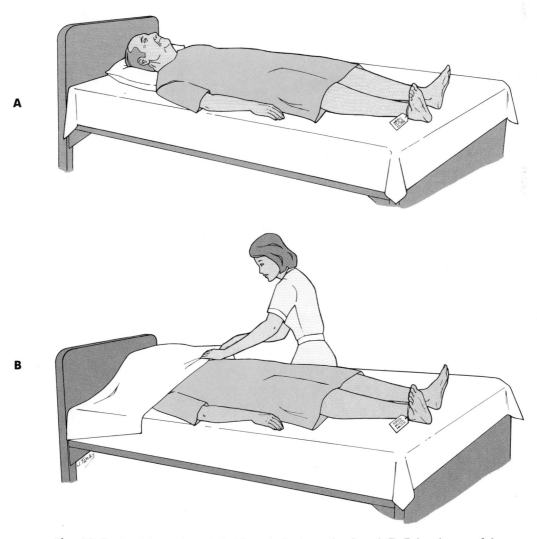

Fig. 30-2   Applying a shroud. **A,** Place the body on the shroud. **B,** Bring the top of the shroud down over the head.

Continued.

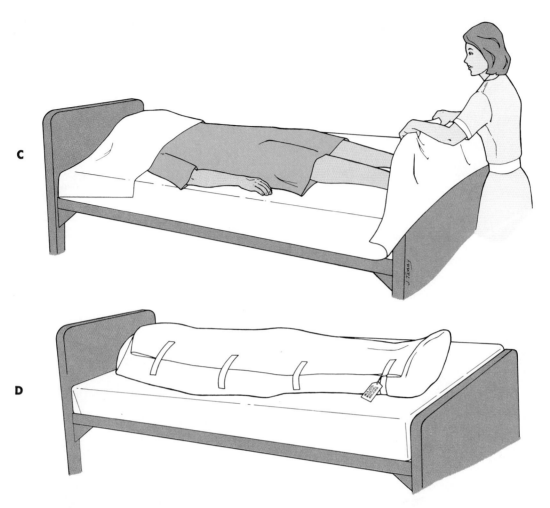

Fig. 30-2 cont'd C, Fold the bottom over the feet. **D,** Fold the sides over the body, tape or pin the sides together, and attach the identification tag.

condition weakens, the nursing team is needed more and more for care and comfort. Even though the person is dying, basic needs continue.

The health team is concerned with the dying person's psychological, social, and spiritual comfort. Visits from the clergy are often appreciated. The dying person also likes when staff members visit often, sit quietly at the bedside, and use touch. Remember that silence and touch are very effective ways to communicate with the patient and family. The patient's right to privacy also needs your attention. The right to privacy is protected before and after death.

Postmortem care is given after death. Each facility has its own policies and procedures about care of the body after death. Postmortem care always includes treating the body with dignity and respect, and respecting the right to privacy.

REVIEW QUESTIONS

Circle the best *answer.*

1 Which is *true?*
   a Death from terminal illness is sudden and un-expected.
   b Doctors know when death will occur.
   c An illness is terminal when there is no reasonable hope of recovery.
   d All severe injuries result in death.

2 Which psychological forces influence living and dying?
   a Hope and the will to live
   b Reincarnation and belief in the afterlife
   c Denial and anger
   d Bargaining and depression

3 These statements relate to attitudes about death. Which is *false?*
   a Dying people are often cared for in health facilities.
   b Attitudes about death are influenced by religion.
   c Infants and toddlers understand death.
   d Young children often blame themselves when someone dies.

4 Reincarnation is the belief that
   a There is no afterlife
   b The spirit or soul is reborn into another human body or another form of life
   c The body keeps its physical form in the afterlife
   d Only the spirit or soul is present in the afterlife

5 Children between the ages of 5 and 7 view death as
   a Temporary
   b Final
   c Adults do
   d Going to sleep

6 Adults and the elderly usually fear
   a Dying alone
   b Punishment for sins
   c Reincarnation
   d The five stages of dying

7 Persons in the stage of denial
   a Are angry
   b Make "deals" with God
   c Are sad and quiet
   d Refuse to believe they are dying

8 The dying person tries to gain more time during
   a Anger
   b Bargaining
   c Depression
   d Acceptance

9 When caring for the dying patient, you should
   a Use touch and listening
   b Do most of the talking
   c Keep the room darkened
   d Speak in a loud voice

10 As death nears, the last sense to be lost is
   a Sight
   b Taste
   c Smell
   d Hearing

11 Care of the dying patient includes the following *except*
   a Eye care
   b Mouth care
   c Active range-of-motion exercises
   d Position changes

12 The dying patient is positioned in
   a The supine position
   b The Fowler's position
   c Good body alignment
   d The dorsal recumbent position

13 A "do not resuscitate" order has been written. This means that
   a CPR will not be done
   b The person has a living will
   c Life-prolonging measures will be carried out
   d The person will be kept alive as long as possible

14 Which are *not* signs of approaching death?
   a Increased body temperature and rapid pulse
   b Loss of movement and muscle tone
   c Increased pain and blood pressure
   d Cheyne-Stokes respirations and the "death rattle"

15 The signs of death are
   a Convulsions and incontinence
   b No pulse, respirations, or blood pressure
   c Loss of consciousness and convulsions
   d The eyes stay open, there are no muscle movements, and the body is rigid

16 Postmortem care is done
   a After rigor mortis sets in
   b After the doctor pronounces the person dead
   c When the funeral director arrives for the body
   d After the family has viewed the body

Answers

				6	a
16	b	11	c	5	b
15	b	10	d	4	b
14	c	9	a	3	c
13	a	8	b	2	a
12	c	7	d	1	c

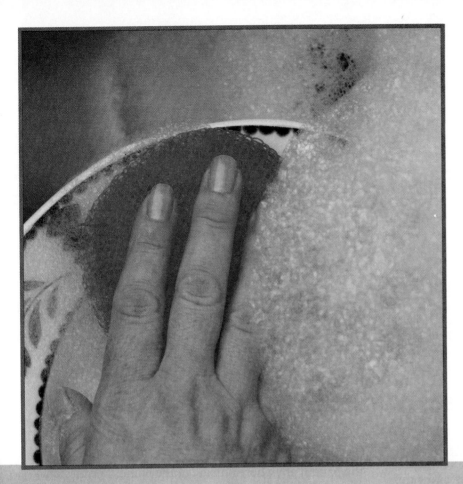

The Home Health Care Assistant

31

OBJECTIVES

- Describe home health care and the agencies that employ home health care assistants
- Describe the responsibilities of home health care assistants
- Describe the qualities and characteristics of the home health care assistant
- List the emergency phone numbers to be kept near the phone
- Identify aspects of the home environment and family relationships that need consideration
- Describe how to save time when doing housekeeping
- Identify infection control measures to be practiced in the home
- Explain how to keep the kitchen and bathroom clean
- Describe the responsibilities of home health care assistants in preparing meals and shopping
- Explain how laundry should be done
- Identify what to record and report to the nurse

Many chronically ill and disabled people are cared for at home. Home care is often preferred for many reasons. The cost of care in hospitals and nursing facilities is high. Inadequate care is given in many nursing facilities. There is a more important reason for home health care. Most people are happier and more secure in their own homes.

"Home health care aide," "home health aide," and "home health care assistant" refer to the nursing assistant employed to give home care.

HOME HEALTH CARE

The home-bound person is given the necessary assistance to meet basic needs. Housekeeping, laundry, shopping, and meal preparation may also be provided. Visiting Nurse Associations, public health departments, some hospitals, and social service agencies provide home care. Home health agencies may be owned by corporations or private companies. You may work for one of these groups. You may also be hired privately by families.

You must always work under the supervision of RNs or doctors. The same ethical and legal guidelines must be followed when working in a hospital, nursing facility, or private home. The procedures and rules presented in this book can be practiced in the home. However, they are performed as directed by the RN or physician.

You may be needed in the home for many reasons. The family may need help giving physical care. Help may be needed to turn, reposition, transfer, or ambulate the patient. The family may be unable to give care. Work responsibilities and small children may take the family's time. The spouse or family members may also have physical limitations. They may be unable to give care. You may tend to all of the individual's personal care needs. The assignment may also include providing a safe, clean living area.

You may be assigned to the same person in one home every day. The assignment may involve 2 or 3 people in different homes. The amount of care and housekeeping required influences the assignment.

The home-bound patient may be any age. Infants, young children, teenagers, adults, and elderly persons may need home care (Fig. 31-1). The diseases, disabilities, and conditions of home care patients vary. The problems may be acute or chronic. Home care may be needed for a short or long time.

THE HOME HEALTH CARE ASSISTANT

The home health care assistant provides patient care and home services. The extent of the home services depends on the needs of the patient and family.

Responsibilities

You are advised to review the roles, responsibilities, and the legal and ethical guidelines described in Chapter 2. Besides patient care, you may be assigned to:

1. Perform light housekeeping so that rooms are clean and neat.
2. Do laundry. The patient's clothing and linens are washed, ironed, and mended as needed. Family laundry may also be done.
3. Shop for groceries and other household items as needed and directed.
4. Prepare and serve nutritious meals. This includes planning menus, following special diets, and feeding the patient if necessary.
5. Clean and use home appliances to perform personal care and housekeeping duties.

There are limitations to the services provided by home health care assistants. Heavy housekeeping is not done. This includes moving heavy furniture, waxing floors, shampooing carpets, washing windows, cleaning rugs or drapes, and carrying firewood, coal, or ash containers. It may be necessary to take the patient to the doctor's office or to other appointments. The supervisor's permission is needed before taking the patient anywhere outside of the home. Permission is also needed for providing transportation or running errands for the patient or family.

Qualities and Characteristics

Home health care assistants must have the qualities and characteristics described in Chapter 2. Working in the home is different from working in a health facility. You work alone in the home. An RN is available by phone. Occasionally the RN visits the patient in the home. However, an RN is not immediately

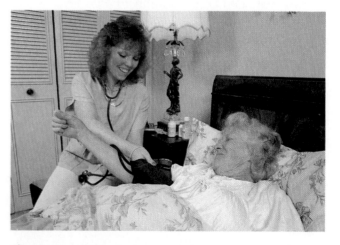

Fig. 31-1 A home health care assistant caring for a patient in the home.

available to give help at the bedside or to handle emergencies.

You must understand the patient's needs. Personal care activities and other procedures must be performed skillfully and safely. You must be able to work alone without supervision. Self-discipline is essential. You must arrive at homes on time. Activities are organized so that personal care needs and housekeeping tasks are fulfilled. Temptations are avoided. Watching television, talking on the telephone, and stopping to have an extra cup of coffee are avoided. Time is spent completing assignments rather than visiting with the patient or family. Efficient use of time is necessary.

Home health care presents certain situations that are not found in health facilities. You may be responsible for shopping. Therefore the patient's money is handled. Honesty and thriftiness must be practiced. The items purchased, the cost, the total amount spent, and the amount of money returned are accurately reported to the patient or family. Nursing assistants handle valuables and personal possessions in health facilities. However, access to the patient's property is far greater in the home. Home furnishings, appliances, linens, and household items are used for personal care and housekeeping duties. The property of the patient and family must be treated with respect. Damage must be prevented. The manufacturer's instructions should be read before using any appliance. The appliance is cleaned after use.

A home care assignment must be fulfilled. You must never leave in the middle of an assignment. Unfortunately, conflicts or problems may develop in caring for the patient or doing housekeeping. Every effort must be made to finish the assignment. The problem should be explained to your supervisor. The supervisor will try to make any needed changes in the situation. You must not walk out on the patient. To do so would leave the patient in an unsafe situation. Walking out is a most unethical behavior.

Ability to Handle Emergency Situations

Emergencies may occur. You must handle emergencies calmly. Basic first aid or emergency care must be given (see Chapter 29). The appropriate people must be notified. The following telephone numbers are kept by the phone:
1. Fire department
2. Police department
3. Ambulance
4. Supervisor
5. Doctor
6. Hospital
7. Responsible family member (home and work numbers)
8. Poison control center

The urgency and nature of the situation determines who is notified first. Some situations require simple first aid. Others threaten the life of the patient and those in the home. You need to learn the differences between simple and life-threatening emergencies.

Safety hazards in the home must be identified. The supervisor and appropriate family members are notified of the safety hazards. You must be ready to act in the event of a fire. Identify exits from the home at the start of the assignment. You also need to know how to move the patient out of the home. Chapter 8 describes fire safety and accident prevention in the home.

THE HOME ENVIRONMENT

Homes vary in size, cleanliness, and furnishings. The type and amount of equipment available for care and housekeeping also varies. Some homes are luxurious in construction and furnishings. Others reflect the poverty of those who live there. Whether rich or poor, each patient and family is treated with respect, kindness, and dignity. Judgments are not made about the patient's life-style, habits, religion, or culture. Whenever possible, the patient's cultural and religious practices are included when planning and preparing meals (see Chapter 16). They are also included when planning care (see Chapter 5).

Family Relationships

Home health care provides opportunities to interact with families. The personalities and attitudes of family members influence the mood in the home. Many family relationships are happy and supportive. However, poor relationships do exist. Mental illness, alcoholism, drug addiction, unemployment, delinquency, and physical illness may affect the family. Some families have difficulty adjusting to or accepting the patient's illness or disability.

Your supervisor will explain the nature of any family problems to you. Care must be taken not to get involved with family problems. You must always maintain a professional manner. Understanding and empathy can be shown to family members. However, you should not give advice, take sides, or make judgments about family conflicts.

The Patient's Room

The home-bound patient may be confined to one room or a section of the home. The patient may be able to move about with assistive devices. Home adjustments may be needed to meet the patient's needs. A patient may be unable to climb stairs in a two-story home. The person's bedroom must be moved downstairs. A hospital bed, commode, overbed table, and other hospital furnishings can be bought or rented. A nurse can advise and assist the family in making changes and in obtaining equipment.

Modern health care equipment and conveniences are missing in home care. Substitutes may be needed for plastic drawsheets, bath basins, supportive devices, trays, and other equipment. The nurse will give guidance and advice about obtaining substitutes. Imagination and creativity can produce many items for personal care and other procedures.

HOUSEKEEPING SERVICES

Organizing patient care and housekeeping responsibilities is important. Patient care is your first priority. However, assigned housekeeping duties cannot be neglected. Careful planning is necessary. A list is made of all the patient care activities and tasks to be done each day. Housekeeping tasks can be done while the patient is sleeping, visiting with family or friends, or watching television.

Cleaning the Home

Housekeeping responsibilities include cleaning the patient's room, the kitchen, bathroom, and other rooms. Some tasks are done weekly. These include vacuuming, washing floors, polishing furniture, and changing bed linens (Fig. 31-2). Certain tasks are done daily or several times a day to keep the home neat and orderly. Newspapers, toys, and magazines are picked up as needed. Ashtrays and wastebaskets are emptied as indicated. Beds are made and furniture is dusted daily. Daily cleaning should take about an hour. Cleaning time depends on the size of the home. Cleaning can be done after patient care. It can also be done when the patient is sleeping or doing other activities.

Helpful Hints

Home health care may include cleaning, shopping, and preparing meals. The following hints will help you save time and work more efficiently.

1. Collect all supplies and equipment needed for a patient care activity or housekeeping task.
2. Use a pail, tray, shopping bag, or laundry basket to carry supplies and equipment from one room to another (Fig. 31-3).
3. Keep paper and pencil in your pocket. Jot down items that must be bought or replaced.
4. Secure a shopping list to a bulletin board, refrigerator door, or other convenient location. Note food, cleaning supplies, paper products, and other items that must be bought. Encourage family members to use the list.
5. Wipe up spills and crumbs as soon as possible. Hardened spills and foods are more difficult to remove.
6. Plan major tasks for certain days. Do not try to shop, do laundry, vacuum, and wash floors all on the same day.
7. Use time efficiently. Patient care can be given, a meal prepared, or the kitchen cleaned while clothes are in the washer or dryer.

Infection Control

You are responsible for preventing the spread of microorganisms in the home. The patient must also be protected from microbes brought into the home. If the patient has an infection, measures are taken to prevent its spread (see Chapter 9). Handwashing is very important. Hands are washed before and after each patient contact and at other appropriate times. Universal precautions are used to prevent contact with the patient's body fluids or body substances. You also need to practice these measures to prevent

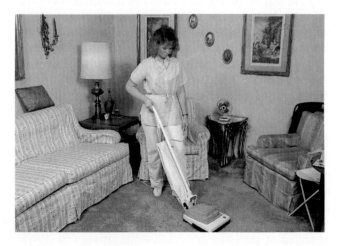

Fig. 31-2 Some house cleaning tasks are done weekly.

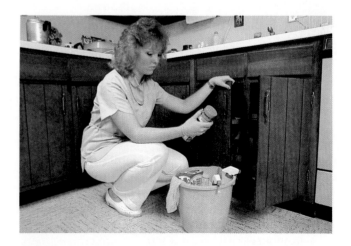

Fig. 31-3 A pail is used to carry cleaning supplies from one room to another.

the spread of microorganisms:

1. Wash dishes and other eating and cooking utensils
2. Clean kitchen appliances, counters, tables, and other surfaces
3. Dust furniture
4. Vacuum and mop floors
5. Wash clothes and linens
6. Clean bathroom fixtures
7. Dispose of garbage, leftover food, and other soiled supplies
8. Wash fruits and vegetables before storing and eating them
9. Cook meats and poultry adequately
10. Sterilize baby bottles

The Kitchen

The kitchen is cleaned more often than any other room. You should clean up after each meal. Cleaning the kitchen should not be left until the end of the day. Housekeeping responsibilities involve disposing of garbage, storing leftovers, washing dishes, and wiping surfaces. Cleaning floors, cabinets, and drawers is also included.

Garbage consisting of paper, boxes, and cans is placed in either a paper or plastic bag. Garbage consisting of food or wet articles is placed in a container lined with a plastic bag. If available, a garbage disposal is ideal for food and liquid garbage. Bones are not put in the garbage disposal. Garbage is emptied at least once a day. Some homes have trash compactors. They save storage space by crushing garbage. Trash compactors help keep kitchens fresh and clean and keep garbage hidden from view. Some states and communities recycle paper, glass, plastic, and other substances. You need to follow recycling procedures if they apply where the patient lives.

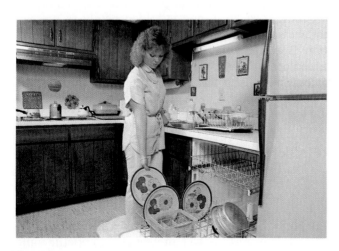

Fig. 31-4 Dishes are rinsed and then stacked in the dishwasher.

Leftover food is placed in small containers. The containers are covered with lids, foil, or plastic wrap. They are refrigerated as soon as possible and used within the next 2 to 3 days.

Dishwashing is a method of infection control. If a dishwasher is not available, dishes are washed by hand with liquid detergent and hot water. Glasses and cups are washed first. They are followed by silverware, plates, and bowls, and then pots and pans. Dishes and other utensils are rinsed well with hot water. Then they are placed in a drainer to dry. If a dishwasher is used, dishes are rinsed before being loaded into the dishwasher (Fig. 31-4). Special dishwasher detergent is used. You should wait until there is a full load before turning on the wash cycle. This saves water and electricity. Pots and pans are not put in the dishwasher. Cast iron, wood, and most plastic items cannot be washed in a dishwasher. Dishes are put away after they have dried.

Countertops, tables, the stove, and the refrigerator are wiped clean. A sponge or dishcloth moistened with warm water and a detergent is used. Grease, spills, and splashes from cooking are thoroughly removed. Some people also use liquid surface cleaners after wiping the surfaces. The sink is cleaned with a scouring powder.

Uncarpeted floors are damp-mopped at least once a week. Spills are wiped up immediately. A dust mop or broom is used for routine sweeping. A dustpan is used to collect dust and crumbs. Sweeping is done daily or more often if needed.

Kitchen drawers and cabinets and the items in them are cleaned 3 or 4 times a year. Drawers and cabinets can be kept neat and orderly by storing and putting items away neatly. The outside surfaces of cabinets and drawers are wiped clean weekly.

The Bathroom

The bathroom is a good place for the growth and spread of microorganisms. Therefore you must be very careful to maintain a clean bathroom.

Every family member has a role in keeping the bathroom clean. Aseptic measures must be practiced whenever the bathroom is used. The toilet is flushed after each use. The sink is rinsed after washing, shaving, or oral hygiene. The tub or shower is wiped out after each use. Hair is removed from the sink, tub, or shower. Towels are hung out to dry or placed in a hamper. Water spills are wiped up.

The bathroom is cleaned every day. All surfaces are cleaned (Fig. 31-5). A disinfectant or a solution of water and detergent is used. The surfaces to be cleaned include:

1. The toilet bowl, seat, and outside areas
2. The floor
3. The sides, walls, and curtain or door of the shower or tub

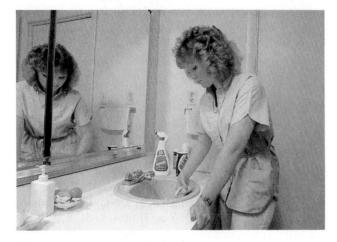

Fig. 31-5 Bathroom surfaces are cleaned daily to control the spread of microorganisms.

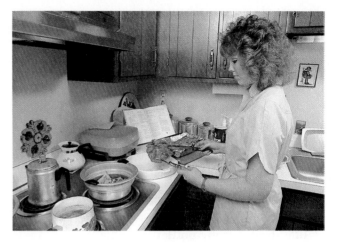

Fig. 31-6 The patient's special needs are considered when preparing meals.

4. Towel racks
5. Toilet tissue, toothbrush, and soap holders
6. The mirror
7. The sink
8. Windowsills

The floor is mopped (or vacuumed if carpeted). The wastebasket is emptied. Clean towels and washcloths are placed on the towel racks. Bathroom windows may be opened for a short time, and air freshener may be used. These help to eliminate odors and give a fresh smell to the bathroom. Bath mats, the wastebasket, and the laundry hamper or basket are washed weekly. Finally, toilet and facial tissue are replaced whenever needed.

Preparing Meals and Shopping

You may be responsible for menu planning and shopping for groceries. Certain factors are considered when planning menus and preparing shopping lists. They include the patient's diet, food preferences, and how much money is available for groceries. Menus are planned for the full week. Recipes are checked to make sure all of the ingredients are on hand or are included on the shopping list. Money can be saved by checking newpapers for sales and using coupons. All grocery receipts are saved for the patient or family member.

Foods must be properly stored as soon as you return from the store. Dairy products and most fresh fruits and vegetables are refrigerated right away. Meats, poultry, fish, and frozen foods are put in the freezer if they are not going to be used immediately. Dried, packaged, canned, and bottled foods keep well in cabinets.

Meal preparation requires knowledge of the four food groups and basic nutrition. A review of Chapter 16 is advised. You should also review the foods al-

lowed and forbidden on the patient's diet. Special eating and digestive problems due to illness, injury, or aging are considered when preparing and serving meals (Fig. 31-6). A good cookbook is a helpful guide to have when preparing meals.

Laundry

Laundry needs special attention to protect items from damage or discoloration. The patient and family are consulted about using detergents, bleaches, and fabric softeners. Clothing labels are checked for washing instructions. Labels also indicate the need for dry cleaning or handwashing.

Clothes are sorted before washing. White clothes, blends, and dark clothes are separated. Towels and sheets are usually washed separately. Items are checked for spots or stains. Pockets are checked for money, pens, pencils, tissues, and other items. Clothes are buttoned or zipped. Belts and adornments are removed if possible to prevent loss or damage.

Clothing to be ironed is folded neatly to prevent unnecessary wrinkling and creasing. Permanent press items are promptly removed from the dryer and are folded or hung on hangers. Clothing is mended when necessary. Freshly laundered and ironed clothing and linens are promptly and neatly returned to drawers and closets.

REPORTING AND RECORDING

Home health care assistants must make accurate observations. The observations are reported to the nurse and recorded on the patients' records (see Chapter 3). Observations include vital signs, treatments, intake and output, bowel movements, appetite, and skin condition.

You need to keep a record of your activities. The

nurse will explain what records to keep and how to complete the forms. Some agencies require mileage records. They are necessary if agency cars are used or if nursing assistants are reimbursed for mileage. Records are also kept of the following:

1. The time of arrival at the patient's home
2. The time a patient care activity or housekeeping task was started and finished
3. The time you left the patient's home
4. The time it took to travel to the next home

SUMMARY

Home health care offers many challenges. An RN directs and supervises your work. However, the RN is not in the home to provide immediate guidance and assistance. You must be able to work independently, without the help of others. Patient care procedures are performed the same way in the home as in health facilities. However, modern and convenient equipment may not be available. You must be creative. Equipment on hand is used for patient care and housekeeping.

Patient care is your first priority. Housekeeping responsibilities may be part of your assignment. Activities are organized to allow enough time for patient care and housekeeping tasks. A safe, clean living environment is maintained for the patient. The patient's home and property are treated with care and respect. The home is not reorganized and rearranged to meet your needs and preferences.

The patient's family also deserves consideration. Family relationships can be loving and healthy. Sometimes there are conflicts among family members. You need to be aware of any family problems. However, you should not get personally involved with the family or their problems.

REVIEW QUESTIONS

Circle the best *answer.*

1 Home health care involves
  a Patient care and housekeeping activities
  b Emergency medical care and rehabilitation
  c Housekeeping and laundry services
  d Patient care and babysitting services

2 The home health care assistant does *not*
  a Do light housekeeping
  b Give medications
  c Do the laundry
  d Prepare meals

3 The home health care assistant
  a Does heavy housework
  b Does family errands
  c Provides family members with transportation
  d Shops for groceries

4 The home health care assistant must be
  a Able to solve family quarrels
  b Honest and able to work alone
  c Able to meet all of the needs of the patient and family
  d Able to give advice about family matters

5 Which is *false?*
  a Each patient and family member is treated with respect, kindness, and dignity.
  b Cultural and religious practices are respected.
  c You should get involved with family problems.
  d You should be aware of family problems.

6 Which will *not* save time when doing housekeeping?
  a Collecting all necessary supplies and equipment for a particular activity
  b Keeping a shopping list
  c Cleaning spills, surfaces, and dishes at the end of the day
  d Planning major tasks for certain days

7 Infection control measures include
  a Handwashing and washing dishes
  b Dusting and vacuuming
  c Doing the laundry and cleaning the bathroom
  d All of the above

8 The best way to dispose of food and liquid garbage is to
  a Put it in a trash compactor
  b Put it in a garbage disposal
  c Put it in a paper bag
  d Flush it down the toilet

9 Which is *true?*
  a Leftovers are kept warm on the stove.
  b Dishes are washed in cold water.
  c Any detergent can be used in a dishwasher.
  d Kitchen surfaces are wiped clean as often as necessary.

10 Daily bathroom cleaning does *not* include
  a Cleaning all bathroom surfaces
  b Cleaning the bath mat, wastebasket, and laundry hamper
  c Damp-mopping the floor
  d Replacing soiled towels

11 When shopping for groceries, consider
  a The patient's diet
  b Food preferences
  c The amount of money available for food
  d All of the above

12 When doing laundry,
  a Wash light and dark clothes together
  b Always use bleach
  c Always check labels for washing instructions
  d All of the above

Answers

12	c	8	b	4	b
11	d	7	d	3	d
10	b	6	c	2	b
9	d	5	c	1	a

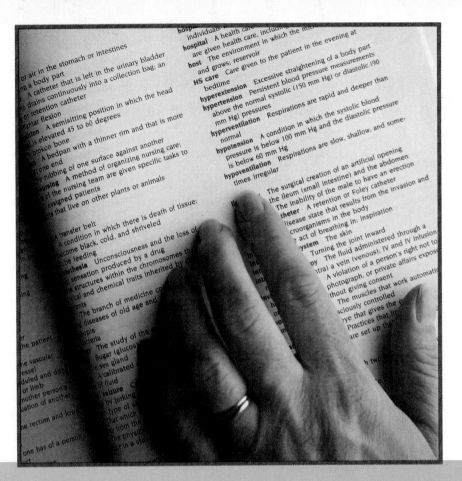

Medical Terminology

OBJECTIVES

- Define the key terms listed in this chapter
- Identify three word elements used in medical terms
- Translate Greek and Latin prefixes and suffixes into English
- Combine word elements into medical terms
- Translate medical terms into English
- Identify the four abdominal regions
- Define the directional terms used to describe the positions of the body in relation to other body parts
- Identify the abbreviations used in health care and their meanings

32

abbreviation A shortened form of a word or phrase

combining vowel A vowel added between two roots or a root and a suffix to make pronunciation easier

prefix A word element placed at the beginning of a word to change the meaning of the word

root A word element containing the basic meaning of the word

suffix A word element placed at the end of a root to change the meaning of the word

word element A part of a word

Many people think the language of medicine is mysterious and secretive—the private language of doctors and nurses. Yet people use medical terms every day. You probably know the terms *flu, diarrhea, cancer, appendectomy, cardiac,* and *pneumonia.* Health and medicine receive a great deal of attention on television and in newspapers and magazines. Because of greater news coverage, medical terms are used and understood more now than in the past.

Learning medical terminology is important for nursing assistants. As you gain more knowledge and experience, you will understand and use medical terms with ease and frequency. Learning medical terms for illnesses, diseases, and common things like bruises, baldness, and a "runny nose" can be fun and educational. This chapter introduces medical terminology and the common abbreviations used in health care.

THE WORD ELEMENTS OF MEDICAL TERMS

Like all words, medical terms are made up of parts or *word elements.* These elements are combined in various ways to form medical terms. A term can be translated by separating the word into its elements. Important word elements are prefixes, roots, and suffixes.

Prefixes

A *prefix* is a word element placed at the beginning of a word. A prefix changes the meaning of the word. The prefix "olig" (scanty, small amount) can be placed before the word "uria" (urine) to make "oliguria," meaning a scanty amount of urine. Prefixes are always combined with other word elements and are never used alone. Most prefixes are Greek or Latin. You need to learn the following prefixes to begin understanding medical terminology.

Prefix	Meaning
a-, an-	without or not
ab-	away from
ad-	toward
ante-	before, forward
anti-	against
auto-	self
bi-	double, two
brady-	slow
circum-	around
contra-	against, opposite
de-	down, from, away from, not
dia-	across, through, apart
dis-	separation, away from
dys-	bad, difficult, abnormal
ecto-	outer, outside
en-	in, into, within
endo-	inner, inside
epi-	over, on, upon
eryth-	red
ex-	out, out of, from, away from
hemi-	half
hyper-	excessive, too much, high
hypo-	under, decreased, less than normal
in-	in, into, within, not
inter-	between
intra-	within
intro-	into, within
leuk-	white
macro-	large
mal-	bad, illness, disease
mega-	large
micro-	small
mono-	one, single
neo-	new
non-	not
olig-	small, scanty
para-	abnormal
per-	by, through
peri-	around
poly-	many, much
post-	after, behind
pre-	before, in front of, prior to
pro-	before, in front of
re-	again
retro-	backward
semi-	half
sub-	under
super-	above, over, excess
supra-	above, over
tachy-	fast, rapid
trans-	across
uni-	one

Roots

The *root* contains the basic meaning of the word. It can be combined with another root, with prefixes, and with suffixes in various combinations to form a medical term. Like prefixes, roots are mainly from the Greek and Latin languages.

A vowel may be added when two roots are combined, or when a suffix is added to a root. The vowel is called a *combining vowel* and is usually an "o." An "i" is sometimes used. An "i" is used when there is no vowel between the two combined roots or between the root and the suffix. A combining vowel makes pronunciation easier.

The most common roots and their combining vowels are listed here.

Root (combining vowel)	Meaning
abdomin (o)	abdomen
aden (o)	gland
adren (o)	adrenal gland
angi (o)	vessel
arterio	artery
arthr (o)	joint
broncho	bronchus, bronchi
card, cardi (o)	heart
cephal (o)	head
chole, chol(o)	bile
chondr (o)	cartilage
colo	colon, large intestine
cost (o)	rib
crani (o)	skull
cyan (o)	blue
cyst (o)	bladder, cyst
cyt (o)	cell
dent (o)	tooth
derma	skin
duoden (o)	duodenum
encephal (o)	brain
enter (o)	intestines
fibr (o)	fiber, fibrous
gastr (o)	stomach
gloss (o)	tongue
gluc (o)	sweetness, glucose
glyc (o)	sugar
gyn, gyne, gyneco-	woman
hem, hema, hemo, hemat (o)	blood
hepat (o)	liver
hydr (o)	water
hyster (o)	uterus
ile (o), ili (o)	ileum
laparo	abdomen, loin, or flank
laryng (o)	larynx
lith (o)	stone
mamm (o)	breast, mammary gland
mast (o)	mammary gland, breast
meno	menstruation

Root (combining vowel)	Meaning
my (o)	muscle
myel (o)	spinal cord, bone marrow
necro	death
nephr (o)	kidney
neur (o)	nerve
ocul (o)	eye
oophor (o)	ovary
ophthalm (o)	eye
orth (o)	straight, normal, correct
oste (o)	bone
ot (o)	ear
ped (o)	child, foot
pharyng (o)	pharynx
phleb (o)	vein
pnea	breathing, respiration
pneum (o)	lung, air, gas
proct (o)	rectum
psych (o)	mind
pulmo	lung
py (o)	pus
rect (o)	rectum
rhin (o)	nose
salping (o)	eustachian tube, uterine tube
splen (o)	spleen
sten (o)	narrow, constriction
stern (o)	sternum
stomat (o)	mouth
therm (o)	heat
thoraco	chest
thromb (o)	clot, thrombus
thyr (o)	thyroid
toxo	poison
toxic (o)	poison, poisonous
trache (o)	trachea
uro	urine, urinary tract, urination
urethr (o)	urethra
urin (o)	urine
uter (o)	uterus
vas (o)	blood vessel, vas deferens
ven (o)	vein
vertebr (o)	spine, vertebrae

Suffixes

A *suffix* is placed at the end of a root to change the meaning of the word. Suffixes cannot be used alone. Like prefixes and roots, they are from Greek and Latin. When translating medical terms, you should begin with the suffix.

A combining vowel is needed if the root ends with a consonant. If the root ends with a vowel and the suffix begins with a vowel, the vowel at the end of the root is dropped. For example, the term "nephritis" means inflammation of the kidney. It was formed by combining "nephro" (kidney) and "itis" (inflammation). The "o" in "nephro" was dropped because the suffix began with a vowel.

You need to learn the suffixes listed in this chapter.

Suffix	Meaning
-algia	pain
-asis	condition, usually abnormal
-cele	hernia, herniation, pouching
-centesis	puncture and aspiration of
-cyte	cell
-ectasis	dilation, stretching
-ectomy	excision, removal of
-emia	blood condition
-genesis	development, production, creation
-genic	producing, causing
-gram	record
-graph	a diagram, a recording instrument
-graphy	making a recording
-iasis	condition of
-ism	a condition
-itis	inflammation
-logy	the study of
-lysis	destruction of, decomposition
-megaly	enlargement
-meter	measuring instrument
-metry	measurement
-oma	tumor
-osis	condition
-pathy	disease
-penia	lack, deficiency
-phasia	speaking
-phobia	an exaggerated fear
-plasty	surgical repair or reshaping
-plegia	paralysis
-ptosis	falling, sagging, dropping, down
-rrhage, -rrhagia	excessive flow
-rrhaphy	stitching, suturing
-rrhea	profuse flow, discharge
-scope	examination instrument
-scopy	examination using a scope
-stasis	maintenance, maintaining a constant level
-stomy, -ostomy	creation of an opening
-tomy, -otomy	incision, cutting into
-uria	condition of the urine

Combining Word Elements

Medical terms are formed by combining word elements. A root can be combined with prefixes, roots, or suffixes. The prefix "dys" (difficult) can be combined with the root "pnea" (breathing). This forms the term "dyspnea," meaning difficulty in breathing.

Roots can be combined with suffixes. The root "mast" (breast) combined with the suffix "ectomy" (excision or removal) forms the term "mastectomy." It means the removal of a breast.

Combining a prefix, root, and suffix is another way to form medical terms. "Endocarditis" consists of the prefix "endo" (inner), the root "card" (heart), and the suffix "itis" (inflammation). "Endocarditis" means inflammation of the inner part of the heart.

There are more complex combinations of prefixes, roots, and suffixes. There may be two prefixes, a root, and a suffix. Or there may be a prefix, two roots, and a suffix. Another pattern involves two roots and a suffix. The important things to remember are that prefixes always come before roots and suffixes always come after roots. You can practice forming medical terms by combining the word elements listed in this chapter.

ABDOMINAL REGIONS

The abdomen is divided into regions in order to help describe the location of body structures, pain, or discomfort. The four regions (quadrants) are shown in Figure 32-1. The regions are the right upper quadrant, left upper quadrant, right lower quadrant, and left lower quadrant.

DIRECTIONAL TERMS

Certain terms are often used to describe the position of one body part in relation to another. These terms give the direction of the body part when a person is standing and facing forward. The following directional terms are derived from some of the prefixes listed in this chapter:

1. *Anterior (ventral)*—located at or toward the front of the body or body part.
2. *Distal*—the part farthest from the center or from the point of attachment.
3. *Lateral*—relating to or located at the side of the body or body part.
4. *Medial*—relating to or located at or near the middle or midline of the body or body part.
5. *Posterior (dorsal)*—located at or toward the back of the body or body part.
6. *Proximal*—the part nearest to the center or to the point of origin.

ABBREVIATIONS

Abbreviations are shortened forms of words or phrases. They are used primarily in written communication to save time and space. Some facilities use abbreviations other than the ones listed here. Most facilities have a list of the abbreviations they accept. You should obtain the list when you are hired and use only the abbreviations accepted by that facility. If you are unsure if an abbreviation is acceptable, write the term out in full to communicate accurately.

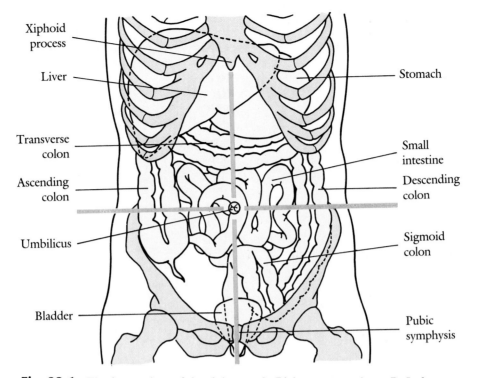

Fig. 32-1 The four regions of the abdomen. **A,** Right upper quadrant. **B,** Left upper quadrant. **C,** Right lower quadrant. **D,** Left lower quadrant.

Abbreviation	Meaning
abd	Abdomen
a.c.	Before meals
ADL	Activities of daily living
ad lib	As desired
Adm (adm)	Admitted or admission
AM (am)	Morning
amb	Ambulatory
amt	Amount
ap	Apical
approx	Approximately
b.i.d.	Twice a day
BM (bm)	Bowel movement
BP	Blood pressure
BRP	Bathroom privileges
c̄	With
C	Centigrade
Ca	Cancer
Cath	Catheter
CBC	Complete blood count
CBR	Complete bed rest
cc	Cubic centimeter
CCU	Coronary care unit
c/o	Complains of
CPR	Cardiopulmonary resuscitation
CVA	Cerebrovascular accident, stroke
dc (d/c)	Discontinue

Abbreviation	Meaning
DOA	Dead on arrival
DON	Director of nursing
drsg	Dressing
Dx	Diagnosis
ECG (EKG)	Electrocardiogram
EEG	Electroencephalogram
ER	Emergency room
F	Fahrenheit
FBS	Fasting blood sugar
FF	Force fluids
fld	Fluid
ft	Foot or feet
gal	Gallon
GI	Gastrointestinal
h (hr)	Hour
H_2O	Water
H.S. (h.s.)	Hour of sleep
ht	Height
ICU	Intensive care unit
in	Inch
I&O	Intake and output
IV	Intravenous
L	Liter
Lab	Laboratory
lb	Pound
liq	Liquid
LLQ	Left lower quadrant
LMP	Last menstrual period
LPN	Licensed practical nurse

Abbreviation	Meaning
lt	Left
LVN	Licensed vocational nurse
LUQ	Left upper quadrant
meds	Medications
mid noc	Midnight
min	Minute
ml	Milliliter
NA	Nursing assistant
neg	Negative
nil	None
no	Number
noc	Night
NPO	Nothing by mouth
O_2	Oxygen
OB	Obstetrics
OJ	Orange juice
OOB	Out of bed
OR	Operating room
Ord	Orderly
OT	Occupational therapy
oz (Oz)	Ounce
PAR	Postanesthesia room
p.c.	After meals
Peds	Pediatrics
per	By, through
PM (pm)	after noon
p.o. (per os)	By mouth
postop (post op)	Postoperative
preop (pre op)	Preoperative
prep	Preparation
p.r.n.	When necessary
Pt (pt)	Patient
PT	Physical therapy
q	Every
q.d.	Every day
q.h.	Every hour
q2h, q3h, etc.	Every 2 hours, every 3 hours, etc.
q.h.s.	Every night at bedtime
q.i.d.	Four times a day
q.o.d.	Every other day

Abbreviation	Meaning
R	Rectal temperature
RLQ	Right lower quadrant
RN	Registered nurse
ROM	Range of motion
RR	Recovery room
RUQ	Right upper quadrant
$\bar{s}$	Without
Spec (spec)	Specimen
SSE	Soap suds enema
stat	At once, immediately
Surg	Surgery
tbsp	Tablespoon
t.i.d.	Three times a day
TLC	Tender loving care
TPR	Temperature, pulse, and respirations
tsp	Teaspoon
U/a (U/A, u/a)	Urinalysis
VS (vs)	Vital signs
WBC	White blood cell count
w/c	Wheelchair
wt	Weight

SUMMARY

Medical terminology involves the use of word elements derived mainly from Greek and Latin. Word elements are prefixes, roots, and suffixes. They are combined in various ways to form medical words. Prefixes go before roots, and suffixes go after roots. They are never used alone. You can practice forming and translating medical words by learning the word elements listed in this chapter. Use a nursing dictionary to check your accuracy.

Knowing the commonly accepted abbreviations will also help you communicate with other health workers. Abbreviations save time and space when you make notes about assignments and patient observations. If you are allowed to chart in the patient's record, use abbreviations accepted by your facility whenever possible.

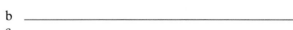

REVIEW QUESTIONS

Fill in the blanks.

1 Word elements used in medical terminology are
   a _____
   b _____
   c _____

2 A _____ is placed at the beginning of a word to change the meaning of the word.

3 A _____ is placed at the end of a word to change the meaning of the word.

4 The four regions of the abdomen are
   a _____
   b _____
   c _____
   d _____

Match the item in column A with the item in column B.

Column A		Column B
5 __ Distal	a	The part nearest to the center or point of origin
6 __ Proximal	b	Relating to or located at the side of the body or body part

Column A		Column B
7 ___ Anterior (ventral)	c	Located at or toward the front part of the body or body part
8 ___ Medial	d	The part farthest from the center or point of attachment
9 ___ Posterior (dorsal)	e	Located at or toward the back of the body or body part
10 ___ Lateral	f	Relating to or located at or near the middle or the midline of the body or body part

Write the definition of the following prefixes

11 a- _____
12 dys- _____
13 bi- _____
14 ab- _____
15 trans- _____
16 post- _____
17 olig- _____
18 hyper- _____
19 pre- _____
20 hemi- _____
21 hypo- _____
22 ad- _____

Write the definition of the following suffixes.

23 -algia _____
24 -itis _____
25 -ostomy _____
26 -ectomy _____
27 -emia _____
28 -osis _____
29 -rrhage _____
30 -penia _____
31 -pathy _____
32 -otomy _____
33 -rrhea _____
34 -plasty _____

Write the definition of the following roots.

35 cranio _____
36 cardio _____
37 mammo _____
38 veno _____
39 urino _____
40 pnea _____
41 cyano _____
42 arterio _____
43 colo _____
44 arthro _____
45 litho _____
46 gastro _____
47 encephalo _____
48 gluco _____
49 hemo _____
50 hystero _____
51 hepato _____
52 myo _____
53 nephro _____
54 phlebo _____
55 oculo _____
56 osteo _____
57 neuro _____

58 pneumo _____
59 toxico _____
60 psycho _____
61 thoraco _____

Match the item in column A with the item in column B.

Column A		Column B
62 ___ Intravenous	a	Inflammation of a joint
63 ___ Apnea	b	Blood in the urine
64 ___ Hemiplegia	c	Excessive flow of blood
65 ___ Thoracotomy	d	Paralysis on one side
66 ___ Arthritis	e	Surgical removal of the uterus
67 ___ Bronchitis	f	No breathing
68 ___ Anuria	g	Inflammation of the bronchi
69 ___ Hematuria	h	Incision into the chest
70 ___ Hysterectomy	i	No urine
71 ___ Hemorrhage	j	Within a vein

Write the abbreviation for the following terms.

72 Bathroom privileges _____
73 As desired _____
74 Complains of _____
75 Twice a day _____
76 Hour of sleep _____
77 Intake and output _____
78 Nothing by mouth _____
79 When necessary _____
80 Postoperative _____
81 Every _____
82 Wheelchair _____
83 At once, immediately _____

Answers

1 a Prefix
  b Root
  c Suffix
2 Prefix
3 Suffix
4 a Right upper quadrant
  b Left upper quadrant
  c Right lower quadrant
  d Left lower quadrant
5 d
6 a
7 c
8 f
9 e
10 b
11 Without or not
12 Bad, difficult, abnormal
13 Double, two
14 Away from
15 Across, over
16 After, behind
17 Scanty, small
18 Excessive, too much
19 Before, prior to
20 Half
21 Decreased, less than normal
22 Toward

23	Pain	54	Vein
24	Inflammation	55	Eye
25	Creation of an opening	56	Bone
26	Removal of, excision	57	Nerve
27	Blood condition	58	Lung
28	Condition	59	Poison
29	Excessive flow	60	Mind
30	Lack, deficiency	61	Chest
31	Disease	62	j
32	Incision, cutting into	63	f
33	Profuse flow, discharge	64	d
34	Surgical repair or reshaping	65	h
35	Skull	66	a
36	Heart	67	g
37	Breast	68	i
38	Vein	69	b
39	Urine	70	e
40	Breathing, respiration	71	c
41	Blue	72	BRP
42	Artery	73	ad lib
43	Colon, large intestine	74	c/o
44	Joint	75	b.i.d.
45	Stone	76	H.S. (h.s.)
46	Stomach	77	I&O
47	Brain	78	NPO
48	Glucose, sweetness	79	p.r.n.
49	Blood	80	postop (post op)
50	Uterus	81	q
51	Liver	82	w/c
52	Muscle	83	stat
53	Kidney		

Glossary

abbreviation A shortened form of a word or phrase

abduction Moving a body part away from the body

acetone Ketone bodies that appear in the urine because of the rapid breakdown of fat for energy

activities of daily living Those self-care activities a person needs to perform daily to remain independent and function in society

acute illness An illness that occurs suddenly and from which the patient is expected to recover

adduction Moving a body part toward the body

alimentary canal The long tube extending from the mouth to the anus; also called the gastrointestinal tract

AM care The routine care performed before breakfast; early morning care

amputation The removal of all or part of an extremity

anal incontinence The inability to control the passage of feces and gas through the anus

anesthesia The loss of feeling or sensation produced by a drug that is given before surgery

anesthesiologist A doctor who specializes in the administration of anesthetics

anorexia Loss of appetite

antiperspirant A skin care product that reduces the amount of perspiration

aphasia The loss of or inability (a) to speak (phasia)

apical-radial pulse Taking the apical pulse and the radial pulse at the same time; two workers are needed for the procedure

apnea The lack or absence of (a) breathing (pnea)

artery A blood vessel that carries blood away from the heart

arthritis Joint (arthr) inflammation (itis)

asepsis The absence of pathogens

aspiration The breathing of fluid or an object into the lungs

assault Intentionally attempting or threatening to touch the body of another person without the person's consent

atelectasis The collapse of a portion of the lung

atrophy A decrease in size or a wasting away of tissue

autoclave A pressurized steam sterilizer

autonomic nervous system A division of the peripheral nervous system; the system controls involuntary muscles and functions that occur without conscious effort

bacteria Microscopic one-celled plant life that multiplies rapidly; germs

base of support The area on which an object rests

bath blanket A thin, light-weight cotton blanket used to cover the patient during the bath; it absorbs water and provides warmth during the bath; it is used to cover the patient during many other procedures

battery The actual unauthorized touching of another person's body without the person's consent

bedsore A decubitus ulcer; a pressure sore

benign tumor A tumor that grows slowly and within a localized area; benign tumors usually do not cause death

bisexual An individual who is attracted to people of both sexes

blood pressure The amount of force exerted against the walls of an artery by the blood

491

body alignment The way the body segments are aligned with one another; posture

body language Facial expressions, gestures, posture, and other body movements that send messages to others

body mechanics Using the body in an efficient and careful way

body temperature The amount of heat in the body that is a balance between the amount of heat produced and the amount lost by the body

bone marrow The substance within the hollow center of bones that manufactures blood cells

bradypnea Slow (brady) breathing (pnea); the respiratory rate is less than 10 respirations per minute

braille A method of writing for the blind; raised dots are arranged to represent each letter of the alphabet; the first ten letters also represent the numbers 0 through 9

calorie The amount of energy produced from the burning of food for energy

capillary The smallest blood vessel; food, oxygen, and other substances pass from the capillaries to the cells

cardiac arrest The sudden stoppage of breathing and heart action

carrier A human being or animal that is a reservoir for microorganisms but does not have the signs and symptoms of an infection

cartilage The connective tissue at the end of long bones

caster A small wheel made of rubber or plastic

catheter A tube used to drain or inject fluid through a body opening

catheterization The process of inserting a catheter

cell The basic unit of body structure

cell membrane The outer covering that encloses the cell and helps the cell hold its shape

central nervous system One of two main divisions of the nervous system; made up of the brain and spinal cord

cerebrospinal fluid The fluid that circulates around the brain and spinal cord

cerumen The waxy substance secreted in the ear

chart Another term for the patient's record

Cheyne-Stokes A pattern for breathing in which respirations gradually increase in rate and depth and then become shallow and slow; breathing may stop (apnea) for 10 to 20 seconds

chromosomes The threadlike structures in the cell nucleus

chronic illness An illness that is slow or gradual in onset and for which there is no known cure; it can be controlled, and complications can be prevented

chyme Partially digested food and fluids that pass from the stomach into the small intestine

civil law Laws concerned with the relationships among people; private law

clean technique A term for medical asepsis

closed fracture A fracture in which the bone is broken but the skin is intact; a simple fracture

colostomy The surgical creation of an artificial opening between the colon and abdomen

coma A state of being completely unaware of one's surroundings; the individual is unable to react or respond to people, places, or things

combining vowel A vowel that is added between two roots or between a root and a suffix to make pronunciation easier

communicable disease A disease caused by pathogens that are spread easily; a contagious disease

communication The exchange of information; a message is sent, and it is received and interpreted by the intended person

complete bed bath Washing the entire body of a patient who is in bed

compound fracture An open fracture; the bone is broken and the bone has come through the skin

constipation The passage of a hard, dry stool

constrict To narrow

contagious disease A communicable disease

contamination The process by which an object or area becomes unclean

contracture The abnormal shortening of a muscle

convulsion Violent and sudden contractions or tremors of muscles; a seizure

crime An act that is a violation of a criminal law

criminal law Laws concerned with offenses against the public and society in general; criminal law is also called public law

culture The values, beliefs, habits, likes, dislikes, customs, and characteristics of a group that are passed from one generation to the next

cytoplasm The portion of the cell that surrounds the nucleus

dangling Sitting on the side of the bed; sitting on the side of the bed and moving the legs back and forth and around in circles

decubitus ulcer An area where the skin and underlying tissues are eroded as a result of a lack of blood flow; a bedsore or pressure sore

defamation Injuring the name and reputation of another person by making false statements to a third person

defecation The process of excreting feces from the rectum through the anus; a bowel movement

dehydration A decrease in the amount of water in body tissues

delusion A false belief

dementia The term used to describe mental disorders caused by changes in the brain

deodorant A preparation that masks and controls body odors

dermis The inner layer of the skin

development Changes in a person's psychological and social functioning

developmental task That which the individual must accomplish during a stage of development

diabetes mellitus A chronic disease in which the pancreas fails to secrete enough insulin; the body is prevented from using sugar for energy

diarrhea The frequent passage of liquid stools

diastole The resting phase of heart action during which the heart fills with blood; the period of heart muscle relaxation

diastolic pressure The pressure in the arteries when the heart is at rest

digestion The process of physically and chemically breaking down food so that it can be absorbed for use by the cells of the body

dilate To expand or open wider

disaster A sudden, catastrophic event in which many people are injured or killed and property is destroyed

disinfection The process by which pathogens are destroyed

dorsal recumbent position The back-lying or supine position

dorsiflexion Bending backward

drawsheet A sheet, smaller in size than a bottom or top sheet, that is placed over the middle of the bottom sheet; it helps keep the mattress and bottom linens clean and dry; it can also be used to turn and move patients in bed; it is sometimes called the "cotton drawsheet"

dysphagia Difficulty or discomfort (dys) in swallowing (phagia)

dyspnea Difficult, labored, or painful (dys) breathing (pnea)

dysuria Painful or difficult (dys) urination (uria)

early morning care AM care

edema The swelling of body tissues with water

elective surgery Scheduled surgery; surgery the patient chooses to have at a particular time

embolus A blood clot that travels through the vascular system until it lodges in a distant blood vessel

emergency surgery Surgery that is unscheduled and is done immediately to save the individual's life or limb

empathy The ability to see things from another person's point of view; putting yourself in the situation of another

endometrium The lining of the uterus

enema The introduction of fluid into the rectum and lower colon

epidermis The outer layer of the skin

esteem The worth, value, or opinion one has of a person

ethics What is right and wrong conduct

exhalation The act of breathing out; expiration

extension Straightening of a body part

external rotation Turning the joint outward

face mask A device used in the administration of oxygen; it covers the nose and mouth

fainting The sudden loss of consciousness caused by an inadequate blood supply to the brain

false imprisonment The unlawful restraint or restriction of another person's movement

fecal impaction The prolonged retention and accumulation of fecal material in the rectum

feces The semisolid mass of waste products in the colon

fertilization The process whereby the male sex cell (sperm) unites with the female sex cell (ovum) to form one cell

first aid Emergency care given to an ill or injured person before medical help arrives

flatulence The excessive formation of gas in the stomach and intestines

flatus The gas or air in the stomach or intestines

flexion Bending a body part

Foley catheter A catheter that is left in the urinary bladder so that urine drains continuously into a collection bag; an indwelling or retention catheter

footdrop Plantar flexion

Fowler's position A semi-sitting position in which the head of the bed is elevated 45 to 60 degrees

fracture A broken bone

fracture pan A bedpan that has a thin rim and is more shallow at one end than a normal bedpan

friction The rubbing of one surface against another

functional nursing A method of organizing nursing care; members of the nursing team are given specific tasks to do for all assigned patients

fungi Plants that live on other plants or animals

gait belt A transfer belt

gangrene A condition in which there is death of tissue; tissues become black, cold, and shriveled

gastrostomy Surgically created opening in the stomach that allows feeding

gavage Tube feeding

general anesthesia Unconsciousness and the loss of feeling and sensation that is produced by a drug

genes The structures within the chromosomes that control the physical and chemical traits inherited by children from their parents

geriatrics The branch of medicine concerned with problems and diseases of old age and the elderly; the care of aging people

germs Bacteria

gerontology The study of the aging process

glucosuria Sugar (glucos) in the urine (uria)

gonad The sex gland

graduate A calibrated container used to measure amounts of fluid

ground That which carries leaking electricity to the earth and away from the electrical appliance

growth The physical changes that can be measured and that occur in a steady, orderly manner

hallucination Seeing, hearing, or feeling something that is not real

health team A variety of health care workers who work together to provide health care for patients

hearing aid An instrument that amplifies sound

hemiplegia Paralysis on one side of the body

hemoglobin The substance in red blood cells that gives blood its color; hemoglobin carries oxygen in the blood

hemorrhage The excessive loss of blood from a blood vessel

heterosexual A person who is attracted to members of the opposite sex

home health agency An agency that provides nursing care and assistance to patients in their homes

homosexual An individual who has a strong attraction to members of the same sex

horizontal recumbent position The supine or back-lying examination position; the legs are together

hormone A chemical substance secreted by glands into the bloodstream

hospice A health care facility or program designed for individuals who are dying of terminal illness

hospital A health care facility where ill and injured persons are given health care, including medical and nursing care

host The environment in which the microorganism lives and grows; reservoir

hs care Care given to the patient in the evening at bedtime

hyperextension Excessive straightening of a body part

hypertension Persistent blood pressure measurements above the normal systolic (150 mm Hg) or diastolic (90 mm Hg) pressures

hyperventilation Repirations are rapid and deeper than normal

hypotension A condition in which the systolic blood pressure is below 100 mm Hg and the diastolic pressure is below 60 mm Hg

hypoventilation Respirations are slow, shallow, and sometimes irregular

ileostomy The surgical creation of an artificial opening between the ileum (small intestine) and the abdomen

impotence The inability of the male to have an erection

indwelling cathether A retention, or Foley, catheter

infection A disease state that results from the invasion and growth of microorganisms in the body

infection precautions Practices that limit the spread of pathogens; barriers are set up that prevent the escape of the pathogen

inhalation The act of breathing in; inspiration

integumentary system The skin

internal rotation Turning the joint inward

intravenous therapy The fluid administered through a needle within (intra) a vein (venous); IV and IV infusion

invasion of privacy A violation of a person's right not to have one's name, photograph, or private affairs exposed or made public without giving consent

involuntary muscles The muscles that work automatically and cannot be consciously controlled

iris The part of the eye that gives the eye its color

joint The point at which two or more bones meet

Kardex A type of card file that summarizes the information contained in the patient's record; medications, treatments, diagnosis, routine care measures, and special equipment needed by the patient are included

ketone body Acetone; it appears in the urine because of the rapid breakdown of fat for energy

knee-chest position The patient kneels and rests the body on the knees and chest; the head is turned to one side, the arms are above the head or flexed at the elbows, the back is straight, and the body is flexed about 90 degrees at the hips

laryngeal mirror An instrument used to examine the mouth, teeth, and throat

lateral position The side-lying position

law A rule of conduct made by a government body

legal That which pertains to a law

liable Being responsible for one's own action

libel Defamation through written statements

licensed practical nurse (LPN) An individual who has completed a 1-year nursing program and has passed the licensing examination for practical nurses; the LPN assists the registered nurse in planning, giving, and evaluating nursing care; licensed vocational nurse (LVN) is the title used in some states

ligament A strong band of connective tissue that holds bones together

lithotomy position The patient's hips are brought down to the edge of the examination table, the knees are flexed, the hips are externally rotated, and the feet are supported in stirrups

logrolling Turning the patient as a unit, in alignment, with one motion

long-term care facility A broad term used to describe a health care facility in which individuals live and are given nursing care; most residents are elderly and unable to care for themselves because of aging or illness

malignant tumor A tumor that grows rapidly and invades other tissues; malignant tumors will cause death if not treated

malpractice Negligence by a professional person

meatus The opening at the end of the urethra

medical asepsis The techniques and practices used to prevent the spread of pathogens from one person or place to another person or place; clean technique

menarche The time when menstruation first begins

meninges The connective tissue that covers and protects the brain and spinal cord; there are three layers: the outer layer called the dura mater, the middle layer called the arachnoid, and the inner layer called the pia mater

menopause The time when menstruation stops; it marks the end of the woman's reproductive years

menstruation The process in which the endometrium of the uterus breaks up and is discharged from the body through the vagina

mental health hospital A hospital for persons who are mentally ill

metabolism The burning of food for heat and energy for use by the cells

metastasis The spread of cancer to other parts of the body

microbe A microorganism

microorganism A small living plant or animal that cannot be seen without the aid of a microscope; a microbe

micturition The process of emptying the bladder; urination or voiding

mitered corner A way of tucking linens under the mattress to keep the linens straight and smooth

mitosis The process of cell division

morning care Care that is given after breakfast; cleanliness and skin care measures are more thorough at this time

nasal cannula A two-pronged device used in the administration of oxygen; the prongs are inserted a short distance into the nostrils

nasal catheter A device used in the administration of oxygen; it is inserted through the nostril to the back of the throat

nasal speculum An instrument used to examine the inside of the nose

need That which is necessary or desirable for maintaining life and mental well-being

negligence An unintentional wrong in which a person fails to act in a reasonable and prudent manner and thereby causes harm to another person or the person's property

nephron The basic working unit of the kidney

neuron The nerve cell; the basic unit of the nervous system

nonpathogen A microorganism that does not usually cause an infection

nonverbal communication Communication that does not involve the use of words

normal flora Microorganisms that usually live and grow in a certain location

nucleus The control center of the cell that directs the cell's activities

nursing assistant An individual who gives simple, basic nursing care under the supervision of an RN or LPN; training may be received through a nursing assistant course, in-service program, or on-the-job training; other titles are nurse's aide, nursing attendant, and patient care assistant; a male nursing assistant is called an orderly

nursing care plan A written guide that gives direction about the care a patient should receive

nursing team The individuals involved in providing nursing care; RNs, LPNs, and nursing assistants make up the nursing team

nutrient A substance that is ingested, digested, absorbed, and used by the body

nutrition The many processes involved in the ingestion, digestion, absorption, and use of foods and fluids by the body

objective data Information observed about a patient that can be seen, heard, felt, or smelled by another person; signs

observation Using the senses of sight, hearing, touch, and smell to collect information about the patient

obstetrics The branch of medicine concerned with the care of women during pregnancy, labor, and childbirth, and for 6 to 8 weeks after birth

open fracture A fracture in which the bone is broken and the bone has come through the skin; a compound fracture

ophthalmoscope A lighted instrument used to examine the internal structures of the eye

oral hygiene The measures that are performed to keep the mouth and teeth clean; mouth care

orderly A male nursing assistant

organ Groups of tissues with the same function

ostomy The surgical creation of an artificial opening

otoscope A lighted instrument used to examine the external ear and the eardrum (tympanic membrane)

ovary The female sex gland

ovulation The process whereby an ovum is released by an ovary

ovum The female sex cell

oxygen tent A device used to administer oxygen; the tent is made of clear plastic and covers all or the upper part of the bed

paraplegia Paralysis from the waist down

parasympathetic nervous system A division of the autonomic nervous system; the system tends to slow down functions

partial bed bath Bathing the patient's face, hands, axillae, genital area, back, and buttocks

pathogen A microorganism that is harmful and is capable of causing an infection

patient record A written account of the patient's illness and response to the treatment and care given by members of the health team; it is commonly referred to as a chart

patient pack Personal care equipment provided by the health care facility; the pack generally includes a wash basin, emesis or kidney basin, bedpan, urinal, water pitcher and glass, soap, and a soap dish

patient unit The furniture and equipment provided for the individual by the health care facility

pediatrics The branch of medicine concerned with the growth, development, and care of children ranging from the newborn to the adolescent

percussion hammer An instrument used to tap body parts for the purpose of testing reflexes

pericare Perineal care

perineal care Cleansing the genital and anal areas of the body

periosteum The membrane that covers the bones

peristalsis Involuntary muscle contractions in the digestive system that move food through the alimentary canal; the alternating contraction and relaxation of the intestinal muscles

phantom limb pain A sensation causing the patient to complain of pain in an amputated part; it may feel as if the part is still there

plantar flexion The foot (plantar) is bent (flexion); footdrop

plasma The fluid portion of the blood

plastic drawsheet A drawsheet made of plastic, placed between the bottom sheet and the cotton drawsheet; it helps keep the mattress and bottom linens clean and dry; some are made of rubber and are called "rubber drawsheets"

postmortem After (post) death (mortem)

postoperative After the operation or surgery

posture The way the body segments are aligned with one another; body alignment

prefix A word element that is placed at the beginning of a word to change the meaning of the word

preoperative Before the operation or surgery

pressure sore A decubitus ulcer; a bedsore

primary caregiver The individual in the child's environment who is mainly responsible for providing or assisting with the child's basic needs

primary nursing A method of organizing nursing care in which the RN is responsible for the total care of patients on a 24-hour basis

pronation Turning downward

prosthesis An artificial replacement for a missing body part

protoplasm A term that refers to all of the structures, substances, and water within the cell

protozoa Microscopic one-celled animals

psychiatry The branch of medicine concerned with the diagnosis and treatment of people with mental health problems

puberty The period during which the reproductive organs begin to function and secondary sex characteristics appear

pulse The beat of the heart felt at an artery as a wave of blood passes through the artery

pulse deficit The difference between the apical and radial pulse rates

pulse rate The number of heartbeats or pulses felt in 1 minute

pupil The opening in the middle of the eye

quadriplegia Paralysis from the neck down; paralysis of the arms, legs, and trunk

range of motion The movement of a joint to the extent possible without causing pain

reality orientation A form of rehabilitation aimed at promoting or maintaining awareness of person, time, and place

recording Writing or charting patient care and observations

reflex An involuntary movement

regional anesthesia The loss of sensation or feeling in a particular part of the body produced by the injection of a drug; the patient does not lose consciousness

registered nurse (RN) An individual who has studied nursing for 2, 3, or 4 years and has passed a licensing examination; the RN is responsible for assessing, planning, implementing, and evaluating nursing care

rehabilitation The process of restoring the disabled individual to the highest level of physical, psychological, social, and economic functioning possible

reincarnation The belief that the spirit or soul is reborn into another human body or into another form of life

religion Spiritual beliefs, needs, and practices

reporting A verbal account of patient care and observations

reservoir The environment in which microorganisms live and grow; the host

respiration The process of supplying the cells with oxygen and removing carbon dioxide from them; the act of breathing air into (inhalation) and out of (exhalation) the lungs

respiratory arrest Condition in which breathing stops but the heart continues to pump for several minutes

responsibility A duty; an obligation to perform some act or function; being able to answer for one's actions

retention catheter A Foley or indwelling catheter

reverse Trendelenburg's position The head of the bed is elevated and the foot of the bed is lowered

rickettsiae Microscopic forms of life found in the tissues of fleas, lice, ticks, and other insects

rigor mortis The stiffness or rigidity (rigor) of skeletal muscles the occurs after death (mortis)

root A word element that contains the basic meaning of the word

sclera The white of the eye

seizure A convulsion

self-actualization Experiencing one's potential

semi-Fowler's position The head of the bed is elevated 45 degrees and the knee portion is elevated 15 degrees; or the head of the bed is elevated 30 degrees and the knee portion is not elevated

sex The physical activities involving the organs of reproduction; the activities are done for pleasure or to produce children

sexuality That which relates to one's sex; those physical, psychological, social, culture, and spiritual factors that affect a person's feelings and attitudes about his or her sex

shock A condition that results when there is an inadequate blood supply to the organs and tissues of the body

side-lying position The lateral position

signs Objective data

simple fracture A closed fracture; the bone is broken but the skin is intact

Sims' position A side-lying position in which the upper leg is sharply flexed so that it is not resting on the lower leg, and the lower arm is behind the patient

slander Defamation through oral statements

sperm The male sex cell

sphygmomanometer The instrument used to measure blood pressure that consists of a cuff (which is applied to the upper arm) and a measuring device

spore A bacterium protected by a hard shell that forms around the microorganism

sputum Mucus secreted by the lungs, bronchi, and trachea during respiratory illnesses or disorders

sterile The absence of all microorganisms, both pathogenic and nonpathogenic

sterilization The process by which all microorganisms are destroyed

stethoscope An instrument used to listen to the sounds produced by the heart, lungs, and other body organs

stoma An opening; see *colostomy* and *ileostomy*

stomatitis Inflammation (itis) of the mouth (stomat)

stool Feces that have been excreted

stroke A cerebrovascular accident; blood supply to a part of the brain is suddenly interrupted

subjective data Information reported by the patient that the health care worker cannot observe by using the senses; symptoms are subjective data

suction The process of withdrawing or sucking up fluids

suffix A word element placed at the end of a root to change the meaning of the word

suffocation The termination of breathing that results from lack of oxygen

sundowning Condition in which signs, symptoms, and behaviors that are characteristic of Alzheimer's disease increase during hours of darkness

supination Turning upward

supine position The back-lying or dorsal recumbent position

suppository A cone-shaped solid medication that is inserted into a body opening; the medication melts at body temperature

sympathetic nervous system A division of the autonomic nervous system; the system tends to speed up functions

symptoms Subjective data

synovial fluid The fluid excreted by the synovial membrane that acts as a lubricant; the fluid allows the joint to move smoothly

synovial membrane The membrane that lines the joints

system Organs that work together to perform special functions

systole The phase of heart action during which the heart contracts; the period of heart muscle contraction

systolic pressure The amount of force it takes to pump blood out of the heart into the arterial circulation

tachypnea Rapid (tachy) breathing (pnea); the respiratory rate is greater than 24 respirations per minute

team nursing A method of organizing nursing care in which an RN serves as a team leader; the team leader assigns other RNs, LPNs, and nursing assistants to care for certain patients

tendons The tough connective tissue that connects muscles to bones

terminal illness An illness or injury for which there is no reasonable expectation of recovery

testis The male sex gland

tetany A state of severe muscle contraction and spasm that can cause death if untreated

thrombus A blood clot

tissue Groups of cells with the same function

toothette A piece of spongy foam attached to a stick that is used for giving oral hygiene

tort A wrong committed against another person or the person's property

transfer belt A belt used to hold onto a patient during a transfer or when walking with the patient; a gait belt

transsexual An individual who believes that he or she is really a member of the opposite sex

transvestite An individual who becomes sexually excited by dressing in the clothes appropriate to the opposite sex

Trendelenburg's position The head of the bed is lowered and the foot of the bed is raised

tumor A new growth of cells; tumors can be benign or malignant

tuning fork An instrument used to test hearing

turning sheet A flat sheet folded in half, or a draw-sheet, that is used to lift, turn, or move a patient in bed; a lift or pull sheet

urethra The structure through which urine passes from the bladder and is eliminated from the body

urinary incontinence The inability to control the passage of urine from the bladder

urination The process of emptying the bladder; micturition or voiding

vaginal speculum An instrument used to open the vagina so that it and the cervix can be examined

vein A blood vessel that carries blood back to the heart

verbal communication Communication that uses the written or spoken word

virus An extremely small microscopic organism that grows in living cells

vital signs Temperature, pulse, respirations, and blood pressure

voiding Urination or micturition

voluntary muscles The muscles that can be consciously controlled; skeletal muscles

vomiting The act of expelling stomach contents through the mouth

will A legal declaration of how an individual wishes to have property distributed after death

word element A part of a word

Index

Tub bath
  assisting patient with, 207, 208
  for infant, 441, 442
  shampooing patient's hair during, 215, 216
Tube
  eustachian, 62
  fallopian, 71
  gastrostomy, 282
  nasogastric, 282, 283
    for suctioning, 358
  rectal, 259-260
Tube feedings, 282, 283
Tuberculosis, 411
Tubing, drainage, for catheter, 236
Tubule
  collecting, 69
  convoluted, 67
Tumors, 392-393
Tuning fork, 336, 337
Tunnel vision, 403
Turning of patient, 154
Turning sheet, 148
  moving patient up in bed using, 152
24-hour urine specimen, collecting, 242
Tympanic membrane, 62
Type and crossmatch, 368

U

Ulcers, decubitus, 194, 221-225
  from bed rest, 306
Umbilical cord, 430
  care of, 438, 439
Unconscious patient, mouth care for, 198, 199
Understanding of patients, 37-47
Undressing patients, 326-329
  for physical examination, 337
Universal precautions, 134, 136, 137
Upper airway suctioning, 357
Ureter, 69
Urethra, 69
  male, 70
Urinals, 233-235
Urinalysis
  routine, 240
  before surgery, 368
Urinary drainage bag, emptying, 238
Urinary elimination, 229-249
Urinary incontinence, 230, 235
  bladder training for, 239-240
  of dying patient, 468
Urinary system, 67, 69
  physical changes of aging and, 98, 99
Urination, 69, 230
  lack of control over, 235
  normal, 230
    maintaining, 230-235
  before physical examination, 337
  reporting about, 230-231
Urine, 69
  acetone in, 230, 243
    testing for, 243, 246, 247

Urine—cont'd
  observation of, 230-231
  stones in, 246, 248
  straining, 246, 248
  sugar in, testing for, 243, 245, 246
  testing, 242
Urine sample, random, 240
Urine specimen
  clean-catch, 242
    collecting, 241
  clean-voided, 242
  collection of
    general rules for, 240
    and testing of, 240-248
  double-voided, 243
  fresh-fractional, 241
    collecting, 243
  from infant or child, collecting, 241
  midstream, 242
  routine, collecting, 240, 241, 242
  24-hour, 241
    collecting, 243
Utensils, eating, for individuals with special
    needs, 382, 383
Uterus, 71

V

Vagina, 72
  irrigation of, 362, 363-364
Vaginal speculum, 336, 337
Valuables
  kept at bedside, 326
  listing of, on admission, 325-326
  removal and storage of, before surgery, 368
Valuables envelope, 325-326
Valves of heart, 62
Varicella, 410
Vas deferens, 70
Vegetables and fruits food group, 269
Veins, 50, 63, 65
Vena cava, inferior and superior, 63-64
Venereal warts, 426
Ventilation in patient unit, 172
Ventral, 486
Ventricles of heart, 62
Venules, 63
Verbal abuse of elderly, 105
Verbal communication, 38, 44
Vesicle, seminal, 70
Vessels, blood, 63-64
Villi, 67
Virus(es), 128
  AIDS, universal precautions to prevent
      spread of, 134
Vision
  of dying patient, 468
  nursing assistant and, 17
  poor, and need for safe environment, 111
  problems with, 403-404
  receptors for, 60
  tunnel, 403

Visitors, patient's, 45-46
Vital signs, measurement of, 285-304
  and reporting of, 287
Vitamins, 270
Vitreous body, 60
Voice box, 64
Voiding, 230
Voluntary muscles, 55
Vomiting, care for, 461
Vowel, combining, 484, 485
Vulva, 72

W

Walkers, 316, 317
Walking
  aids for, 314, 315-317
  with blind person, 405
  with cane, 316
  helping patient with, 312, 313
  with walker, 317
Wall oxygen outlet, 358
Wall suction, 357
Warmth during physical examination, 337
Warts, venereal, 426
Washcloth, mitted, making and using, 203
Water
  boiling, for disinfection, 132
  drinking, providing, 281
  normal requirements for, 275-276
Water balance, 275-278
Water bed to prevent decubitus ulcers, 224
Weight, measuring, on admission, 325, 326
Wet cast, support for, 395
Wheelchair
  teaching transfers to and from, 382, 386,
      387, 388
  transferring patient to, 158, 160-163
  transport of discharged patient via, 332, 333
White blood cells, 62
Whooping cough, 410
Wills, 12, 21
  "living," 469
Windpipe, 64
Word elements, 484
  combining, 486
  of medical terms, 484-486
Wound suctioning, 358
Wrist, range-of-motion exercises for, 310, 311
Wrist and ankle restraints, 117
  applying, 118
Writing notes as verbal communication, 44
Written competency evaluation for nursing as-
    sistant, 18

X

X-ray examination, chest, before surgery, 368

Y

Young adulthood, 90-91